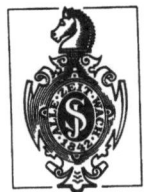

Luigi Allegra · Pier Carlo Braga
Roberto Dal Negro (Eds.)

Methods
in Asthmology

With 107 Figures and 53 Tables

Springer-Verlag
Berlin Heidelberg New York
London Paris Tokyo
Hong Kong Barcelona
Budapest

Luigi Allegra, M.D.
Istituto di Malattie Respiratorie
Policlinico – Pad. Litta, Via F. Sforza, 35
20100 Milano, Italy

Pier Carlo Braga, M.D.
Centro di Farmacologia Respiratoria
Via Vanvitelli, 32, 20129 Milano, Italy

Roberto Dal Negro, M.D.
Servizio di Fisiopatologia Respiratoria
Ospedale di Bussolengo, Via Ospedale, 2
37012 Bussolengo (Verona), Italy

ISBN 978-88-470-2265-2   ISBN 978-88-470-2263-8 (eBook)
DOI 10.1007/978-88-470-2263-8

65/31 45-5 4 3 2 1 0 – Printed on acid-free paper

Preface

Bronchial asthma is a multifactorial disease. Cooperation between pneumologists, physiologists, immunologists, pharmacologists, psychologists, and pediatricians is frequently needed for the complete investigation of an asthma case. This means that a physician in general practice cannot alone assess all the aspects of asthma and must frequently refer patients to a variety of specialists employing different techniques to manage this disease.

In keeping with the original meaning of $\sigma \acute{v} \nu$-$\delta \rho \acute{o} \mu o \varsigma$, asthma has long been viewed as a syndrome, as a "con-course" of several different causal and mediating factors. A correct approach to examination should clarify all of these more or less evident aspects. The aim of the present book is to provide a collection of articles detailing current knowledge on the most important techniques and methods, as this information to date has usually been scattered in papers from different cultural and scientific areas. We thus hope that this book will provide physicians with a unique source on the principal methods which can be used to analyze individual cases of asthma and a helpful reference source for better understanding the multiple pathways to the disease.

LUIGI ALLEGRA
PIER CARLO BRAGA
ROBERTO DAL NEGRO

Contents

VIII   Contents

List of Contributors

ALLEGRA, L.; Institute of Respiratory Diseases, School of Medicine,
University of Milan, Milano, Italy

ANDERSON, S.; Department of Respiratory Medicine, Royal Prince
Alfred Hospital, Camperdown, NSW, Australia

BANFI, P.; Department of Pneumology, S. Corona Hospital,
Garbagnate (MI), Italy

BENTI, R.; Department of Nuclear Medicine, IRCCS, Ospedale
Maggiore, Milano, Italy

BERNI, F.; Department of Pneumology, S. Corona Hospital,
Garbagnate (MI) Italy

BOSSI, R.; Institute of Respiratory Diseases, School of Medicine,
University of Milan, Milano, Italy

BRAGA, P. C.; Center for Respiratory Pharmacology,
School of Medicine, University of Milan, Milano, Italy

BRUNO, A.; Department of Nuclear Medicine, IRCCS, Ospedale
Maggiore, Milano, Italy

CENTANNI, S.; Institute of Respiratory Diseases, School of Medicine,
University of Milan, Milano, Italy

CIACCIA, A.; Institute of Infections and Respiratory Diseases,
School of Medicine, University of Ferrara, Ferrara, Italy

DAL NEGRO, R.; Department of Lung Pathophysiology,
General Hospital, Bussolengo (VR), Italy

DAMATO, S.; Institute of Respiratory Diseases, School of Medicine,
University of Milan, Milano, Italy

DEL BONO, L.; Centro per lo Studio dell'Asma e delle Allergopatie
Respiratorie, Cisanello, Pisa, Italy

DEL BONO, N.; Centro per lo Studio dell'Asma e delle Allergopatie
Respiratorie, Cisanello, Pisa, Italy

FABBRI, L.; Institute of Infections and Respiratory Diseases,
School of Medicine, University of Ferrara, Ferrara, Italy

FLOREANI, A. A.; Department of Internal Medicine, Pulmonary
and Critical Care, University of Nebraska, Omaha, NB, U.S.A.

GERUNDINI, P.; Department of Nuclear Medicine, IRCCS, Ospedale
Maggiore, Milano, Italy

HARGREAVE, F. E.; Firestone Regional Chest and Allergy Unit,
St. Joseph's Hospital, Hamilton, Ontario, Canada
LINDER, J.; Department of Internal Medicine, Pulmonary and Critical
Care, University of Nebraska, Omaha, NB, U.S.A.
McGRANAGHAN, S.; Department of Internal Medicine, Pulmonary
and Critical Care, University of Nebraska, Omaha, NB, U.S.A.
MAGYAR, P.; Department of Pulmunology, Semmelweis
Medical University, Budapest, Hungary
MALO, J. L.; Department of Chest Medicine, Hôpital du Sacre-Coeur,
Montreal, Canada
MAPP, C. E.; Institute of Occupational Medicine, School of Medicine,
University of Padova, Padova, Italy
MOAVERO, N. E.; Institute of Respiratory Diseases, School of Medicine,
University of Milan, Milano, Italy
NIZANKOWSKA, E.; Department of Medicine, Copernicus Academy
of Medicine, Kraków, Poland
ORIE, N. G. M.; Department of Internal Medicine,
University of Groningen, The Netherlands
PAPI, A.; Institute of Infections and Respiratory Diseases,
School of Medicine, University of Ferrara, Ferrara, Italy
PIATTI, G.; Institute of Respiratory Diseases, School of Medicine,
University of Milan, Milano, Italy
POMARI, C.; Department of Lung Pathophysiology, General Hospital,
Bussolengo (VR), Italy
RENNARD, S. I.; Department of Internal Medicine, Pulmonary
and Critical Care, University of Nebraska, Omaha, NB, U.S.A.
SMITH, C. M.; Department of Allergy and Allied Respiratory
Disorders, Guy's Hospital, London, United Kingdom
SPURZEM, J. R.; Department of Internal Medicine, Pulmonary
and Critical Care, University of Nebraska, Omaha, NB, U.S.A.
SZCZEKLIK, A.; Department of Medicine,
Copernicus Academy of Medicine, Kraków, Poland
TESSIER, P.; Department of Chest Medicine, Hôpital du Sacre-Coeur,
Montreal, Canada
THOMPSON, A. B.; Department of Internal Medicine, Pulmonary
and Critical Care, University of Nebraska, Omaha, NB, U.S.A.
TURCO, P.; Department of Lung Pathophysiology, General Hospital,
Bussolengo (VR), Italy
WANNER, A.; Pulmonary Division, School of Medicine,
University of Miami, Miami, FL, U.S.A.
WONG, B. J. O.; Firestone Regional Chest and Allergy Unit,
St. Joseph's Hospital, Hamilton, Ontario, Canada
ZIMENT, I.; Department of Medicine, Olive View Medical Center,
UCLA School of Medicine, Sylmar, CA, U.S.A.

Part I
Basic Aspects

Definition and Classification of Asthma

N. G. M. ORIE

Professor emeritus of Pulmonary Diseases, Pneumonology Section,
Department of Internal Medicine, University of Groningen, The Netherlands

Motto: Sometimes we cannot see the woods for the trees

Introduction

The history of the semantics of generalized reversible airway obstruction, "asthma," is rather complex, but perhaps this is not so surprising. There are few conditions in which so many variables, endogenous and exogenous in nature, are involved, and these can provoke an immense variability in the phenotype of asthma.

Short-term variability of an endogenous nature exists mainly as a result of circadian rhythm. Exogenous variations, resulting from the presence or absence of allergens or nonallergic irritants, may also change the clinical picture over short periods of time. Depending on the nature and duration of the exposure and the type of the reaction (early and late allergic reaction) the symptoms may vary to a considerable extent.

The clinical picture is also markedly influenced throughout life by the (endogenous) natural history of allergy and nonallergic bronchial hyperreactivity. Exogenous changes over long periods of time, such as changes in the exposure to allergens, changes in the climate as a result of moving to a new location, and changes in the types of air pollution, can cause symptoms to improve or deteriorate, particularly in situations that are related to industrial or occupational factors.

Complications and complicating factors of an acute or chronic nature can again provoke immense short- and long-term variability.

Finally, due to the avalanche of therapeutic possibilities in the last 40 years, such as bronchodilators and anti-inflammatory drugs, comparison of the clinical pictures of contemporary cohorts with those of an age-matched similar series in longitudinal studies has become an awkward proposition. The same holds true for the changes brought about as a result of preventive (vaccination) and therapeutic (antimicrobial) measures.

This implies that both cross-sectional and longitudinal studies will have, by necessity, a considerable number of biases.

The longitudinal study by Van der Lende started 20 years ago [43] tells us how a child born in 1940 developed between the ages of 30–50. It teaches us quite a bit about the relationship between earlier signs and symptoms and the patient's present condition. However, this fate will not be representative for the child born in 1960 let alone for the child that is born today. In the same way cross-sectional studies will sometimes show important regional and ethnic differences, but again the predictive value for the future of present day childhood studies will be extremely limited.

"The bronchitic child is father to the bronchitic man" is probably very true [69] but it must be remembered that each present day man has a father quite different from future fathers being born today although endogenous patterns may be the same. The best approach is probably comparison of cross-sectional and longitudinal data.

In publications before and shortly after the second world war the description of asthma was rather vague and the knowledge of the disorder was often taken for granted. Doctors "assume that all sensible doctors must have the same views as themselves and will understand what they mean" [21]. Most of us realize that this is rarely true.

Coinciding with the publication of a *Ciba Guest Symposium* on emphysema [13] and some papers dealing in particular with epidemiological, problems in "bronchitis" [15], Scadding [73, 74] reflected on the principles of definition in medicine and particularly in asthma. Fletcher suggested a concise but clear terminology in the field of chronic nonspecific lung diseases, which still has much in common with the one currently in use [21]. The same holds true for the definitions of the American Thoracic Society (ATS), published in 1962 [2]. Since then, many other (excellent) definitions or amendments have been proposed [87] and assessed in clinical practice [66], but it is virtually impossible to discuss them all separately. They are not fundamentally different; one cannot see the woods for the trees.

In discussing this issue in 1992, it seems logical to take the 1962 suggestions of the ATS and Scadding's considerations [54, 55] as a starting point. The discussions of the 1971 Ciba conference on the identification of asthma [14] and the suggestions published in 1987 by the ATS in its second statement on the definition of chronic obstructive pulmonary disease (COPD) and asthma [3] can then be taken into account. COPD was used as the cover term for bronchitis, emphysema, and peripheral (small) airway disease. The latter statement stresses our point that a discussion on the validity of the separation of the obstructive airway diseases into asthma and COPD cannot be avoided (for an overview, see Fig. 1).

In 1961 and 1964 we suggested [54, 55] that most cases of asthma and COPD should be considered as primarily originating from the same source, fruits of the same tree. The individual phenotypes, i.e., the differences in clinical appearance and behavior, were considered to be the result of endogenous and exogenous variables, mainly of a quantitative nature and also as a result of complications and complicating disease(s). The basic mechanism for both asthma and COPD was held to be of a hereditary nature expressing it-

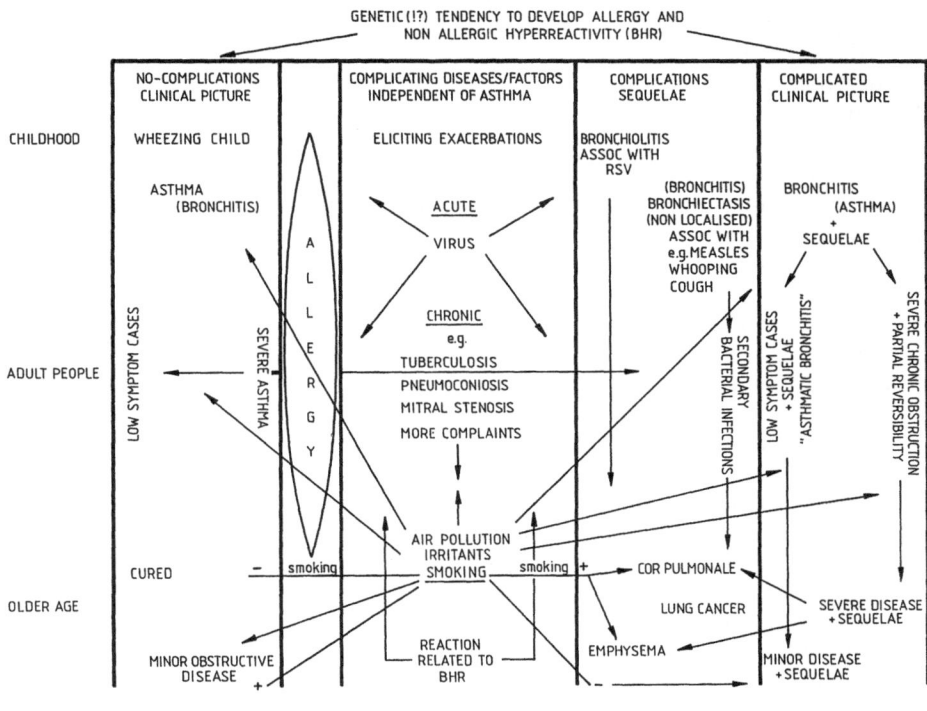

Fig. 1. Suggested classification. Complications are rapidly disappearing from the Western world, but are still seen in older people and are common in developing countries

self in an increased (tendency to develop) allergy and bronchial hyperreactivity (BHR) to nonallergic irritants. As long as a genetic defect has not been demonstrated, this issue must remain in the realm of speculation and hypothesis [22]. Nevertheless we feel that presently available circumstantial evidence may very well fit into this "umbrella" concept. This issue was recently the topic of two papers that discussed the pros and cons in detail [80, 87].

Definition and Classification of Asthma

According to Scadding [74 p. 1], who gave a very lucid and important analysis of the problem, the definition of a disease is: "the sum of the abnormal phenomena displayed by a group of living organisms in association with a specific common characteristic by which they differ from the norm for their species in a biologically disadvantageous way." (The abnormality may also have advantageous implications [1].) That common characteristic is called "the defining characteristic." This may be "of several sorts depending on the point which has been reached in a diagnostic process which moves towards, but frequently stops short of causation, its desirable end point." Scadding points out that such a characteristic can be, for example, a syndrome or a functional or anatomical phenomenon.

As a primary definition of asthma ([74] p. 5) he suggests: "… a disease characterized by wide variations over short periods of time in resistance to flow in intrapulmonary airways." This definition has much in common with the 1962 ATS definition [2]. It also fits in well with the classic example of the "disease" asthma: a girl or young woman who develops a severe generalized bronchial obstruction after contact with a cat and who responds within a few minutes to the application of a β-mimetic drug.

The first difficulty arising from Scadding's definition is the use of the expressions "wide variations" and "short periods of time," which, of course, are open to a wide range of interpretations, for example, regarding the issue of reversibility in differentiating the many cases of emphysema [59] or "irreversible" asthma [83]. Moreover, marked differences in bronchus obstruction, in particular when they arise over several days or weeks, may go almost completely unnoticed by the patient. An additional difficulty, particularly when trying to separate the "normal" individual from the "patient," is the frequency with which these variations ("attacks") occur.

Different borderline values for "wide variations" or "short periods of time" and for the incidence of attacks may considerably influence prevalence figures. This probably explains, at least in part, the tremendous variability in prevalence found in different countries and the allocation of similar patients to different disease categories in different studies [31, 66]. It is only by using identical borderline values that real similarities or differences between countries [31] and ethnic groups [94] can be separated from differences due to inclusion or exclusion of minor degrees of disease. (The question arises whether we do not, in fact, have a gradual transition from severe disease, via moderate and minimal disease, to normalility concomitant with an increased resistance to mediators and irritants in the "supranormal" part of the population.) However, it may well be that for different purposes, for example, outpatient facilities, number of hospital beds, or vaccination programs, prevalence figures of different degrees of severity should be used. This aspect is as yet largely unexplored.

In discussing the problem of borderline cases, Scadding remarks that although this is a real difficulty, it is a problem that is also found in other diseases.

Nevertheless it seems useful to discuss in some detail a few of the many exogenous and endogenous factors that are responsible for variations in and distortion of the clinical picture of asthma and which may also explain quite a few of the borderline cases. There is short-term variability, both endogenous (e.g., the circadian rhythm) and exogenous (e.g., allergenic load, intensity of irritants, virus infections). In addition, long-term endogenous and exogenous variations occur that change the reaction pattern of the patients and thus the phenotype of the asthma [75, 97, 98].

In childhood, for example, there is usually a high incidence of asthmatic symptoms which often decrease rather sharply around the age of 6–8 years [23, 67, 97]. Moreover, in young children there is a preponderance of boys with asthma, but in adolescence girls are slightly in excess [75, 97, 98] (see also below). More boys "outgrow" their asthma although remnants are often left [24, 40].

In older patients the gradual decrease of allergic symptoms [76], allergic skin reactions (Fig. 2) [4, 46], and levels of circulating antibody [92] is probably another example of these endogenous changes. BHR probably also decreases with age [5, 91] (Fig. 3) as does the histamine skin reaction [77]. In childhood the situation is less clear [25, 62].

Other important (endogenous) factors in females include changes as a result of menarche, menstruation, menopause, and pregnancy (and comparable changes in males ?).

There are also many examples of long-term exogenous variations that cause changes in the clinical expression of asthma. Some of these variations are predictable, such as the occurrence and intensity of allergenic load (pollens, fungus, house mite); others are more or less unpredictable, for example, upper and lower respiratory tract viral infections or industrial pollution.

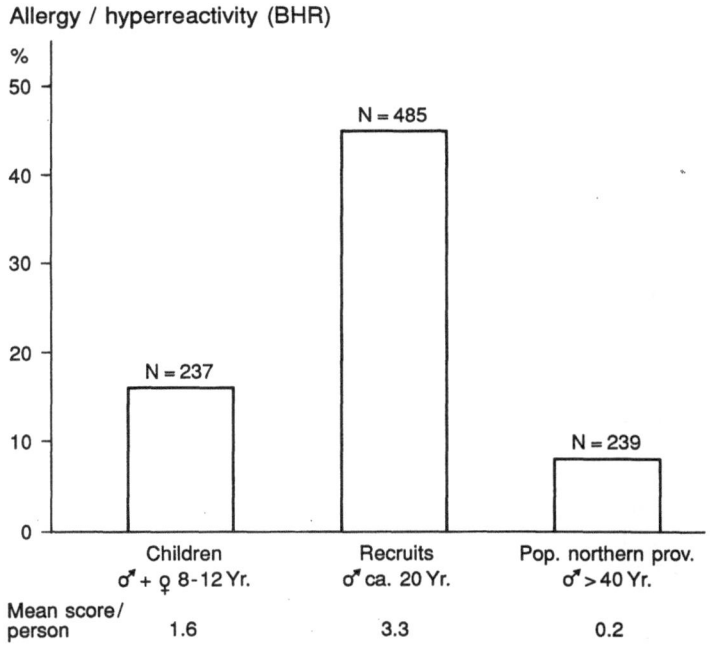

Fig. 2. Immediate type skin reactions is response to inhalation allergens in random samples of patients of different age. The late allergic reaction shows an even more clear regression in older age

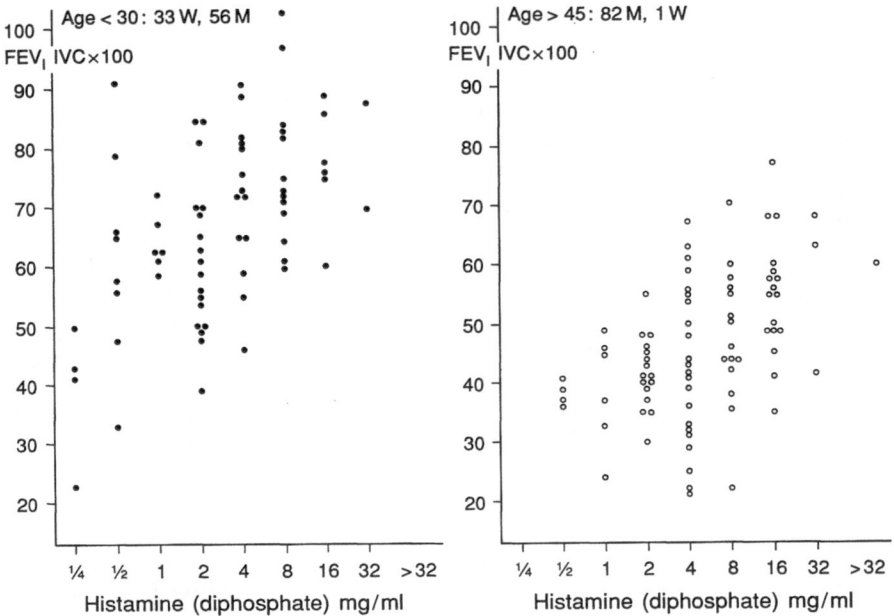

Fig. 3. Histamine reactivity (BHR) in relation to age and lung function

Moreover, there is the important influence of smoking and complicating diseases such as tuberculosis, pneumoconiosis, and mitral stenosis. Although it is often suggested that the bronchial obstruction in a number of patients with tuberculosis, pneumoconiosis, or mitral stenosis is the result of these diseases, there is support for the suggestion that the obstruction is at least partly independent of these disease [9, 27, 41, 88] although there is also a reciprocal action.

Bacterial infections, usually secondary to viral or allergic inflammation, probably have no adverse effect on bronchial obstruction except during the obstructive period resulting from the initial provoking factor in predisposed individuals (see Table 1; see also "Bacterial Bronchial Infection" p. 11) [30, 70].

The above discussion centered around the relatively simple definitions given by the ATS [2] and Scadding [73, 74]. The recent (1987) definition of the ATS [3] poses more problems. In addition to fluctuation of airways obstruction, it stresses hyperresponsiveness of the bronchial tree and, to a lesser extent ("in fatal cases"), inflammation. Formerly, allergy and hyperreactivity were mentioned as essential mechanisms. One might wonder whether the introduction of the term "inflammation" instead of late allergic reaction, which describes more precisely the eosinophilic type of inflammation, is not a step backwards. This definition, however, does not affect the problem of the borderline cases between normals and asthmatics or the separation between asthma and COPD (see below). Although the presence of BHR can

Table 1. Characteristics of bronchopulmonary infections classified as primary (predisposing factors not predominant) and secondary conditional (predisposing factors predominant, local defect)

Primary infections (e.g. influenza)	Conditional infections (e.g. H influenzae-infections)
Mostly viruses, sometimes bacteria or fungi	Mostly bacteria or fungi
Subjects are equally susceptible	Only in predisposed subjects
Recurrences are rare	Recurrences are common
Major parts of the respiratory tract are usually involved	Generally a localized process
Agent not previously present in the patient	Agent usually present in the patient (oropharynx, bronchial tree)
Treatment (if possible) against micro-organisms	Treatment (also) directed against predisposing factor (corticosteroids)
Often provoke general airway obstruction	Rarely provoke general airway obstruction
Incidence: all ages	Mostly in childhood and older age

often be suspected from the history of the patient, its formal assessment is not an examination room procedure; no exact reference values for inflammation are as yet available. Thus the new definition offers no advantages from a semantic point of view.

The definition mentions the fact that asthma may develop into a condition in which the airways obstruction shows little or no reversibility and also that COPD patients may have significant reversibility after treatment. We do not agree with the view that such overlap occurs only occasionally [6, 71], or that it is seen only after treatment.

In summary, the ATS definitions have inherent shortcomings that may influence the data on the percentage of patients in a population to a considerable extent. These shortcomings are very hard to avoid. Only careful description may help. Moreover, they – and other – definitions stress real differences with other varieties of generalized airway disease without considering whether these differences can be explained by the natural history of the basic provoking factors and the difference in exogenous and endogenous factors and complications and complicating diseases. Therefore the separation of asthma from related diseases or syndromes (if they can be separated) remains difficult.

Other Definitions and Categories of Asthma

Clinical Categories

Scadding ([74] p. 6) differentiated between several clinical, categories such as extrinsic atopic asthma, extrinsic nonatopic asthma, intrinsic asthma (1977) (later called cryptogenetic asthma [74] p. 7), exercise-induced asthma, and asthma associated with chronic bronchopulmonary disease (tuberculosis, pneumoconiosis). Other authors have added other categories: infectious asthma, gastric asthma, and other varieties in which a certain provoking factor is particularly manifest. In several of these "disease entities," specific pathogenetic factors are stressed such as "IgE production as a 'causal factor', the presence of non-IgE related immunological mechanisms, or the absence of demonstrable immunological mechanisms combined with specific patient characteristics: infantile eczema, age, and sex" ([74] p. 6).

These classifications need further analysis and confirmation. They are of interest when considering prevention and treatment for the same reason that it is important to know the cause of an increased glucose level in a diabetic (such as diet and infection). They are, however, only important for pathophysiological considerations or classification if they represent clearly different entities. We will discuss one category, intrinsic asthma, in more detail.

Intrinsic Asthma (Cryptogenetic Asthma)

There are undoubtedly patients with clear-cut asthma in whom no specific external factors or immunological abnormalities can be demonstrated; prevalence figures are usually not given.

A simple explanation would, of course, be the presence of a hitherto unknown or neglected allergen (e.g., *Trichopyton* [89], or a new mite [32]). It may also be that we are dealing with an allergen that was suspected, but for which no suitable test method existed, e.g., *Didymella exitialis* [11]. Scadding ([74] p. 7) suggests that "Among patients with 'cryptogenic asthma' there is a group characterized by nonseasonal incidence, possibility of onset without previous respiratory symptoms at any age (especially later in life than usual in extrinsic atopic asthma), tendency to persistence with variations in severity rather than complete remission of symptoms, in some patients high but usually variable eosinophilia in blood and bronchial secretions, and in many an unsatisfactory response to therapeutic measures short of corticosteroids, to which the response is often dramatic." There are several other differences between intrinsic asthma, so defined, and extrinsic atopic asthma. Whether auto-antibodies to smooth muscle and, among women, thyroid and gastric antibodies and antinuclear factor are specific for this group is still unsettled.

It seems probable that one or more independent units can be identified in this intrinsic group. But in the majority of patients with so-called intrinsic asthma with an apparently late onset of features, the explanation might well be that the childhood phase of the disease has been forgotten or is insufficiently inquired about.

This may be illustrated by a comparison of figures from a survey of childhood asthma/bronchitis and the history of a random sample of older people from the same region. In a survey in children in the northern part of the Netherlands, Knol et al. [39] found that approximately 25% of the children of 8–12 years suffered from chronic obstructive respiratory disease; in a random sample of an older male population (ages 45–70), van der Wal found that of 8.7% had had childhood respiratory disease [64]. There is no reason to expect such a tremendous increase in incidence in contemporary children. If one also takes into consideration the age-dependent decrease in allergic reactions (skin reactivity of IgE [60, 92]), then the majority of so-called older intrinsic cases may be explained. Whereas the natural history of allergy is well known, the natural history of nonallergic hyperreactivity (BHR) is more controversial and has not been introduced in Fig. 1. The biologic curve may resemble the allergic hyperreactivity curve, but the BHR, particularly in its clinical manifestation, is much more influenced by exogenous allergic and anatomical factors. The history of childhood complications of asthma (sinus disease, pneumonia), which is sometimes also found in intrinsic cases, also points to a close relationship of these cases with the "common" variety of asthma.

Other Categories

Whether or not infectious asthma, gastric asthma, excercise-induced asthma, and hyperventilation asthma are different well-defined entities remains to be decided. For the time being we consider them as expressions of the same, as yet basically unexplained, mechanism(s). This also holds true for generalized airways obstruction after respiratory viral infections [21] which is found predominantly in predisposed patients [30, 35, 44, 45, 57]. A similar observation has been made for exercise-induced asthma in children in whom it is usually a part of the "common" asthma pattern [49, 74 p. 3].

Many of the semantic problems might be avoided by adhering to the suggestion of the Ciba Foundation report on asthma: to give a very precise and detailed description of the population involved in a study [14 p. 174]. This means age, sex, childhood and family history, results of clinical, radiological, and laboratory examination, and data on type and degree of allergy, BHR, and lung function, including circadian rhythm and reactions to several drugs. The information should also include data on a number of characteristics which may be related to the type of patients described (skin abnormalities, upper and lower airway respiratory infections).

Finally, in some cases the results of more sophisticated investigational methods may assist in elucidating the disease process, e.g., the presence of different kinds of circulating antibodies and data on mediators or cellular components detected in bronchial lavage fluid [99, 100].

Bacterial Bronchial Infection

We have suggested the following classification of bronchopulmonary infection:

Primary infections: the microorganism is the direct cause of the infection, predisposing factors probably being of less importance pathogenetically
Secondary infections: predisposing factors are essential in the pathogenesis.
1. Opportunistic: defect in the systemic/phagocytic/immunologic defense
2. Conditional: local defect; no defect in the systemic/phagocytic/immunologic defense

There are several pathogenetic mechanisms responsible for bronchopulmonary infections. In current clinical practice, however, bacterial infections are usually of the conditional type, being associated with reversible bronchial obstruction, often with minor or major anatomical bronchial lesions [58, 82]. They therefore very often occur in patients with a tendency to bronchial obstruction and are often initiated by a virus infection. There are many data to support this point of view [29, 61]. It provides an answer to the question that is being raised over and again in the literature e.g., in a excellent Editorial in the *Lancet* [19]: why are the results of antibiotic therapy so disappointing in these cases.

The treatment of the bronchial obstruction – in most cases by corticosteroids – has to be the first and most important step, not the prescription of antibiotics. This is probably true in childhood as well as in adult life. We are dealing here with a specific example of a well-known general phenomenon: bacterial infections in many organs of the human body, e.g., urinary bladder, gall bladder, and probably ear and nasal sinuses, are often provoked by obstruction.

Asthma and Chronic Obstructive Pulmonary Disease

In the context of this discussion it seems appropriate to discuss in somewhat more detail the 1987 ATS recommendation to separate the whole group of obstructive airways disease(s) into two subgroups: asthma and COPD [3]. COPD is the general collective term for bronchitis, peripheral airways disease, and emphysema. Is there sufficient reason for this separation?

Many important experiments to answer this question – already mentioned in the discussion about the definition and subclassification of asthma – were recently summarized in a state of the art meeting chaired by Woolcock [95].

Chronic Bronchitis

The definitions of chronic bronchitis by the British Research council (1965) and the ATS (1987) [3, 15] center around the presence of mucus and therefore of sputum production and cough. A precise delineation of duration and frequency of the episodes of cough and/or sputum was made for epidemiological purposes. This certainly will increase the comparability of groups, but not the specificity of the diagnosis. Although there is, to the best of my knowledge, no exact information, experience suggests that many cases, in particular the not so severe ones, do not fit the narrow limitation of the definition of chronic: "occurring on most days for at least three months of the year for at least two successive years" and disappear from the affected population.

The 1987 ATS definition stresses that airway obstruction is found very often.

Although not explicitly stated in the 1962 definition, it was generally held that excess mucus production is an important cause of airflow obstruction and "chronic bronchitis has been commonly used to mean expiratory airflow obstruction." Many patients with COPD have excess sputum production as well as hyperplasia of the mucus glands of the trachea and large bronchi. Both abnormalities have been linked etiologically to cigarette smoking.

It is, of course, quite impossible to consider this interesting but extremely complicated problem in more detail in this short introductory chapter.

In childhood, asthma and bronchitis cannot be very well distinguished from each other [26, 93, 48]. The hereditary data in asthma and bronchitis seem to be essentially the same [16, 48, 88]. The exact mechanisms that determine the obstructive manifestation of the presumably genetic trend are unknown, although infections will provoke part of the exacerbations [28]. They also provoke complications such as peripheral airway disease [52] and bronchiectasis [49, 90], especially in predisposed individuals.

In adolescence, when many children for reasons still unknown "outgrow" their childhood disease, a considerable number of children are probably left with the remnants of the aforementioned complications: peripheral airway disease and bronchiectasis [24, 40]. Many children will become adolescent patients with no or minor symptoms and variable degrees of allergy and BHR [24]; some will become severe asthmatics with strong allergic characteristics and (partly secondary to the allergy?) often also severe BHR.

Given the declining impact of allergy with advanced age (e.g., hay fever) [24, 60, 92] and the fact that the majority of adult bronchitics are much older than the asthmatics, it seems reasonable to assume that the severity of the allergic component will be considerably diminished in bronchitic patients, even if both groups should have the same allergic tendency. Another consequence of the age dependency of allergy is that eosinophilia, and probably also the number of other reactor cells that provoke the inflammatory reaction after allergic exposition, will diminish. The same is true for the BHR which probably diminishes concurrently [5, 38, 64]. However, whereas this biologic (primary) BHR decreases along with the secondary variety which results from allergic (and maybe other kinds of) inflammation, the strength of the reaction we actually observe in the BHR test may often increase as a result of anatomical factors: diminished elastic retractile forces of the lung and damage to the interstitial tissue, both of which may be the result of smoking [72, 81] and industrial pollution. In these patients, BHR is now more strongly related to the initial lung function, in particular to the forced spirometric values [11, 68] (Fig. 3). Moreover, deterioration of the anatomical structure is seen particularly in patients with (the anatomical sequelae of their) childhood asthma [71, 78].

It is not surprising therefore that in young adulthood the clear-cut allergic picture dominates, whereas in older individuals the allergic characteristics diminish and the influence of anatomical lesions in childhood becomes more important. The preexisting lesions, peripheral airway disease and, not strictly localized bronchiectasis which are mainly found in asthmatic children [37, 49, 52] may also explain the cough and sputum production and the susceptibility to bacterial infections [44].

The fact that major, not strictly localized bronchiectasis is virtually disappearing from the list of common pulmonary diagnoses (to the best of my knowledge no exact figure is available but the trend is obvious) but not in developing countries [36, 53] might lend support to the fact that bronchiectasis is the main source of sputum production in a patient. This does not deny the existence of a generalized bronchial hypersecretion, but it is doubtful whether hypersecretion can be diagnosed from the amount of sputum produced, except in some very severe situations in asthma. Coughing is not easily explained by the anatomical lesions in the major bronchi which do not essentially differ in asthma and bronchitis [18].

Another approach to the problem of the relationship between asthma and bronchitis is the comparison of those features that are considered essential in diagnosing asthma and bronchitis. We have already discussed the question of whether some of the essential asthmatic features, heredity, allergy and eosinophilia, and BHR, may not also be found in bronchitics, where they may be considered as remnants of childhood and adult allergic asthmatic disease which initiated the childhood complications and cooperated in producing the specific (adult) bronchitic features.

A few words, finally, on other characteristic features of bronchitis: (ir)reversibility, pathology, and treatment. Here the comments, are of a different nature.

Reversibility

In patients with so-called irreversible airway obstruction, considerable reversibility may still be demonstrated when studying *inspiratory* spirometric data [42]. The same holds true for the body-box studies during quiet breathing [84]. A major part of the *expiratory* irreversibility – which is, moreover, often far from absolute (Rouing see [59, 6]) – is therefore certainly due to airway collapse caused by the loss of elastic recoil and to changes in the characteristics of the interstitial lung tissue. Twelve out of 36 "classic" emphysema patients have an increase in inspiratory vital capacity of 600 ml, and seven of 36 even of over 900 ml ([71], see also [59] fig. 164).

Pathology

Anatomical differences have long been considered as one of the hallmarks of the difference between asthma and bronchitis. The work of Dunnill et al. [18] has shown, however, that both in asthmatic and in bronchitic patients there is a proliferation of mucus-secreting goblet cells and hypertrophy of mucous glands in the airways. The main difference is the bronchial smooth muscle thickness, which is greater in asthma than in bronchitis. The latter might be explained by the lower frequency and intensity of the muscle contractions during the attacks in older patients.

Therapy

It is evident that the therapies for asthma and bronchitis are gradually but steadily coming closer together. The differences between the patients, e.g., with respect to age, degree of allergy and BHR, and complications, will have their repercussions on the therapeutic approach [56, 63, 65].

Peripheral Airway Disease, Bronchiectasis, and Emphysema

The chain of reasoning in the discussion on the relationship between asthma and peripheral airways disease bronchiectasis, and emphysema is essentially the same as that between asthma and bronchitis. These lesions are preferentially found in the majority of patients (and their families) with a clear (hereditary?) trend to generalized airways obstruction, asthma, or bronchitis [37, 49, 52]. The factors that provoke these specific complications in predisposed patients are, however, different, and operate at a different age.

One of these is, for instance, respiratory syncytial virus (RSV) infection, which affects virtually every child in the first 2 years of its life. In particular, *peripheral airway disease* is recognized as a complication of RSV infection in predisposed infants [52]. *Bronchiectasis* of the diffuse, not strictly localized type probably has a similar origin, but develops as a rule somewhat later, mainly as a result of complications of measles or whooping cough, again predominantly in predisposed children [37]. In this situation, postviral bacterial superinfection, predominantly with *Haemophilus influenzae*, will settle in the affected bronchi [33, 34], thus playing a role in exacerbations [50, 51], which are usually precipitated by allergic or viral obstruction [30, 44, 70].

Many of the cases of *emphysema* are related to smoking. The anatomical sequelae from childhood suggest why only relatively few smokers are considerably affected, i.e., those with an asthmatic background and especially those with the anatomical sequelae [71] often (approximately 20% of patients) found also in emphysema [81, p. 204]. This is in accordance with recently published data [47] that the difference between smokers and nonsmokers disappears if the cases with poor lung function are eliminated in such a comparison.

The above reasoning may explain why gross bronchiectasis as described in older textbooks is rapidly disappearing, probably mainly due to vaccination and antibiotics, and due to this it still exists in developing countries (36, 53) and is comparable to our situation 40 years ago. It also explains why complicating diseases (pneumoconiosis) or complicating factors (smoking) affect only a minority of the people exposed. It also provokes two more suggestions. Is the increase in asthma a real phenomenon or does it just mean that the elimination of some of the complications mentioned above causes the clinical picture of bronchitis to switch to the uncomplicated (pure asthmatic) variety. The higher prevalence of asthma in children who had childhood respiratory disease and therefore loss of lung function [28, 46] could thus be explained as consequence of the preexisting (genetic or familiar) trend already present in the child and which provoked the earlier respiratory disease.

Final Remarks

The data obtained in a very recent study, an investigation on the use of the different terms "asthma" and "COPD" in different countries that is very interesting for several reasons, show clearly that two problems remain [66]. The first is the meaning of the different terms which are obviously, very often considered as having been defined satisfactorily; an opinion which is, however, not reflected in this and other papers. In this respect it is remarkable that the label "chronic nonspecific lung disease" is considered to be badly defined. I wonder if that should be interpreted as meaning that it cannot be used in clinical practice? This is of course correct (which may serve as the basis for a more detailed description). The second problem is that a close relationship of asthma with COPD seems, as a rule, not to be supported by a survey of specialists.

There is no clear and direct answer, but the choice of terminology and the subsequent desire for further analysis seem to result in a negative answer. Reversibility is considered as being infrequent in the three nonasthmatic items of COPD. There is no recommendation to get more complete and reliable information from the patient about events in earlier stages of life or family history.

The lack of hesitation to accept a reltionship between asthma and COPD is also reflected in the rather limited use of (inhalation) steroids in nonasthmatic patients (but remarkably enough also in patients with classic asthma).

So it is clear that further epidemiological, clinical pathological and fundamental research will be necessary to provide a final answer. But an analysis of the semantic problems is not complete if it does not mention factors that may have confused or invalidated the issue in earlier work. In each of the three research fields there are some examples that seem worth while mentioning.

A first point, already briefly mentioned, is the question of – sometimes considerable – increase in the prevalence of asthma [93]. In such studies the fact that death from respiratory illness in childhood has virtually disappeared in developed countries is often neglected, which means that a considerable number of prospective cases is added to the population. Moreover, the shift in symptomatology as a result of the elimination of bronchiectasis will again tend to cause an increase in the number of noninfected "pure" asthmatics.

In clinicopathological studies another point is relevant. Part of the basis of the theory that anatomical bronchitic lesions – in particular small airway disease – is the result of smoking may find its origin in the fact that anatomical data, used in comparing smokers and nonsmokers, are often obtained from post-mortem specimens of patients with suspected or proved bronchial

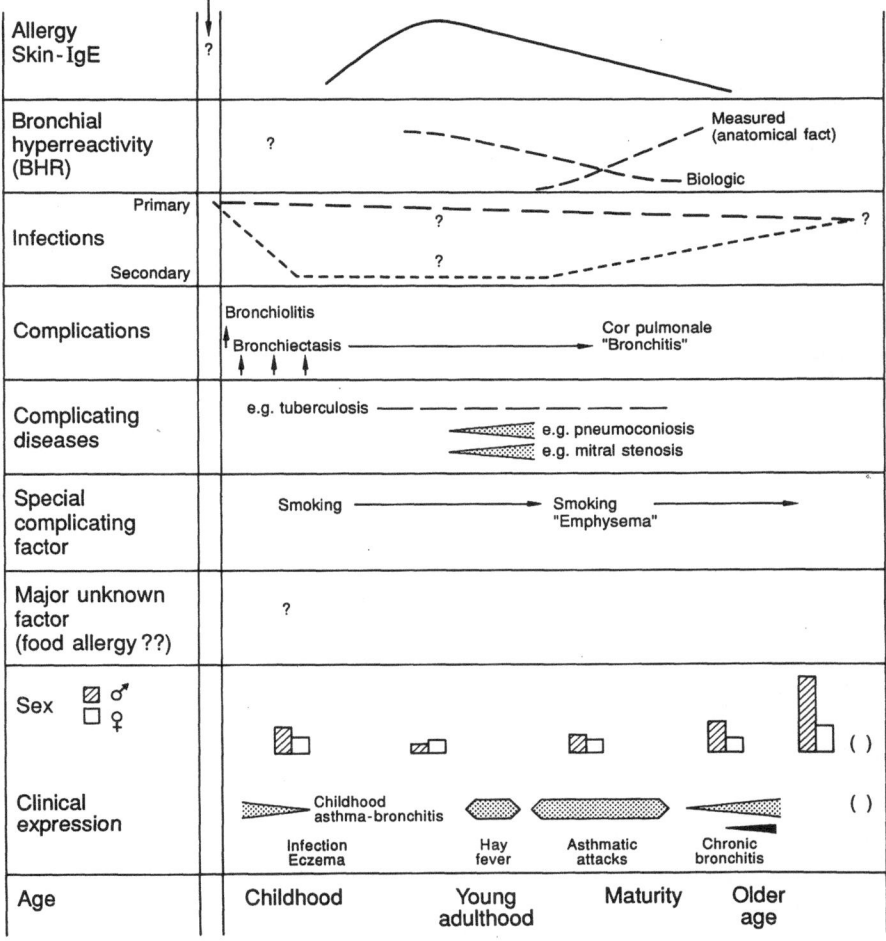

Fig. 4. Effort to present a schematic description of isolated factors and their natural history that, superimposed in many various ways, affect the clincial picture of asthma

carcinoma [96]. If we accept that the development of bronchogenic carcinoma is closely linked to the existence of "bronchitis" [17, 85], the following situation arises. Smoking patients in whom a localized pulmonary growth is diagnosed will quite often have a bronchogenic carcinoma. In nonsmoking patients this will only exceptionally be the case. Therefore, in comparing smoking and nonsmoking patients one compares at the same time a group with a high risk for carcinoma to a group in which carcinoma will be an exception. But it also means that we compare a group with a high percentage of "bronchitis" [16, 88] to a group in which this percentage will not be above average.

The remarkable coincidence in time of some of the changes in clinical behavior related to age and gender with the onset of the production of adrenal or gonadal sex hormones stresses the need for further study of this relationship. The fact that boys are affected twice as often as girls in early youth in particular [75, 80, 96] is still unexplained. That it should be the result of geometric differences in the bronchial tree is not very probable because these differences are also seen in infantile eczema and in food allergy.

Conclusion

A brief summary of the semantics of asthma and generalized airway obstruction has been given. The pros and cons of considering asthma, bronchitis, and emphysema as the outcome of genetically based hypersensitivity of an allergic or nonallergic nature which is molded by many endogenous and exogenous factors have been presented.

Although it is impossible to mention the vast amount or literature that supports or invalidates the unifying hypothesis, it may be good to remember that if we combine the data on the nature of childhood asthma and bronchitis with the data on their sequelae in later life [37, 40, 52] and the life expectancy for the affected adult group [10], this integrated scheme fits the analysis of Burrows [8] very well, even if there are certain differences in the estimate of the relative importance of the factors involved (which in fact may be different in different countries and ethnic populations).

It is certainly not my intention to lump all patients with diffuse airways obstruction together. On the contrary, as research continues many clear-cut apparently autonomous diseases will probably be isolated and identified. There are already at present such separate disease entities, e.g., anti-protease deficiency, the immotile cilia syndrome, and the yellow nail syndrome. For other diseases this is less evident but still a possibility, e.g., Kartagener's syndrome (perhaps identical with the immotile cilia syndrome) and MacLeod's syndrome.

Certainly in the future more subgroups will be separated from the large, group of obstructive airways disease as more facts become known [95]. However, existing evidence supports the "umbrella" philosophy (Fig. 4) in most cases [66, 80].

Labels are immaterial; provoking factors and complications are important. Therefore, as long as no *causal* definition can be given, a careful description of all patients with diffuse obstructive airways disease remains vital.

Acknowledgements. I am much indebted to Prof. H. J. Sluiter for his many
valuable suggestions. I am also grateful for the secretarial assistance of Wil-
ma Gremmer, Hanneke Bosma, Petra Wetterauw, and A. de Vries-Bos.

References

1. Alderson M (1975) Mortality from malignant disease in patients with asthma.
   Lancet 2:1475
2. American Thoracic Society (1962) Chronic bronchitis, asthma, and pulmonary
   emphysema. Am Rev Respir Dis 85:762–768
3. American Thoracic Society (1987) Standards for the diagnosis and care of patients with chronic obstructive pulmonary disease (COPD) and asthma. Am Rev
   Respir Dis I-130:225–243
4. Barbee RA, Kaltenborg W, Lebowitz MD, Burrows B (1987) Longitudinal
   changes in allergen skin test reactivity in a community population sample. J Allergy Clin Immunol 79:16–24
5. Booy-Noord H (1973) Discussion. Troisième session de la Groupe de Travail:
   Function respiratoire en epidémiologie. Societas Europaea Physiologiae Clinicae
   Respiratoriaea, Lanaken. In: Les tests de bronchocontriction en epidémiologie.
   Rev Inst Hyg Mines 28:205–210
6. Bork LE van (1983) Pharmacodynamics of thiazinamium methylsulphate and
   oxyphenonium bromide an the differences in effects between an aerosol of oxyphenonium bromide or ipratropium bromide and a metered aerosol of ipratropium bromide. In: Schultze-Wenninghaus G, Widdicombe JG (eds) Role of anticholinergic drugs in obstructive airway disease. Gedon and Reuss, Munich
7. Burrows B, Knudson RJ, Cline MG, Lebowitz MD (1977) Quantitative Relationships between Cigarette Smoking and Ventilatory Function. Am Rev Resp Dis
   115:195–205
8. Burrows B, Bloom JW, Gayle A, Traver MSN, Cline MG (1987) The course and
   prognosis of different forms of chronic airways obstruction in a sample from the
   general population. N Engl J Med 317 (21):1309–1314
9. Cabanes LR, Weber SN, Matran R et al. (1989) Bronchial hyperresponsiveness to
   methacholine in patients with impaired left ventricular function. N Engl J Med
   320 (20):1317–1322
10. Carpenter L, Beral V, Strachan D et al. (1989) Respiratory symptoms as predic-
    tors of 27 years mortality in a representative sample of British adults. Br Med J
    299 (6695):357–361
11. Cayley GR, Harries MG, Lacey J, Newman Taylor AJ, Tee RD (1985) Didymel-
    la exitialis and late summer asthma. Lancet 1 (8437):1063–1066
12. Charpin D, Badier M, Orehek J (1985) Dose-response curves to inhaled carba-
    chol in asthma and chronic bronchitis. Bull Eur Physiopathol Respir 21:417–420
13. Ciba Guest Symposium (1959) Terminology, definitions, and classification of
    chronic pulmonary emphysema and related conditions. Thorax 14:286–299
14. Ciba Foundation Study Group No. 38 (1971) Identification of asthma (edited by
    Porter R and Birch J). Churchill Livingstone, Edingburgh
15. Committee on the Aetiology of Chronic Bronchitis (1965) Definition and classifi-
    cation of chronic bronchitis for clinical and epidemiological purposes. Lancet
    775–779

16. Doeleman F (1957) Sociaal-geneeskundige studies over asthma bronchiale. Royal VanGorcum, Assen
17. Doll R, Bradford Hill A (1952) A study of the aetiology of carcinoma of the lung. B Med J 2:1271
18. Dunnill MS, Anderson JA, Masarella GR (1969) A comparison of the quantitive anatomy of the bronchi in normal subjects, in status asthmaticus, in chronic bronchitis and emphysema. Thorax 24:176–185
19. Editorial (1987) Antibiotics for exacerbations of chronic bronchitis? Lancet 2: 23–24
20. Empey DW, Gold WM, Jacobs L, Laitinen LA, Nadel JA (1976) Mechanisms of bronchial hyperreactivity in normal subjects after URTI. Am Rev Respir Dis 133: 131–139
21. Fletcher CM (1961) Definition and classification of bronchitis, asthma and emphysema. In: Orie NGM, Sluiter HJ (eds) Bronchitis: an international symposium, 27–29 Apr 1960. Royal VanGorcum, Assen, pp 273–278
22. Fletcher CM, Pride NB (1984) Definitions of emphysema, chronic bronchitis, asthma and airflow obstruction. Thorax 39:81–85
23. Fry J (1961) The catharral child. Butterworths, London, p 106
24. Gerritsen J, Koëter GH, Knol K, Postma DS (1989) Athma from childhood to early adult life. In: Sluiter HJ, van der Lende R, Gerritsen J, Postma DS (eds) Bronchitis IV. Royal VanGorcum Assen, pp 337–347
25. Gerritsen J, Koëter GH, Postma DS, Schouten JP, Knol K (1989) Prognosis of Asthma from Childhood to Adulthood. Am Rev Respir Dis 140:1325–1330
26. Godfrey S (1977) Childhood asthma. In: Clark TJH, Godfrey S (eds) Asthma. Chapman and Hall, London, pp 324–366
27. Goei JT, Tammeling GJ, Nieveen J (1962) Longfunctie – onderzoek bij mitralistenose. Ned Tijdschr Geneeskd 106:1789
28. Gold DR, Tager IB, Weiss ST et al. (1989) Acute lower respiratory illnesss as a predictor of lung function and chronic respiratory symptoms. Am Rev Respir Dis 140 (4):877–884
29. Gregg I (1975) The role of viral infection in asthma and bronchitis. In: Proudfoot AT (ed) Symposium viral diseases. The Royal College of Physicians, publication 46, p 87
30. Gregg I (1977) Infection. In: Clark TJK, Godfrey S (eds) Asthma. Chapman and Hall, London, pp 162–176
31. Gregg I (1983) Epidemiological aspects. In: Clark TJH, Godfrey S (eds) Asthma. Chapman and Hall, London, pp 242–284
32. Hage-Hamsten M van, Johansson SGO (1989) Clinical significance and allergenic cross-reactivity of Euroglyphus maynei and other nonpyroglyphid mites. J Allergy Clin Immunol 83 (3):581–589
33. Hers JFPh (1955) The histopathology of the respiratory tract in human influenza. Thesis, University of Leiden
34. Hers JFPh (1961) The pathology of chronic relapsing mucopurulent bronchitis with and without bronchiectasis. In: Orie NGM, Sluiter HJ (eds) Bronchitis. Royal VanGorcum, Assen, pp 149–159
35. Horn M, Gregg I (1973) Role of viral infection and host factors in acute episodes of asthma and chronic bronchitis. Chest 63 [Suppl]:445–485
36. Ip MSM, So SI, Lam WK, Liong E (1992) High prevelance of asthma in patients with bronchiectasis in Hong Kong. Eur Resp J 5:418–423
37. Israëls AA, Warringa RJ, Löwenberg A (1961) Bronchiectasis. In: Orie NGM, Sluiter HJ (eds) Bronchitis. Royal VanGorcum, Assen, pp 171–175
38. Joos GF (1988) The role of neuropeptides in the pathogenesis of asthma. Thesis, State University of Gent
39. Knol K (1965) Een klinisch en epidemiologisch onderzoek naar de betekenis van bronchiale hyperreactiviteit bij kinderen met chronische aspecifieke respiratoire aandoeningen (CARA). Thesis, University of Groningen

40. Kraepelien S (1959) Respiratory studies in asthmatic children during symptom-free periods. Thesis, University of Stockholm
41. Kreukniet J, Orie NGM (1961) Chronic bronchitis, bronchial asthma, a host factor in patients with pulmonary tuberculosis. All Asthma 7:200
42. Labadie H (1961) Certain patho-physiological differences between bronchial asthma and pulmonary emphysema. In: Functional exploration of the respiratory and cardiovascular system in asthma, emphysema and related disorders. Proceedings of the small meeting, Barcelona 1960. Stenfoert-Kroeze, Leiden, p 83
43. Lende R van der (1969) Epidemiology of chronic nonspecific lung disease (chronic bronchitis). Thesis, University of Groningen
44. Löwenberg A, Orie NGM (1976) Viral, mycoplasma and bacterial infections in nurses with symptoms of respiratory diseases. Scand J Respir Dis 57:290–300
45. Löwenberg A, Orie NGM, Sluiter HJ (1973) Über die Bakteriellen Infektionen der tieferen Luftwege und der Lunge. Prax Pneumol 27:393–402
46. Martinez FD, Wayne J, Morgan J, Wright AL, Holberg CJ, Taussig LM et al. (1988) Dimished lung function as a predisposing factor for wheezing respiratory illness in infants. N Engl J Med 319:1112–1117
47. Matsuda K, Shirakusa T, Kuwano K, Hayashi S, Shigematsu N (1987) Small airway disease in patients without chronic airflow limitation. Am Rev Resp Dis 136:1106–1111
48. McNicol KN, Williams H (1969) Prevalence, natural history, and relationship of wheezy bronchitis and asthma in children. An epidemiological study. Br Med J 4:321–325
49. Milner AD (1987) Specific asthma problems. In: Tinkelman S et al. (eds) Childhood asthma. Dunitz, London, p 10
50. Mulder J (1938) Haemophilusinfluenzae (Pfeiffer) as an ubiquitous cause of common acute and chronic purulent bronchitis. Acta Med Scand 94:98
51. Mulder J, Goslings WRO, Plas MC van der, Cardozo PL (1952) Studies on treatment with antibacterial drugs of acute and chronic mucopurulent bronchitis caused by Haemophilus influenzae. Acta Med Scand 143:32
52. Nagayama Y, Nakahara T, Sakurai N et al. (1987) Allergic predisposition among infants with bronchiolitis. J Asthma 24:9–17
53. Ongki AS (1987) Severe acute lower respiratory infections in Gunung Wenang General Hospital, Manado Indonesia. Paediatrica Indonesia 27 (9):169–176
54. Orie NGM (1961) Discussion by invitation. In: Orie NGM, Sluiter HJ (eds) Bronchitis. Royal VanGorcum, Assen, pp 285–286
55. Orie NGM (1964) Appendix on terminology of bronchitis. In: Orie NGM, Sluiter HJ (eds) Bronchitis II. Royal VanGorcum, Assen, p 398
56. Orie NGM (1980) Clinical Managemant of Asthma. Prog Resp Res 14:248–260, Karger, Basel
57. Orie NGM, Löwenberg A (1977) Erreger, Wirt und Terrain: Über den Begriff der Pathogenität im Bereich des Respirations-Traktus. Tatsachen und Hypothesen. Praxis und Klinik der Pneumonologie 5:532–538
58. Orie NGM, Huizinga E, Israëls AA, Geelen EEM, Sluiter HJ, Warringa RJ (1955) Relation entre bronchiectasie et allergie. Bronches 5:95–109
59. Orie NGM, Sluiter HJ, Tammeling GJ, Vries de K, Wal van der AM (1964) The fight against Bronchitis². In: Orie NGM, Sluiter HJ (eds) Bronchitis II. Royal VanGorcum, Assen, pp 354–356
60. Orie NGM, Vries K de, Weller HH, Lende R van der, Grobler NJ, Booy-Noord H, Tammeling GJ, Sluiter HJ (1967) Maladie bronchopulmonaire obstructive. Bull Soc Med Hauteville 34:1
61. Orie NGM, Sluiter HJ, Löwenberg A (1980) Luchtweg obstructie (CARA) en luchtweginfectie. In: Vandepitte J en Yourassowky E (eds) Recente ontwikkelingen in de infectieuze respiratoire pathologie. Excerpta Medica, Amsterdam–Oxford–Princeton 63–77
62. Pee S de, Timmers MC, Hermans J, Duiverman EJ, Sterk PJ (1991) Comparison

of maximal airway narrowing to methacholine between children and adults. Eur Respir J 4:421–428

63. Postma DS, Peters I, Steenhuis EJ, Sluiter HJ (1988) Moderately severe chronic airflow obstruction. Can corticosteroids slow down obstruction? Eur Resp J 1:22–26
64. Postma DS, Koëter GH, Sluiter HJ (1989) Pathophysiology or airway hyperresponsiveness. In: Weiss S, Sparrow D (eds) Airway responsiveness and atopy in the development of chronic lung disease, Raven, New York, pp 21–71
65. Postma DS, Renkema TEJ, Koëter GH (1990) Effects of corticosteroids in "chronic bronchitis" and "chronic obstructive airway disease". AAS 30: Inflammatory indices in chronic bronchitis. Birkhauser Verlag Basel
66. Pride NB, Allegra L, Vermeire P (1989) Diagnostic labels applied to model case histories of chronic airflow obstruction. Responses to a questionnaire in 11 North American and Western European countries. Eur J Respir Dis 2:702–609
67. Pullan CR, Rey EW (1982) Wheezing asthma and pulmonary dysfunction ten years after infection with respiratory syncythal virus in infancy. Br Med J 284: 1665–1669
68. Ramsdale EH, Morris MM, Roberts RS, Hargreave FE (1984) Bronchial responsiveness to methacholine in chronic bronchitis: relationship to airflow obstruction and cold air responsiveness. Thorax 39:912–918
69. Reid DD (1969) The beginning of bronchitis. Proc R Soc Med 62:311–316
70. Roldaan AC, Masurel N (1983) Virusinfectie van de luchtwegen en influenzavaccinatie bij patienten met CARA. Ned Tijdschr Geneeskd 137:489
71. Rouing PJE (1960) Hypoxemia, erythropoëse en hemolyse. Thesis, University of Groningen
72. Rijder RC, Dunnill MS, Anderson JA (1971) A quantitative study of bronchial mucous gland volume, emphysema and smoking in a necropsy population. J Pathol 104:59–71
73. Scadding JG (1963) Principles of definition. Br Med J 1423–1430
74. Scadding JG (1983) Definitions and clinical categories of asthma. In: Clark TJH, Godfrey S (eds) Asthma. Chapman and Hall, London, pp 1–11
75. Selander P (1960) Asthmatic symptoms in the first year of life. Acta Paediatr 49:265
76. Serafini U (1950) La pollinosi. EMES, Roma
77. Skassa-Brociek W, Manderscheid JC, Michel FB, Bousquet J (1987) Skin test reactivity of histamine from infancy to old age. J Allergy Clin Immunol 80:711–716
78. Sluiter HJ (1955) Cor pulmonale. Thesis, University of Groningen
79. Sluiter HJ, Van der Lende R (1989) Bronchitis IV. Closing words, p 382, Royal VanGorcum Assen, The Netherland
80. Sluiter HJ, Koëter GH, De Monchy JGR, Postma DS, De Vries K, Orie NGM (1991) The Dutch Hypothesis (chronic non-specific lunt disease) revisited. Eur Resp J 4:479–489
81. Thurlbeck WM (1963) A clinico-pathological study of emphysema in an American hospital. Thorax 18:59–67
82. Thurlbeck WM (1976) Chronic Airflow Obstruction in Lung Disease. Saunders, Philadelphia–London–Toronto 129:898–902
83. Turner-Warwick M (1977) On observing patterns of airflow. Obstruction in chronic asthma. Chest 71:73–86
84. Ulmer WT (1970) Analysis of changes in airways resistance during quiet breathing in obstructive lung dissease. In: Orie NGM, van der Lende R (eds) Bronchitis III. Royal VanGorcum, Assen, pp 231–235
85. Wal van der AM (1964) Chronische aspecifieke respiratoire aandoeningen (Cara) als voorwaarde voor het ontstaan van bronchuscarcinoom. Thesis, University of Groningen (summary in English)
86. Van der Wal AM, Huizinga E, Orie NGM, Sluiter HJ, De Vries K (1966) Cancer and Non-specific Lung Disease (C.N.S.L.D.). Scand J Resp Dis 47:161–172, 146: 888–894

87. Vermeire PA, Pride NB (1991) A "splitting" look at chronic nonspecific lung disease (CNSLD): common features but diverse pathogenesis. Eur Resp J 4: 490–496
88. Vries K de, Orie NGM, Mey AVM (1960) Asthmatic factors in chest complaints of miners. Acta Med Scand 167: 301–308
89. Ward GW, Karlsson G, Rose, G, Platts-Mill TAE (1989) Trichophyton asthma: sensitistation of bronchi and upper airways to dermatophyte antigen. Lancet i: 859–862
90. Warringa RJ (1955) Over bronchiectasie. Thesis, Groningen.
91. Weiss ST, Tager IB, Woodrow Weiss J, Munoz A, Speizer FE, Ingram RH (1984) Airways Responsiveness in a Population Sample of Adults and Children. Am Rev Respir Dis 129: 898–902
92. Wittig HJ, Belloit J, De Filippi I, Royal G (1980) Age-related serum immunoglobulin E levels in healthy subjects and in patients with allergic disease. J Allergy 66: 305–313
93. Williams MH (1989) Increasing severity of asthma from 1960 to 1987. The New Engl J of Med 320 (15): 1015–1016
94. Woolcock AJ, Peat JK, Keena V, Smith D, Molloy C, Simpson A, Middleton P, Vallance P, Alpers M, Green W (1989) Asthma and chronic airflow limitation in the Highlands of Papua New Guinea: low prevelance of asthma in the Asaro Valley. Eur Respir J 2: 822–827
95. Woolcock AJ (1988) State of the Art/Conference Summary. Asthma – What are the important experiments? Am Rev Respir Dis 138: 730–744
96. Wright JL, Lawson LM, Pare PD, Wiggs BJ, Kennedy S, Hogg JC (1983) Morphology of pheriferal airways in current smokers and ex-smokers. Am Rev Respir Dis 127: 474–477
97. Yunginger JW, Reed CE, O'Connell EJ, Melton LJ, O'Fallon WM, Silverstein MD (1992) A Community-based Study of the Epidemiology of Asthma. Am Rev Respir Dis 148: 888–894
98. Zuiderweg A (1962) Over het voorkomen van asthma (chronische aspecifieke respiratoire aandoeningen) in een huisartsenpraktijk in Z.-O. Groningen. Thesis, University of Groningen (summary in English)
99. Aalbers R et al (1993) Bronchial lavage and bronchoalveolar lavage in allergen-induced single early and dual asthmatic responders. Am Rev Resp (in press)
100. Aalbers R et al (1993) Allergen-induced recruitment of inflammatory cells 3 and 24 h after challenge in allergic asthmatic lungs. Chest (in press)

Physiology of the Airways

S. DAMATO

Institute of Respiratory Diseases, School of Medicine, University of Milan, Milano, Italy

Introduction

The lung's total nonelastic resistance is the sum of the airways resistance to airflow (R_{aw}) and the frictional resistance of the lung tissues to respiratory movements. The latter significantly contribute to total nonelastic pulmonary resistance in patients with interstitial lung diseases, but in normals their contribution approaches only 15% [50].

During inspiration, the rib cage expands and the pressure in the pleural space (P_{pl}) decreases. However, the change in lung volume (ΔV) is also dependent upon its elastic recoil or compliance (C); as a consequence, the decrease of the alveolar pressure (P_{alv}) will be smaller than P_{pl}, the transpulmonary pressure ($P_{pl} - P_{alv}$) being a measure of the elastic recoil of the lung tissue. Given a static condition, open glottis and breath holding, P_{alv} equilibrates with P_{pl}, which is therefore a measure of the static elastic recoil of the lung tissue (P_{stl}). As P_{alv} decreases, a pressure difference, the driving pressure (DP), will arise with respect to the ambient pressure at the mouth (P_{mo}). A proportional flow is generated towards the alveoli during inspiration and the opposite during expiration, P_{alv} now being the sum of P_{pl} and elastic lung recoil. The driving pressure is related to both R_{aw} and gas inertance (I_{aw}) within the airways:

$$DP = R_{aw}\dot{V} + I_{aw}\ddot{V}$$

where $\dot{V}$ is the flow rate and $\ddot{V}$ is the acceleration. At low frequencies inertial phenomena can be neglected.

Assuming a uniform respiratory system and homogeneous flow rate distribution, it is possible to combine all the mechanical events in a single equation:

$$P_L = (\Delta V/C) + (\dot{V}R)$$

where P_L is the pressure applied to the lungs ($P_{mo} - P_{pl}$), ΔV is the lung volume change, C is the compliance value correspondent to that lung volume change, V is the flow rate and R is resistance. This equation [33] can express the whole system, omitting its inertia and assuming that resistance does not change with lung volume or the airflow regime in the airways.

The bronchial tree is not only involved in the mechanical behavior of the respiratory system, rather, through its structural arrangement, the bronchial tree is also involved, both in health and in disease, in the lungs' defense mechanisms in response to noxious agents and in other nonrespiratory functions. Let us consider now in greater detail the physiology of the bronchial tree, analyzing the various factors involved in its determination: the driving pressure–flow relation, the airways caliber, the volume–pressure–flow relation, the site of airways resistance, the structure–function relation, and the morphometry–function relation.

Driving Pressure–Flow Relation

The resistance to airflow along the bronchial tree is the driving pressure (DP) to flow rate ratio; normally, it is nearly 2 cm H_2O l^{-1} s. This relation is a complex one since the airways are ducts which are neither rigid, nor perfectly circular, nor regularly branching. However, let us disregard for the moment the above mentioned objections. The DP along the airways overcomes friction and accelerates the molecules with time (local acceleration) producing airflow, with the DP depending on rate and pattern of airflow. Laminar flow is the most simple pattern and it is characterized by streamlines that parallel the sides of the tube, the central ones moving faster than those closest to the walls; therefore, the flow profile is a parabolic one. When the pattern of airflow generated is a laminar one, DP is directly proportional to flow rate ($\dot{V}$), gas mixture viscosity (η) and to the length of the tube (l), while it is inversely proportional to the radius (r), according to Poiseuille's equation [33]:

$$\Delta P = 8\,\eta\,\mathrm{l}\,\dot{V}/\pi\,r^4$$

so that by halving the airway radius there will be a 16-fold increase of DP to maintain a given flow rate.

The airflow through the bronchial tree remains laminar until reaching a critical condition in the airways corresponding to that described by a Reynolds number greater than 2000. The Reynolds number (Re), which is dimensionless, is directly proportional to $\dot{V}$, tube diameter (d), and density of the gas mixture (δ), while it is inversely proportional to the viscosity (η) according to the following equation:

$$Re = \dot{V}\delta\,d/\eta$$

that is, the higher the values of flow rate and airways diameter, the higher the Reynolds number. The flow pattern will become turbulent, due to complete disorganization of streamlines, when the Reynolds number is greater than 2000. In this case DP generating airflow is directly and exponentially proportional to $\dot{V}$, according to the following equation:

$$DP = \delta l \dot{V}^2/2\,\delta$$

density (δ), and not viscosity, being the influential characteristic of the gas mixture.

In a simple tubing model of the bronchial tree the flow rate is high at the level of the trachea, having as a consequence a probable turbulent pattern. Since the cross-sectional area increases enormously down the airways, the flow rate will become extremely low and probably have, consequently, a laminar pattern at the level of the peripheral airways. However, since the bronchial tree is a branching system, the consequent formation of eddies, especially during expiration, will mix the two flow patterns generating a transitional pattern whose corresponding DP will be dependent both on density (turbulent flow) and viscosity (laminar flow) of the gas mixture.

Furthermore, during expiration, the gas mixture flows along a tubing compartment having a high cross-sectional area, i.e., the alveolar ducts, toward a compartment having a small cross-sectional area, i.e., the main bronchi. As a consequence, the gas molecules, with the converging of the tubes, will accelerate with distance while flow with time is unchanged; this convective acceleration is responsible for some degree of DP decay along the airways [36] which is not due to friction and which produces local air acceleration. The opposite, a convective deceleration, will occcur during inspiration [49].

Airways Caliber

The size of the airways does not depend only upon their quantitative and qualitative anatomical features; their own elastic characteristics and those of the surrounding lung tissue are also involved.

The airways caliber is continuously determined in static and dynamic conditions by the pressure difference across their walls (transmural pressure). The pressure gradient along the airways, from alveoli to mouth, is small during quiet breathing, at the lung volume level of functional residual capacity (FRC). Therefore, the transmural pressure along the airways is similar to that measured in a static condition. The pressure inside the airways is atmospheric along all the airways, as is also the case for the pressure outside their extrathoracic portion, transmural pressure being nearly zero and the airways caliber being anatomically determined. For the intrathoracic but extraparenchymal airways the pressure outside the bronchial wall is that in the pleural space (P_{pl}); therefore the transmural pressure is positive and corresponds to the distending pressure of the lungs at that lung volume. For the intraparenchymal airways, the pressure outside the bronchial wall still approximates P_{pl} [37] but it is not homogeneously distributed, since gravity [40] interferes with P_{pl} through the curvilinear relation between changes of transpulmonary pressure ($P_{pl} - P_{alv}$) and lung volume. Pleural pressure is less negative in the more gravity-dependent areas of the lungs (base) or in those areas having smaller elastic recoil as a consequence the transmural pressure will decrease. However, the net effect of the transmural pressure will depend upon the structure of the bronchial walls and the smooth muscle tone, the airways compliance; cartilage rings or plates in the bronchial wall will give rigidity to the structure and avoid the collapse of the airway when the transmural pressure is negative.

The caliber of the intraparenchymal airways is also directly proportional to lung volume; since the volume changes during breathing, the airways caliber changes correspondingly. However, the lung volume interferes with airways also through its influence on P_{pl}. Moving the respiratory level from FRC to residual volume (RV) will increase P_{pl} toward positive values, especially at the lung base, and the transmural pressure will become negative. Through the action of the pleural pressure distending the lung, the airways caliber is affected by primary lung tissue diseases such as emphysema.

Other factors can directly influence the airways caliber such as contraction or release of bronchial musculature, mucosal edema, hypertrophy and/or hyperplasia of mucous glands, increased mucus production, and smooth muscle hypertrophy.

Volume–Pressure–Flow Relation

More relevant information about the flow resistive properties of the airways can be obtained studying the relation between flow rate, pleural pressure, and lung volume during a maximal inspiration–expiration maneuver [26, 27].

The maneuver (Fig. 1) first requires fast and complete inspiration from the resting respiratory lung volume level (FRC) until reaching the total lung capacity (TLC) level. After 1 or 2 s of breath holding, an expiration is required as sudden, rapid, complete and continuously forceful as possible until reaching the RV pulmonary level. The volume expired from TLC to RV level is the forced vital capacity (FVC). From the RV level new inspiration-expiration maneuvers can be done with different levels of effort.

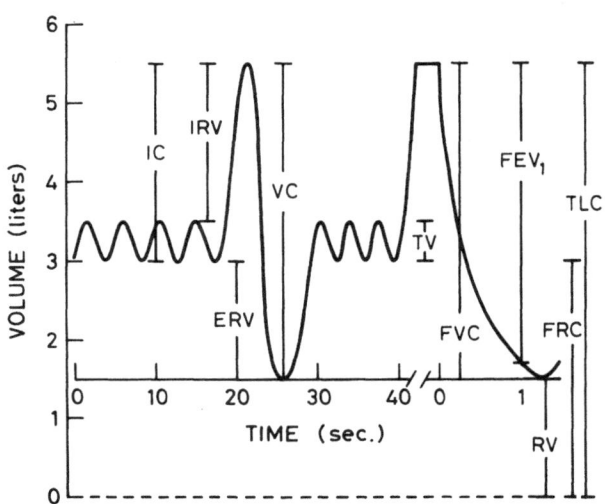

Fig. 1. Spirographic tracing. *ERV*, expiratory reserve volume; *FEV₁*, forced expired volume in 1 s; *FRC*, functional residual capacity; *IC*, inspiratory capacity; *IRV*, inspiratory reserve volume; *RV*, residual volume; *TLC*, total lung capacity; *TV*, tidal volume; *VC*, vital capacity

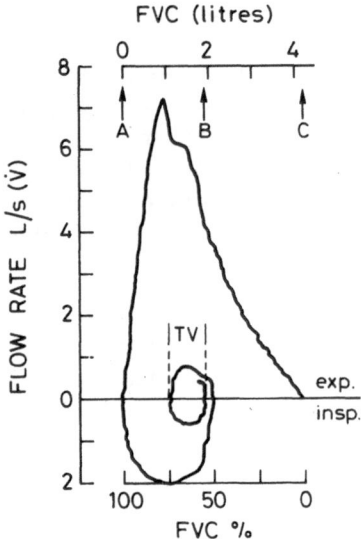

Fig. 2. Maximal expiratory flow volume (MEFV) curve. Original flow rate and volume signals stored on digital magnetic tape and replayed at slow speed on an analog plotter. *FVC*, forced vital capacity; *TV*, tidal volume; *insp*, inspiration; *exp*, expiration; *A*, total lung capacity breathing level; *B*, functional residual capacity level; *C*, residual volume level

The volume changes during this maneuver can be reported with respect to time (Fig. 2), the classic spirogram, or with respect to the contemporary maximal flow rate ($\dot{V}_{max}$) (Fig. 2), the so-called maximal expired flow volume curve (MEFV). Before the first 25% of VC has been expired, the flow rate reaches a maximum (FEF$_{max}$), or peak expiratory flow (PEF); further on, in spite of the persisting maximal effort, the flow rate gradually decreases, usually describing a slight curve toward the volume axis. Fig. 3 shows the contemporary representation of acceleration.

It is now useful to analyze the same events measuring P_{pl}, together with airflow and lung volume. It will be possible to differentiate the effects deter-

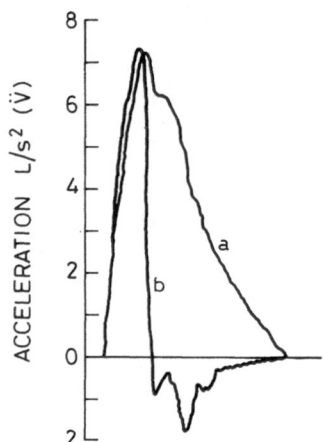

Fig. 3. Acceleration tracing along the MEFV curve. Original signals stored on digital magnetic tape and replayed at slow speed on an analog plotter. Line *a* is the flow rate trace; line *b* is the acceleration trace

mined on the MEFV curve by: (a) the degree of expiratory effort, (b) the change in resistance with decreasing lung volume, and (c) the dynamic regulation of the airways caliber. This analysis is based upon the isovolume pressure–flow curves (Fig. 4), requiring forced expiration maneuvers at different lung volume levels, with different degrees of effort and related P_{pl} values [18]. There are three important features:

1. At lung volumes approaching TLC, $\dot{V}_{max}$ increases, increasing P_{pl}; therefore within this lung volume range the flow rate is effort-dependent.

2. Decreasing lung volume, P_{pl} being the same, the flow rate decreases, showing the effect of the lung volume on airways caliber and resistance.

3. At lung volume lower than 80 % of TLC or 70 % of FVC, a $\dot{V}_{max}$ plateau is observed in spite of increasing effort and P_{pl}; therefore, within this lung volume range the flow rate is effort-independent and increasing P_{pl} equally increases airways resistance.

The effort-independent airflow limitation does not only depend on lung volume but it also has a dynamic component. This is shown considering a family of forced inspired-expired flow volume curves with different degrees of effort (Fig. 5). Again, there are three important features:

1. During expiration, whatever the degree of effort, the curves are superimposed on the maximal one at intermediate and low lung volumes. This pattern clearly shows some degree of airflow limitation, effort-independent, during forced expiration.

2. During inspiration, the different degree effort flow volume curves do not superimpose both at low and intermediate lung volumes. This pattern does not show any effort-independent flow limitation during inspiration.

3. At the 75 % FVC lung volume level the expiratory flow is slightly higher than the inspiratory one; this difference is in the opposite direction at 50 % and 25 % FVC lung volume levels.

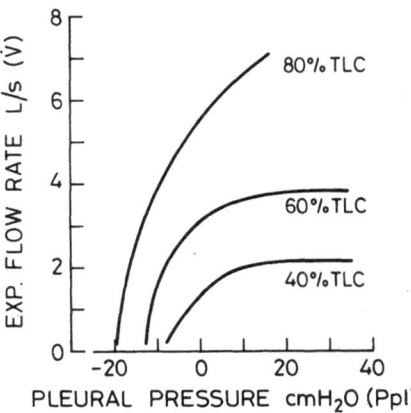

Fig. 4. Isovolume pressure–flow curves during forced expiration; *TLC*, total lung capacity. Pleural pressure increases with increasing effort. A decreasing lung volume level causes an airflow rate decrease for the same degree of effort. The airflow plateau for a specific lung volume level indicates the effort-independent flow rate range

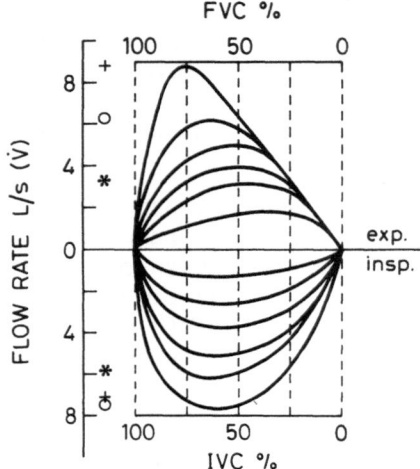

Fig. 5. A series of inspiratory-expiratory flow volume loops repeated at different levels of effort. The outer loop represents the highest effort level. *FVC*, forced expired vital capacity; *IVC*, inspired vital capacity; *exp*, expiration; *insp*, inspiration. ∗, flow rate at 25% FVC remaining to be expired or 25% IVC; ○, flow rate at 50% FVC remaining to be expired or 50% IVC; +, flow rate at 75% FVC remaining to be expired or 75% IVC

The airways flow resistive properties seem different during maximal inspiration with respect to expiration. During inspiration, since P_{pl} is markedly negative, the transmural airway pressure is largely positive and the bronchi are wider; consequently, flow rate is high. Increasing lung volume, as inspiration continues, the airways caliber further increases, the flow rate being high over a large proportion of VC in spite of the decreasing force generated by the inspiratory muscles as they shorten.

It is evident that during expiration there is a dynamic airway flow limitation at intermediate-low lung volumes. The mechanism of this dynamic airflow limitation is not known precisely, but a hypothesis has been made [36], which is based upon a mechanical lung model. Alveoli, represented by an elastic sac, and intrathoracic airways, represented by a compressible tube, are both enclosed in the pleural space. Normally P_{pl} is negative, P_{alv} being the sum of P_{pl} and P_{stl} (Fig. 6 A); P_{alv} is positive with respect to ambient pressure and an airflow is present through the airways toward the mouth. The P_{alv} value is not preserved along the airways, since it is consumed by airways resistance. A spectrum of decreasing pressure values will be present along the airways (P_{aw}), toward the mouth; since transmural pressure is positive along the entire system, airflow will continue.

During forced expiration (Fig. 6 B), P_{pl} is positive, P_{alv} still being the sum of P_{pl} and P_{stl}. Along the tubing a decreasing spectrum of P_{aw} will again develop. Since P_{pl} is positive, it will be possible that in an airway segment P_{pl} exceeds P_{aw} and, the transmural pressure being negative, the airway segment would collapse and airflow would stop. However, as the tube goes into compression, its caliber will decrease as a function of its own wall compliance and P_{aw} will increase reaching equilibrium with P_{pl}. Airflow will continue till when transmural pressure remains positive.

The above described condition is defined as the equal pressure point (EPP) or as dynamic compression of the airways, the model's theory having

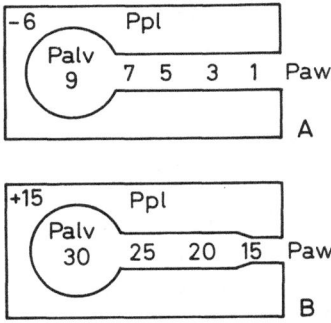

Fig. 6. The expiratory dynamic airways compression or equal pressure point concept. Schematic distribution of pleural (P_{pl}), alveolar (P_{alv}), and airways (P_{aw}) pressure values (cm H_2O) during quiet expiration (A) and during forced expiration (B). Elastic recoil pressure is 15 cm H_2O

the same name. In normal subjects, at lung volume above FRC level, this compression involves the segmentary bronchi; in extreme chronic bronchitis, it is possible at bronchoscopy to directly observe dynamic expiratory compression already during tidal breathing. Once the maximum expiratory flow is achieved, the EPP position becomes fixed and a further P_{pl} increase, i.e., increasing effort, simply produces more compression on the airways segment from the EPP toward the mouth; the flow rate from alveoli to EPP no longer being influenced.

The EPP therefore divides the bronchial tree into two segments: (1) peripheral to the EPP toward the alveoli, the upstream segment, having positive transmural pressure, (2) central to the EPP, toward the mouth, the downstream segment, having P_{aw} equal to P_{pl} by definition. Since the two segments are arranged in series, $\dot{V}_{max}$ at the mouth is that of the upstream segment [36]. The DP which overcomes resistance in the upstream segment (R_{us}) corresponds to the lung elastic recoil pressure (P_{stl}); in fact, P_{alv} is equal to P_{pl} plus P_{stl}, and the pressure value at EPP is by definition P_{pl}. $\dot{V}_{max}$ can therefore be expressed in terms of elastic lung recoil pressure and resistance in the upstream segment as follows:

$$\dot{V}_{max} = P_{stl}/R_{us}$$

This is a dinamic way through which lung tissue diseases influence $\dot{V}_{max}$. Diseases such as primary lung emphysema could limit airflow rate under effort without a primary disease involving the structure of the airways.

The upstream segment does not really correspond to a predetermined segment of the bronchial tree, since its extension is a function of lung volume. During forced expiration lung volume decreases and the EPP moves toward the alveoli. This situation is determined by these local sequential events: airways caliber reduction, airways resistance increase, faster decay of DP along the airways, EPP condition nearer to the alveoli. Therefore, as forced expiration proceeds, it will increase the contribution of more peripheral airways to $\dot{V}_{max}$ determined at the mouth. Finally, with the movement of EPP toward alveoli, the airways segments involved have greater wall compliance and a bronchial collapse could happen, followed by air trapping in the involved lung areas and possible significant reduction of forced expiratory

32   S. Damato

VC with respect to a slow expiratory VC. This mechanism can contribute to a functional amputation of lung volume during effort, when it is most necessary for oxygen supply.

Unfortunately the EPP is only a theory, and other theories have attempted to explain the expiratory effort-independent dynamic airflow limitation. For example the wave-speed theory [14, 41] proposes that flow is limited by the velocity of propagation of pressure waves along the wall of the airways; at a site where the flow rate equals the propagation velocity of pressure waves, a choke point develops, preventing further increases of flow rate.

The measurements of $\dot{V}_{max}$ in relation to lung volume are widely used to evaluate the flow resistive properties of the lung. It is clear, however, that $\dot{V}_{max}$ depends upon several factors: the lung volume, the expiratory effort degree, the lung tissue recoil pressure, the cross-sectional area distribution along the bronchial tree, and the airways resistance.

With intraparenchymal airways obstruction, as occurs in chronic obstructive pulmonary disease (COPD), airways resistance increases; with increasing airways obstruction $\dot{V}_{max}$ at FRC level is even more near to the flow rate measured during tidal breathing (Fig. 7). In such circumstances increasing expiratory effort will not have any relevant effect in increasing flow rate and ventilation. This mainly expiratory limitation to increase airflow is counterbalanced by a prolongation of expiratory time with respect to the inspiratory one; therefore, depending on frequency and amplitude of tidal breathing,

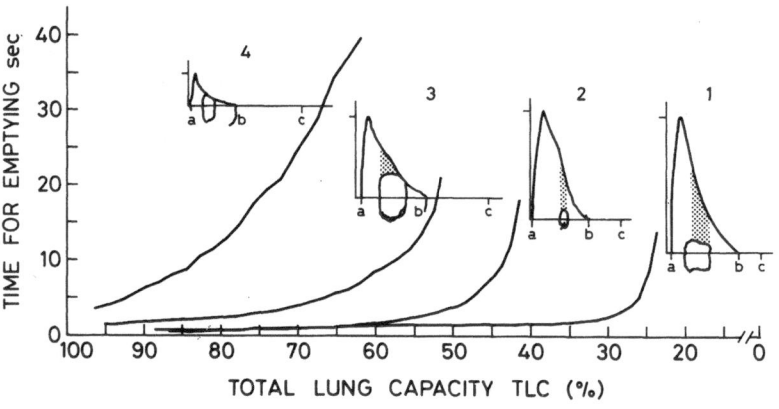

Fig. 7. MEFV curves (volume as liters on *abscissa* and flow rate as 1 s^{-1} on *ordinate*) have been transformed in the forced decay of the total lung capacity (*TLC*), as percent on *abscissa*, with respect to time for forced lung volume emptying, calculated at 100 ml volume intervals, as absolute value on *ordinate*. Time for emptying is the ratio between lung volume and instantaneous forced expired flow rate; assuming a lung volume of 4 l and a flow rate of 4 l/s, the expected time for emptying the lungs is equal to 1 s. Subject *1*, normal; Subject *2*, smoker; Subject *3*, asthmatic; Subject *4*, affected by chronic bronchitis–emphysema complex. Subject's lung function data are reported in Table 1. *a–b*, forced vital capacity; *b–c*, residual volume, *a–c*, total lung capacity

the inspiratory to total breath time ratio (T_i/T_{tot}) will decrease and the mean inspiratory flow or drive (VT/T_i) will increase. If expiratory time is not prolonged enough in proportion to obstruction, the resting breathing level rises and the contributions of FRC and RV to TLC will both increase; this has been clearly shown during asthma and has been also attributed to the continued action of inspired muscles during exiration [35]. By raising the resting lung volume, the airways are distended and the flow rate could increase. The stress for the respiratory muscles is the automatic limitation for this compensation mechanism, since at high lung volume the inspiratory muscle pressure required to inflate the lung increases [7]. At a certain limit, the respiratory muscles' work becomes unbearable and too expensive, the subject no longer increases the breathing level and is not able to produce the ventilation needed for effort of even decreasing intensity. Further increases of FRC/TLC or RV/TLC will take place if a parenchymal problem is also present or air trapping takes place; the reduction in elastic lung recoil will dynamically further increase the expiratory airflow obstruction.

In Fig. 7, the time problem is also shown in greater detail, transforming the MEFV curve into the decay of TLC with respect to the time for forced lung emptying [11]. Since the proportion of RV with respect to TLC increases with obstruction, the curves move toward the TLC level from normal subject to patient with COPD. In the normal subject the time for emptying is nearly 2 s along the maneuver, increasing very slightly, but linearly, until the level of FRC; above that point the time increases faster toward infinity at RV level. For the asthmatic subject, whose obstruction is mainly airways determined, the curve shows significantly higher time for emptying values with respect to the normal subject for comparable proportions of TLC, the difference becoming greater with decreasing lung volume. Furthermore, in the asthmatic subject the relation between lung volume and time for forced emptying is curvilinear along the entire maneuver. In the COPD patient there is a mixture of primary bronchial obstruction and emphysema; at comparable proportions of TLC, both airflow limitation on the MEFV curve and time for forced emptying of lung volume are increased with respect to the normal

Table 1. Lung function data for subjects in Fig. 7

Subject	Age	Weight	Height	Sex	TLC	RV/RLC	FVC	FEV_1/FVC	sG_{aw}
1	25	78	180	m	8.8	17.8	7.2	79.0	0.180
2	57	88	180	m	8.3	36.2	5.3	75.0	0.180
3	53	60	163	f	7.0	47.0	3.70	38.0	0.030
	a.b.					38.0		62.0	0.057
4	70	60	165	m	5.8	57.3	2.45	36.7	0.040
	a.b.					56.0		39.2	0.042

Age in years; weight in kilograms; height in centimeters; total lung capacity (TLC) in liters; forced vital capacity (FVC) in liters; residual volume (RV) to TLC ratio as a percentage; forced expired volume in 1 s (FEV_1) to FVC ratio as a percentage; sG_{aw}, specific airways conductance; a.b., after salbutamol

condition. The relation in COPD is steeper than in the normal subject but nearly linear in shape.

In the obstructive pattern generated by prevalent airways dynamic expiratory compression, the EPP moves rapidly toward the alveoli during forced expiration and it divides the bronchial tree in segments arranged in series. $\dot{V}_{max}$ at the mouth decreases since the airways caliber of the upstream segment also decreases. As the segments are arranged in series, the airways resistance will increase and flow rate will decrease with a linear pattern after compression takes place. The same linear pattern would be followed by the increased time for emptying. However, normally the flow rate along the bronchial tree is not homogeneously distributed because of anatomical and mechanical factors; this inhomogeneity is accentuated in intrinsic airways obstruction such as occurs in asthma. The bronchial tree is subdivided into parallel segments and in this distribution pattern the EPP is also not homogeneously distributed along the bronchial tree. In this case the conductance, which is the reverse of resistance, of the system will be the sum of the conductance of the single segments; changing resistance in one segment would have a nonlinear effect on the total. This explains the nonlinear pattern of $\dot{V}_{max}$ as it decreases during forced expiration and the configuration of the MEFV curve [38, 39], whose convexity toward the volume axis increases in asthma with airways obstruction. The time for forced TLC emptying will also not linearly increase during forced expiration in prevalent intrinsic airways obstruction.

One last point needs some clarification: the possible interference of airways obstruction on ventilation and, as a consequence, on oxygen supply to alveoli and blood. Let us assume that the degree of ventilation is only a function of the change in lung volume, produced by respiration, with time. The volume change, for changes in pleural pressure, of each ventilatory unit will be a function [45] of its mechanical characters (compliance and resistance) and of the time available (which is a function of the frequency of breathing). If we multiply the units of compliance by those of resistance, the product has, in fact, the dimension of time (the mechanical time constant); in fact compliance $= 1 \times cm\ H_2O^{-1}$ (normal value 0.2) and resistance $= cm\ H_2O \times l^{-1} \times s$ (normal value 2.0).

If lung regions had resistance or compliance markedly different from others, then this property of altered time constants might produce differences in regional ventilation. In normal lungs the mechanical time constant is 0.4 s; only when the time available is smaller than that, does the change in volume and the ventilation decrease. This condition corresponds to a frequency of breathing which is equal to 60/0.4 or 150/min. Let us imagine now a lung unit, whatever its size, having very high resistance, for instance 12 cm H_2O l^{-1} s; its mechanical time constant will be equal to 2.4 s and, therefore, at a breathing rate above 25/min that unit will not be mechanically ventilated in proportion to pressures applied by respiratory muscles. If we consider a contemporary comparable increase in compliance, the mechanical time constant would be 14.4 s and the critical frequency would be 4.2/min. Both the above conditions are extreme. If we consider a reasonable range of compliance and resistance alteration, it will appear that in most clinical situations, during resting conditions, the mechanical characteristics, on their own, are not able to interfere significantly with the overall ventilation, providing that the respiratory musculature is efficient enough to produce adequate pressure changes. The degree of gas exchange impairment in fact is often not directly comparable with the mechanical impairment, the same degree of impairment being not necessarily associated with evident gas exchange impairment at rest.

Site of Airways Resistance

In normals, larynx and pharynx account for nearly 40% of R_{aw}; only 20% is determined by airways having a diameter smaller than 2–3 mm [32, 50]. Let us consider that a normal R_{aw} value is 1.2 cm H_2O l^{-1} s; in order to increase R_{aw} to the value of 2, the resistance in the peripheral airways would have to increase nearly fivefold. The contribution of the peripheral airways to R_{aw} is even lower at volumes near TLC, but it increases as lung volume is reduced below FRC. The measurements of $\dot{V}_{max}$ will mainly reflect the dimensions of central intrathoracic airways, whilst only below FRC will the values reflect to a greater extent the dimension of the more peripheral airways. Since direct measurement of R_{aw} is done at a volume level above FRC, these values are relatively insensitive to the contribution of the peripheral airways in normal subjects.

The question of the contribution of smaller airways to R_{aw} has also been analyzed using the difference in flow regime between larger and smaller airways. MEFV curves have been studied in normals and during breathing of a mixture having a significantly lower density than ambient air. The most commonly used mixture has been helium (He) 80% plus oxygen (O_2), with a density of 0.178 compared to 1.2 for ambient air [52]. Turbulent flow, as stated above, is density dependent and is the prevalent flow regime in the larger airways; laminar flow is density independent and is prevalent in the smaller airways. The $\dot{V}_{max}$ values will be higher during He-O_2 breathing, compared to ambient air, when the flow measured at the mouth is mainly dependent on the dimensions of the larger airways. The greater the contribution of smaller airways to R_{aw}, and consequently to the decrease in $\dot{V}_{max}$, the smaller the difference in measured values between He-O_2 and ambient air. The MEFV curves, during breathing of the two different gas mixtures, are represented in Fig. 8; the contribution of the smaller airways to R_{aw} would be represented by the proportion of FVC having isoflow [29]. The high variability and the technical difficulties of this measurement have been shown [15]; however, it is usually accepted that in normals less than 15% of FVC is expired with flow rates mainly determined by resistance in smaller airways. In one study [34], the isoflow volume was 13% in normal nonsmokers and 24% in normal smokers.

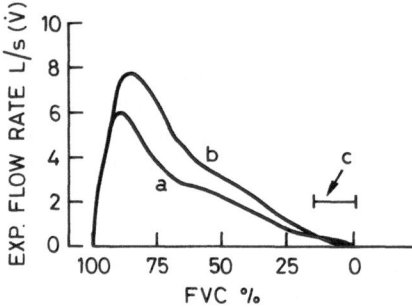

Fig. 8. MEFV curve during ambient air (*line a*) and helium–oxygen (*line b*) breathing. *FVC*, forced expired vital capacity; *c*, volume, as percent of FVC, having the same flow rate in both conditions $(V_{iso}\dot{V})$

The situation in disease is completely different, as has been shown [23] studying the site of intrinsic narrowing of the bronchial tree in postmortem lung preparations of COPD patients. As a mean, R_{aw} was 5 cm H_2O l^{-1} s and 80% of R_{aw} was in bronchi having diameter less than 2–3 mm. Large airways, although they were the site of mucous glands hypertrophy, did not account for much of the increased R_{aw}. Only in evident COPD is the measurement of R_{aw} therefore an evaluation index of smaller airways involvement. Any other test used for evaluating the function of the smaller airways in that condition would be equivalent to plethysmographic R_{aw} measurements, e.g., the more simple and economic test of forced expiration. This last test gives, after all, information about the smaller and larger airways; the indexes about the former are expected to be much more altered than those of the latter, as can be easily seen in clinical lung physiology practice. In asthma, the changes in MEFV curves on breathing He-O_2 are variable [13], suggesting that the site of predominant airways narrowing and expiratory airflow limitation is in the small airways in some patients while others have more widespread narrowing.

Structure–Function Relation

The trachea is a single airway divided into extra- and intrathoracic segments and having a reversed U shape; its caliber varies between 15 and 20 mm, the length being approximately 12 cm. It is subdivided into two main bronchi whose cumulative cross-sectional area can be smaller than the parent branch, in contrast to the pattern shown further on along the bronchial tree. The main bronchi also have a reversed U shape; they are intrathoracic but extraparenchymal airways and generate five lobar bronchi. Lobar bronchi are followed by 19 segmentary bronchi, corresponding to parenchymal segments having autonomous bronchial and vascular supports. Above here the cross-sectional area increases with branching, while the diameter of each generated branch decreases [58]. After some further subdivisions, the segmentary bronchi become bronchioles, whose most peripheral branches are the terminal bronchioles.

The airways generated by the terminal bronchioles, the respiratory bronchioles, have a variable number of alveoli along their wall, the terminal bronchioles being the borderline between the conducting airways and the gas exchange airways. Some authors do not recognize such a clear division, since alveoli are seldom found proximal to the borderline [56]. Distal to terminal bronchioles are three generations of respiratory bronchioles and several generations of alveolar sacs and ducts [20, 21], each successive branch containing an increasing number of alveoli. The respiratory bronchioles have a limited number of alveoli and, for this reason, Weibel [58] considers those structures as the transition area from conducting to gas exchange airways. The lung parenchyma relative to each terminal bronchiole is defined as an

Table 2. Subdivision and structural features of conducting airways

Large bronchi

  Airways: trachea, main bronchi, inferior lobar bronchi
  Relation with lung: outside lung tissue
  Diameter: between 16 and 7 mm
  Wall: U-shaped cartilage
  Muscle: posterior transverse bands
  Mucous glands: between cartilage rings and into muscular layer
  Epithelium: apparently 4–6 layers, pseudostratified; goblet and ciliated cells

Medium bronchi

  Airways: other lobar bronchi and segmentary bronchi
  Relation with lung: separated by a peribronchial sheath
  Diameter: between 7 and 4 mm
  Wall: cartilage plates
  Muscle: bidirectional spiral bands
  Mucous glands: many
  Epithelium: apparently 3–4 layers, pseudostratified; goblet and ciliated cells

Small bronchi

  Airways: intrasegmental bronchi
  Relation with lung: separated by a peribronchial sheath
  Diameter: between 4 and 1 mm
  Wall: small cartilage plates
  Muscle: more steeply bidirectional bands
  Mucous glands: few
  Epithelium: apparently 2–3 layers, pseudostratified; goblet, ciliated, and a few Clara cells

Bronchioles

  Airways: bronchioles down to terminal bronchioles
  Relation with lung: attached to surrounding lung tissue
  Diameter: between 1 and 0.5 mm
  Wall: no cartilage
  Muscle: thickest band in relation to wall thickness
  Mucous glands: none
  Epithelium: one cuboidal layer; ciliated, Clara, and a few goblet cells

acinus or a terminal ventilatory unit; their total number is about 30000, each one having a pyramidal shape and receiving the airway and the artery from the apex.

The conducting airways may be divided (Table 2) into large bronchi, medium bronchi, small bronchi, and bronchioles. Their structure is characterized by the following concentric layers, from within outwards: the mucous membrane, the submucosa, the fibrocartilaginous layer, and the peribronchial tissue.

The Mucous Membrane

The mucosa has three main components: the epithelium, a basement membrane, and the lamina propria.

The epithelial cells are provided with a tuft of kinocilia at their apical cell face; kinocilia are organelles of movement that are known to beat rhythmically into a periciliary fluid in a given direction and at about 20 Hz frequency. The epithelial cells not only have a simple barrier function but they are able to synthesize and transform several substances interfering with the bronchial smooth muscle response to bronchoconstrictive agents [16]. Another important function is the regulation of the osmolarity of the periciliary fluid and of the perireceptorial space; this function is performed through the ion exchanges determined by the cell's polarity [1], which decreases toward the periphery of the bronchial tree. On the epithelial cell surface there are β_2 receptors of the adrenergic autonomic nervous system [2], regulating cell functions together with mechanical, inflammatory, and osmotic stimuli.

The goblet cells, together with the submucosal mucous glands, participate in airway mucus production. The ciliated cells and the secretory apparatus constitute a system for mucociliary clearance [57] along the bronchial tree; its efficiency depending upon the kinetics of the cilia and the qualitative-quantitative secretion characteristics. At the large bronchi level the goblet-ciliated cell ratio is $1:5$, while it increases to $1:30$ in medium and small bronchi. At the bronchiole level the goblet cells are replaced by the Clara cells protruding in the bronchial lumen over the ciliated cells; it seems that the Clara cells produce a secretion which has both glycoprotein (mucus) and lipoprotein (surfactant) properties.

Between the basement membrane and the epithelium there are mast cells along the entire length of the human airways; some of them are found in the epithelium, abutting into the lumen [30]. These cells are obtained by bronchoalveolar lavage and constitute between 0.1 % and 1.0 % of cells recovered [17]. When the cells are activated, there is secretion of mediators, mainly histamine, through microtubules that move toward the cell membrane; the control of secretion is complex and lipid metabolism is involved [51].

The lamina propria has two main layers: (a) internally, a cellular layer in which lymphocytes, nerves and a capillary network are found and (b) externally, a fibrous layer with reticulin, which is connected with basement membrane, and collagen-elastic fibers linked with surrounding lung tissue at the bronchiole level.

Lymphoid nodules may be seen in the mucosal membrane at the level of large and medium bronchi. These occur as follicles without capsules and germinal centers (bronchial-associated lymphoid tissue) and contain small and medium-sized lymphocytes. The nodules are covered by a single layer of nonciliated epithelium and are involved in local and systemic immune responses to damage and infection.

The fast adapting irritant receptors are into and under the epithelium layer; they respond to a heterogeneous series of mechanical, chemical, and physical stimuli. The cough receptors are similar to the irritant receptors; the former are mainly situated at the tracheal level, while the irritant receptors are in the large airways. Their stimulation is transmitted, through myelinated fibers, to the vagus nuclei. Some other sensory nerve endings, analogous to irritant receptors, are localized in the epithelial layer, and stimulation reaches the vagus nuclei through nonmyelinated C fibers. These pass through the parasympathetic ganglia and can produce, with efferent postganglionic fibers, a reflex arc shorter than the one through the vagal nuclei. The stimulation of irritant receptors produces hyperventilation, cough, bronchoconstriction, and mucus secretion. These effects are largely, but not completely, mediated by the release of acetylcholine (cholinergic reflex) and inhibited by atropine; the remaining portion of the effects is mediated by the local release of neuropeptides, e.g., substance P, which also promotes inflammation (local neurogenic inflammation) with hyperemia, increased vascular permeability, and edema [3, 19, 31].

The Submucosa

This layer is generally made up of loose tissue containing the secretory portion of the mucous glands, smooth bronchial musculature, nerves, and lymphatics.

Mucous acinar glands are composed primarily of serous and mucous cells, the former producing neutral glycoproteins and the latter acidic glycoproteins. The secretions are carried to the airway surface through the gland ducts, which have a ciliated nonsecretory surface epithelium. The mucous gland layer is nearly 35% of the wall in a normal main bronchus; this ratio is usually referred to as the Reid index. The glands are mainly located in the wall of large and medium bronchi; as inflammation takes place there is gland hypertrophy and mucus hypersecretion. Gland secretion of fluid and mucus is under parasympathetic, adrenergic, and peptidergic neural control. In addition, gland secretion is mediated by local inflammatory mediators released from mast cells and neutrophils and having an effect on histamine, prostaglandins, and leukotrienes [44].

The smooth muscle layer, relative to the diameter of the bronchus, increases in thickness passing down the airways; as a proportion of the wall thickness, the muscle layer reaches its maximum in the terminal bronchioles. The muscle fibers at the bronchiole level are situated in the fibrous layer and are connected with the surrounding lung tissue smooth muscle fibers.

Numerous receptors have been demonstrated on the surface of smooth muscle fibers. Acetylcholine receptors [42] account for most of the muscle contraction following activation of the vagal reflex [43], the cholinergic bronchomotor excitation system, with the mediator being released by the parasympathetic efferent fibers. An analogue of acetylcholine, metacholine, is used for experimental bronchoconstriction; larger inhaled doses being required in normals than in patients with bronchial hyperresponsiveness [59]. In spite of the lack of evidence for direct sympathetic innervation, the bronchial tree musculature is rich in β_2-adrenergic receptors which mediate dilatation, the β-adrenergic bronchomotor inhibitory system; these receptors are triggered by circulating catecholamines rather than by neurotransmitters released from nerve terminals [2]. However, the physiological role of β-receptors in inhibiting induced bronchoconstriction is minor, demonstrating the existence of a nonadrenergic inhibitory system in human airways; the neurotransmitter involved has not been identified but several neuropeptides, e.g., vasoactive intestinal polypeptide (VIP) and adenosine, have been proposed [3]. There is also evidence of α-adrenoreceptors on bronchial smooth muscle, whose activity in normal subjects is obscured by the much higher density of β-receptors; only in asthma and airways inflammation may their stimulation cause airway narrowing [54]. Specific humoral receptors for histamine, prostaglandins and leukotrienes are also present on human bronchial smooth muscle [4].

Within the smooth muscle of the airways there are stretch receptors which show a slowly adapting response to maintained lung inflation; their highest density is in the more proximal airways. These receptors, connected to the vagus nuclei through myelinated afferent fibers, are involved in the Hering-Breuer reflex and in the postinspiratory bronchodilatation observed in subjects after induced bronchoconstriction.

The Fibrocartilaginous Membrane

This layer includes the cartilaginous structures and the fibrous membrane.

Cartilages have a reversed U shape in the trachea and the main bronchi. Further along the bronchial tree they become plates, being even smaller and less numerous toward the periphery and disappearing at the bronchiole level.

Outside the cartilaginous layer there is a nervous plexus containing vagal fibers (parasympathetic autonomic system), sympathetic fibers (from the first thoracic ganglia), and most of the parasympathetic ganglia, along the entire bronchial tree [48]. The postganglionic vagal fibers reach the target cells; the predominant neurotransmitter at both the preganglionic and postganglionic sites is acetylcholine. It has been demonstrated the presence of sympathetic nerve terminals in human parasympathetic ganglia [48].

The fibrous membrane consists of mainly longitudinal bundles of elastic and collagen fibers connecting together the cartilaginous plates; there are numerous openings for connective tissue, fat, gland ducts, vessels, and nerves. In the small bronchi oblique fibers pass from the fibrocartilaginous layer into the mucous membrane. At the bronchiole level, the fibrous membrane loses its separate identity and the connective tissue elements are in direct continuity with those of the surrounding lung tissue.

The Peribronchial Tissue

It is composed of fibrous tissue, fat, lymphatic tissue, nerves, vessels, and bronchial glands. This tissue ensheaths the bronchi as far as the origin of the bronchioles, where the bronchial tree becomes continuous with the surrounding lung tissue. There is a virtual space between the bronchi and the peribronchial tissue which can fill with fluid or air. The peribronchial tissue connects with the perivascular tissue, the interlobular septa, and the pleura, and it is thus part of the lung connective tissue framework.

The Gas Exchange Airways

At the gas-exchange airways level, the respiratory bronchioles are lined with cuboidal epithelium, which becomes flatter and thinner peripherally until it joins the alveolar epithelium. Under the basement membrane there are smooth muscle fibers which decrease toward the periphery. Alveolar ducts are surrounded by a network of connective tissue containing reticulin together with collagen, elastic, and muscle fibers, whose number decreases toward the alveolar sacs. Lymphoid aggregates are concentrated in the distal airways, especially at the bronchoalveolar junctions. Alveoli are blind sacs arising from the walls of the respiratory bronchioles and alveolar ducts. They are flexible polyhedric structures which change shape during breathing or bronchiole contraction. The alveolar walls are supported by a broad three-dimensional network containing reticulin with collagen and elastic fibers, which is responsible for the elastic properties of the lung tissue. The lining alveolar epithelium is composed of two cell types supported by the basement membrane. The cytoplasm of the type I epithelial cells covers 90% of the alveolar surface. The type II cells are more compact and contain characteristic inclusions which represent surfactant; this substance covers the epithelium and minimizes the alveolar surface tension forces at different lung inflations. Some other important cell populations comprise the alveolar lining. Lymphocytes represent 7%–10% of the 10×10^6 cells in a bronchoalveolar lavage sample [28], 70% being T lymphocytes (45% T helper and 25% T suppressor). The alveolar macrophages are important in healthy lungs, since they act as scavenger cells, process foreign antigens for presentation to lymphocytes, and secrete a peptide that causes mediator release from mast cells [53].

Some functional considerations arise from the structural arrangement described above:

1. The bronchioles are roots anchored in the lung parenchyma, transmitting the respiratory movements to the remaining bronchial tree which runs inward and outward along the virtual peribronchial space. Thus the bronchioles are subjected to parenchymal traction or compression; moreover, the forces are transmitted across the virtual peribronchial space in just the same way as they are across the pleural space. When fluids fill the peribronchial space, the retractive forces fail to hold the bronchi open and some degree of obstruction will be evident, for instance, during chronic or acute pulmonary edema.

2. Large bronchi have small dynamic caliber changes. In case of compression they only reduce the diameter by invagination of the posterior membranous walls. On muscular contraction the ends of the cartilages are drawn together, resulting only in a small reduction of the cross-sectional area. The medium bronchi are mainly supported by the retractive forces, the cartilage plates giving some stiffness; on muscular contraction the plates come together allowing the lumen to diminish. On smooth muscle contraction at the bronchiole level, the surrounding lung tissue is distorted and adjacent alveoli become elongated; since the muscle layer is at its thickest in relation to the bronchial wall, its contraction induces a relatively greater reduction of the original bronchial lumen than in the remaining bronchial tree.

3. The pulmonary defense mechanisms at the conducting airways level are mainly of a mechanical nature (humidification, dilution produced by secretions, aerodynamic filtration produced by airways branching, mucociliary clearance); at this level IgA, locally secreted by plasma cells, and other substances, secreted when specific target cells are stimulated, are involved. At the gas exchange airways level the main defense mechanisms are cellular and humoral in nature.

4. Under physiological conditions there is a resting smooth muscle bronchial, or bronchomotor, tone. This is maintained by tonic vagal output, as demonstrated by the marked bronchodilatation which occurs following bilateral vagotomy or by the bronchoconstriction that occurs following the administration of an anticholinesterase. Bilateral vagal stimulation causes marked constriction of the central airways but has little influence on bronchioles. The major role of sympathetic innervation may be the modulation of parasympathetic neurotransmission. Some bronchodilatation is achieved by stimulating the β_2-adrenoreceptors [22]. Several neuropeptides, e.g., substance P, are involved in the noncholinergic excitation system of bronchomotor tone, while others, e.g., VIP, are involved in the inhibitory system. Specific humoral regulation of bronchomotor tone is mediated by histamine, prostaglandins, and leukotrienes.

Morphometry–Function Relation

The quantitative morphology (morphometry) of the branching of the airways can be described as the generations [58] on a resin plastic cast of the human bronchial tree, assuming that it is symmetrical and that the simple law of dichotomy can be applied. This implies that the number of branches in each generation is given by 2^z, where z is the number of generations. In this model the airways are numbered beginning at the trachea and the generation number will increase with successive branches. As the trachea is the airway having generation number zero, the two main bronchi will correspond to generation number one, the 65536 terminal bronchioles would have generation number 16, and the 8388608 forth generation alveolar ducts, successive to three generations of respiratory bronchioles, would have generation number 23. Therefore, in this model there will be 65536 acini, 240 alveolar ducts per acinus, and 15.73×10^6 alveolar ducts. By fitting the model to the data, the number of terminal bronchioles is too high and this structure will be better represented by generation number 14 or 15; at the same time there are too few alveolar ducts [20, 21]. As was appreciated by its authors, this model misses the asymmetry of the bronchial tree.

The asymmetry of the system mainly stems from the conducting airways, since it is known that at the respiratory bronchiole level the law of regular dichotomy applies [20, 21, 47]. Within each of the 30000 acini counted in the lungs, there are three generations of respiratory bronchioles plus three to nine generations of alveolar ducts. An important feature of the respiratory bronchioles is that the diameter of the daughter branches does not decrease compared to the parent branch, as is the case in the conducting airways. As a consequence the cross-sectional area will increase at a higher rate during branching.

In order to overcome the difficulties in describing the asymmetry, the river branching study system, described by Strahler [55], has been applied [24] in counting and measuring the conducting airways in a resin cast of the bronchial tree. The smallest stream, or airway, is identified as the branch having 0.7 mm diameter and pruning the cast beyond that level. The remaining proximal bronchial tree is numbered by orders, the smallest branches having order number one; within each order the number of branches can be counted and their dimensions can be measured.

The main point in the Strahler model is that the branches are numbered beginning from the periphery toward the central airways. The order number of each branch increases only when the two joining branches have the same order number; otherwise, the order number would be the highest order between the two joining branches. Therefore, we have a branch number six only when there is confluence of two branches having order number five. The pruned bronchial tree is described by 17 Strahler order numbers, the trachea being the order number 17. There is a close relation between (Fig. 9) the logarithm of the number of branches and the Strahler order, the slope of the linear relation being 2.74. This means that in this ordering system each

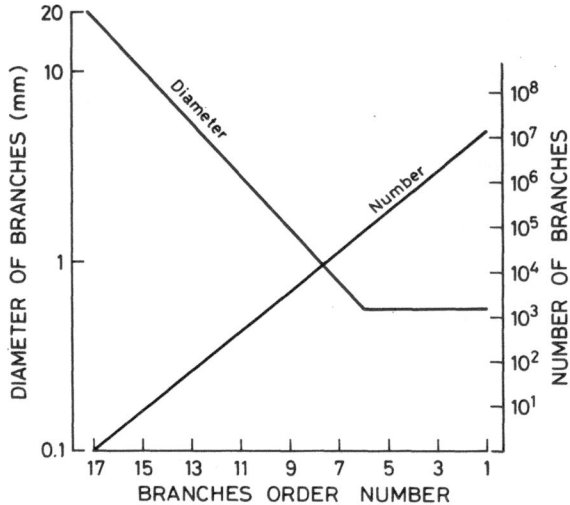

Fig. 9. Morphometric features of bronchial branching. *Abscissa*, Strahler order number; *ordinate*, number of branches on the *right* side and diameter of branches on the *left* side. At the trachea level, order number 17, there is the lowest number of branches and the largest diameter. Number of branches increases with decreasing order number toward the alveoli, whilst the diameter decreases. Above order number six, the number of branches further increases but the diameter remains unchanged. (Original data from [24])

branch gives rise, as a mean, to 2.74 daughter branches; this number is called the common ratio of geometric branching progression. The simple relation existing between the number of branches and their order number is also present for the branches' dimensions (diameter and length). However, the most important point is that in the airways the law of increase of diameter with increasing order is exactly one half of the branching law (2.74/2 = 1.37). The change in diameter in the airways is only applicable down to the level of branches having order number six (Fig. 9); beyond that level the branching is no longer associated with a decrease in branch diameter, as is the case for the respiratory bronchioles. The system considers the terminal bronchioles as the branches having order number 6, but this is not the real case and there will be a slight underestimation of the number of such branches (28000 instead of 30000). Nonetheless the system has the advantage of describing the bron-chial tree in functional terms, since the branch having order number six is a marker of a change in function along the bronchial tree.

During these morphometric analyses of the bronchial tree it has been possible to measure the overall airways dimensions at different sections of the branching system. Their consequences in terms of end cross-sectional area, linear distance, and volume can be reported (Table 3) for five morphometric compartments.

Only 5% of the lung volume, approximated to 4000 ml, is in the conducting airways, the remaining being in the respiratory zone including the transition zone of the respiratory bronchioles. The system therefore makes a compromise between the need to maintain as small as possible the size of the conducting airways and the opposite requirement of maintaining as low as possible the resistance to airflow along the conducting airways. The system applies the biological principle of minimum work for convective flow [25]; in

Table 3. Dimensions of bronchial tree morphometric compartments

Region	Distance (mm)	Volume (ml)	Cross-section (cm^2)
A	220	80	2
B	130	71	14
C	5	43	79
D	3.6	865	281
E	2.6	3000	7×10^5

A, upper airways; B, compartment between carina and lobular bronchioles; C, compartment between lobular and terminal bronchioles; D, respiratory bronchioles transition zone; E, alveolar ducts and sacs

fact, the Strahler ordering system of the conductive airways corresponds to the theoretical condition, which requires the law branching diameter to be one half of the coefficient of subdivision.

Let us consider a tidal volume of 600 ml, inspired during 3 s, the mean inspiratory flow being 200 ml/s. Since there are nearly 30000 terminal bronchioles, the flow through each branch is 0.00067 ml/s. Furthermore, we must consider that the cross-sectional area increases from trachea to terminal bronchioles by 40-fold (Table 3); therefore the flow in the terminal bronchioles would decrease by the same amount and the flow rate at that level of airways would be very low indeed. Considering the possibility of hyperventilation and consequent higher flow rate, it has in any case to be taken into account that the airflow, passing from terminal to respiratory bronchioles, would further decrease by a factor of 3.5, due to an equal increase in cross-sectional area (Table 3).

Since the rate of increase of cross-sectional area is greater peripherally, the flow rate will progressively decrease until the force moving the gas molecules will be the passive diffusion in the gas phase (gas mixing). The efficiency of diffusion requires different conditions with respect to the mass transport of molecules [9, 10, 12]. Diffusion will require both a large surface between the two diffusing components and, because of the crucial importance of linear distance, the smallest linear distance for the biggest proportion of lung volume. This condition is met by the bronchial tree, changing the morphometric characteristics at the level of the terminal bronchioles. Some 75% of lung volume is in the respiratory zone, within a mean linear distance of 2.6 mm and distributed in a very large cross-sectional area (7×10^5 cm^2); each of the 30000 acini will have a volume of 0.2 ml. A one mm linear movement of inspired O_2 molecules in this zone corresponds to complete mixing of nearly one half of the alveolar volume involved.

The slope change of the relation between branches diameter and order number (Fig. 9) is an expression of an airways function change. The transition between mass transport and gas mixing is represented by the concept of the stationary interface [46]. It corresponds to the point along the bronchial tree where the gas molecules do not progress any further because of mass transport and diffusion takes place. This interface, during tidal breathing, is probably at the level of a third order respiratory bronchiole. Since the number of orders of alveolar ducts and sacs varies between three and nine, the linear distance for diffusion will be between 2 and 11 mm. The degree of mixing and, as a consequence, of gas concentration between alveolar units will be variable indeed. This would explain the marked inefficiency of gas mixing observed in diseased lungs [5, 6].

The main lesson, in terms of airways function, which stems from the morphometric study of the bronchial tree is that the process of gas concentration conditioning at the alveolar level (ventilation as gas mixing) is largely independent of the resistance to airflow along the conducting airways. The consequences of airways obstruction on the amount of oxygen available at the alveolar level will be dependent upon the positioning of the stationary interface and the obstruction distribution factor. The less homogeneous the distribution of airways resistance the greater is the effect on gas mixing inefficiency. The same decrease of FEV_1 in an asthmatic patient would have different consequences on alveolar mixing, represented by different degrees of hypoventilation in terms of alveolar O_2 concentration. The net effect on blood oxygenation will depend on the combination of: degree and distribution of obstruction, lung tissue damage as occurs in emphysema, impairment of gas mixing, predetermined individual morphometric characteristics such as the prevalence of small airways in the bronchial tree [8], and local alveolar distribution of ventilation perfusion ratios.

Furthermore, monitoring arterial blood oxygenation during induced asthma or in chronic asthma would give results not strictly related to FEV_1 measurements but still related to quantity and quality of obstruction. It has to be taken into account that in asthmatic subjects with normal base lung function tests (peripheral $\dot{V}_{max}$ excluded), changes in peripheral airways resistance would be able to damage alveolar gas mixing and gas exchange efficiency without detectably significant chan-ges in R_{aw} and FEV_1.

References

1. Al-Bazzaz FJ (1986) Regulation of salt and water transport across airway mucosa. Clin Chest Med 77:259–272
2. Barnes P, Karliner JS, Dollery CT (1980) Human lung adrenoceptors studied by radioligand binding. Clin Sci 58:457–461
3. Barnes P (1987) Neuropeptides in the lung: localizing, function and pathophysiologic implications. J Allergy Clin Immunol 79:285–295
4. Black J (1986) Receptors on human airway smooth muscle. Bull Eur Physiopathol Respir 22 [Suppl 7]:162–170
5. Bowes CL, Cumming G, Horsfield K, Loughhead J, Preston S (1982) Gas mixing in a model of the pulmonary acinus with asymmetrical alveolar ducts. J Appl Physiol 52:624–633
6. Bowes CL, Richardson JD, Cumming G, Horsfield K (1985) Effect of breathing pattern on gas mixing in a model with asymmetrical alveolar ducts. J Appl Physiol 58:18–26

7. Campbell EJM, Agostoni E, Davis JN (1970) The respiratory muscles: mechanics and neural control, 2nd edn. Saunders, Philadelphia
8. Cosio MG, Hale KA, Niewoehner DE (1980) Morphologic and morphometric effect of prolonged cigarette smoking on the small airways. Am Rev Respir Dis 121:265–271
9. Cumming G, Crank J, Horsfield K, Preston SB (1966) Gaseous diffusion in the airways of the human lung. Respir Physiol 1:58–74
10. Cumming G, Guyatt AR (1982) Alveolar gas mixing efficiency in the human lung. Clin Sci 62:541–547
11. Damato S, Bianco S, Allegra L (1980) The decay of thoracic gas volume during forced expiration. Respiration 40:9–12
12. Damato S, Cumming G (1989) Tidal volume change and gas mixing in the lung. Respiration 56:173–181
13. Despas PJ, Leroux M, Macklem PT (1972) Site of airway obstruction in asthma as determined by measuring maximal expiratory flow breathing air and a helium-oxygen mixture. J Clin Invest 51:3235–3241
14. Dowson SV, Elliot EA (1977) Wave-speed limitation on expiratory flow – a unifying concept. J Appl Physiol; Respirat Environ Exercise Physiol 43:498–515
15. Dull WL, Secker-Walker RH (1979) Helium oxygen flow volume curve in young healthy adults. Respiration 38:18–26
16. Flavahn NA, Vanhouette PM (1985) The respiratory epithelium releases a smooth muscle relaxing factor. Chest 87:189S–190S
17. Flint KC, Leung KBP, Pearce FL, Hudspith BN, Brostoff J, Johnson NMcI (1985) Human mast cells recovered by bronchoalveolar lavage: their morphology, histamine release and the effects of sodium cromoglycate. Clin Sci 68:427–432
18. Fry DL, Hyatt RE (1960) Pulmonary mechanics: a unified analysis of the relationship between pressure, volume and gas flow in the lungs of normal and diseased human subjects. Am J Med 29:672–689
19. Hakanson R, Sunder F, Moghimzadeh E, Leander S (1983) Peptide containing nerve fibres in the airways: distribution and functional implications. Eur J Respir Dis 131:115–146
20. Hansen JE, Ampaya EP (1975) Human air space shapes, sizes, areas and volumes. J Appl Physiol 38:990–995
21. Hansen JE, Ampaya EP, Bryant GH, Navin JJ (1975) Branching pattern of airways and air spaces of a single human terminal bronchiole. J Appl Physiol 38:983–989
22. Hensley MJ, O'Cain CF, McFadden ER Jr, Ingram RH Jr (1978) Distribution of bronchodilatation in normal subjects: beta agonist versus atropine. J Appl Physiol 45:778–782
23. Hogg JC, Macklem PT, Thurlbeck WM (1968) Site and nature of airway obstruction in chronic obstructive lung disease. N Engl J Med 278:1355–1360
24. Horsfield K, Cumming G (1968) Morphology of the bronchial tree in man. J Appl Physiol 24:373–383
25. Horsfield K (1977) Morphology of branching trees related to entropy. Respir Physiol 29:179–188
26. Hyatt RE, Schilder DP, Fry DL (1958) Relationship between maximum expiratory flow and degree of lung inflation. J Appl Physiol 13:331–336
27. Hyatt RE, Black LF (1973) The flow volume curve: a current perspective. Am Rev Respir Dis 107:191–199
28. Hunninghake GW, Crystal RG (1981) Pulmonary sarcoidosis: a disorder mediated by excess helper T-lymphocyte activity at sites of disease activity. N Engl J Med 305:429–434
29. Hutcheon M, Griffin P, Levison H, Zamel N (1974) Volume of isoflow. A new test in detection of mild abnormalities of lung mechanics. Am Rev Respir Dis 110:458–465
30. Jeffrey PK, Corrin B (1984) Structural analysis of the respiratory tract. In: Bie-

nenstock J (ed) Immunology of the lung and upper respiratory tract. McGraw-Hill, New York, pp 1–27

31. Laitinen A (1985) Autonomic innervation of the human respiratory tract as revealed by histochemical and ultrastructural methods. Eur J Respir Dis 66:7–42

32. Macklem PT, Mead J (1967) Resistance of central and peripheral airways measured by a retrograde catheter. J Appl Physiol 22:395–401

33. Macklem PT, Mead J (eds) (1986) Handbook of physiology, sect 3: the respiratory system, vol 3: mechanics of breathing. American Physiological Society, Bethesda

34. Malo JL, Leblanc P (1975) Functional abnormalities in young asymptomatic smokers with special reference to flow volume curves breathing various gasses. Am Rev Respir Dis 111:623–629

35. Martin J, Powell E, Shore S, Emrich J, Engel LA (1980) The role of the respiratory muscles in the hyperinflation of bronchial asthma. Am Rev Respir Dis 121:441–447

36. Mead J, Turner JM, Macklem PT, Little JB (1967) Significance of the relationship between lung recoil and maximum expiratory flow. J Appl Physiol 22:95–108

37. Mead J, Takishima T, Leith D (1970) Stress distribution in lungs: a model of pulmonary elasticity. J Appl Physiol 28:596–608

38. Mead J (1978) Analysis of the configuration of maximum expiratory flow volume curves. J Appl Physiol 44:156–165

39. Melissinos CG, Webster P, Tien YK, Mead J (1977) Time dependence of maximum flow as an index of nonuniform emptying. J Appl Physiol 47:1043–1050

40. Milic-Emili J, Henderson JAM, Dolovich MB, Trop D, Kaneko K (1966) Regional distribution of inspired gas in the lung. J Appl Physiol 21:749–759

41. Mink SN, Wood LDH (1980) How does HeO_2 increase maximum expiratory flow in human lungs. J Clin Invest 66:720–729

42. Murlas C, Nadel JA, Roberts JM (1982) The muscarinic receptors of airway smooth muscle: their characterization in vitro. J Appl Physiol 52:1084–1091

43. Nadel JA (1980) Autonomic regulation of airway smooth muscle. In: Nadel JA (ed) Physiology and pharmacology of the airways. Dekker, New York, pp 217–257

44. Nadel JA, Widdicombe JH, Peatfiled AC (1985) Regulation of airways secretions, ion transport and water movement. In: Fishman AP, Fisher AB (eds) Handbook of physiology, sect 3: the respiratory system, vol. 1: circulatory and nonrespiratory functions. American Physiological Society, Bethesda, pp 419–445

45. Otis AB, McKerrow CB, Bartlett RA, Mead J, McIlroy MB, Selverstone NJ, Radford EP (1956) Mechanical factors in distribution of pulmonary ventilation. J Appl Physiol 8:427–443

46. Paiva M (1973) Gas transport in the human lung. J Appl Physiol 35:401–410

47. Parker H, Horsfield K, Cumming G (1971) Morphology of distal airways in the human lung. J Appl Physiol 31:386–391

48. Partanen M, Laitinen A, Hervonen A, Toivanen M, Laitinen LA (1982) Catecholamine and acetyl cholinesterase containing nerves in human lower respiratory tract. Histochemistry 76:175–188

49. Pedley TJ, Schroter RC, Sudlow MF (1978) Gas flow and mixing in the airways. In: West J (ed) Bioengineering aspects of the lung. Dekker, New York, pp 163–265

50. Pride NB (1971) The assessment of airflow obstruction: role of measurement of airways resistance and of tests of forced expiration. Br J Dis Chest 65:135–169

51. Robinson C, Holgate ST (1985) Mast cell-dependent inflammatory mediators and their putative role in bronchial asthma. Clin Sci 68:103–112

52. Schilder DP, Roberts A, Fry DL (1963) Effect of gas density and viscosity on the maximal expiratory flow volume relationship. J Clin Invest 42:1705–1713

53. Schulman ES, Liu MC, Proud D, MacGlashan DW Jr, Lichtenstein LM, Plaut M

(1985) Human lung macrophages induce histamine release from basophils and mast cells. Am Rev Respir Dis 131:230–235
54. Snashall PD, Boother FA, Sterling GM (1978) The effect of alpha-adrenoreceptor stimulation on the airways of normal and asthmatic man. Clin Sci Mol Med 54:283–289
55. Strahler AN (1950) Equilibrium theory of erosional slopes approached by distribution analysis. Am J Sci 248:673–696
56. Thurlbeck WM, Wang NS (1974) The structure of the lungs. In: Widdecombe JG (ed) MTP international reviews of science: respiration physiology series 1, vol 2. Butterworths, London
57. Wanner A (1988) Mucus transport in vivo. In: Braga PC, Allegra L (eds) Methods in bronchial mucology. Raven, New York, pp 279–289
58. Weibel ER (1963) Morphometry of the human lung. Springer, Berlin Heidelberg New York
59. Woolcock AJ (1985) Expression of results of airway hyperresponsiveness. In: Hargrave FG, Woolcock AJ (eds) Airway responsiveness measurement and interpretation. Astra Pharmaceutical Canada, Missisauga, pp 80–85

Asthma: Origin, Mechanisms, and Clinical Aspects

I. ZIMENT

Department of Medicine, Olive View Medical Center, UCLA School of Medicine, Sylmar, CA, USA

Introduction

Although asthma responds to therapy directed at changes in the airways of the bronchial tree, the cause of the asthmatic response may lie elsewhere. Thus, treatment may need to be directed at the specific causative factor and at any organ or tissue that is primarily responsible. It is not possible to provide an accurate breakdown of the frequency with which other sites are etiologically involved, but in a large proportion of asthmatic patients infectious disorders in the upper respiratory tract appear to initiate the bronchospastic reaction. A relatively small proportion of cases of asthma are attributable as secondary reactions to primary diseases located in various organs of the body, including the lungs themselves.

The mechanisms by which specific primary factors cause the asthmatic reaction are complex and cannot be fully explained by simple analysis. The airway response can be mediated directly by mucosal and submucosal neurochemical reactions or indirectly through autonomic reflexes that are, in turn, modulated by further interactions of neurochemical mechanisms. The total system is reduplicative, allowing separate but loosely integrated pathways to mediate the bronchospastic response. Several different classes of pharmacologic agents are able to intervene in the causative mechanisms or to negate the asthmatic response at various levels in the nervous system and the respiratory tract.

The major extrapulmonary causes of asthma and their mechanisms will be described individually.

Nasal Diseases and Asthma

The relationship between the nose and the lungs is clearly seen in asthma patients who also suffer from hay fever, particularly in those subjects who develop rhinorrhea and bronchospasm as a joint response to a specific allergen. Indeed, the relationship between hay fever and asthma was formerly stressed by the term "hay asthma," although it is now obvious that hay is rarely the exciting factor, and fever is not manifested as part of the basic response whether the nose or the lungs are affected. The nasal disease corresponding to asthma is allergic rhinitis: both are common in families with a strong history of atopy, and each may occur in the same patient and may also be associated with eczema.

Allergic Rhinitis

Smith et al. [36] evaluated 1125 patients with allergy; 78% with extrinsic asthma also had nasal symptoms, while asthma occurred in 38% of patients whose primary problem was allergic rhinitis. The underlying atopic tendency appears to have a genetic basis, and a common HLA distribution may account for a liability to allergic rhinitis associated with asthma and eczema. A clone of T lymphocytes infiltrates the nasal mucosa and appears to underlie the cellular reactions that cause the manifestations of rhinitis [35].

Allergic rhinitis tends to appear in childhood and is less likely to remit than is asthma. The presence of allergic rhinitis at a young age may be followed by the development of troublesome chronic asthma, but this is thought to occur in only 5%–10% of patients [35]. However, since allergic rhinitis may occur in 10% of children and 20%–30% of adolescents [32], a considerable number of adult asthmatic patients may have a history of "hay fever" earlier in life; indeed, as many as 85% of patients with asthma give a history of prior allergic rhinitis [3]. This can sometimes be recognized by the persistence of a nasal crease (from the frequent rubbing of the allergic nose during childhood) or by darkening of the skin of the lower eyelids.

Aeroallergens are presumed to be the major cause of both rhinitis and asthma in atopic subjects, who have a genetic predisposition to produce excessive amounts of immunoglobulin E (IgE) in response to repeated antigenic stimulation [16]. Presumably, similar reponse mechanisms exist in the lung and the nose, but nasal allergy is more prevalent because of the greater susceptibility of the nasal mucosa to deposition of inhaled antigens during inhalation. In the atopic individual, production of IgE is eventually followed by binding of the antibody to receptors on sensitized mast cells [23]. The activated cells will liberate inflammatory mediators when exposed to antigenic stimulus under suitable circumstances. It is probable that in addition to macrophages and eosinophils, basophils also play a prominent role in mediating the late obstructive response that characterizes persisting allergic rhinitis [17].

The exact relationship between allergic rhinitis and allergic asthma varies between different populations and with the specific antigen. Thus, patients who are allergic to ragweed pollen may develop severe rhinitis, but this antigen rarely causes asthma. In contrast, antigens such as cat salivary protein may cause both rhinitis and asthma in a susceptible individual, with the nasal response predominating early in life. If a child has both asthma and allergic rhinitis, there is a much greater chance that the asthma will persist into adulthood than is the risk for the asthmatic child without rhinitis; the likelihood of persistence is still greater if there is a family history of atopy. Local mechanisms that determine antigen deposition and penetration of the mucosa, as well as mediator release, differ in the nose and lung as an outcome of anatomic and physiologic individuality.

Sinusitis

In Galen's time it was believed that catarrhal secretion dripping from the pituitary gland into the lung caused pulmonary disease. This theory of pituitous catarrh was denounced by van Helmont, but was recently resurrected in modern terms with the concept that the flux of phlegm comes from the paranasal sinuses rather than from the pituitary. Old and new evidence has been presented by Slavin in support of a vagally mediated nasobronchial reflex form of bronchospasm that can be initiated by sinusitis [34]. Infection may stimulate paranasal sinus receptors from which reflex vagal activation causes an increase in lower airway muscle tone. Slavin and colleagues have evaluated numerous patients in whom sinusitis preceded the appearance of asthma; a causal relationship was suggested by lack of both atopy and corticosteroid dependency, and a marked improvement in the asthma following appropriate treatment of the patients' sinusitis [33]. However, the abnormal sinus radiographs that are frequent in patients with asthma may represent noninfectious inflammation, since cultures of sinus material are often negative for bacteria, fungi, and viruses.

The association of asthma and sinusitis appears to be common. Thus it is possible that about 50% of asthmatic patients will have abnormal sinus findings if these are sought by appropriate radiologic evaluation [1]. However, personal experience suggests that the finding of sinus disease in asthma may be considered to be coincidental in many cases; indeed, in the general population a causal relationship is difficult to demonstrate, and the nature of the association still requires further evaluation [15]. In some patients, the asthma improves when the sinusitis is effectively treated with mucosal constrictors and antibiotics. It is reasonable to follow Slavin's advice to consider the possible presence of sinus disease when asthma is difficult to control and to direct vigorous specific therapy at any suggestion of sinus infection and congestion that may be found [33].

When sinusitis is suspected as a possible cause of asthma, various techniques can be used to evaluate the sinuses [8]. These include plain radiography, plain tomograms, computerized tomography (CT), nuclear magnetic resonance imaging (which is particularly useful for detecting fungal infection), thermography, positron emission tomography, xenon-enhanced dynamic CT (to assess sinus ventilation), evaluation of smears and cultures from the nose or of fluid from antral puncture, sinuscopy or fiberoptic rhinoscopy, and nasal cytology. Ultrasonography and transillumination are of little value, while nasal plethysmography is only useful as a research tool. A

Waters view on radiography or selective CT scans can provide clear evidence of sinus disease in most cases. Therapeutic approaches include standard medical therapy with antibiotics, vasoconstrictors, and corticosteroids; if necessary, surgical intervention is used to improve sinus drainage. Endoscopic sinus surgery offers more precise intervention.

Nasal Polyposis

Settipane and Chaffee reviewed nearly 5000 patients seen in an adult allergy practice [29]. Nasal polyposis was diagnosed in 4.2%; asthmatic patients had a higher incidence (6.7%) than patients with rhinitis alone (2.2%). The non-allergic asthmatic population had an even higher incidence (12.5%), and of the 211 patients with polyps, 71% had asthma. There is a clear association of aspirin intolerance resulting in severe asthma in patients with polyposis; in the series of Settipane and Chaffee, 14% of the patients with polyps had aspirin intolerance. The association of nasal polyps and asthma in children was rare in these authors' experience. A large proportion of patients will show evidence of allergy, and there is a significant increase in haplotype HLA A1/B8 in asthmatic patients with polyps [33]. The disease also occurs in cystic fibrosis and with chronic nasal or sinus infection. Patients with polyps sometimes show bronchial hyperreactivity in the absence of overt asthma. In general populations, the association of asthma with polyps will be far less evident than in a selected group of allergic patients, but the relationship nevertheless appears to be significant.

It is not certain in any individual patient that therapeutic maneuvers directed at polyps will have a beneficial effect on asthma. Indeed, it had previously been thought that bronchial hyperreactivity could be increased as a consequence of polypectomy, although this does not generally appear to be the case. Thus, it is appropriate to evaluate and treat polyps on the basis of the need to control nasal symptoms and to not be influenced by the fact that the patient has concomitant asthma. Most polyps arise from the ethmoid sinuses, and endoscopic instrumentation of the nose is usually required to visualize them – although large ones may be readily seen through a nasal speculum. Appropriate radiologic studies may display their anatomy, with CT being more revealing.

Aspirin Hypersensitivity

There is a well known association of aspirin hypersensitivity with asthma. The relationship probably occurs in less than 5% of patients with asthma, but some series report that up to 25% of asthmatic patients suffer from hypersensitivity to aspirin or other nonsteroidal anti-inflammatory agents. The mechanism appears to involve mediator release, but no fully satisfactory explanation has been elucidated. About a quarter of all patients with aspirin-induced asthma have polyps, and it has been claimed that polypectomy may improve the asthma in up to 84 % of these patients [10]. Other asthmatic patients may have symptoms of rhinitis or sinusitis, which may be exacerbated by aspirin in the absence of polyps.

Asthma induced by aspirin or nonsteroidal anti-inflammatory agents may appear within minutes following ingestion of the drug; the response may be severe and life-threatening. Other dyes and sensitizers, such as paraben, tartrazine, and sulfites, may have a similar effect, but this appears to occur rarely with dyes and sulfites and more commonly with parabens. The mechanisms for these reactions has not been determined, although at least six theories have been proposed [38]. The disorder can be difficult to demonstrate with challenge studies, and desensitization is not generally practiced although it may prove to be successful. If the relationship is suspected in an asthmatic patient, aspirin containing drug products and other nonsteroidal analgesics should be avoided.

Mechanisms Linking Nose Disease and Asthma

Rhinitis, sinusitis, and polyposis can occur in patients with an allergic diathesis, and these subjects may also develop immunologically mediated asthma. Many children with allergic nasal disorders may show bronchial hyperreactivity, and in later life asthmatic symptoms may predominate. Impaired nasal breathing can force the patient to breathe through the mouth, and this results in poor humidification of the inspired air; this relatively dry air may irritate the tracheobronchial tree and result in a tendency to asthma. Inhalation of mucus from the abnormal upper airway, or passive postnasal drip, may also cause irritation of the lower airways and can introduce infection into the bronchial passages, which could possibly predispose to bronchitis and to β-adrenergic blockade [1]. The relationship between the nose and asthma may be traced through a reflex involving the afferent trigeminal entry into the reticular formation and the dorsal vagal nuclei, with the efferent arc being completed through the vagal supply to the lower airways [34].

Irritants placed in the nose can cause reflex bronchospasm in susceptible subjects, and this effect can be blocked by atropine. Shim and Williams [31] have demonstrated that strong or irritating odors (such as insecticide, household cleaning agents, cigarette smoke, perfumes, fresh paint, car exhaust, and cooking foods) may induce bronchospasm in asthmatics. Anosmic patients can experience the reaction, suggesting that a direct immunologic reaction in the nasal mucosa results in the bronchospasm either through a mediator or neural response: however, the odor molecules do not function as antigens. Shim and Williams speculate that a psychologic factor may also be involved. There is uncertainty about the frequency of the causal relationship between nonspecific provocation of the nose and asthma.

Laryngeal Asthma

Wheezing can be produced by a voluntary or semivoluntary adduction of the vocal cords. Some asthmatics with their disease in remission can produce a voluntary wheeze during a forced exhalation, or they can deliberately exhale in such a way as to avoid wheezing. This differs from functional laryngeal wheezing as an episodic event in which the patient and the physician may believe that the subject has true asthma. A variety of names have been given to this syndrome of "laryngeal asthma," including nonorganic acute (or functional) upper airway obstruction, episodic laryngeal dyskinesia, emotional laryngeal wheezing, Munchausen's stridor, factitious asthma, and glottic dysfunction. Goldman and Muers, in a recent review, suggest that the name for this entity should be vocal cord dysfunction presenting as asthma [12].

The typical patient is a woman under 40 with rapid breathing at low lung volume, absence of hyperinflation, and wheezing heard best over the laryngeal area on auscultation. Spirometric tracings in these subjects tend to be poorly reproducible and may be mostly normal; there is a lack of bronchial responsiveness to provocative stimuli. The flow-volume loop may show a variable extrathoracic obstruction pattern with fluttering of the inspiratory limb [26], and laryngoscopy may show adduction of the true and false vocal cords during various phases of the respiratory cycle [22]. The "asthma"' may improve with sedation, and control of symptoms may be achieved by working with a speech therapist to reduce the tendency to adduct the vocal cords. However, the patient with a correctable emotional problem underlying the disorder is unlikely to improve unless she can be made aware of the benign nature of the problem, since the disorder so closely mimics asthma and thus causes the anxiety that this diagnosis engenders [22]. Simple explanation and reassurance may suffice in the mildly depressed or anxious patient, whereas psychotherapeutic management will be required in more serious cases [26].

Psychologic Causes of Asthma

The role of the vagus nerves in the mechanisms of asthma have been intensively demonstrated at a distal level, but the central controls have not been so closely evaluated [13]. The neural interrelationship of the vagal nuclei are extensive and include pathways from the cerebral cortex. Psychic conditions have a ready access through vagal efferents to various visceral organs and thus can have a profound effect upon cardiac, pulmonary, and gastrointestinal function. The psychosomatic mechanisms underlying many disorders are well recognized, and the psychic component can have a major interacting role in most vagally controlled organ dysfunctions.

There is undoubtedly a cerebrovagal pathway that can influence the manifestations of asthma, and in some patients this is of domineering relevance. These patients may suffer from psychically induced exacerbations of asthma, and, even when other mechanisms are accountable for bronchospastic attacks, psychosomatic control may modulate the response. Thus, patients who are highly allergic to a specific allergen, such as a cat, may develop asthmatic symptoms when thinking about or viewing a picture of a cat. Similarly, asthmatic children who are emotionally stressed may develop an asthma attack that will respond to reassurance and comforting rather than to pharmacologic agents. In extreme cases, children improve when subjected to a "parentectomy," and sent to an asthma hospital or summer camp that encourages independence from the oversolicitous concern of an anxious parent.

In many cases, it is very evident that psychologic factors are involved in causing a patient's exacerbation of asthma. Thus, an acute emotional disturbance may trigger an attack, or stressful events may culminate in a progressive worsening of the asthma. The respiratory response may serve to shield the patient from an unwelcome situation, and thus the asthma may provide secondary gain or help the victim control their environmental situation. The physician who takes a careful history or perceives the interaction of the patient with their household, school, or work may be able to discern the role of psychologic events in the fluctuation of the asthmatic symptoms. Furthermore, the chain-reaction of the fear of dyspnea causing panic that worsens the breathing pattern may be a major factor in the evolution of an emotional patient's asthmatic condition.

Hyperventilation can be either a cause or a symptom of psychic discomfort, and it may precede or accompany asthma in some patients [7]. Indeed, the apparent distress seen in hyperventilation may mimic asthma, but the variability of symptoms and the lack of evidence of bronchospasm on pulmonary function testing can help make the diagnosis. If hyperventilation is a precursor of an asthmatic reaction, the patient is liable to manifest other features of anxiety with both psychic and somatic findings. Yellowlees and Kalucy postulate that hyperventilation may lead to a parahippocampal abnormality that may depend on genetic susceptibility, and this can interact with a propensity to panic reaction thus causing a worsening of the respiratory symptoms [41]. It is therefore important to recognize that asthmatics whose attacks are preceded by or present with complaints such as palpitations, paresthesiae, muscle spasms or cramps, visual disturbances, auditory disturbances, or near-syncope may have a hyperventilation-anxiety syndrome [7]; this may be confirmed by measuring the arterial blood gas and finding hypocapnia with good oxygenation. Any asthmatic patient with such findings may be considered to have a major component of anxiety that merits specific therapy.

In addition to anxiety and panic reactions, patients with asthma may have underlying depression that can have a profound effect on their ability to cope with their respiratory problem and their reponse to anti-asthma therapy. Anxiety and depression may coexist and may be accompanied by other psychologic disorders such as hysteria, hypochondriasis, character disorder, dependency, obsessive behavior, or repression [14]. The asthmatic syndrome may become a necessary part of the patient's life, and it may be used to manipulate interactions with others for secondary gain. Such patients are liable to respond poorly to standard therapy and they are likely to both underuse and overuse their bronchodilators and to be noncompliant. In these cases, periodic overuse of sympathomimetics, theophylline, and steroids may compound the symptoms of anxiety and psychologic distress and can endanger the patient's life.

When a psychologic component is suspected as a cause of asthma, a detailed evaluation should be made and, if necessary, psychiatric consultation should be arranged. Standard psychologic testing my be needed, including interview, questionnaires, Minnesota Multiphasic Personality Inventory, Eysenck Personality Inventory, Mill Hill Vocabulary Scale, and so forth [14]. A variety of therapeutic options have been described; tranquilizers can help control the hyperventilation syndrome, while imipramine or other antidepressants may be very beneficial for asthma that is related to depression. The prescribing of psychotherapeutic drugs is more clearly indicated when the patient's dyspnea is associated with a blood gas profile of adequate oxygenation accompanied by hypercapnea. Many techniques have been reported to be useful for anxiety and panic, including yoga, meditation, hypnosis, behavior modification, and verbal desensitization. Unfortunately, the benefits of such techniques are liable to be short-lasting since the typical patient may lack the motivation or resources to persist with the therapy.

Other Upper Airway Causes of Nonasthmatic Wheezing

Wheezing can be produced by other forms of upper airway obstruction, caused in particular by infection, spasm, or mechanical impingement upon the airway [2].

Infections

Any bacterial, viral, or fungal infection of the throat, larynx, or trachea can produce wheezing as an early manifestation; as the disease advances, stridor can develop, and this presages complete obstruction of the airway lumen. Throat infections, such as Vincent's angina, are generally obvious on physical examination. Epiglottitis and laryngeal infection usually affect the voice and are readily recognized from the clinical presentation. Tracheitis and bronchitis may be accompanied by fever, cough, purulent sputum, and retrosternal discomfort or pain. All these conditions may be accompanied by other evidence of infection, such as a leukocytosis, and they respond poorly to bronchodilator therapy.

Spasm

Spasm of the throat or larynx is a very rare cause of wheezing. This may occur in tetany, tetanus or rabies, and in anaphylactic reactions [2]. There is usually a suggestive history and evidence of extrapulmonary involvement in these disorders. Psychogenic spasm of the laryngeal muscles can occur as an extreme variant of laryngeal asthma and will present with obstructive findings, including stridor, in a patient with a very disordered psyche.

Airway Impingement

This can occur with intrinsic organic lesions or extrinsic growths. Intrinsic lesions include foreign bodies in the larynx, trachea, or major bronchi and their presence may be suggested by a history of aspiration. Neoplasms, both benign and malignant, can produce wheezing; if arising in the bronchus of a lobe of the lung, localized wheezing will be heard. Edema or stenosis of the airway can occur from mechanical, chemical, inflammatory, or traumatic injury, and the history will usually suggest the causation. Extrinsic lesions include thyromegaly, lymphoma, other neoplasms, hemorrhage, or aortic aneurysm. The associated physical abnormalities or clinical findings should suggest the presence of such lesions.

In all cases of nonasthmatic wheezing, physical examination, chest X-rays and CT scanning should delineate the causative lesion. Appropriate pulmonary function studies for tracheal lesions reveal an abnormal inspiratory component of the flow-volume curve. Laryngoscopy or bronchoscopy will usually enable the diagnosis to be established, but extrinsic lesions may require surgical exploration for definitive evaluation.

Aspiration

Recurrent wheezing or intractable cough occurring repetitively can cause aspiration of fluids or solids [24]. This may happen as a consequence of swallowing disorders [9], cricopharyngeal dysfunction, [37], mechanical lesions in the esophagus, or gastroesophageal reflux [21]. The abnormality will usually be suggested by history and physical examination and may be confirmed by endoscopy or an esophagram; the latter may need to be accompanied by tilting maneuvers to display reflux from the stomach into the esophagus. The mechanism by which reflux causes bronchospasm is not always clear, but it may be as a direct outcome of airway irritation from microaspiration or secondary to a reflex initiated by the reflux of acid into the esophagus [4, 21]. It has been suggested that 24 h monitoring of intraesophageal pH may be helpful; a causal relationship is suggested if wheezing is shown to be associated with a fall of pH to less than 4. For most patients, a history of heartburn, nocturnal bronchospasm or hoarseness, or wheezing developing while lying flat may provide the clue that vigorous therapy directed at relieving or treating the reflux may benefit the respiratory symptoms. In children, the following features may suggest reflux as a cause of asthma: difficult to control asthma, recurrent atelectasis or pneumonia, asthma occurring 1–2 h after going to sleep, repeated vomiting associated with cough or wheeze, postprandial indigestion or eructations [30]. In these younger patients, similar evaluation (including the use of a pH probe to test for acid reflux) and therapy to that advised for adults may be appropriate. Theophylline, which can relax the gastroesophageal sphincter, should be avoided or doses of the drug should be lowered if its use is correlated with evidence of reflux.

Lower Airway Causes of Wheezing

Diseases affecting lower airways may present as asthma, and definitive therapy requires precise diagnosis. The major categories of disorder to consider are tropical lung diseases, aspergillosis, collagen vascular diseases, and pulmonary embolization.

Eosinophilic Lung Diseases

Numerous parasitic disorders can cause paroxysmal cough, dyspnea and wheezing, and this may result in a form of asthma that is not uncommon in some tropical countries [19]. The cardinal sign is peripheral eosinophilia that can exceed 20% of the total white cells or an absolute count of 3000 per cu/mm [11]. The major cause of tropical eosinophilia is filariasis. Filaria are transmitted by mosquito from human to human or animal to human. Other parasite disorders include dirofilariasis, ascariasis (the historical cause of Loeffler's syndrome), strongyloidiasis, hookworm, paragonamiasis, schistosomiasis, echinococcosis, toxocariasis, and capillariasis. Precise diagnosis may be difficult unless the parasite is recovered from the bowel, blood, lymph nodes, or airways. Bronchoalveolar lavage may show eosinophilia, while a lung biopsy may show early inflammatory changes with eosinophils, which are later replaced by lymphocytes, epitheloid cells, and multinucleated giant cells [27]. The physical examination may suggest parasitosis, with anemia, hepatomegaly, splenomegaly, lymphadenopathy, or occult blood in the stool as possible findings. The chest X-ray may show various patterns of diffuse infiltrates or haziness, particularly in the basilar and midzones of the lungs; these may show a migratory quality over time. In filariasis, serum IgE is markedly elevated and antifilarial antibodies can be found. Similar nonspecific and specific findings have been reported in other parasitic diseases.

Several other causes of pulmonary eosinophilia can be considered, in which eosinophils are found in lung infiltrates and in the blood in association with accompanying cough, dyspnea, and wheezing. Nonparasitic causes of pulmonary eosinophilia include miliary tuberculosis, Wegener's granulomatosis, sarcoidosis, and drug reactions. The most important cause is drug allergy: the main agents that have been implicated are penicillin, sulfonamides, acetylsalicylic acid, tolbutamide, methotrexate, gold salts, and, rarely, cromolyn [11]. Nitrofurantoin may result in either an acute reaction that may resolve in a month or a chronic reaction that may progress to pulmonary fibrosis. Chronic eosinophilic pneumonia is characterized by a characteristic peripheral localization of the pulmonary infiltrate and by rapid clearing with steroid therapy. In contrast, the variable infiltrates in the rare hypereosinophilic syndrome do not resolve so readily with steroid administration. Diagnosis will require a careful history and physical examination, radiologic studies, bronchoscopy and, usually, lung or lymph node biopsy, with appropriate microbiologic studies. Sarcoidosis will be suggested by the finding of anergy and an elevated serum angiotensin-converring enzyme (ACE) level.

Allergic Bronchopulmonary Aspergillosis

This causes a particularly resistant form of asthma that may require prolonged therapy with large doses of steroids for control of the symptoms. Transient or persistent perihilar or more peripheral lung infiltrates may be accompanied by mucoid impaction and central bronchiectasis, which are readily displayed on routine radiographs or by CT. There is eosinophilia in the blood, and elevated levels of serum IgE occur in association with precipitating antibodies against *Aspergillus fumigatus* and a positive skin test reaction to aspergillin. In some patients, the disease is associated with the development of bronchocentric granulomatosis; this can be seen on lung biopsy. The sputum may reveal dark brown plugs containing fungal elements, which may be seen on microscopy and can be grown in culture.

Collagen Vascular Diseases

These do not often cause wheezing, but on occasion the findings of the physical, radiologic, and serologic features of rheumatoid arthritis, lupus erythematosus, or vasculitis may be accompanied by the apparent development of asthma. The most important vasculitic syndrome that is associated with asthma is the allergic granulomatosis and angiitis described by Churg and Strauss [5]. Victims are adults who often give a history of childhood asthma, and they present with lesions that may involve the skin, the nervous system, the heart, and the gastrointestinal tract in addition to the lungs. Typically, patients exhibit fever, anemia, weight loss, cough, wheezing, and peripheral eosinophilia. As the necrotizing vasculitis progresses, the asthmatic symptoms tend to decrease [5, 11]. Diagnosis usually requires a tissue biopsy. The rheumatologic disorder and the wheezing generally respond to steroid therapy but may require other immunosuppressive agents.

Cardiac Asthma

This term was first introduced to describe the sudden onset of nocturnal dyspnea in cardiac failure [39]. Currently, the diagnosis is restricted to patients who respond with coughing and wheezing secondary to left ventricular failure. In most of these subjects, there may be underlying bronchial hyperresponsiveness, and they show the same increased response to inhaled methacholine that is demonstrated in asthma, with partial reversal following inhaled bronchodilator. Thus, patients with cardiac asthma may benefit from bronchodilator drugs in addition to therapy directed at the heart. It is important to recognize the presence of heart failure in older patients with cardiac asthma, since administration of morphine may be uniquely effective, whereas it is contraindicated in noncardiac asthma.

Drugs

Heroin [18], cocaine [28], and other drugs, when taken by inhalation, can provoke asthma, possibly by releasing histamine or other mediators; or else they may result in the adult respiratory distress syndrome. It is not known what factors determine whether an individual will develop an asthmatic reaction or an alternative response to a specific insult. This emphasizes that careful evaluation is often required to establish whether a wheezing patient has conventional asthma or an unconventional response to another disorder or cause.

Pulmonary Emboli

Although persistent or recurrent attacks of wheezing may suggest repeated small emboli in patients with peripheral vascular disease, the documentation of such a relationship is rare [25, 40]. However, the association can be investigated by standard methods such as inhalation/perfusion scans, Doppler tests, venography, and angiography. If pulmonary embolic disease is diagnosed and anticoagulation therapy appears to rapidly relieve the wheezing, it is reasonable to conclude that the asthmatic response is caused by mediators released by the emboli.

Carcinoid Syndrome

This is a rare disorder characterized by flushing, diarrhea, changes in blood pressure, dyspnea, and wheezing: other manifestations may occur such as right heart valve lesions. The diagnosis is confirmed by finding high levels of urinary 5-hydroxy-indoleacetic acid and by discovering the tumor – which is usually abdominal in situation – on computerized scanning.

α-1-Antitrypsin Deficiency

Puerto Rican children have an increased prevalence of asthma in New York, and this has been correlated with variant phenotypes of α-1-antitrypsin (AAT). A particularly high incidence of abnormal S and Z heterozygous phenotypes was recently reported [6]. Thus, in some asthmatics, abnormal AAT levels may be found, and this may eventually lead to specific therapy designed to correct the abnormality.

Wheezing in Children

Asthma is common in childhood and should always be considered as an explanation for wheezing accompanied by cough and dyspnea [30]. The differential diagnosis includes numerous other causes, particularly in children under the age of two; in the age group of 6–12 months, more than 30% develop wheezy illnesses such as bronchiolitis. The most common causes are respiratory viral infections due to respiratory syncytial virus, parainfluenza viruses, influenza viruses, adenoviruses, and rhinoviruses. Bacterial infections rarely cause wheezing, but chlamydia and mycoplasma infections may occasionally affect infants.

Nontinfectious causes of wheezing include anatomical abnormalities such as congenital tracheoesophageal fistula, congenital heart disease, and anomalies of the great vessels. Gastroesophageal reflux can occur at all ages, as can aspiration of foreign bodies. Childhood disorders that cause wheezing include bronchopulmonary dysplasia, cystic fibrosis, and bronchiectasis; very unusual causes include bronchomalacia and bronchial isomerism [20]. As with adults, human immunodeficiency virus (HIV) infection may present with numerous pulmonary manifestations including wheezing. Other forms of congenital or acquired immunodeficiency may present in childhood with wheezing as a consequence of lung infection. Pulmonary edema of any causation and various interstitial lung disorders – such as lymphocytic interstitial pneumonia, desquamative interstitial pneumonia – need to be considered as possibilities in both children and adults when the wheezing is associated with a radiograph suggesting an interstitial edema or pneumonitis. As is the situation with all forms of asthma, wheezing in children may be provoked by inhaled irritants, or by drug or other insults that release histamine, by exercise and by emotional distress.

Investigations into persisting wheezing in infants and children may be difficult to pursue, and thus many patients may be treated as having intractable asthma, since a true explanation for the symptoms remains elusive. Modern techniques in radiologic evaluation and sophisticated pulmonary function tests may be required if a thorough history, physical examination, and routine radiographs fail to reveal the cause and full treatment for bronchospasm, inflammation, and infection fail to provide relief.

References

1. Adinoff AD, Cummings NP (1988) Sinusitis and its relationship to asthma. Am J Asthma Allergy Ped 1:93–99
2. Amin NM (1986) Unusual causes of wheezing in adults. Immunol Allergy Pract 8:154–162
3. Boyd G (1989) Allergic conditions of the nose in asthmatic patients. In: Mackay IS (ed) Rhinitis. Mechanisms and management. Royal Society of Medicine Services, London, pp 225–230
4. Castel DO (1989) Asthma and gastroesophageal reflux. Chest 96:2–3
5. Chumbley LC, Harrison EG, DeRemee RA (1977) Allergic granulomatosis and angiitis (Churg-Strauss syndrome): report and analysis of 30 cases. Mayo Clin Proc 52:477–484
6. Colp C, Pappas J, Vernali C, Lieberman J (1991) Alpha-1-antitrypsin studies in Puerto Rican children with asthma. Chest 100 [Suppl]:58S
7. Demetier SL, Cordasco EM (1986) Hyperventilation syndrome and asthma. Am J Med 81:989–994
8. Druce HM (1991) Emerging techniques in the diagnosis of sinusitis. Ann Allergy 66:132–136
9. Editorial (1990) Reflux and respiratory symptoms. Lancet 336:282–283
10. English GM (1986) Nasal polypectomy and sinus surgery in patients with asthma and aspirin idiosyncrasy. Laryngoscope 96:374–380
11. Enright T, Chua S, Lim DT (1989) Pulmonary eosinophilic syndromes. Ann Allergy 62:277–283
12. Goldman J, Muers M (1991) Vocal cord dysfunction and wheezing. Thorax 46:401–404
13. Gorman JM (1990) Psychobiological aspects of asthma and the consequent research implications. Chest 97:514–515
14. Griffith DE, Kronenberg RS (1991) Psychologic, neuropsychologic, and social aspects of COPD. In: Cherniack NS (ed) Chronic obstructive pulmonary disease. Saunders, Philadelphia, pp 568–575
15. Herrera AM, deShazo RD (1990) Sinusitis: its association with asthma. Postgrad Med 87:153–164
16. Holgate ST (1990) Mediator and cellular mechanisms in asthma. J R Coll Physicians Lond 24:304–312
17. Howarth P (1989) The immunopharmacology of rhinitis. In: Mackay IS (ed) Rhinitis. Mechanisms and management. Royal Society of Medicine Services, London, pp 33–51
18. Hughes S, Calverley PMA (1988) Heroin inhalation and asthma. Br Med J 297:1511–1512
19. Lal C, Sharma OP (1989) Everything that wheezes is not asthma. Chest 96:1418–1419
20. Lee P, Bush A, Warner JO (1991) Left bronchial isomerism associated with bronchomalacia, presenting with intractable wheeze. Thorax 46:459–461
21. Mays EE (1976) Intrinsic asthma in adults. Association with gastroesophageal reflux. JAMA 236:2626–2628
22. McFadden ER Jr (1987) Glottic function and dysfunction. J Allergy Clin Immunol 79:707–710
23. Naclerio RM (1991) Allergic rhinitis. N Engl. J Med 325:860–869
24. Nelson HS (1990) Is gastroesophageal reflux worsening your patient's asthma? J Respir Dis 11:827–844
25. Olazabul F, Roman-Irizarry LA, Oms JD, Conde L, Marchand EJ (1968) Pulmonary emboli masquerading as asthma. N Engl J Med 278:999–1001
26. Ramirez-R J, Leon I, Rivera LM (1986) Episodic laryngeal dyskinesia. Clinical and psychiatric characterization. Chest 90:716–721

27. Rohatgi PK, Smirniotopoulos TT (1991) Tropical eosinophilia. Semin Respir Med 12 (2):98–106
28. Ruben RB, Neugarten J (1990) Cocaine-associated asthma. Am J Med 88: 438–439
29. Settipane GA, Chaffee FH (1977) Nasal polyps in asthma and rhinitis. J Allergy Clin Immunol 59:17–21
30. Siegel SC, Rachelefsky GS (1985) Asthma in infants and children. J Allergy Clin Immunol 76:1–14
31. Shim C, Williams MH Jr (1986) Effect of odors in asthma. Am J Med 80:18–22
32. Slater JE, Kaliner MA (1989) Allergic rhinitis. Am J Asthma Allergy Ped 2: 101–106
33. Slavin RG (1988) Nasal polyps and sinusitis. In: Middleton E Jr, Reed CE, Ellis EF, Adkinson NF Jr, Yunginger JW (eds) Allergy: principles and practice, 3rd edn. Mosby, St. Louis, pp 1291–1303
34. Slavin RG (1985) Upper respiratory tract disease. In: Weiss EB, Segal MS, Stein M (eds) Bronchial asthma: mechanisms and therapeutics, 2nd edn. Little Brown, Boston, pp 400–409
35. Smith JM (1988) Epidemiology and natural history of asthma, allergic rhinitis and atopic dermatitis (eczema). In: Middleton E Jr, Reed CE, Ellis EF, Adkinson NF Jr, Yunginger JW (eds) Allergy: principles and practice, 3rd edn. Mosby, St. Louis, pp 891–929
36. Smith JM, Knowler AL (1965) Epidemiology of asthma and allergic rhinitis. I. In a rural area. II. In a university centered community. Am Rev Respir Dis 92: 16–30, 31–38
37. Stein M, Williams AJ, Grossman F, Weinberg A, Zuckerbraun L (1990) Crico-pharyngeal dysfunction in chronic obstructive pulmonary disease. Chest 97: 347–352
38. Stevenson DD, Simon RA (1988) Aspirin sensitivity: respiratory and cutaneous manifestations. In: Middleton E Jr, Reed CE, Ellis EF, Adkinson NF Jr, Yunginger JW (eds) Allergy: principles and practice, 3rd edn. Mosby, St. Louis, pp 1537–1554
39. Swineford O Jr (1971) Asthma and hayfever. Thomas, Springfield, chap 13
40. Windebank WJ, Boyd G, Moran F (1973) Pulmonary thromboembolism presenting as asthma. Br Med J 1:90–94
41. Yellowless PM, Kalucy RS (1990) Psychobiological aspects of asthma and the consequent research implications. Chest 97:628–634

Part II
Conditions Leading to Asthma

Genetic Predisposition in Asthma

C. POMARI and P. TURCO

Department of Lung Pathophysiology, Bussolengo General Hospital, Verona, Italy

In 1921, Prausnitz demonstrated that the intradermal injection of serum from donors sensitive to a number of proteins caused skin sensitization to these proteins in the recipients [2]. In 1923, the serum factor responsible for this reaction was called "reagin" by the two American researchers, Coca and Cooke [5]. The latter also later coined the term "atopy" to indicate a number of clinical forms characterized by fever and bronchial asthma occurring in certain individuals when exposed to hay dust.

The observations of that period led to the hypothesis that sensitization to certain environmental proteins could be transmitted from one indiviudual to another and, what is more, prompted the claim that apparently inert substances were able to cause what was defined as an "allergic" response only in a minority of genetically predisposed subjects [5].

Some 50 years or so later, in 1967, it was discovered that the factor responsible for the allergic reaction was an antibody, which was called immunoglobulin E (IgE) [14].

It later became clear that reagins, though belonging to the immunoglobulin class, had characteristics which differed from those of the antibodies active against microorgansisms: they were not detected in serum by normal precipitation reactions, were thermolabile, and presented the particular property of fixing themselves to the skin, producing typical reactions such as edema and erythema [14].

Today, IgEs are known to be produced by plasma cells in the lung and gastrointestinal regions and constitute less than 0.001% of circulating immunoglobulins. Their synthesis is stimulated by exposure to "allergenic" substances and persists for lengthy periods of time despite elimination of the stimulus.

Atopic subjects thus appear to respond to daily exposure to small amounts of allergens with the continuous production of IgE-type antibodies [17].

For several years now there has been a continual succession of clinico-epidemiological observations aimed at demonstrating a possible familial transmission of the atopic condition.

One of the basic tenets of genetics states that different gene loci are independently assorted during the transformation of the gamete, except when they are strongly aligned in a particular chromosome.

On the basis of this principle, a number of English investigators recently demonstrated the existence of a cotransmission of alleles in the vicinity of gene loci responsible for IgE-mediated hyperresponsiveness in atopy. Starting with the isolation of chains of deoxyribonucleic acid (DNA) of white blood cells from subjects belonging to various family groups, they showed that IgE-mediated hyperresponsiveness is significantly cotransmitted by a genetic variable, whose marker is situated on the long arm of chromosome 11 [12].

On the basis of this finding, it was thus postulated that the atopic state is probably related to hereditary chromosomal transmission of the autosomal dominant type [11].

Agosti et al. [1], after transplanting bone marrow from an allergic asthmatic donor in a nonasthmatic recipient, observed a specific IgE-mediated hyperresponsiveness in the latter with subsequent development of asthma.

The atopic condition is frequently found concomitantly alongside a number of disease forms regarded as clinical expressions of allergy, such as rhinitis, airway hyperreactivity, and bronchial asthma [25]. However, whereas in atopic asthma the interaction between the antigens inhaled and the IgEs sensitized on the mast cells of the bronchial mucosa is regarded as the most important mechanism for release of mediators of anaphylaxis, no single all-embracing theory justifying a direct relationship between bronchial asthma and atopy has yet been formulated [23].

The findings reported in the literature show a significant correlation between severity of asthma and presence of atopic disease, in that IgE levels have been found to vary in relation to the degree of severity of the asthma [16, 18].

Nevertheless, the atopic condition in itself would not appear capable of accounting for the development of the associated clinical forms [26]. Numerous other factors would seem to be jointly responsible for the severity and incidence both of atopy and of bronchial asthma: environmental allergen levels, diet, and cigarette smoking may play an important role [19, 20].

In the view of certain authors, lower respiratory tract infections (syncitial respiratory virus, parainfluenza virus) contracted during the early years of life constitute a further important risk factor [9].

According to Kaliner, moreover, an imbalance between the components of the autonomic nervous system may also play a major role in the pathogenesis of asthma [15]. Quite apart from the direct effect which the autonomic system has on regulation of airway caliber, the very release of mediators from mast cells induced by an immunological stimulus may also be affected by the neurohormonal system. This would appear to be borne out indirectly by the finding that β- or parasympathomimetic drugs may be capable of influencing the release of mediators from mast cells. β_2-Adrenergic agonists appear, in fact, to be capable of inhibiting mast cell degranulation, while α-adrenergic and cholinergic drugs would appear to increase such degranulation [15].

Numerous epidemiological studies on the influence of familial predisposition, studies on the presence of asthma in twin populations, and studies on genetic markers have been conducted with a view to identifying and better characterizing the role of various factors possibly capable of contributing to the development of asthma.

A family predisposition to asthma has been found in all studies in which this factor has been investigated [9].

Twin studies have confirmed a greater frequency of atopy and asthma in monozygotic (19%) than in heterozygotic twins (4%), while Higgins and Keller have found evidence that the incidence of asthma in infancy is greater in those with a family history of atopy (18.3%) than in those with no such history (7.4%) [3, 9, 10, 13].

However, the finding of a low incidence of correlated family history and asthma in monozygotic twins (only 19%) is such that we are strongly prompted to postulate that the onset of clinical symptoms is exclusively related to the phenotypic expression of this disease [3]. Whereas demonstration of asthma in a family group may represent the effect of a genetic factor, it may equally well be the expression of a common environmental stimulus [9, 21].

Certain investigators, in fact, have postulated that the finding of a greater incidence of asthma in family groups may be related to common exposure to environmental stimuli rather than merely to familial genetic predisposition [9, 21].

One of the factors which has been studied as a possible cause of predisposition to allergic disease is that related to a particular genetic set of class II histocompatibility antigens. The precise function of this group of antigens is to act as "identity markers" on the surface of various cells; T lymphocytes, via their receptors, must interact with these markers in order to perform their specific immunity functions. The major histocompatibility complex (MHC) in humans is known as HLA (human leukocyte group A) antigen [22].

Turton et al., however, typed the HLA system loci in 122 asthmatics in comparison with 167 controls and found no significant difference, thus confirming the hypothesis that the different degrees of expression of the immune response in family groups are affected by environmental stimuli rather than by the genetic set related to the HLA system [18].

All in all, then, it seems likely that several different pathogenetic mechanisms may contribute to the development of asthma symptoms.

It has recently been postulated that various genetic conditions may contribute to the development of atopy and bronchial asthma and that atopy may increase the likelihood of developing asthma only when there already exists a genetic condition capable of promoting development of the disease [24].

The molecular biology studies conducted by Cookson and Hopkin have shown that, of subjects presenting IgE-mediated hypersensitivity related to a common genetic variant on chromosome 11, 80% had only an atopic condition and 60% a history of bronchospasm, while 20% were already diagnosed as suffering from bronchial asthma [6, 7].

The finding that not all atopic subjects are asthmatics might therefore suggest that atopic status in itself is probably not enough to cause a hyperreactive bronchial response or the classic symptoms of asthma [8].

Moreover, objections have recently been raised as to the usefulness of distinguishing asthma on the basis of IgE-mediated hypersensitivity, since this mechanism appears to present in both atopic and nonatopic forms [4]. In many epidemiological studies, it would appear that asthma does correlate significantly with high IgE levels, whereas there is a characteristic correlation between positive allergic skin tests and rhinitis [11].

Another advance in our knowledge of the causes of bronchial asthma may come from a recent hypothesis put forward by Corrigan and Kay [8], who claim that T lymphocytes may play a major role in the development of asthma. Different subsets of T helper lymphocytes may be activated in asthmatic subjects, irrespective of the presence of atopy. It would appear that the production of IgEs by plasma cells may be regulated by a lymphokine (IL4) produced by the T helper lymphocytes (TH2 cells), which, in response to an immunological stimulus, may be capable of releasing lymphokine (IL4) capable of producing specific IgEs and of playing an important role in recruiting numerous cells (mast cells, eosinophils, neutrophils, etc.) in the bronchial mucosa [8, 11]. The cell recruitment itself, however, appears to be regulated by another lymphokine (IL2) and by γ-interferon, produced by a further subset of T lymphocytes (TH1 cells), which may also be stimulated by nonimmunological mechanisms [8].

This hypothesis, which is related to the discovery that chromosome 11q is capable of transporting a number of genes for the T lymphocyte surface antigens, may therefore suggest that a hereditary chromosomal dysfunction of autosomal dominant type may cause an alteration in the lymphocyte cell line [11].

If, as Corrigan and Kay claim [8], the T lymphocytes are capable of affecting the level of circulatory IgEs and of recruiting and activating numerous cells in the airway mucosa in response to various stimuli, it is therefore possible that the intervention of the latter may be of basic importance in the pathogenesis of the bronchial hyperreactive response and in the development of the symptoms typical of bronchial asthma.

These recent theories may thus open up new horizons in the progress of our knowledge of the pathogenesis of asthma and may orient future research towards the quest for increasingly sophisticated diagnostic means.

The hypothesis that asthma may be a hereditary disease and that its expression and clinical course may depend on the effects of various environmental factors [16] would make its early diagnosis even more important with a view to achieving prompter and more effective management of the disease.

References

1. Agosti JM, Sprenger JD, Lum LG (1988) Transfer of allergen-specific IgE-mediated hypersensitivity with allogenic bone marrow transplants. N Engl J Med 319: 1623–1628
2. Avenberg KM, Harper DS, Larsson BL (1980) Footnotes on allergy. Pharmacia, Uppsala, pp 1–103
3. Barnes PJ, Rodger IW, Thomson NC (1988) Pathogenesis of asthma. In: Barnes PJ, Rodger IW, Thomson NC (eds) Asthma: basic mechanisms and clinical management. Academic, London, pp 415–444
4. Burrows B, Martinez FD, Halonen M (1989) Association of asthma with serum IgE levels and skin-test reactivity to allergens. N Engl J Med 320:271–277
5. Coca AF, Cooke RA (1923) On the classification of the phenomena of hypersensitivities. J Immunol 8:163
6. Cookson WOCM, Hopkin JM (1988) Dominant inheritance of immunoglobulin-E responsiveness. Lancet 1:86–87
7. Cookson WOCM, Sharp P, Faux J, Hopkin JM (1989) Linkage between immunoglobulin-E responses underlying asthma and rhinitis and chromosome 11q. Lancet 1:1292–1294
8. Corrigan CJ, Kay AB (1990) CD4 T-lymphocyte activation in acute severe asthma. Am Rev Respir Dis 141:970–977
9. Coultras DB, Samet JM (1987) Epidemiology and natural history of childhood asthma. In: Tinkelman DG, Falliers CJ, Naspitz CK (eds) Childhood asthma: pathophysiology and treatment. Dekker, New York, pp 131–157
10. Fife D, Speizer FE (1981) Epidemiology of asthma. In: Gershwin ME (ed) Bronchial asthma: principles of diagnosis and treatment. Grune and Stratton, New York, pp 1–11
11. Higginbottom T, Varna N (1989) Asthma: an inherited dysfunction of bone marrow cells? Eur Respir J 2:921–922
12. Hopkin JM (1990) A genetic approach to atopy. Eur Respir J 3:851–852
13. Hopp RJ, Bewtra AK, Watt GD, Nair NM, Townley RG (1984) Genetic analysis of allergic disease in twins. J Allergy Clin Immunol 73:265–270
14. Ishizaka K, Ishizaka T, Hornbrook MM (1966) Physicochemical properties of reaginic antibody. Correlation of reaginic activity with mcE globulin and reaginic antibody. J Immunol 97:840
15. Kaliner M, Shelhamer JH, Pamela BD, Smith LJ, Venter JG (1982) Autonomic nervous system abnormalities and allergy. Ann Intern Med 96:349–357
16. Kelly WJW, Hudson I, Phelan PD, Pain MCF, Olinsky A (1990) Atopy in subjects with asthma followed to the age of 28 years. J Allergy Clin Immunol 85: 548–557
17. Kus J, Tse KS, Enarson D, Grybowski S, Chan-Yeung M (1984) Lymphocyte subpopulation in patient with allergic rhinitis. Allergy 39:509–514
18. Marsh DG (1987) Genetic factors of allergy. In: Michel FB, Bousquet J, Godard P (eds) Highlights in asthmology. Springer, Berlin Heidelberg New York, pp 31–36
19. Pauwels R (1987) Pathogenic mechanisms in childhood asthma. Triangle 1:13–18
20. Peat JK, Salomone CM, Woodcock AJ (1990) Longitudinal changes in atopy during a 4-year period: relation to bronchial hyperresponsiveness and respiratory symptoms in a population sample of Australian schoolchildren. J Allergy Clin Immunol 85:65–74
21. Reed CE (1975) Epidemiology and natural history. In: Stein M (ed) New directions in asthma. American College of Chest Physicians, Park Ridge, pp 291–300
22. Ricci M, Rossi O (1989) Compendio di allergologia. Collana Scientifica Eurospital, Aosta, pp 19–74
23. Russel JH, Townley RG, Biven RE, Bewtra AK, Nair NM (1990) The presence of airway reactivity before the development of asthma. Am Rev Respir Dis 141:2–8

24. Sibbald B, Horn MEC, Brain EA, Gregg R (1980) Genetic factors in childhood asthma. Thorax 35:671–674
25. Zimmerman B, Chambers C, Forsyth S (1988) Allergy in asthma. II. The highly atopic infant and chronic asthma. J Allergy Clin Immunol 1:71–77
26. Zimmerman B, Feanny S, Reisman J, Hak H, Rashed N, McLaughlin FJ, Levison H (1988) Allergy in asthma. I. The dose relationship of allergy to severity of childhood asthma. J Allergy Clin Immunol 1:63–70

Endocrinological Changes and Asthma

G. PIATTI and S. CENTANNI

Institute of Respiratory Diseases, School of Medicine, University of Milan, Milano, Italy

Introduction

It is well known that the pathogenesis of bronchial asthma is multifactorial. However, fluctuations in sex hormones can also modulate bronchomotor tone, although there is not always agreement on hormonal effects on the airways and in vitro results often conflict with in vivo observations.

There is an intrinsic weakness in the study of relationship between hormones and airways function due to the lack of pharmacologic demonstration of bronchial receptors for sex hormones and sex hormone-specific induced effects [1].

The age-related endocrinological changes occurring in the body are important determinants for bronchial asthma. In fact, puberty may have an influence on asthma, similar to menses, pregnancy, and menopause.

Sex, Puberty, and Athma

The onset of asthmatic disease is often earlier and more frequent in the male child than in the female [2]; therefore, during adolescence the males may improve while females often just begin to suffer [3]; thus the male-female ratio inverts around puberty and asthma becomes more common in adult women than men.

Premenstrual Asthma

Asthma is affected by menstrual cycle as evidenced by the phenomenon of premenstrual asthma (PMA). Approximately 34% of women suffer premenstrual deterioration of their athma [1, 4–6] as confirmed by serial peak flow measurements; these women have both more severe asthma [7] and more severe dysmenorrhea than other asthmatic women [8, 9]. Their PMA seems to be linked to the fall in the late luteal phase progesterone concentration [10–12] which acts as a smooth muscle relaxant in the gut, genitourinary tract, vascular system, and in the bronchial tree as well, although the change in serum progesterone between the follicular and luteal phases (30 ng/ml) seems insufficient to alter airways responsiveness to methacholine [13].

In vitro and in vivo data have shown that 17-β-estradiol and progesterone potentiate, up to 14 fold, the relaxing effect of isoproterenol on bronchial smooth muscle [14]. Therefore, a decrease in estrogen levels occurring in women both before ovulation and before menstruation may also be responsible for the increase in bronchial tone. The latter is a result of the decreased levels of endogenous catecholamines due, in turn, to estrogens and progesterone. This situation is similar to that occurring in patients with steroid-dependent asthma when corticosteroids are stopped [15].

Variations in the levels of endogenously synthesized prostaglandins, and particularly prostaglandin PG $F_{2\alpha}$, may be involved in the mechanism of PMA [8, 9, 15, 16]. Furthermore, oral contraceptives can worsen asthmatic symptoms [13, 17].

Pregnancy and Asthma

Pregnancy affects bronchial asthma in a controversial way: although it often acts in reducing asthmatic symptoms [18], in some patients symptoms are unchanged or markedly increased [19–22]. Thus, it is best to treat the disease, minimize the acute episodes, and reduce the adverse effect of asthma on pregnancy [23, 26]; in any case asthmatic exacerbations are most frequent in the last trimester [27, 28].

The course of asthma during pregnancy is related to its severity before pregnancy: in fact, mild asthma is generally unaffected by pregnancy while patients with serious asthma usually do worse [22]. Repeated pregnancies have the same effect as the first: women whose asthma improved during the first pregnancy also experience an improvement at the second pregnancy and vice versa [3, 29].

Placenta-produced estrogens and progesterone, which markedly increase during the second and third trimester [26] and the increased release of corticosteroids (plasma free cortisol is two to three times the normal level are the most important factors related to the improvement of asthma during pregnancy) [3, 22–24]. Nevertheless, other considerations must be made for women whose asthma worsens: pulmonary refractoriness to cortisol effects due to competitive binding to glucocorticosteroid receptors by progesterone, aldosterone, or deoxycorticosterone may lead to an effective decrease in β-adrenergic receptor number or responsiveness.

The increased PG $F_{2\alpha}$-mediated bronchoconstriction and the increased gastroesophageal reflux-induced asthma [18] are also important factors that may lead to a worsening of asthma during pregnancy [24].

In addition, data on increased preterm births in pregnant asthmatic women suggest a relationship between bronchial and uterine smooth muscle lability in patients with asthma.

Menopause and Asthma

Mensopause generally worsens a preexisting asthma; however, in females around the age of 50 years old, the mean age of menopause, there is a peak in the onset of asthmatic disease [2]. When asthma begins at this time, without asthmatic or atopic precedings, can be referred to as "perimenopausal asthma".

We have been able to observe, in these women, some changes in hormonal patterns, with increased levels of estrogens such as those found during the reproductive age. Estrogens, in turn, stimulate the release of PG $F_{2\alpha}$, altering the PGF/PGE ratio and inducing bronchoconstriction [30, 31]. These effects are probably related to an increased formation of gap junctions in the bronchial smooth muscle, as demonstrated in the uterus [32].

Conclusions

Hormones other than sex hormones seem to play a role in triggering at least some types of asthma, e.g., recent data suggest a relationship between hyperthyroidism and asthma [3]. Correlations between bronchial asthma and endocrinological changes remain, at the present, poorly investigated. The importance of individual factors as determinants for athma probably varies from individual to individual and their combined effect must be considered.

References

1. Valerio G, Lella A, Fanizza G, Barbanente P, Atimonelli R, Carnimeo N (1987) Airway hyperreactivity and menstrual cycle in asthmatic patients. Allergol Immunopathol (Madr) 15 (6):379–381
2. Bonner JR (1983) The epidemiology and natural history of asthma. Clin Chest Med 5:557–565
3. Falliers, CJ (1981) Developmental and endocrine aspects of respiratory allergy. J Asthma 18:17–21
4. Gibbs CJ, Coutts II, Lock R, Finnegan OC, White RJ (1984) Premenstrual exacerbation of asthma. Thorax 39:833–836
5. Stokes DN (1988) Premenstrual asthma (letter). Anaesthesia 43 (7):601–602
6. Eliasson O, Scherzer HH (1984) Recurrent respiratory failure in premenstrual asthma. Conn Med 48:777–778
7. Eliasson O, DeGraff-Ac JR (1987) A cautionary tale about investigations of the effect of the menstrual cycle on asthma. Am Rev Respir Dis 136:1515–1516
8. Eliasson O, Scherzer HH, DeGraff-Ac JR (1986) Morbidity in asthma in relation to the menstrual cycle. J Allergy Clin Immunol 77 (1):87–94
9. Eliasson O, Longo M, Dore-Duffy P, Densmore MJ, DeGraff-Ac JR (1986) Serum 13–14 di OH-15-Keto-prostaglandin F2 alpha and airway response to meclofenamate and metaproterenol in relation to the menstrual cycle. J Asthma 23 (6):309–319
10. Dalton K (1988) Progesterone for premenstrual exacerbations of asthma (letter). Lancet 17 (2):684

11. Beynon HL, Garbett ND, Barnes PJ (1988) Severe premenstrual exacerbations of asthma: effect of intramuscular progesterone. Lancet 13 (2):370–372
12. Chen HI, Tang YR (1989) Effects on the menstrual cycle on respiratory muscle function. Am Rev Respir Dis 140:1359–1362
13. Juniper EF, Kline PA, Roberts RS, Hargreave FE, Daniel EE (1987) Airway responsiveness to metacholine during the natural menstrual cycle and the effect to oral contraceptives. Am Rev Respir Dis 135:1039–1042
14. Foster PS, Goldie RG, Paterson JW (1983) Effect of steroids on beta-adrenoceptor-mediated relaxation of pig bronchus. Br J Pharmacol 78:441–445
15. Eliasson O, Densmore MJ, Scherzer HH, DeGraff-Ac JR (1987) The effect of sodium meclofenamate in premenstrual asthma: a controlled clinical trial. J Allergy Clin Immunol 79:909–918
16. Lenoir RJ (1987) Severe acute asthma and the menstrual cycle. Anaesthesia 42:1287–1290
17. Pelikan Z (1978) Possible immediate hypersensitivity reaction of the nasal mucosa to oral contraceptives. Ann. Allergy 40:211–219
18. Juniper EF, Daniel EE, Roberts RS, Kline PA, Hargreave FE, Hewhouse HT (1989) Improvement in airway responsiveness and asthma severity during pregnancy. A prospective study. Am Rev Respir Dis 140:924–931
19. Cohendy R, Godard, P, Bousquet J, Aubas P, Michel FB (1988) Pregnancy and asthma. Rev Mal Respir 5 (3):261–267
20. Huff RW (1989) Asthma in pregnancy. Med Clin North Am 73 (3):653–660
21. Guerin JM, Meyer P, Habib Y (1987) Asthma during pregnancy. Rev Pneumol Clin 43 (3):156–159
22. Gluck JC, Gluck PA (1976) The effects of pregnancy on asthma: a prospective study. Ann Allergy 37:164–168
23. Di Marco AF (1989) Asthma in the pregnant patient: a review. Ann Allergy 62 (6):527–533
24. Schatz M, Hoffman C (1987) Interrelationships between asthma and pregnancy: clinical and mechanistic considerations. Clin Rev Allergy 5 (4):301–315
25. Weber RW, Nelson HS (1986) Immunologic and atopic aspects of pregnancy and lactation. Ann Allergy 57 (3):159–166
26. Spector SL (1984) Reciprocal relationship between pregnancy and pulmonary disease. State of the art. Chest 86:1S–5S
27. Greenberger PA (1985) Asthma in pregnancy. Clin Perinatol 12 (3):571–584
28. Harman EM (1985) Pulmonary problems of pregnancy. Compr Ther 11 (5):26–32
29. Schatz M, Harden K, Forsythe A, Chilingar L, Hoffman C, Sperling W (1988) The course of asthma during pregnancy post-partum and with successive pregnancies; a prospective analysis. J Allergy Clin Immunol 81 (3):509–517
30. Farina F, Colombi S, Cantone R, Pastore M, Centanni S, Galimberti M (1986) Studio degli ormoni ipofiso-gonadici in alcuni casi di asma bronchiale. Min Med 77:243–247
31. Farina F, Francioni S, Galimberti M, Pastore M, Centanni S, Anomalie ormonali in un caso di asma bronchiale ad insorgenza perimenopausale. GIMT 37:145–148
32. Garfield RE, Kannan MS, Daniel EE (1980) Gap-junction formation in myometrium: control by estrogens, progesterone and prostaglandins. Am J Physiol 238:C81–89

Psychogenic Factors in Asthma

R. Bossi*, P. Banfi and F. Berni

* Institute of Respiratory Diseases, School of Medicine, University of Milan, Milano, Italy
Department of Pneumology, S. Corona Garbagnate Hospital, Milano, Italy

"The symbolic processes are the basis for the somatic symptoms arising ..."
G. Groddeck, The Book of ES

Introduction

Emotional factors can cause both the onset and the outburst of an asthmatic crisis. The pathogenesis of all organic or psychic diseases influenced by psychic factors takes root in an emotional conflict. The response to the emotional conflict differs from subject to subject:

1. The person solves the conflict.
2. The person reacts with anxiety, anguish, depression and even tachycardia, tachypnea and insomnia.
3. The person fails to solve the emotional conflict, becomes involved in a state of neurosis, and sometimes develops an out and out organic disease.

In practice, the passage from the psychic to the physical sphere may entail a process of evolution, still poorly understoad, mediated by the autonomic nervous system.

Respiratory disorders, and asthma in particular, are likely to be perceived by the patient at different levels. The act of breathing is experienced as an act of participation and exchange with the environment.

According to certain authors [5, 6, 9, 13], every psychosomatic disorder corresponds to a certain kind of personality. The asthmatic subject would seem to be particularly dependent on his mother and, later, on the person who takes her place. According to other authors [1–4], the development pattern of the somatic disease in the adult would suggest that symptoms are mediated by the neurovegetative sympathetic and parasympathetic systems [11, 33]. In asthma, peptic ulcer and other intestinal disorders, a major role is played by the parasympathetic system. In the case of arterial hypertension, cephalalgia, and arthritis, it is the sympathetic nervous system that comes into play.

The Clinical and Psychological Pattern of Bronchial Asthma

Bronchial asthma is characterized by an impaired respiratory function. The asthmatic attack can arise all of a sudden and its main clinical symptom is dyspnea often associated with sneezing fits, rhinorrhea, cough, and a sense of chest oppression. The auxiliary muscles of respiration are contracted during the attack, especially those of the neck.

Recent hypotheses associate mucosal inflammation with three other common symptoms: bronchospasm, edema, and hypersecretion. When the attack is over, these disappear, following a variable order. The severity of the disease is more or less dependent on the incidence of relapses, which are likely to occur because of pollens (seasonal allergies), dust, molds, drugs, paints, foods, respiratory virus-related diseases, or without apparent cause (Fig. 1). At a psychological level, it can often be clinically observed that, on recognizing the premonitory symptoms of an asthma attach, the patient is seized by a state of agitation and anxiety, which can easily be perceived from the patient's facial expression and state of paleness, cyanosis, cold perspiration, and psychic tension.

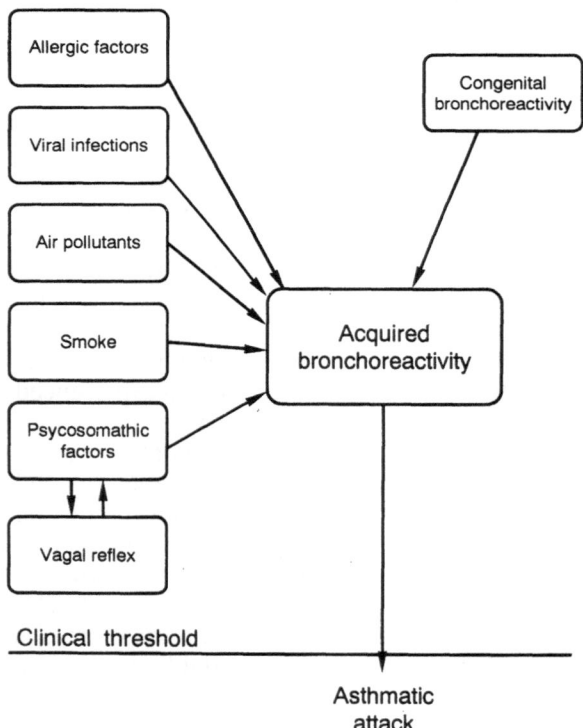

Fig. 1. Risk factors in asthma

The incidence of asthma in the population varies according to the different studies that have been carried out. According to the WHO, 12%–14% of newborns are atopic. In any case, considering the different forms of disability reported in patients below age 17, asthma accounts for one third of all the cases considered.

It is interesting to observe that generally the number of hospitalizations due to bronchial asthma decreases significantly as age increases. By contrast, hospital admissions for chronic bronchitis follow an opposite trend, as if asthma underwent a transformation due to the weakening of immune defenses or to the somatopsychic evolution of the patient [3], particularly the anxiety-inducing component, which is an essential characteristic of the asthmatic patient. Ader [1] suggested that the immune response may be influenced by emotional factors, which play an important role in modulating the relationship between the central nervous system and the immune system. Neuropeptides in particular are thought to be the mediators through which emotions are transmitted [6, 10, 34].

Benson et al. [7] found that the somatopsychic changes in a previously relaxed subject are likely to stimulate the immune system. An observation of this kind would justify some other treatment of the asthmatic patient besides organic therapies. From the pneumological, allergological, and psychophysiological viewpoints, bronchial asthma can be defined as a deregulation of bronchial tone with hyperreactivity and excessive amplification of the responses to specific and nonspecific stimuli of different nature, since the modulation of breathing can be modified by humoral or nervous chemical routes. From the psychophysiological viewpoint, bronchial hyperreactivity may be considered as the somatic synthesis of two factors:

1. From the *physiological* viewpoint, bronchial hyperreactivity can be observed for different reasons, including inflammation, hyperventilation, stimulation due to allergens, inhalation of fog, chemicals, or simply cold air.

2. From the *psychological* viewpoint, hyperreactivity can be triggered by emotional tension or anxiety and therefore depends on the mental state of the person at a given time [14].

These two factors – physiological and psychological – are related to the environment and to the individual's adjustment effort. As a matter of fact, they play a relatively important role in the outburst of an asthma attack. Stress-inducing adjustment problems created by the social and familiar environments may, to a certain extent, act as factors able to predispose one to or trigger an asthma attack.

Psychogenic Asthma

Studies carried out by the supporters of psychosomatic medicine [12] have often tried to develop a research system able to highlight the dualisity (organic and psychic) nature of asthma. Indeed, the synergic action of organic and psychic changes contributes to the onset of asthma. Table 1 is a schematic representation fo the physical and psychological factors involved in asthma. Del Bono et al. [11] have shown that bronchial nonstriated muscle is regulated by the vagas nerve and by the sympathetic nervous system which, in turn, can be influenced by cortical and subcortical activity.

Psychosomatic studies [4, 5, 8, 9, 15] stressed that there are several neuropsychic etiopathogenic factors whereby:

1. A psychic stimulus (stress, anxiety, or fear) is enough to trigger an asthma attack (merely psychic phenomenon).

2. Psychic symptoms appear in a subject already suffering from asthma.

3. The psychic influence (psychosocial factors, stress, environmental and cultural conditioning) may predispose to asthma.

According to studies that examined the overall status of the individual, alteration of bronchial tone is a problem of psychological evolution that is linked to the processes of knowledge and experience in the individual, whereas other studies consider the relationship of the subject with reality and with the capacity to physically adjust to psychological stress. Certain theories assume that several psychosomatic diseases, including asthma, become established in target organs characterized by weak resistance. According to other studies, asthma is a disease linked to an impaired psychobiological adjustment. Such an adjustment is said to start quite early, with the very first experiences with the outer world, and seems to be conditioned by one's parents [17].

In establishing a relationship with the mother [5] (seen as an object of total attention) or with the mother's breast (object of partial attention) [2], the child goes through either gratifying or frustrating experiences, which will influence future personality development. Environmental stimuli eventually play a major role during the psychophysical growth of the individual so long as certain response mechanisms can be activated through conditioning [16]. It was demonstrated that asthmatic reactions can also be triggered in animals

Table 1. Physical and psychological factors in asthma

Well known factors (physical factors)	Poorly known factors (psychological factors)
Reagins	Stress
Effects of β_2 stimulants	Anxiety
Therapeutic concentration of theophylline	Anger
Parasympathetic ganglia	Fear
Substance P	Excitement
Allergens	Love
C fibers	Happiness
β-Adrenoreceptors of lymphocytes	

through a pattern of conditioning, e.g., in goats and sheep by Liddal [16] and in guinea pigs by Ottenberg [26]. As for humans, as early as 1886 McKenzie [23] described the case of a female patient, whose asthma attacks were triggered if she came in contact with roses, who had an asthma attack when she saw roses made of cloth.

Among the factors able to induce an asthma attack, a major role is played by stress. In the 1960s, Tiffeneau [32] suggested that an emotional stress was able to trigger an asthma attack in subjects with a low excitability threshold.

McFadden [22] administered an aerosol of a physiological salt solution to a group of asthmatic subjects lotting them believe that the inhaled substance was an allergen to which they were sensitive. Measurements were taken of specific airways conductance (sG_{aw}), which underwent significant changes in 50% of subjects (called "reactors") and no changes at all in the remaining 50% ("nonreactors").

Eventually, "reactors" received a broncodilator but they were told that it was an allergen and no response was observed, unlike with "nonreactors". This type of response persuaded the authors that the sympathetic nervous system played a secondary role in the regulation of bronchial tone.

The patients with dyspnea eventually received placebo as bronchodilator and conductance was back to baseline values. Intravenous administration of atropine suppressed the response to suggestion owing to its pharmacological effect. Although the study was not carried out a double-blind, this study showed that suggestion acts through a central mechanism without any stimulation of afferent tracts, that the stimulus was mediated by cholinergic tracts and therefore modified by the administration of atropine, and that not all asthmatic patients were sensitive to suggestion [14].

In 1970, Luparello [18] carried out a double-blind study on asthmatic subjects with reversible bronchoconstriction. Specific conductance (sG_{aw}) was measured after administration of a substance presented initially as a bronchodilator and later as a bronchoconstrictor, which confirmed the action of suggestion on the respiratory tract. In 1971, Mathé and Knapp [20] used a distressing, frightening film and a mathematical problem to be solved under difficult conditions as stress-inducing factors in silent asthmatic patients and in control subjects. Comparing the data obtained with baseline values, they observed the following: (a) increase in heart rate; (b) increase in arterial pressure; and (c) increase in plasma cortisol and noradrenaline urine excretion. Under stress, a reduction of sG_{aw} values but not of adrenaline was observed in asthma sufferers.

In 1976, Spector et al. [30] observed in a group of asthmatic subjects that the parameter most sensitive to respiratory functional changes in the methacholine test was sG_{aw}. Although linked to the effects of suggestion, sG_{aw} is manifests its action especially on proximal airways rather than peripheral airways; the involvement of the vagus nerve is also possible.

In 1978, Horton et al. [14] observed a correlation between suggestion-induced bronchoconstriction measured by means of a plethysmograph and bronchial hyperreactivity measured after histamine and methacholine tests.

The Personality of the Asthmatic Subject

Most clinical studies on the personality of the asthmatic subject observed the existence of "inhibitory" or "regressive" defense mechanisms.

As early as in 1941, French and Alexander [13] suggested that the roots of psychosomatic asthma were to be sought in the childhood of the asthmatic subject and, more precisely, in the "fear of losing motherly love." The asthmatic child lives an ambivalent relationship with his mother [21], which turns into a real phobic neurosis and, according to the authors, the asthmatic subject also lives in a situation of dependence on his mother.

Several possibilities of variation and modulation of breathing have been schematized. These include interruption of respiration while speaking or singing; deep inspiration with brief expirations while laughing or crying; prolonged expiration while sighing; and frequent breathing during fear or excitement.

The main feature of the personality of the asthmatic subject is insecurity, so much so that Alexander [2] compared asthma to vegetative neuroses. Certain authors [19, 25, 33] interpreted asthma as a psychosomatic and allergic disease and, in their view, the personality of allergic subjects is emotionally unstable, inclined towards hysteria and phobia, and even towards the repression of sexuality.

The literature describes various kinds of asthmatic personality in which the names of famous personages are linked to a particular type of asthma: Proust's asthma, triggered by images; Trousseau's asthma, triggered by anger; and Jacquelin's asthma, triggered by certain dreams.

Steiner et al. [31] identified asthma as the representation of the somatization of the thirst for air experienced as an introjection defense system.

As a rule, most of these studies attribute a central role in the pathogenesis of asthma to the mother, towards whom the asthmatic subject develops an emotional affective dualism. The repression and regression mechanisms in the asthmatic subject are coupled by somatization as a defense mechanism. When tested clinically, the ego of the asthmatic subject is characterized by a state of anxiety, tendency to aggressiveness, inclination towards emotions, and block of sexual drives. With respect to the relationship with the mother, Azzario [4, 5] defines two types of mothers: (1) the present mother who is hyperprotective, thoughtful, anxious, and suffocating and (2) the missing mother who is unable to offer enough affection, warmth, and protection to the child. These maternal figure create a state of emotional instability and anxiety in the subject, which has its equivalent in the asthmatic state. The asthma attack is indeed said to express a peak of emotional tension. A further distinction has been made between "spoilt" asthmatic children and "neglected" asthmatic children. The former are not able to express aggressiveness and the latter tend to suppress it for fear of jeopardizing their relationship with others. Pinkus et al. [29] revealed through psychodiagnostic tests that asthmatic subjects tend to underestimate the image of themselves as bodies and suppress any emotional, ideational, or mental sign according to a conformistic social pattern of behavior.

Elements fundamental to a psychosomatic interpretation of asthma are: stress, emotionality, and anxiety, which is the most important factor since it is the expression of an emotionally [25, 27] disturbed life and causes a continuous waste of energy through stress. The fear of dying, experienced by the asthmatic patient during an attack, is to be interpreted as an element of further uncertainty that conditions the patient's life. The more the patient suffers from asthma attacks, the more his or her mind and personality will be seized by a vicious circle leading to organic bronchial and emotional hyperreactivity. The asthmatic subject continuously shifts from states of anxiety and depression [24] when suffering from asthma attacks, with a tendency towards isolation from everything and everybody, to states of euphoria when in a phase of respiratory well-being, which leads to underestimating the disease and even discontinuing treatment, with risks and consequences that can easily be imagined.

The Social Relationships of the Asthmatic Subject

It is widely known that the asthmatic patient tends to establish a relationship of psychic dependence with his or her doctor and psychotherapist and an attachment related to expectations of recovery. The expression of the influence exerted by the doctor on the asthmatic patient raches its peak when the administration of placebo brings about a beneficial effect (bronchodilation or, in any case, the regression of symptoms).

Research carried out by Pappagallo et al. [28], on the influence of the family on the emotional personality of the asthmatic subject, suggested the following:

1. The father of an asthmatic subject is a secondary figure.
2. The mother often gives up her job in order to look after her asthmatic child.
3. There is often a conflictual relationship between the parents of an asthmatic child.
4. Older asthmatic children often reject drugs if administered by their mothers.
5. The patient is often dependent on his or her doctor whether a pediatrician, pneumologist, allergologist, or psychologist.

The hypothesis has been put forward that the asthmatic symptom is an attempt by the subject at independence and is seen as a way to establish a relationship between his or her own self and others. In other words, the asthmatic subject suffering from an asthma attack is thought to express aggressiveness and the attempt to rebel against the surrounding environment in order to dominate it.

To sum up, the personality of the asthmatic subject seems to suffer from a situation of unbalance between the desire for independence from the mother and the wish to depend on her. Thus, the asthmatic patient seems to experience a dual role as "victim" and "persecutor", who conditions the attention and behavior of the family by means of his or her disease and asthma attacks.

Conclusions

There are various interesting factors in the psychosomatic genesis of asthma, including family relations, especially with the mother; stress; emotionality; anxiety; and environmental conditioning. All these factors, combined with organic causes (allergies to pollens, dust, molds, herbs, foods, drugs, various chemicals, etc.), contribute to triggering asthma attacks, which confines the personality of the asthmatic in a spiral of emotional instability. As time goes by, this situation further exacerbates the physical conditions of the patient and pharmacological treatment becomes extremely difficult or even inefective if the psychosomatic and psychogenic components of the disease are underestimated. It is our opinion that a multispecialist approach towards the asthmatic patient, especially in early childhood, is advisable for the future. Indeed, psychotherapy combined with a pharmacological treatment is likely to obtain optimal results.

References

1. Ader R (1981) Psychoimmunology. Academic, New York
2. Alexander R (1984) Medicina psicosomatica. Giunti Barbera, Florence
3. Aronsonn G, Koivunen E (1985) Differences in personality between parents of asthmatic children and non asthmatic children. J Psychosom Res 29 (2):177–182
4. Azzario P (1968) L'asma quando è malattia psicosomatica. Med Psicosom 3:309
5. Azzario P (1969) La sindrome asmatica quando è psicosomatica. La figura della madre quale fattore ambientale. Med Psicosom 4:421
6. Bengttson W (1969) Emotions and asthma. Eur J Respir Dis [Suppl] 136 (65):123–129
7. Benson E (1988) Progress in neuroendocrin immunology. Fidia, Abano Terme
8. Burki NK, Mitchell K, Chaudhary BA, Zechman FW (1978) The ability of asthmatics to detect added resistive loads. Am Rev Respir Dis 117:171–175
9. Carone M, Bettinardi O, Patessio A, Bertolotti G, Rossi MD, Zotti AM, Donner CP (1989) Valutazione della reattività psicofisiologica allo stress in soggetti asmatici. Rassegna Pat App Respir 4:159–170
10. Chiari G, Foschino Barbaro GM, Nuzzo ML, Pecci L, Rossi R (1987) Individual knowledge of emotions in asthmatic children. J Psychosom Res 31:341–350
11. Del Bono N (1981) Importanza del SNV nella patogenesi del broncospasmo. Atti 8° Congr Naz SIMP, pp 657–666
12. Dunbar A (1966) Mind and body, psychosomatic medicine. New England edition
13. French IM, Alexander R (1941) Psychogenic factors in bronchial asthma. Med Monogr IV:1–2 (National Research Council, Washington)

14. Horton DJ, Suda WL, Kisman KA, Souhrada J, Spector SL (1978) Bronchocon-strictive suggestion in athmatic role for airways hyperreactivity and emotions. Am Rev Respir Dis 117:1029
15. Huddel DW, Cooperson Dennis M, Kisman RA (1982) Recognition of added re-sistive lods in asthma. Am Rev Respir Dis 126:121–125
16. Liddel H (1951) The influence of experimental neuroses on respiratory function. In: Abramson H (ed) Somatic and psychiatric treatment of asthma. William and Wilkins, Baltimore
17. Liebman C (1979) Il ruolo della famiglia nel trattamento delle forme croniche di asma. Ter Fam 2:81–99
18. Luparello ET, Lyons HA, Bleeker ER, McFadden ER (1968) Influence of sug-gestion on airway reactivity in asthmatic subjects. Psychosom Med 30:819–825
19. Marty D (1968) La rélation d'objet allergique. Rev Franc Psychoanal 1:32–37
20. Mathé AA, Knapp PH (1971) Emotional and adrenal reactions to stress in bron-chial asthma. Psychosom Med 33:323
21. Marx D, Zofel C, Linden U, Bonher H, Franzen V, Florin I (1986) Expression of emotion in asthmatic children and their mothers. J Psychosom Res 30 (5): 609–616
22. Mc Fadden ER, Luparello ET, Lyons HA, Bleeker ER (1968) The mechanism of action of suggestion in the induction of acute asthma attacks. Psychosom Med 11:134–143
23. Mc Kenzie JM (1886) The production of rose asthma by an artificial rose. Am J Med Sci 91:45
24. Miller BD (1987) Depression and asthma: a potentially letal mixture. J Allergy Clin Immunol 80:481–487
25. Orlandelli E, Fischietto B (1979) Influenza dei fattori emozionali nella risposta bronchiale a stimoli aspecifici e specifici. Folia Allergol Immunol Clin 26: 541–544
26. Ottenberg I (1958) Learned asthma in guinea pigs. Psychosom Res 20:395–400
27. Pancheri P, Bonini S, Connolly A, Romeo F, Simonetta A, Pede P (1977) Metod-ologia psicodiagnostica nell'asma bronchiale. Folia Allergol Immunol Clin 24: 582–587
28. Pappagallo Damato S (1981) Sintomo asmatico e ottica relazionale. Atti 8° Congr Naz SIMP, pp 723–730
29. Pinkus L (1980) L'asma bronchiale: un conflitto di identità. Med Psicosom 25 (1):3–8
30. Spector S, Luparello TJ, Kopetzky MI, Souhrada J, Kinsman RA (1976) Re-sponse of asthmatics to methacoline. Psychosom Med 113:43–50
31. Steiner H, Higgs C, Gregory KF, Laszlo G, Harvey JE (1987) Defense style and perception of asthma. Psychosom Med 49 (1):35–44
32. Tiffeneau R (1961) Stimuli psycosomatiques asthmogènes. Mesure de leur intensité. Presse Med 68::115–119
33. Thoren R (1967) Psychosomatic approach to bronchial asthma. Acta Allergol XXII:145–173
34. Tunsater A (1984) Emotions and asthma. Eur J Respir Dis [Suppl] 136 (165): 131–137

Part III

Assessment of Respiratory Functions: Methodology

Volume, Flow, and Resistance Assessment in Asthma

S. DAMATO

Institute of Respiratory Diseases, School of Medicine, University of Milan, Milano, Italy

Introduction

The assessment of lung function in the asthmatic patient has the following main targets:

1. Evaluation of the degree and prevalent location of lung function impairment during symptom-free periods, these being not available in all patients and depending on asthma definition

2. Evaluation of lung function during stable asthma, while the patient is undergoing optimal treatment including protection and/or therapy, on the basis of asthma pathogenesis and patient compliance with all possible indicated therapeutical interventions

3. Evaluation of lung function before and after administration of drugs, mediators, or physical stimuli in order to quantify their possible constrictor, dilatator, or protective effects in asthmatic patients or subjects suspected to be asthmatics

4. Monitoring of lung function during the day and day to day with respect to symptoms and to adjustment of treatment.

In this chapter, airways patency is the aspect of lung function that is considered; lung function tests, procedures, evaluation parameters, and interpretation of results are largely dependent upon the specific target of the lung function study, as stated above. More technical, but still crucial, points are reported in the Appendices A, B and C, while information concerning technical problems in lung function evaluation are available in the literature [20, 22, 89, 117]. For clarity and in the attempt to limit the length of this chapter, a discussion of some of the more unusual or troublesome procedures is omitted. The symbols and units used are presented in Table 1.

Lung Volumes

Tidal volume (TV) is the volume of gas which is inspired or expired during a respiratory cycle (Fig. 1). For measurements during tidal breathing, a resolu-

Table 1. Main symbols and units in volume, flow, and resistance assessment

Symbol	Quantity		Unit	Definition
m	Length		Meter	
kg	Mass		Kilogram	
s	Time		Second	
°C	Temperature[a]		Degree Celsius	$t = T - T_0$
Hz	Frequency		Hertz	s^{-1}
N	Force		Newton	$m\,kg\,s^{-2}$
kPa[b]	Pressure	(P)	Pascal	$N\,m^{2}\,10^{3}$
l	Volume	(V)	Liter	$10^{-3}\,m^{3}$
$l\,s^{-1}$	Flow	($\dot{V}$)	Time derivative of V	
$l\,s^{-2}$	Acceleration	($\ddot{V}$)	Second time derivative of V	
P	Viscosity	(η)	Poise	Pa s

[a] Celsius temperature (t) is defined as the difference between the thermodynamic temperature T and T_0 ($= -273.15\,°C$)
[b] For conversion factors to mm Hg or cm H_2O multiply by 7.5 or 10.2, respectively, from mm Hg or cm H_2O divide by 0.133 or 0.098.

tion of 10 ml and tolerance of 2% or 20 ml is required [92]; the numerical representation of TV in liters is carried out to three decimal places. The size of TV is determined by the body weight and the metabolism rate, ventilation per minute (VE) being calculated breath by breath or by multiplying expired TV by the frequency of breathing (per minute). Differences between inspired and expired TV are determined by several factors; some of them being dependent upon the correct use of the instrument in relation to ATP or ATPS measurement conditions and BTPS correction (see Appendix C). This difference has to be considered in detail when calculating oxygen (O_2) consumption or carbon dioxide (CO_2) production. TV can be measured by volume displacement equipment (spirometer) or by differential pressure transducers arranged in a pneumotachographic set (pneumotachograph). Using a spirometer, the instrumental response time and frequency response with respect to frequency of breathing are the crucial factors. Using a pneumotachograph, the crucial factors are the accuracy and linearity of the instrument. Ideally, for measuring TV at rest, a number 2 Fleisch head is required, with different calibration factors for inspiration and expiration, while at higher flow rates a number 3 Fleisch head is required, with recalibration of the system.

The specificity of VE in the clinical lung physiology setting for the diagnosis of asthma is low; it could be a parameter to quantify hyperventilation in response to stimuli or a means for standardization of procedures. During tidal breathing it is possible to quantify the pattern of breathing by continuous calculation of respiratory drive (TV/T_{insp}) and timing (T_{insp}/T_{tot}), which can be related to prolongation of expiration in asthma. All these measurements require great accuracy in terms of procedure and equipment arrangement.

Functional residual capacity (FRC) is the volume of air contained in the lungs at the level of end expiration during tidal breathing (Fig. 1); the measurement accuracy required is 50 ml. FRC is a crucial lung volume to be measured, since most of the lung volume subdivisions stem from its measurement, which is based on body plethy smographic or gas dilution techniques.

One gas dilution technique is based upon the closed circuit helium concentration equilibrium between the known gas volume in a spirometer and the unkown FRC. The measurement is usually done with the volume-stabilized method [70]; O_2 is added continuously to the circuit and its flow is adjusted during the procedure to match the subject's O_2 uptake. Once the spirometer is full of the gas mixture, containing air and some proportion of helium, the equipment dead space is filled with the mixture by pushing the spirometer bell while the valve is open to ambient air. The valve is then rotated to close the circuit and the spirometer volume and initial helium meter values are read. The subject is then connected to the mouthpiece and time is allowed to stabilize the resting breathing level and to achieve steady state O_2 consumption. This point is crucial since the resting breathing level is representative of the subject's real FRC. The subject is instructed to perform a complete inspiration followed by a complete expiration and then breath quietly for a while in order to reach the physiological level; in fact when the subject is first connected to the equipment, the resting breathing level is altered by the position change, the momentary apnea, and many other subjective and objective factors. The breathing valve is switched to the closed circuit when the subject is at end normal expiration; this point is checked by ob-

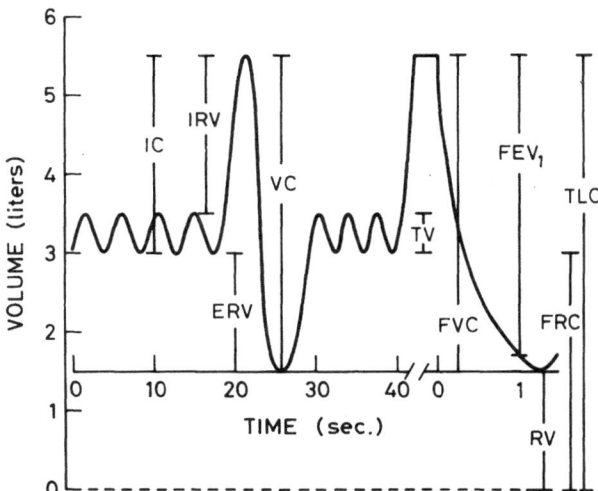

Fig. 1. Spirometer volume trace during breathing maneuvers. ERV, expiratory reserve volume; FEV_1, forced expiratory volume in 1 s; FRC, functional residual capacity; FVC, forced vital capacity; IC, inspiratory capacity; IRV, inspiratory reserve volume; RV, residual volume; TLC, total lung capacity; TV, tidal volume; VC, vital capacity

servation of the rib cage or by detection of no flow at the valve. Errors may occur in switching subjects into the closed circuit system; subjects may also exhibit irregular breathing patterns, which may complicate the procedure. The test is interrupted after 10 min or at the point when there is no helium concentration change greater than 0.05 % over a 1 min interval [92]. Incorporating inspiratory capacity maneuvers which require full inspiration from FRC level followed by expiration to FRC level, shortens the period required for equilibration and may increase the accuracy of the measurement [87]. It has to be considered that, during such maneuvers, the resting breathing level may be altered if the subject has not been trained in advance.

FRC, in the closed circuit helium method, is calculated from the following equation:

$$FRC = \{[(F_1 - F_2) + V_{kn}]/F_2\} - V_{dmp}$$

where F_1 and F_2 are initial and final helium concentration readings, V_{dmp} is the mouthpiece dead space, and V_{kn} is the volume (air + helium) in the spirometer at the beginning of the procedure. Several corrections may be applied to the calculated FRC: (a) correction from ATPS to BTPS condition, about +8 %; (b) correction for helium absorbed into the bloodstream, the average correction being –60 ml; (c) correction for respiratory quotient, assumed as 0.8, and nitrogen (N_2) increment, the combined correction being –100 ml [87]. The most common problems encountered are leakage of gas between mouth and valve, with the consequence of no trend toward equilibration, and an exhausted CO_2 absorber, which causes changes in respiratory pattern and some error in helium meter readings. The published standard deviation of repeated helium dilution measurements range from 90 to 160 ml, the system variability accounting for nearly 80 ml; the 95 % tolerance limit for detecting a real change in FRC is estimated at 340 ml, based on two sets of duplicate measurements [98].

Another gas dilution technique is the open circuit method, in which a resident gas, N_2, is eliminated during breathing of 100 % O_2 or a mixture containing 21 % O_2 plus argon (N_2 multibreath washout). The total amount of expired N_2 (mixed expired N_2 concentration multiplied by the cumulated volume of gas expired) is nearly 79 % of the air volume contained in the lung at the beginning of the washout. This method requires a fast N_2 analyzer, an open circuit system with a bag in box assembly, and a pneumotachograph or a spirometer assembly. Since many calculations and corrections of real measurements are required, the equipment is computer assisted and requires special care and technical knowledge. It is designed for gas mixing studies [9, 88] rather than for lung volume measurements alone.

FRC measurements with both gas dilution methods are time-consuming. In airways obstruction, as occurs in asthma, the inefficiency of alveolar gas mixing would be responsible for very long equilibration or washout times. Some compartments of the lung may partially or entirely fail to equilibrate with the inspired gas mixture, underestimation of FRC being the consequence [92].

The plethysmograph measures the total compressible gas volume [26] in the thorax (thoracic gas volume, TGV), whose correspondance to FRC depends upon that of the breathing level, too. Its accuracy is not affected by the presence of poorly ventilated zones, which often cause the gas dilution techniques to underestimate the volume. The difference between the TGV and the dilution FRC would give an estimate of the inefficiency of alveolar ventilation in asthma, this measurement being useful to quantify and qualify the lung dysfunction. The subject is seated in the plethysmograph allowing for temperature equilibration once the cabin has been closed. He is then connected to the special mouthpiece-shutter assembly and special care is taken to reach the resting breathing FRC level, following the same suggestions given above for the gas dilution methods. At FRC level (end of tidal expiration), the shutter is closed to occlude the mouthpiece, and the subject is asked to rhythmically compress and decompress his TGV by lightly panting against the closed shutter. While the shutter is closed, no airflow occurs within airways, so mouth pressure changes (ΔP_{mo}) are equal to alveolar pressure changes (ΔP_{alv}); in the meantime, pressure changes in the box (ΔP_{box}) are continuously monitored. The P_{box} changes reflect the TGV changes and have an inverse relation with P_{alv} changes (Fig. 2); the linearity of this inverse relation being preserved by the isothermal conditions. Boyle's law may be applied to these pressure volume (PV) changes:

$$PV = (P + \Delta P)(V + \Delta V)$$

where P is P_{alv} at FRC level (measured as P_{mo} at shutter open, which is ambient or barometric pressure, P_B), ΔP is the change in P_{alv} with panting (measured as ΔP_{mo} while shutter is closed), V is the unknown FRC or TGV

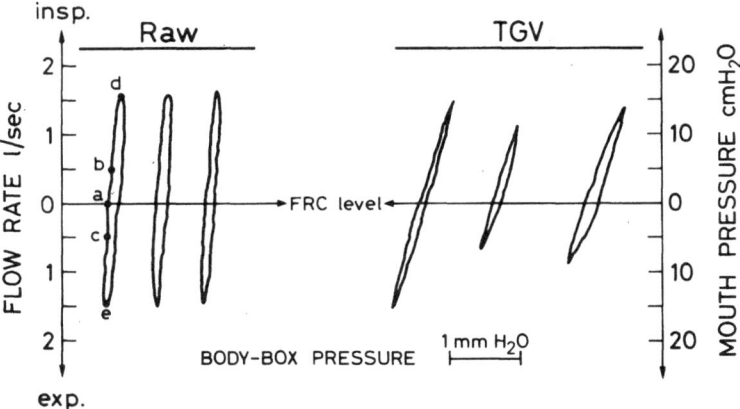

Fig. 2. Plethysmographic thoracic gas volume (TGV) and airway resistance (R_{aw}) plots from a normal subject; exp, expiration; insp, inspiration; FRC, functional residual capacity. a–b, slope for inspiratory R_{aw}; a–c, slope for expiratory R_{aw}; d–e, slope for total R_{aw} calculations

and ΔV is the TGV change during panting (measured as P_{box} changes, ΔP_{box}). Reconsidering the above equation:

$$V = TGV = (P_{box}/\Delta P_{mo})(P_B + \Delta P_{mo})$$

ΔP_{mo} being negligible in comparison to P_B. Considering that the amount of water vapor is constant during gas compression and decompression, P_{H_2O} has to be subtracted from P_B. Therefore the new equation will be:

$$TGV = (\Delta P_{box}/\Delta P_{mo}) P_B - P_{H_2O}$$

the relation between box and mouth pressures being plotted on the oscilloscope or on paper by means of an analogue plotter (Fig. 2). The shutter closed loops are usually linear, although a small hysteresis is occasionally observed. Some studies [14, 41, 95, 96, 100] have shown an overestimation of TGV in asthma because of high airway resistance; this is due to the fact that P_{mo} does not properly reflect P_{alv} at flow interrupted in such a condition. Furthermore, there will be a phase shift between P_{alv}, measured as P_{mo}, and TGV change during compression-decompression, measured as P_{box}. This results in a loop formation on plotted traces, which is not due to instrumental lag time but is an expression of obstruction. The slope of the $\Delta P_{box}/\Delta P_{mo}$ relation is measured as an angle (α) and by calculating its cotangent (ctg). TGV can be calculated applying the following formula:

$$TGV = [(P_{box_c}/P_{box_d})(P_{mo_d}/P_{mo_c})(P_B - P_{H_2O})(SVC)] \, ctg(\alpha)$$

c being the calibration values for pressure (P_{mo}, usually 0.5 kPa) and volume (P_{box}, usually that corresponding to 30 ml change), d being the deflection of the calibration signals (usually set to 50 mm for both signals), ctg being the cotangent of the measured angle α drawn endpoint to endpoint, P_B being atmospheric pressure (101.3 kPa at sea level), P_{H_2O} being water vapor pressure at 37 °C (6.3 kPa). The subject volume correction (SVC) is given by:

$$SVC = [pltvol - (w/0.97)]/pltvol$$

were pltvol is the volume of the plethysmograph in liters, w is the subject's weight in kg and 0.97 is assumed as the density of the human body. Since the calibration and the corresponding deflection values can be simply expressed by calibration factors (cf), the new simplified formula will be:

$$TGV = ctg\,\alpha\,(cf_{box}/cf_{mo}) \cdot SVC \cdot (P_B - P_{H_2O}) - V_D$$

where V_D is the volume between mouth and pneumotachograph. The mean value of four angles is used for the calculations, the coefficient of variation of TGV values being 3.8% in trained and 6.1% in untrained subjects [82]. In some patients accessory muscle painting may result in increased TGV due to inclusion of compressible intra-abdominal gas [6, 15]; but with standard panting techniques this error is usually not significant.

The FRC varies with the level of physical activity, posture (being smaller in supine posture), quantity of body fat, and rib cage-lungs mechanical features (conformation of thorax also being important). Since the resting level of ventilation is increased with obstruction (see Chap. 2), an increase of FRC or TGV is expected in asthma, obstruction being often present also during symptom-free periods or because of concomitant smoking and chronic obstructive pulmonary disease (COPD). Increased FRC, together with increased TLC, has been seen in many in patients with acute or severe attacks of asthma; this is defined as hyperinflation [46, 114, 115]. Elevation of FRC has also been attributed in this condition to the continued action of inspiratory muscles during expiration [65, 76].

The procedure for the measurement of FRC or TGV is completed by supplementary breathing maneuvers [92] that allow measurement of several lung volumes. These can be used for calculating some of the pulmonary capacities (Fig. 1):

1. Expiratory reserve volume (ERV) is the volume that can be maximally expired from the FRC breathing level, reaching the lowest possible lung volume. ERV ist affected by obesity, altered rib cage, incorrect resting breathing level, and dysfunction of the respiratory muscles. It is not used as an independent evaluation parameter, but for the calculation of residual volume from FRC values which have been determined with the helium method.

2. Inspiratory reserve volume (IRV) is the volume that can be maximally inspired from the resting end-inspiratory level, which is FRC + TV.

3. Inspiratory capacity (IC) is the volume that can be inspired from the FRC breathing level; it correspoonds to the sum of TV and IRV. IC is reduced with increasing FRC, as in airways obstruction, unless TLC is not proportionally increased.

4. Vital capacity (VC) is the volume measured at the mouth between the highest and the lowest lung volume levels. It can be measured during inspiration (inspiratory vital capacity, IVC), which is performed from complete expiration or residual volume level to complete inspiration or TLC level; the slow expiratory vital capacity (EVC) being therefore performed from TLC to residual volume levels. The selected value should not exceed the next highest one by more than 300 ml [34]. VC decreases in airways obstruction proportional to the possible increase in residual volume, unless TLC is not increased. A decrease of VC is also due to dynamic compression during expiration, the size of reduction depending on the intensity of the expiratory effort, on the degree of intrinsic airways obstruction, and on the degree of lung parenchyma elasticity impairment. Therefore it is crucial that EVC is measured during slow maneuvers; the timing of the EVC should be indicated in the report for better comparison with the timing of the forced expiration.

5. Residual volume (RV) is the volume of gas remaining in the lung at the end of a complete expiration. RV is not directly measurable; it is calculated by subtracting the ERV from FRC. In airways obstruction, RV increases in proportion of the increase in FRC and the eventual decrease in ERV. The reported intrasubject coefficient of variation is about 8% [101].

6. Total lung capacity (TLC) is the volume of gas in the lung at the end of a complete inspiration. TLC can be calculated as (RV + VC) or (FRC + IC), therefore being influenced by possible errors in measuring FRC, ERV, and IVC. In asthma TLC can be increased both during acute attacks or a long-standing history of COPD. RV/TLC is an expression of the contribution of not ventilated lung to TLC: it is eventually increased in relation to a higher level of resting lung volume and to changes in the elastic recoil of the lungs. An erroneously high FRC level will result in erroneously high RV/TLC; the same would happen if the expiration is to fast, since a forced maneuver might contribute to airways compression and reduce ERV values in airway obstruction. The interpretation of RV/TLC therefore has to be very careful.

Resistances

During breathing, the elastic, frictional, or resistive and inertial features of lungs, airways, and chest wall are the determinants of the pressure difference to be applied to the respiratory system in order to obtain airflow and volume changes [84]. The elastic component is a function of volume (V), the resistive one is a function of flow ($\dot{V}$) and the inertial component is a function of acceleration ($\ddot{V}$). Inertial components are negligible during quiet breathing and the respiratory pressure difference to flow ratio ($P_{rs}/\dot{V}$) is only a function of the total respiratory resistance (R_{rs}), providing that the elastic or volume component is subtracted. This obtained by isovolume measurements of resistance [35] or by simultaneous measurement of the elastic component.

The difference between P_B and P_{mo} (transrespiratory pressure) is the driving pressure for the entire system (airways, lung tissue, and chest wall), the ratio with airflow being defined as total respiratory resistance (R_{rs}), which is the sum of airways (R_{aw}), lung tissue (R_{ti}) and chest wall resistances. Applying sinusoidal pressure variations to the respiratory system, with an external generator at the mouth (loudspeaker, sinusoidal pump), and studying the resulting relation between pressure applied and airflow, it is possible to measure, at a given sinusoidal pressure frequency change, the input impedance of the respiratory system. Several mechanical properties of the system can be studied measuring the input impedance at a number of different frequencies, the influence of a specific property being dependent upon the frequency [28, 86]. The elastic and inertial components are eliminated either by making the measurements at the frequency at which they cancel each other out (resonant frequency) or by measuring that particular component. The pseudorandom noise forced oscillation technique [57, 77] is based upon the simultaneous application at the mouth of inputs with a large frequency content and on the measurement of the resulting flow and pressure; both signals at the mouth are analyzed by means of computer based equipment. Changes of R_{rs} have been investigated in different conditions, including asthma and COPD [109, 110]. Input impedance, in the opinion of the authors, can be used as an alternative for plethysmograph R_{aw} measurements, gives complementary information with respect to the forced expired volume in 1 s (FEV_1), and is more sensitive than the measurements of specific airways conductance (sG_{aw}) during bronchial challenge tests in asthmatic patients. This method seems very promising in situations in which the subject is uncooperative, e.g., an infant [25].

The pressure difference between lung surface, the pleural pressure (P_{pl}), and mouth (P_{mo}) is the driving pressure which defines the lung resistance (R_L) for a given flow rate ($\dot{V}$):

$$R_L = (P_{pl} - P_{mo})/\dot{V} = kPa\ l^{-1}\ s$$

The $P_{pl} - P_{alv}$ difference is determined by R_{ti}, whilst the $P_{alv} - P_{mo}$ difference is determined by R_{aw}, R_L being equal to $R_{ti} + R_{aw}$. P_{pl} is measured in upright posture as esophageal pressure [75] by means of a catheter-balloon system introduced through a nare into the lower third of the esophagus. The catheter is usually 1 m long, has a 2 mm external diameter, and is connected to a differential pressure transducer. Airflow and volume at the mouth are measured by means of a pneumotachograph. The three variables, P_{pl}, P_{mo}, and $\dot{V}$, are recorded during spontaneous breathing with respect to time, P_{pl} and $\dot{V}$ measured at the same volume during both inspiration and expiration. The signals have to be in phase; instrumental phase lag can usually be avoided if the frequency response of the equipment is flat up to at least 10 Hz. Computation can be speeded up by using an oscilloscope and subtracting from the measured esophageal pressure a signal proportional to the volume in order to cancel the elastic component and obtain a single valued relation between pressure and flow [72]. RL measurements by means of esophageal pressure tend to be about 20% higher than plethysmograph R_{aw} measurements, the difference being attributed to R_{ti}.

The determination of airway resistance (R_{aw}) requires measurement of the pressure drop, or driving pressure, between alveoli (P_{alv}) and mouth (P_{mo}), related to airflow, at a given lung volume. P_{alv} can be measured by the interruptor method [73]. During transient interruption of airflow, P_{alv} will equilibrate rapidly with P_{mo}. Provided that occlusion is sufficiently rapid and assuming no influence of the respiratory muscles, P_{mo} immediately after occlusion will approximate P_{alv} immediately before occlusion. Since inertia and airways compliance interfere with pressure equilibration along the bronchial tree, an estimate of P_{alv} can be obtained by measuring P_{mo} some time after occlusion and back extrapolating to a time close to the occlusion time [19]. The measurement is usually done during a series of interruptions at regular intervals for a short period of time (80–150 ms), which is virtually imperceptible to the subject, while he is breathing spontaneously through a pneumotachograph equipped with an electronic flow interruptor device. The pressure is measured continuously; at open airways the pressure (P_o) is a measure of flow rate, while at airflow interruption (P_i) it is a measure of the pressure required to offset the resistance of airways and equipment (K). R_{aw} is obtained by the relation:

$$R_{aw} = [(P_i - P_o)/P_o] \cdot K$$

The equipment is easily portable and relatively cheap, and the method does not require much cooperation from the subject. Unfortunately the assumptions are not completely acceptable when lung diseases delay equilibrium between P_{alv} and P_{mo}, as is the case in airways obstruction, e.g., acute asthma attacks, with substantial differences of results compared to other R_{aw} measuring methods.

The standard method for measuring airway resistance is based upon the technique of two stage panting within a plethysmograph [27]. The principle of P_{alv} determination is similar to that of TGV determination in isothermic conditions: the changes in lung volume during compression and decompression maneuvers are expressed by P_{box} changes in the volume-constant plethysmograph and are proportional to P_{alv} (measured as P_{mo} during airways occlusion). The equation for TGV is the basis of the calculation:

$$TGV = (\Delta P_{box}/\Delta P_{mo}) P_B$$
$$\Delta P_{mo} = (\Delta P_{box} P_B)/TGV$$

R_{aw} is equal to the relation between P_{alv} (which is P_{mo} during occlusion) and flow rate $(\dot{V})$ changes:

$$R_{aw} = \Delta P_{mo}/\Delta \dot{V} \quad \text{or} \quad [(\Delta P_{box} P_B)/TGV]/\Delta \dot{V}$$
$$R_{aw} = [(\Delta P_{box} P_B)(\Delta P_{box}/\Delta P_{mo}) P_B]/\Delta \dot{V}$$
$$R_{aw} = (\Delta P_{box}/\Delta \dot{V})(\Delta P_{mo}/\Delta P_{box}) = \Delta P_{mo}/\Delta \dot{V}$$

Therefore the R_{aw} measurement requires a record of the relationship between $\dot{V}$ and P_{box} changes, the slope of which is the tangent (tg) of angle β, and of the relationship between P_{box} and P_{mo} changes during an occluded airways maneuver, the slope of which is the tangent of angle α. The final formula is:

$$R_{aw} = [(tg\,\alpha/tg\,\beta)(P_{mo_c}/P_{mo_d})(\dot{V}_d/\dot{V}_c)] - R_{sys}$$

where R_{sys} is the resistance of the system device, c is the calibration value, d is the deflection of calibration signal for P_{mo} and $\dot{V}$. These last factors can be treated as a constant factor (cf) in the final calculation:

$$R_{aw} = (tg\,\alpha/tg\,\beta\,cf) - R_{sys}$$

R_{aw} is known to normally decrease with increasing lung volume, as airways are distended; the relation is, however, curvilinear [12], while it is linear for the reciprocal of resistance or conductance (G_{aw}; l/s/kPa). To provide a volume standardization G_{aw} is divided by the TGV at which R_{aw} was originally measured, yelding the specific conductance (sG_{aw}; l/s/kPa/l or s^{-1} kPa^{-1}). The reciprocal of sG_{aw} is specific airways resistance (sR_{aw}).

In the plethysmograph method R_{aw} is therefore measured simultaneously with TGV. The subject is seated, closed in the body box at stable temperature and pressure; while connected to the special pneumotachograph shutter system, he is asked to pant or breath normally for the $\Delta\dot{V}/\Delta P_{box}$ plot at first and then against a closed shutter for the $\Delta P_{mo}/\Delta P_{box}$ plot. The mean of four reproducible angles is usually used for the final R_{aw} calculation, as for TGV. Usually the selection of angles for TGV measurement is easy since the slope of $\Delta P_{mo}/\Delta P_{box}$ is straight except in patients with extensive obstruction (see above). A slightly S-shaped curve (Fig. 2) is usually obtained during quiet breathing for the relationship $\Delta\dot{V}/\Delta P_{box}$ in normal subjects, providing the inspired and expired gas volume are both at BTPS conditions. This condition is achieved by warming and humidifying the inspired gas, otherwise variation in TGV is not due exclusively to compression and decompression of alveolar gas, a loop formation of the resistance plot being the consequence. The use of panting maneuvers, instead of normal brathing, reduces loop formation, since the amount of air breathed is small; otherwise the subject has to be connected to a rebreathing bag with gas at BTPS conditions. An electronic correction by subtracting a signal proportional to changes of inspired-expired volume due to BTPS conditions [49, 50] is also possible. The rapid shallow panting method does not require an inspired air heating system and is less sensitive to changes in laryngeal resistance [99] whilst the quiet breathing method requires less instruction.

In asthma, as in other obstructive lung diseases, the pressure-flow plot for R_{aw} calculation has a loop and an accentuated S-shape, especially during expiration (Fig. 3). This is observed also in correct BTPS management and is due to gas compression because of airways closure. Resistance is usually measured by calculating (Fig. 2) the slope during inspiration (inspiratory R_{aw}) or expiration (expiratory R_{aw}), both between 0 and $0.5\ l\,s^{-1}$; it may also be calculated by the lsope obtained tracing a line between the two extremities of the plot (total R_{aw}). In the same subject, R_{aw} is usually a little lower during panting than during quiet breathing [4]. An automated method has

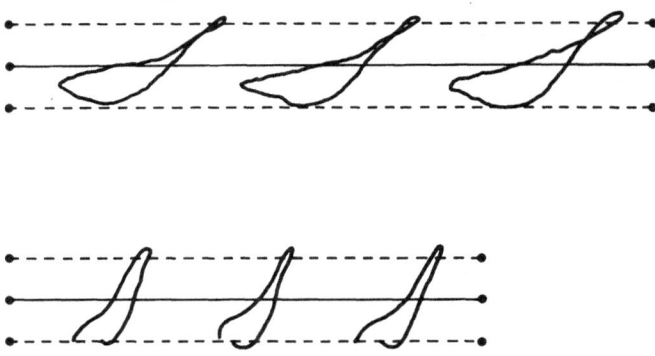

Fig. 3. Plethysmographic R_{aw} plots from an asthmatic subject before (top) and after (bottom) bronchodilatation. Continuous line is zero flow at FRC level; dotted lines are $0.5\ l\,s^{-1}$ flow rate levels during inspiration and expiration. Scales and parameters as in Fig. 2

been proposed [18] for the computer assisted determination of R_{aw}. It calculates an averaged value for inspiratory and expiratory R_{aw} during the plethysmograph panting technique. Since the target of airways resistance determination is an evaluation of airways dimensions, it is reasonable that the most valuable calculation in this respect is that of inspiratory R_{aw}. In choosing reference values, one has to consider the methods used in the reference study concerning procedure and slope calculations. The reported coefficient of variation for sG_{aw} is 10% [82]. The range of R_{aw} is 0–2 kPa l^{-1} s, tolerance being 0.01 kPa l^{-1} s or 5%, whichever is greater [84]. The sG_{aw} values are widely used to monitor airways obstruction in asthma patients since the amount of collaboration required from the patient is limited and it is possible to make several determinations in series, as during bronchial challenge tests in order to calculate the provocative dose at the level of a 35% decrease of sG_{aw} with respect to baseline determination.

Forced Expiration Test: Flow Rates and Dynamic Lung Volumes

Forced expiration is one of the most widely used breathing maneuvers in evaluating airways patency under dynamic conditions. The subject develops the flow rates usually needed to meet the level of ventilation required during effort without metabolic and cardiovascular stress. The test allows measurement and calculation of a number of lung function indices, some of which may also be altered in the absence of breathlessness during the activities of a sedentary life. These indices also enable the clinician to evaluate the degree of obstructive airflow limitation.

The functional information is obtained by the relation of inspired-expired volume to time, the volume time curve or spirogram (Fig. 4), and by the relationship of the instantaneous maximal expiratory flow rate (MEF) to lung volume, the maximal flow volume (MEFV) curve. The volume in the MEFV curve, usually on the abscissa, may be reported as an absolute value or as the proportion of both FVC or TLC remaining to be expired (Fig. 5). MEF values on the ordinate may be selected at 75% (MEF_{75}), 50% (MEF_{50}), and 25% (MEF_{25}) of FVC [13, 17, 23, 24, 36, 59, 67, 74, 113] or at 20%, 40%, 60%, and 80% of TLC [13, 23, 43, 113].

The goals of the forced expiration test are: (a) to produce the highest possible flow rate necessary in order to completely empty the lungs in the shortest time and (b) stress the mechanical interplay between lung parenchyma, airways wall compliance, and airways caliber. In order to reach these goals, the forced expiration has to be a real "forced" maneuver which includes these five successive steps: (1) breathing quietly until definitely reaching the FRC breathing level, (2) a complete inspiration performed from FRC until TLC level (3) a breath-holding period of 1–2 s, (4) a sudden, continuously maximal, forced expiration in order to empty the lungs as much as possible and in the shortest time interval, (5) a complete final inspiration.

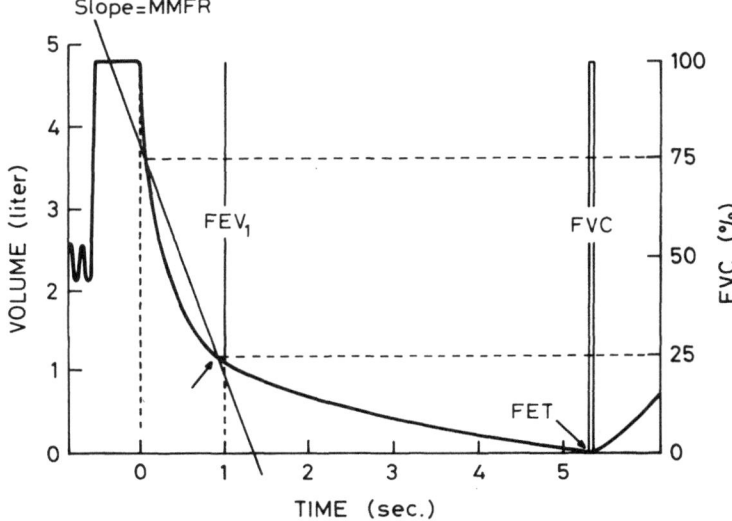

Fig. 4. Volume–time diagram and related indices during forced expiration. FEV_1, forced expired volume in 1 s; FET, forced expiration time; FVC, forced vital capacity; MMFR, Mead maximum expiratory flow rate

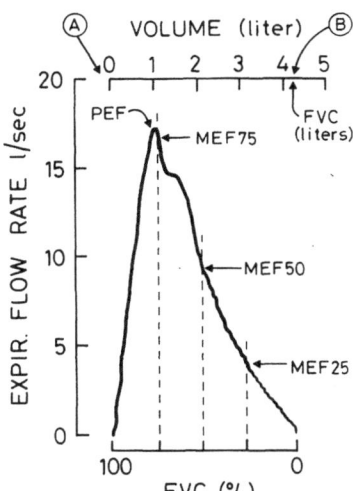

Fig. 5. Flow–volume loop during forced expiration. FVC, forced vital capacity or the volume interval between the total lung capacity (A) and the residual volume (B) levels. PEF, peak expiratory flow; MEF, maximum expiratory flow at 75%, 50%, and 25% of FVC remaining to be expired

Let us justify the previous steps. The first is needed both because the lung volume history to reach TLC may influence the dynamic behavior of the airways and in order to evaluate the subject's remaining capacity to increase flow rate, during effort, at FRC level (see Chap. 2, Fig. 7). In the second step the real TLC level at the beginning of forced expiration is important in order to obtain the maximal initial airways distension and to avoid underestimation of the following FVC. The breath-holding period in the third step is important for real suddeness and highest continuous effort intensity of the following forced expiration. Furthermore the breath-holding period is useful to exactly determine the zero time and the duration of the forced expiration. In the fourth step the completeness and maintenance of the same maximal effort degree during expiration is mandatory in order to avoid underestimation of FVC and to promote the dynamic compression of the intraparenchymal airways. The final complete inspiration in the last step is intended as a maneuver to confirm the level of TLC previously reached.

The test seems very simple; nevertheless it is important that adequate time for testing, operator background preparation in clinical lung physiology, correct instruction of patients, and selection of the acceptable tests are available. Most of the equipment actually in use is computer assisted and it would be easy to obtain and print additional technical data, e.g., the breath-holding period described above and other aspects, discussed below, for each one of the forced expiration tests performed. These supplementary data would help in further standardization and quality control within and between laboratories. Although some of this information could be obtained by visual examination of the original curves, this is not feasible because printing all plots for the tests would be an expensive and time consuming procedure.

The lung volume in the MEFV relationship may be continuously measured by using a plethysmograph and/or by integrating the pneumotachograph flow rate signal at the mouth. During forced expiration the lung volume decreases because of the volume being expired and the TGV being compressed. Only by applying the plethysmograph method is it possible to measure both components and relate all MEFs to the correct remaining lung volume, as a proportion of the initial one. There will be a lag between all MEFs and the correct simultaneous proportion of lung volume remaining to be expired if the effect of the TGV compression is not taken into account, as occurs by measuring volume at the mouth (which is what is usually done). The consequence is an underestimation of all MEFs from the MEFV curve, the error in healthy subjects being on average 5% at the end of the curve and 8% in the middle [118]. It is important ot take into account this underestimation of MEFs and the consequent overestimation, of airflow limitation new paragraph. Furthermore, by using FVC in the MEFV curve, which is the most widely used procedure, it is important to consider that underestimation of FVC, e.g., incomplete inspiration and/or expiration, implies an overestimation of MEFs at a determined proportion of FVC. This error is relevant in the case of incomplete expiration since the missing part of FVC is that expired at lower flow rates. The greater obstructive airflow limitation is, the greater will be the danger of MEFs overestimation and obstruction underestimation toward the end of the test and the need for a precise measurement of the entire possible expirable volume.

Duration of Forced Expiration

The starting and end points of forced expiration may correspond to those in which expiratory flow are under the resolution range of the equipment, which for a pneumotachograph during forced expiration is $0.07 \, \text{l} \, \text{s}^{-1}$ [23]. It must be considered that: (a) in severe obstructive airflow limitation a significant proportion of FVC is expired at a flow rate very nearly approaching the above mentioned value, more time being necessary for volume expiration, (b) the size of FVC is itself important for the correct MEFs selection along the MEFV curve, (c) the size of FVC is one of the selection criteria between the performed forced expirations actually accepted. Taking this into account, the end of forced expiration is, for convenience, defined [23] as occuring when the volume measured during 0.5 s is less than 25 ml. It has been demonstrated, however, that nearly 20% of COPD patients in a study [33] did not meet this condition within 10 s of forced expiration, and thus the data were inadequate for clinical studies. Prolongation of efforts beyond this value has been, however, reported as putting the subject at risk for syncopal episodes during testing [11]. Considering these difficulties, it has been sugested [23], in terms of equipment performance, that the registeration time has to be at least 14 s, including all steps of the forced expiration test. Therefore, in some conditions start-end points determination might be crucial, and it would be useful for the operator to have the facility of a display of the original flow trace and the evidence of the start-end points selected by the computer. The possibility of manipulating these points from the keyboard and of having repeated calculations of all indices should also be available. In fact, there are often subject uncertainties in the beginning or the end of the maneuver, and these cannot always be correctly interpreted by personal computer software. The determination of start-end points allows measurement of the forced expiratory time (FET), which might be useful in selecting the best test, from among a number of forced expiration maneuvers having different FVC and other indices values. However, the correct and reliable FET measurement requires complete interactivity and operator knowledge of the computer-assisted equipment.

Timing of Forced Expiration and MEFs

In order to quantify expiratory effort, suddeness and intensity, it would be useful to measure, on a routine basis, the time interval necessary to achieve the peak expiratory flow (PEF) and the time distance between PEF and the following MEFs. If effort has not been sudden enough, the MEF_{75} will be timed before PEF, which results in an unacceptable test, even if the FVC value makes the test acceptable (see below). The timing also gives one an idea of the relation between the indices measured and calculated during the first second, e.g., FEV_1 and the several flow rate indices. As obstructive airflow limitation proceeds, flow rates generating FEV_1 become a decreasing proportion of those generating FVC.

Best Test and/or Best Indices Selection

There is general agreement about the usefulness of obtaining a number of forced expiration maneuvers from the subject, in order to evaluate a set of technically satisfactory tests and to base the final evaluation on the best test (best real) or the best indices from different acceptable tests (best ideal). Some authors, in their studies involving forced expiration test, asked the subjects to perform two tests [7]; other asked for three [5, 48, 71, 78], five [43, 51, 85, 102, 112], ten [16, 17], or twenty [105]. Usually, if eight maneuvers have all been technically unsatisfactory, it is better to terminate the study, since the results will be of little value [34].

In normal subjects the forced expiration test is highly reproducible; however, patients with obstructive lung disease show greater variability than normal subjects [1]. Usually, functional evaluation is based on the data from the "acceptable forced expiration tests," which are defined as those, from among the technically satisfactory tests, in which either FVC does not differ by more than 5 % from the largest value [7, 11, 23, 38, 47, 62, 63, 74] or FVC variations are within the 200 ml range [5]. It must be considered that, in some patients with hyperreactive airways, e.g., in asthma, the inspiration to TLC may trigger bronchoconstriction so that with consecutive maneuvers obstruction evaluation indices worsen [37].

From among all acceptable expiratory efforts it has been proposed to use either that with the highest FVC [32, 59, 68, 79], that with the highest PEF [43, 63, 113], that with the highest FEV_1 [5, 78], or that with the highest flow rate values [47, 64] as the best test. Others have proposed to use values averaged from two or three acceptable tests [13, 24, 58, 112]. Some studies have been conducted with the forced expiration test using flow rates value into the 95th or 97.5th percentile [53, 54]. Other authors have proposed an averaging and smoothing procedure in order to obtain ideal MEFV curves [51, 105]. Eight different methods of choice of the best test were compared in another study [85], in which the authors proposed superimposing the MEFV curves to achieve a composite maximal curve having the largest FVC, provided that by visual inspection the curve shapes are similar. The American Thoracic Society (ATS) first proposed [2] using the single forced expiration tracing with the largest sum of FVC and FEV_1. More recently, ATS [3] proposed using the highest values of the single indices from three acceptable forced expiration tests. This procedure would ensure a better reproducibility, providing that, determined visually, the MEFV curves have similar overall shapes once they have been superimposed at the TLC initial level [23]. Unfortunately, visual inspection is not possible, since there is currently no equipment on the market which gives, at a reasonable price for routine studies, an on-screen display of the superimposed MEFV curves from the three or five acceptable tests.

The selection criteria of the best test in the evaluation of obstructive airflow limitation is particularly important for the flow rate indices. In this context, the shape of the MEFV curve has to be taken into consideration. In the obstructive condition, the curve's shape might change with small differences in completeness and continuity of maximal effort and consequent differences of FVC recovered in the time allowed to forced expiration. The shape of the MEFV curve is in itself an imortant feature for delineating the obstructive airflow limitation pattern [71] and in defining the important relation between flow rates at the beginning (PEF, MEF_{75}) and at the middle to end of the maneuver (MEF_{50} and MEF_{25}). In some asymptomatic asthmatic patients, it is common to observe MEFs just above the reference value range in the first half of FVC and just below that range in the last half, FEV_1 and MMFR being in the normal range. All single values cannot be considered pathologic on their own; nevertheless this condition is abnormal. The relation between different indices is often more useful in evaluating some patterns of obstruction than is all the numerous single data [104]. In order to observe the relation between MEFs and between them and other obstruction indices, e.g., FEV_1 and FEV_1/FVC, it is crucial that all selected data come from a single real forced expiration test, the "best real test", as, for instance, defined years ago by the ATS [23]. It must also be considered that the need for the selection of best instantaneous flow rate values from different tests stemmed also from the fact that FEV_1 was not usually available for the same test with the previous equipment, which used to draw the flow volume loop [11]. As has been stressed above, MEFs might be overestimated if FVC is underestimated because of incomplete expirations. Some authors [55] have admitted that their failure in demonstrating the concavity of a MEFV curve in older subjects [53], which means relative overestimation of MEF_{50} and MEF_{25} compared to MEF_{75}, might be due to the above mentioned phenomenon, corresponding to the selection of the highest flow rate values between several acceptable tests. The most stringent criterion in the choice of MEFs is that they come from the largest and the fastest test performed; the factors to be considered are FVC, FET, PEF, and FEV_1, the largest sum of FVC and FEV_1 being perhaps an acceptable compromise.

Several studies have been conducted in order to quantify within and between subject variability of indices from the forced expiration test, only some of them being mentioned here [1, 7, 10, 17, 40, 53, 54, 56, 62, 67, 69, 80, 90, 103]. The within subject coefficient of variation for volumes and flow rates from forced expiration tests is significantly less than the between subjects one, all of them being greater in patients with obstructive airflow limitation than in normals. The within subject coefficient is important for longitudinal studies and the between subjects one for cross-sectional evaluation. Unfortunately, the studies are often quite different in the case series, in the equipment used, and in the methods and procedures. It is therefore very compromising to express these coefficients of variations for the different indices with certainty. However, in normals and under the best technical conditions, a reasonable within subject coefficient for volumes such as FEV_1 is 3% and for MEFs nearly 6%; the between subjects coefficients are nearly 15% for FEV_1 and 25% for MEFs. Larger and more standardised studies are needed, especially for the flow rates indices.

Response to Bronchodilators Drugs

Forced expiration is widely used to assess, by means of dynamic lung volumes or flow rates, the change of airflow limitation in response to bronchoactive drugs, usually given by inhalation. In reporting the results, the changes should be related to the average of baseline (X_1) and final (X_2) values. Simple relation only to the initial value leads to errors due to the tendency of any result to regress toward the mean for the law of inital values [23, 97]. This approach is also important if a comparison between changes in different forced expiration indices, having different absolute values (as, for instance, is the case for MEF_{75} and MEF_{25}), is attempted.

Obstruction Evaluation Indices from Forced Expiration Test

Forced Vital Capacity (FVC)

The FVC is the air volume delivered during the forced expiration test. In normal subjects there is no significant difference between FVC and EVC, which is obtained during slow and complete expiration from the same TLC level. In obstructive lung disease FVC may be reduced compared to EVC because of dynamic airway compression at high expiratory flow rates, the difference being a useful index of the pattern of obstructive airflow limitation. In some patients this difference is surprisingly large and might account for effort breathlessness to a larger extent than does bronchoconstriction; it is similar to a partial functional lung amputation, of variable extent, which takes place when a greater proportion of the lung volume needs to be ventilated. It is important that the value of EVC is reported together with all data from forced expiration testing, since FVC, with respect to reference values, might be reduced both in restrictive and obstructive lung dysfunction patterns. In the final report the largest FVC value from among the three acceptable tests is commonly used, even if that value did not come from the same test as the other chosen indices [3, 23].

Timed Forced Expiratory Volume (FEV₁)

This is the volume expired at a selected time interval from the beginning of the forced expiration, usually 1 s (FEV_1). Another conventional time interval used mainly in children, is 0.5 s, because FVC is expired in less than 1 s. Its meaning is the same as for FEV_1 [59] and it decreases compared to reference values both in restrictive and obstructive patterns. Only during restriction is FEV_1 reduction the same as for FVC, with no obstructive airflow limitation being present. However, obstructive airflow limitation confined to the lower half of FVC results in little change in FEV_1 [61]. As is the case for PEF and MEF_{75}, FEV_1 is partly effort-dependent. Furthermore, similar to the increase in plethysmograph R_{aw} values, only in advanced chronic airflow obstruction does the reduction of FEV_1, PEF, and MEF_{75} reflect the severity of peripheral airways obstruction. In fact, in this condition the normal series distribution of airways resistance is reversed, the highest proportion being in the peripheral airways [45].

FEV_1, like FVC, is measured on the volume-time plot or together with the MEFV relation using computer assisted equipment. The FEV_1 value used for the final report is usually the largest of three acceptable tests, as is the case for FVC [3, 23]. In a few patients, it is impossible to obtain a real sudden beginning of forced expiration and therefore the zero time is not available. In this condition the starting point of the forced expiration should be obtained by back-extrapolation to the zero volume of the tangent drawn along the steepest portion (Fig. 6) of the volume-time relation [2], or it may be defined as that point where expiratory flow rate exceeds $0.5 \ 1 \ s^{-1}$ [23]. The value of the extrapolated volume during FEV_1 measurement should be reported along with the other data. In fact, to achieve a reliable zero time the extrapolated volume should be less than 10% of the FVC or 100 ml, whichever is greater [11]. It must be noted that in obstructive airflow limitation it will be very difficult to draw the tangent, since the volume-time plot is virtually a continuous curve. The best that can be done is to obtain a technically acceptable test, by spending more time in explaining what is going on to the patient and by not programming too many lung function tests in the same session.

FEV_1 may be expressed as an absolute value, in liters, or as a percent of VC, the so-called Tiffeneau index. This is used to determine whether FEV_1 reductions are due to restriction or obstruction, the index being normal in restriction since airflow limitation with respect to reference values is primarily

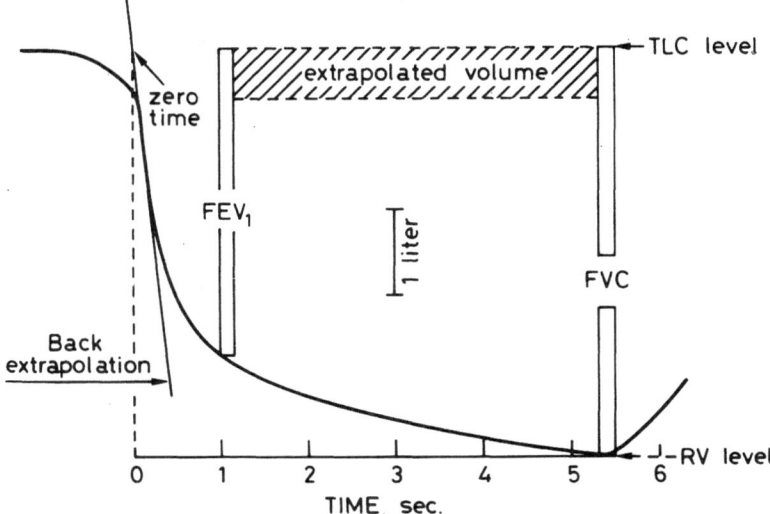

Fig. 6. Back-extrapolation for calculation of zero time, forced expiratory volume in 1 s (FEV_1) and forced vital capacity (FVC) during forced expiration. Volume (liters) on ordinate, time on abscissa. TLC, total lung capacity; RV, residual volume

determined by the lung volume reduction (e.g., in case of pneumonectomy). Whether it is more useful to express FEV_1 as a percent of FVC, EVC, or IVC is a matter of debate. The use of IVC seems inconsistent with the fact that FEV_1 is an index of expiratory obstruction. During expiration the factors influencing airflow through the airways are different than those during inspiration, especially when obstruction is present, in this case the difference between inspiratory and expiratory flow rate being greater (see Chap. 2, Fig. 5). Therefore the ratio FEV_1/IVC would be an expression of this increasing difference during obstruction between inspiratory and expiratory flow rate; it will not be an expression of the expiratory airflow limitation itself. For the same reason there is often a lack of correlation between expiratory obstruction evaluation indices and sG_{aw}, determination of which is made at a low airflow rate and during inspiration. Regarding the possible choice between FVC and EVC in the Tiffeneau index, it has to be considered that FEV_1 was generated by the airflow rates which generated FVC, not by those which generated EVC. The difference between FVC and EVC stems from a wider range of reasons than those involved in the generation of FEV_1 and FVC alone, the supplementary information being primarily present in the real measured values of the two expiratory VCs. Some considerations may be made about the use of the Tiffeneau index:

1. After bronchodilator use it is possible to record modifications of lung volumes, secondary to airways patency change; as a consequence, the FEV_1/FVC values might not be a reliable obstruction reversibility index [93].

2. In case of a severe obstruction and dynamic airway compression, a significant proportion of FVC is expired at very low flow rates and the complete determination of FVC would require a prolonged forced expiration. As a consequence, FEV_1/FVC is not reliable under conditions of severe obstruction, and the absolute value of FEV_1 appears to be the most reliable evaluation and prognostic index in this situation of airflow limitation.

3. During acute asthma attacks, as during stimuli induced bronchoconstriction, there are proportional reductions of FEV_1, FVC, and EVC; the Tiffeneau index therefore being normal [52, 118]. Due to severe obstruction, the FRC level is very high and as a consequence VC is low. If any functional evaluation is possible in this condition for monitoring purposes, the determination of FVC is the most useful, together with gas exchange studies and transcutaneous blood gas monitoring.

In asthmatic patients, FEV_1 is used in all stages of the disease as an obstruction evaluation index, a bronchoconstriction reversibility evaluation, and in drawing dose-response curves during bronchial challenge tests. Most authors identify the provocative agent dose (PD) as that corresponding to a 20% decrease of FEV_1 (PD_{20}) compared to a baseline condition determined by means of three acceptable forced expiration tests [83]. Others have proposed to identify PD by means of an absolute FEV_1 decrease of 500 ml from the baseline condition [18]. PD_{20} has been demonstrated to be related to baseline FEV_1/FVC: the greater the baseline obstruction the lower the PD_{20} [94]. Also, for this reason the bronchial challenge test is usually performed only when FEV_1 is not less than 80% of the reference value. A comparative study has been made between the FEV_1 determination of PD_{20} and the sG_{aw} determination of PD_{35} for histamine; it has been shown that PD_{20} values are able to better discriminate asthmatic from nonasthmatic patients [21]. The use of both indices is recommended since some postinspiratory bronchoconstriction could interfere in asthmatic subjects with the bronchial challenge test.

Not only PD_{20} may be determined during bronchial challenge in asthma. Using FEV_1, it is possible to calculate: (a) sensibility [42], which is the provocative agent threshold dose corresponding to a change greater than two standard deviation of the baseline average FEV_1 value from three acceptable tests and (b) the reactivity [81], which is the slope of the dose-FEV_1 response curve. However, PD_{20} is the most commonly used index.

Maximal Midexpiratory Flow Rate (MMFR)

MMFR is the mean forced expiratory flow during the middle half of the FVC. It is calculated (Fig. 4) from the volume-time relation, using the measured FVC and the time interval between 75% and 25% of FVC remaining to be expired [60]. MMFR is also called the forced expiratory flow during the middle half of FVC ($FEF_{25\%-75\%}$). MMFR decreases, with respect to reference values, with airflow limitation, both from obstruction or restriction; its meaning as an obstructive index depends on the simultaneous consideration of FVC compared to the reference value. MMFR is widely used, has good reproducibility [56], and is relatively independent of expiratory effort. From among the three acceptable forced expiration tests, it is commonly used the highest MMFR value or that from the best test (criteria discussed above). Less commonly used is the forced expiratory flow between 200 and 1200 ml ($FEF_{200-1200}$), which is the average flow for the specified early segment of FVC.

Peak Expiratory Flow Rate (PEF + PEFR)

PEF is the maximal flow during forced expiration and occurs nearly 100 ms after zero time. The required duration of the peak is 10 ms but 30 ms is also acceptable [23]. This index is very much effort-dependent. Providing the effort is a maximal one and FVC is in the normal range, PEF in healthy subjects is an index of the central airways caliber; when obstructive airflow limitation develops, it is increasengly influenced by the caliber of the peripheral airways. PEF is measured with the pneumotachograph and is expressed as $l\,s^{-1}$; the value from the best test or the highest among the acceptable tests is commonly used for comparison with the reference values.

The PEF during forced expiration may also be measured with an airflow meter, first introduced in 1959 [116] and still known as the standard Wright peak flow meter. The instrument provide an index, in 1 min^{-1}, referred to as the peak expiratory flow rate (PEFR). Later, the mini Wright, the pulmonary monitor, and the Assess peak flow meter were introduced. The more recent instruments are portable and inexpensive, making it possible to issue them to patients for home use. Many studies [30, 31, 39, 111] have been performed evaluating different portable peak flow meters, providing reference values for PEFR (the results from different peak flow meters and pneumotachograph equipment not always being comparable), and analyzing their application in the follow-up of airflow-limited patients. The variability of the measurements is satisfactory for longitudinal studies of airflow limitation; usually the instruments are not reliable when the airflow rate is very low, approaching that of tidal breathing. The values measured by the patients are reported in a diary, together with symptoms and drugs administrations. It is therefore possible, providing the instrument has been calibrated and the patient is reliable and well trained, to obtain a clinical assessment of gross obstructive airflow limitation and its pattern in relation to drug administration, symptoms, and physical signs, time of day, season of the year, physical activities, and exposure to pollutants and allergens. Classification of clinical patterns of airflow limitation in chronic asthma by using these instruments has been proposed [107]. The variability of PEFR measurements made every 2 hours for a week has been proposed as an alternative to bronchial reactivity measurements in surveys of subjects suffering from wheezing [44].

Maximal Instantaneous Forced Expiratory Flow (MEF)

MEF (or $\dot{V}_{max}$ or FEF) is the flow rate achieved at the specified proportion of FVC that remains to be expired (MEF$_{75}$, MEF$_{50}$, MEF$_{25}$). Less commonly used are the values referred to TLC, since such a procedure would require the plethysmograph method for flow-volume measurements (see above). MEF values selected for comparison with reference values commonly are the highest from those of the acceptable forced expiration tests [23]. As lung volume decreases during forced expiration, the equal pressure point (see Chap. 2) moves into the periphery of the lung. Therefore MEFs measured at lower lung volume levels better reflect the airflow limitation of more peripheral airways than do MEFs at higher volumes.

MEFs are expressed as 1 s^{-1}; the values may be divided by the observed lung volume (FVC or TLC) yielding "specific" MEF values. This last normalization procedure [118] is useful in children and adolescents since it allows comparison of values in growing subjects of different ages, heights, and lung sizes. It is also useful in patients with suspected obstructive airflow limitation when the relation between the anthropometric parameters and lung size has been changed by a different or the same process that causes the lung disease (e.g., growth defects, overweight, spinal deformity, thalassemia). In fact, there is a direct correlation between flow rate and lung volume: the absolute reduction in flow rate could be dependent on the volume reduction itself, as is the case in pure lung fibrosis or pneumonectomy. When the expired volume decreases because of dynamic airways compression, the specific MEF values are in the normal range of the specific MEF reference values if volume amputation is the only consequence of the lung defect; the gap between EVC and FVC will, of course, be the main indicator of this condition. However, by far the most common condition in the expiratory dynamic compression setting is the presence of volume amputation and airflow limitation during forced expiration. Therefore specific MEFs, compared to predicted specific values, will remain altered to a lesser degree than the nonspecific values, together with the reported EVC-FVC difference.

The coefficients of variation of MEFs, mainly those for MEF_{25} and those referring to the between subjects condition, are high. Nevertheless these indices are widely used in the clinical evaluation of the pattern of airflow limitation and in asthma. An important consideration has to be made regarding the selection of reference values, since the various procedures used for the forced expiration test in the original studies could differ very much from each other and in relation to the equipment and procedures used in one's own lung function evaluation laboratory. A useful criterion applicable to using MEFs in assessing obstructive airflow limitation is this: the obstruction not only produces absolute changes of single values with respect to reference, but also produces a concomitant disproportion between the MEF reductions, compared to normals, at the three levels of FVC. MEF_{25} is more affected than MEF_{50} and MEF_{75}. This pattern usually is also present in the absence of a significant reduction of the Tiffeneau index compared to reference values. As the obstructive airflow limitation becomes more evident, on a careful evaluated clinical basis, FEV_1 reduction also becomes edvident, the MEFs reductions now being enormous compared to that observed for FEV_1.

Many other indices of obstructive airflow limitation might be produced from the forced expiration test, but their use is confined to the most sophisticated lung function evaluation laboratories, or their reproducibility is poor, or the procedure is difficult for the subject and/or the operator; usually, there are no acceptable reference values that are available for routine use.

Appendix A:
Basic Concepts Regarding Measurements and Indices

Accuracy implies that there is a correct value about which repeated measurements are normally distributed or scattered in a Gaussian manner. In a normal distribution 68% of observations lie within ±1 standard deviation (SD), and 95% lie within ±2 SD from the mean. The series of measurements is usually indicated by a single value, such as the mean ($\bar{x}$), the median, or the mode; the three values being equal in case of normal distribution. The arithmetic mean is the sum of the observations divided by the observations number; the median is the middle observation of a series of data arranged in increasing order; the mode is the value corresponding to maximum density of the frequency distribution curve. Accuracy is defined as the degree of conformity to a reference standard, e.g., a calibrating syringe, or a true value over the entire range of values encountered in clinical studies. Acceptable limits of accuracy depend upon: (a) range of values encountered in a population of normals, (b) magnitude of the changes expected to occur with disease, (c) magnitude of changes one wants to detect as a disease improves or worsens. The error in a measurement, which is the inverse of the accuracy, can be partitioned into systematic and random components. The accuracy of an estimate from limited data can be measured by calculating the standard error (SE). It is equal to the standard deviation (SD) of the distribution hypothetically obtained by repetitive measurements (n) with errors. The SE of the mean of n observations being equal to $SD/\sqrt{n}$.

Calibration is the procedure which is used to calculate a calibration factor for the conversion of the analogue (an electrical signal) output of the instrument into a digital (a number) value having the dimension of the physical variable to be measured. The input for the calibration corresponds to a fixed true change of the physical variable, if it is available, or a conventional reference standard.

Frequency response reflects the ability of an instrument to measure the changes in dynamic events within defined levels of accuracy. The response is flat at a given frequency if input and ouput signals are equal.

Hysteresis is the phenomenon exhibited when the reaction of a system to a definite change is dependent upon previous reaction (e.g., inspiration with respect to expiration).

Linearity is the term used to describe the response of an instrument to changes in input signals. The relationship between input and output signals of the system is described by a linear equation. The linearity of an instrument has to be tested over the full operating range. The output values that are outside the limits of linearity could be corrected using a calibration curve.

Normality refers to the lung function condition of a reference population free of pathologic conditions, diseases, or other conditions affecting lung function. Lung function studies in large populations of normal subjects can be used to predict, by means of regression equations a range of normal values for subjects with specific characteristics (environment, sex, age, height, race, etc.). Predictive normal values for lung function parameters are important for their use in clinical interpretation and for increasing sensitivity for the detection of early stages of diseases. Nevertheless, the predictive normal values for many parameters are inadequate for application in the majority of laboratories. The main reasons are differences in procedures, equipment, and population characteristics. The majority of studies in normals are not at all coordinated for homogeneous geographic areas in order to obtain the right amount of information about the required size and composition of the normal population sample. Therefore, it is important for each clinically oriented laboratory to personally choose the predictive normal values from studies performed using the same procedures, which are empirically in agreement with a small sample of their own normal population. Linear equations are usually used to predict normal values. Since computers are widely available, it is now possible to use nonlinear equations; however, in this case the boundaries within which each equation can be used are more stringent. Although a mean value is a valuable element, a more use- ful interpretation often requires knowledge of the lower limits of normal values. If normal values follow a normal distribution, it is possible to express the observed value as a multiple of the SD of the normal population. The lower limit of a normal value, at a confidence level of 95 % of the normal population, would be the mean minus 1.65 SD, while at a confidence limit of 97.5 % it would be the mean minus 1.95 SD. In the second case the number of possible false positives for an abnormal function decreases but the number of false negative may increase. This depends upon the criteria of choice of the normal population studied compared to the risk factors affecting the lung function parameter under study. A possible compromise might be the choice of a higher limit for screening purpose in order to minimize the possibility of false negatives, while a lower limit would be safer in the clinical setting. A review of available equations for prediction of normal values of lung function parameters has been done by Qanjer [90, 91], while Zapletals review [117] is oriented to the lower age range.

Reproducibility is the agreement between repeated measurements, regardless of how close the mean value is to the standard reference of true value; it also implies the concept of measurement precision. The difference, or deviation (d), between the measured value (x) and the mean ($\bar{x}$) is one way of expressing the variation. The variance is the sum (Σ) of the squared deviations of observations $(x - \bar{x})^2$ divided by one less than their number $(n-1)$. The standard deviation (SD) is calculated as the square root of the estimated variance:

$$SD = \sqrt{[(x - \bar{x})^2/(n-1)]}$$

When SD changes in proportion to the mean, it is useful to obtain a dimensionless index by expressing SD as a proportion of the mean ($\bar{x}$) or coefficient of variation (v):

$$v = (SD/\bar{x}) \cdot 100 \%$$

The SD of repeated measurements is commonly used as an estimate of reproducibility; the smaller the SD, the greater the reproducibility. It can be reported with respect to a reference standard (e.g., the calibration syringe) or repeated measurements from patients. In this case it is affected by both patients and instruments as well as by random errors. The number of significant figures required is determined by considering clinical needs. Reliability, stability, and repeatability are also important in the context of an instrument, a method, or a questionnaire.

Resolution defines the minimal change that can be deected, in technical terms, with an instrument.

Response time can be characterized by the time needed by an instrument to react to an input signal equal to 90% of the full range of the measurement scale.

Tolerance defines the maximal deviation allowed from the specified value, usually expressed as a proportion of that absolute value.

Appendix B: Basic Instruments

A *Wheatstone bridge* is used to accurately measure the resistance of a detector component. The bridge has four resistances, across which there is a continuous tension. One is the unknown detector resistance to be measured while two resistances are known, and another is known but variable. A null meter is used for precise determination of when resistances are balanced. The sensor resistor is designed so that changes in input signal, for instance the output signal of a differential pressure transducer connected to a pneumotachographic head, are directly related to the measurerable changes in the sensor resistance. The use of a precise known resistance in the bridge makes the measurements of input signals extremely accurate.

A *transducer* is a sensor that converts one kind of energy into another, in this particular case pressure into an electrical signal. The most common transducer is the variable reluctance pressure transducer, which consists of a stainless steel diaphragm between two coils which creates an equal inductance on both sides of the unflexed diaphragm. By applying pressure, the diaphragm will flex creating an imbalance between the two coils connected in a bridge circuit described above. The output is proportional to differential pressure. The internal volume of the instrument is very small, therefore the transducer has good frequency response.

Volume displacement measuring devices or *spirometers* reflect changes in volume through the physical movement of a collector device, most commonly either an inverted sealed cylinder floating on water (wet type spirometer) or a moveable piston or bellows (dry type spirometer). They can be divided into two main categories: (1) those having gas conditioning facilities and helium concentration measuring devices applicable in the gas dilution techniques and (2) those with mandatory dynamic features in order to measure dynamic lung volumes. Spirometers are very accurate in measuring volume but they do not measure directly flow rate, which can be electronically derived by means of analog signal processing. Measurement of PEF cannot be done with the spirometer since there is a too fast change in flow rate for the frequency response of the instrument. The spirometer should be capable of recording at least 8 liters as a function of time; paper speed should be variable, preferably 3 cm min^{-1} for slow breathing maneuvers and 120 cm min^{-1} for the recording of dynamic lung volumes. The displacement should be linear and capable of being recorded with a tolerance of ±2% of the reading or of ±50 ml, whichever is greater. A change in volume of 25 ml should be detectable (resolution). The timing of the recordings should be accurate to within 2%. Calibration of the equipment should be regularly done by means of a calibrating syringe, at least 1 liter, over the entire volume range. The frequency response of the spirometer, tested with a sinusoidally varying input of more than 1 liter, has to be flat up to 4 Hz in order to be adequate for measuring timed forced expiratory volumes. Tests for leaks should be performed often; temperature meaurements, for volume corrections, should be performed within the spirometer bell.

The *pneumotachograph* is a device that measures the instantaneous air flow rate. The instrument can be based on different physical principles, e.g., ultrasonic or optic flow meters, or a turbine blades device. By far the most commonly used are Lilly (a mesh screen) and Fleisch (parallel short capillary tubes) pneumotachographs. The head of the instrument poses a small resistance to airflow (less than 0.1 kPa l^{-1} s). The pressure drop across the resistance is linearly related to flow rate. The pressure on both sides of the resistance element is transmitted through small diameter tubing to an appropriate differential pressure transducer, whose output is proportional to flow rate ($\dot{V}$), providing there is a laminar flow pattern through the head. In case of turbulent flow the pressure drop would be proportional to $\dot{V}^2$. In order to maintain laminar flow, air flows through the head of the instrument with the interposition of a short truncated conical tubing with increasing cross-sectional area toward the pneumotachograph head. The signal from the transducer is passed through an amplifier and a DC-coupled analogue or a digital integrator, resulting in the continuous monitoring of instantaneous air flow and volume. The resistance element is maintained at 37°–38°C by means of an electrical heating element, to prevent condensation of expired water vapor which would change the resistance of the pneumotachograph head compared to the calibration condition. Since the system is based upon the assumption of a laminar flow pattern, it will be influenced by gas viscosity, which is dependent upon gas composition and temperature (see Appendix C). The reading of the instrument will also be influenced, as will the spirometer, by air temperature through its effect on water vapor (see Appendix C). Tolerance expected for flow measurements is ±4% or ±70 ml s^{-1} (whichever is greater), both during inspiration and expiration. Specifications for volume, calculated by means of flow rate integration, are those of the spirometer. The frequency response of the assembled equipment to sinusoidal flow rate changes has to be flat until 12 Hz in order to measure instantaneous flow rate during forced exspiration [66].

Calibration can be done with flow meter tubes (rotameter) or, if integrating devices are available, by flowing a known volume of air through the pneumotachograph at varying speeds. A 3 liter calibrating syringe is recommended in order to obtain a wide flow rate range sampling from the instrument. It is better to maintain the pneumotachograph head at ambient temperature during the calibration, in view of the viscosity and temperature corrections needed for the actual readings (see Appendix C) and of the not perfect control of the temperature of the gas actually flowing though the instrument head. Separate calibration factors should be measured for flow and volume in each direction if both inspiratory and expiratory flow rate have to be measured or integrated, since some degree of hysteresis might be present in the equipment. It is also important to calibrate the equipment using the actual geometry of the system in which the pneumotachograph is used. In the Lilly system the head is designed to have a linear response to air flow ranging between 0 and $12 \, l \, s^{-1}$, while in the Fleisch system different sized heads are available for a wide variety of applications with greater accuracy and linearity performances for flow rate measurements. This greater accuracy is dependent upon the accuracy of the operator. In fact, it is necessary to change pneumotachograph heads and recalibrate the system depending on the application and the subject's size and performance: measuring flow rate and volume during tidal breathing would require a number 2 Fleisch head, measuring flow rate during forced expiration would require a number 3 Fleisch head if PEF is less than $8 \, l \, s^{-1}$ or a number 4 head if PEF is more than $8 \, l \, s^{-1}$. Continuous monitoring of flow rate during effort testing would require a number 3 Fleisch head. In microprocessor-based equipment the flow rate reading can be corrected by a mathematical expression which reproduces the experimental relation between flow and pressure transducer output. Some linearizing functions have been proposed [29]; but these are only valid for the gas composition and the geometric arrangement for which the system has been tested, otherwise they will magnify the error.

The direct flow calibration of the pneumotachograph by means of calibrating rotameters at three flow rate levels is necessary if the calibration of the integrator is also required. This is achieved by successive blowings of a calibrated volumetric syringe at different speeds. In any case the double calibration procedure makes available calibration factors to be used for periodic check-up of the system from the bottom (pneumotachograph head and pressure transducer) or from the top (digital integrator and software-based equipment readings manipulation). It must also be considered that the volume signal is often unstable because the electric off-set of the flow signal is not constant over a prolonged period of time, but this problem may be overcome by appropriate warming up of the electronic equipment, by thermal isolation of the pneumotachograph head, or by the appropriate software in the computer-based equipment. Another reason for zero volume instability is that the volumes of inspired and expired gas are different, mainly because they have different temperatures, water vapor content, and gas composition. All these factors affect flow measurements; this problem is avoided in the computer-based systems since integration of flow is set to zero at end inspiration-expiration points (zero flow rate) and BTPS correction for inspired volume is applied to each flow rate data point.

The computer-based pneumotachograph is actually the most widely used device for measuring airflow rate and continuously calculating air volume. The software makes the system potentially capable of periodic equipment self-checks, corrections, calculations, comparison with reference values, filing of data and basic interpretation of results. The link between the computer and the equipment is based upon an analogue to digital converter (ADC), which has to be well matched with the equipment in order to maintain the accuracy level required from the original measuring device. First of all, the full range of the ADC has to correspond to that of the equipment, which is $15 \, l \, s^{-1}$ for a number 4 Fleisch head and $10 \, l \, s^{-1}$ for a number 3 head. Each data point is converted by an ADC to an 8-bit binary word. The maximum output of the ADC is $2^8 - 1$ or 255, including positive and negative flows, the positive output being therefore 127. The resolution of the equipment will be insufficient $(15/127 = 0.12 \, l \, s^{-1})$ with a number 4 pneumotachograph Fleisch head but still sufficient for a number 3 head $(10/127 = 0.07 \, l \, s^{-1})$. The accuracy would be improved by using an ADC with greater resolution, e.g., a 10-bit or a 12-bit ADC [8]. The accuracy of the equipment is also affected by the sampling rate of the ADC; in fact, the instantaneous flow rate value is assumed to be the average flow over the time interval between each conversion. Therefore the higher the sampling rate the higher the resolution of the equipment, 100 Hz being the ideal value. Assuming an 8-bit processor and a 12-bit ADC, a forced expiration maneuver would allocate 3000 (3 K) bytes during 20 s, which is a very small amount of memory for the personal computers currently on the market. A problem arises if calculations and monitor display are required on-line during acquisition. In this case, the time interval between conversions would not be enough and the ADC sampling rate would have to be reduced, together with the equipment's measuring accuracy. A compromise has to be found between the cost of the processor, being mainly proportional to its speed, the basic on-line requirements for continuous equipment and respiratory maneuver control, and the level of accuracy required.

The *plethysmograph* or body-box is a large chamber with a volume of 500–1000 liters. It was first applied in clinical lung physiology by DuBois in measuring total compressible gas volume in the thorax (TGV) and airways resistance (R_{aw}). The volume displacement type measures the plethysmograph volume change produced by the breathing of the subject seated into the chamber, pressure being constant. The most commonly used plethysmograph is the constant volume, variable pressure type, in which the plethysmograph pressure changes during breathing while the volume is constant. The instrument is equipped with a pneumotachograph and three transducers, which measure changes in P_{box}, P_{mo}, and $\dot{V}$. Volume (V) at the mouth is continuously obtained by integration of airflow rate. Between mouthpiece and pneumotachograph a shutter is interposed which is closed during TGV panting maneuvers in order to compress and decompress the thoracic gas volume. Some instruments have a plastig bag filled with air at BTPS condition and fitted in the mouthpiece-shutter-pneumotachograph assembly. All signals are continuously displayed on an oscilloscope and eventually plotted against each other depending on the relationship to be quantified.

A requirement is that the volume-constant plethysmograph is vented to the atmosphere in order to deal with the increasing pressure due to heating of air by the subject. An intercom must be available for communication between subject and operator while the plexiglass door of the box is closed.

The pneumotachograph selected for R_{aw} measurements has to be linear over the range of 0.2–1.5 l s^{-1}. Calibration procedure, tolerance, and resolution of flow rate and volume measurements are those specified above for the pneumotachograph equipment. Both solenoid and air-actuated shutter are available in the mouthpiece-flow meter assembly. The shutter, which closes within 0.1 s, is smoothly interfaced with the pneumotachograph to avoid air turbulence. The mouth pressure is measured through a lateral tap in the instrument's shutter assembly by a differential transducer having a range of 2 kPa, a resolution of 0.01 kPa, and a tolerance of ±1% of full scale deflection. The box pressure is measured by a differential pressure transducer that has a range of 0.4 kPa, is very sensitive, and which is designed to minimize artifacts. The frequency response of the plethysmograph has to be flat, and changes in P_{mo} and P_{box} should be in phase up to 10 Hz. The same frequency responce is required for the displaying or recording X-Y devices. Several calibration devices are required: a 10–100 ml motor-driven, airtight syringe for the P_{box} transducer, a manometer or U-tube for the P_{mo} transducer, a rotameter and a calibrating syringe (volume from 1–3 liters) for the pneumotachograph.

An *anemometer* is a sensor measuring the mass flow, which is the number of molecules moving trough the equipped device. Mass flow has no relation to the volume occupied by the molecules. Therefore mass flow does not correspond to volumetric flow and its measurement is not affected by air pressure or temperature. The sensor is a large diameter, low resistance tube equipped with stainless steel wires centered in a laminar flow stream. The two wires are electrically heated to different temperatures and included in a bridge circuit maintained at a constant resistance ratio value. If the hot wire loses heat more rapidly than the cold one, as occurs while air flows across them, a current proportional to the mass flow of the gas must be added to balance the bridge. Since the anemometer electronic output is alinear and shows a greater voltage change at low flows than high flows, a digital linearization algorithm is necessary to maintain accurate readings of both flow and volume, once it has been calibrated. Because of this property, the anemometer has a constant resolution as a percentage of reading, large dynamic range and high signal to noise ratios at low flows. Providing the transducer is computer assisted, it could be possible to perform with the same sensor applications ranging from pediatric to adults exercise testing. The sensor is not affected by system pressure drop or changes in expired gas composition, temperature and humidity.

Appendix C: Measuring Conditions and Conversion Factors

Temperature and Gas Volume

The volume of a quantity of gas varies with the pressure and thermodynamic temperature. There are three main experimental conditions in clinical lung physiology:

1. ATP, which is the volume or flow determined at ambient temperature and barometric pressure, as during calibration of a nonheated pneumotachograph

2. ATPS, which is the volume or flow determined at ambient temperature and barometric pressure and saturated with water vapor as during the calibration of a wet type spirometer

3. BTPS, which is the volume or flow determined at body temperature and barometric pressure and saturated with water vapor. This is the condition of the inspired gas volume into the lungs and of the expired gas volume at the mouth.

The need for corrections of measured flow or volume values to BTPS condition stems from the possible differences between the measuring conditions, the instrument calibration, and the condition of volume or flow into the lungs. Inspired volume, since it is not heated and humidified, needs to be corrected to BTBS condition of the lungs from the ambient measuring conditions. By contrast, expired volume needs to be corrected to BTPS condition only if it is cooled passing from the mouth to the measuring device, the degree of cooling to be measured or assumed.

Considering the condition of a wet spirometer, since inspired and expired air are measured at the spirometer under ambient conditions, the correction has to be applied from ATPS (temperature reading of the spirometer) to both inspired and expired gas. The correction applies to all lung volume subdivisions measured with a spirometer during static and dynamic conditions. However, during forced expiration the cooling of the expired gas in its passage from mouthpiece to spirometer varies with the expiratory flow; as a result there can be significant errors in the calculation of certain dynamic spirometric indices.

Using a pneumotachograph whose head is at the mouth and assuming that cooling of expired gas is avoided, no correction is needed for expired gas, because of the relation between temperture and gas volume, while a correction from ATP to BTPS condition is required for inspired gas measured at the mouth. The pneumotachograph head is heated by a thermostatic electric resistance only in order to prevent condensation of expired water vapor in the capillary tubes, which would change their resistance to air flow with respect to the calibration condition.

The ratio between gas volume at BTPS condition (V_2), temperature being 37 °C, and measuring conditions (V_1), temperature being t, is:

$$V_1/V_2 = [(273+37) \times (P_B - P_{H_2O}(t))] / [(273+t) \times (P_B - P_{H_2O}(37))]$$

where P_B is the barometric pressure in kPa, t is the temperature at the measuring condition, P_{H_2O} is the partial water vapor pressure at temperaure t or at 37 °C. The partial water vapor pressure of a 100% saturated gas at atmospheric pressure (which is 101.3 kPa) can be approximated, between 20°–40 °C, as follows:

$$P_{H_2O} = 1.7603 - 0.806 \, t + 0.0058 \, t^2$$

Table A1. Gas mixture viscosity

Gas	Viscosity gas equation	C_{vis}	E_{vis}
N_2	$167.6 + 0.453 \cdot t$	138.1	137.0
O_2	$200.0 + 0.298 \cdot t$	42.6	32.5
CO_2	$150.7 + 0.465 \cdot t$	0	6.3
H_2O	$132.6 + 0.570 \cdot t$	1.7	9.5

N_2, nitrogen; O_2, oxygen; CO_2, carbon dioxide; H_2O, water vapor; t, temperature in °C; C_{vis}, viscosity (kPa s) of ambient air or pneumotacograph calibration gas mixture (79.1% N_2, 20.9% O_2, 20°C, 50% H_2O saturated, 101.3 kPa barometric pressure); E_{vis}, viscosity of expired gas (79.5% N_2, 16.5% O_2, 4% CO_2, 37°C, 100% H_2O saturated, 101.3 kPa barometric pressure)

Temperature, Gas Composition, and Gas Viscosity

The pneumotachographic mesurement of flow rate is based on the assumption that there is a linear relation between the flow rate and the pressure difference across the pneumotachograph head, applying the equation for pure laminar air flow pattern. Under this condition the air flow rate is inversely proportional to gas viscosity (see Chap. 2), which changes with the gas mixture composition. Viscosity can be calculated on the basis of empirical equation [106], assuming that the viscosity of a pure gas varies with temperature between 20°–40°C as reported in Table A1.

The total viscosity of the pneumotacograph calibrating gas mixture is 182.3 kPa s, while it is 185.3 for the expired gas mixture, as is assumed in Table A1. As a consequence, the gain of the instrument for expired air changes by a factor of 1.016 with respect to calibrating and inspired air. Since air composition into the lung is that of expired gas at the mouth, the actual inspiratory instantaneous flow readings should be devided by this factor, so that they increase by 1.6% compared to the actual readings.

References

1. Afschrift M, Clement J, van de Woestjine KP (1974) Maximum expiratory flows and effort independency in patients with airway obstruction. J Appl Physiol 37: 566–569
2. ATS Statement (1979) Standardization of spirometry. Am Rev Respir Dis 119: 831–838
3. ATS Statement (1987) Standardization of spirometry. Am Rev Respir Dis 136: 1285–1298
4. Barter CE, Campbell AH (1973) Comparison of airways resistance measurements during panting and quiet breathing. Respiration 30:1–11
5. Barter CE, Campbell AH (1976) Relationship of constitutional factors and cigarette smoking to decreased forced expiratory volume in 1 sec. Am Rev Respir Dis 113:305–314
6. Bedell GN, Marshall R, DuBois AB, Harris JH (1956) Measurement of the volume of gas in the gastrointestinal tract. Values in normal subjects and ambulatory patients. J Clin Invest 35:336–345

7. Black LF, Offord K, Hyatt RE (1974) Variabiliy in the maximal expiratory flow volume curve in asymptomatic smokers and non-smokers. Am Rev Respir Dis 110:282–292
8. Black KH, Petusevsky ML, Gaensler EA (1980) A general purpose microprocessor for spirometry. Chest 78:605–612
9. Bouhuys A (1963) Pulmonary nitrogen clearance in relation to age in healthy males. J Appl Physiol 18:297–300
10. Bouhuys A, Mitchell CA (1975) Maximum expiratory flow-volume curves. J Appl Physiol 38:907–912
11. Boushey HA, Dawson A (1982) Spirometry and flow volume curves. In: Clausen JL (ed) Pulmonary function testing – guidelines and controversies. Academic, New York, pp 61–82
12. Briscoe WA, DuBois AB (1958) The relationship between airway resistance, airway conductance and lung volume in subjects of different age and body size. J Clin Invest 37:1279–1285
13. Brooks SM, Zipp T, Barber M, Carson A (1978) Measurement of maximal expiratory flow rates in cigarette smokers and non-smokers using gases of high and low densities. Am Rev Respir Dis 118:75–81
14. Brown R, Ingram JH Jr, McFadden ER Jr (1978) Problems in the plethysmographic assessment of changes in total lung capacity in asthma. Am Rev Respir Dis 118:685–692
15. Brown R, Hoppin FG Jr, Ingram JH Jr, Saunders NA, McFadden E Jr (1978) Influence of abdominal gas on the Boyle's law determination of thoracic gas volume. J Appl Physiol 44:469–473
16. Burki NJ, Dent MC (1976) The forced expiratory time as a measure of small airway resistance. Clin Sci Mol Med 51:53–58
17. Chinn DJ, Lee WR (1977) Within and between-subject variability of indices from the closing volume and flow volume traces. Bull. Eur Physiopathol Respir 13:789–802
18. Chowienczyk PJ, Rees PJ, Payne J, Clark TJK (1981) A new method for computer assisted determination of airways resistance. J Appl Physiol 50:672–678
19. Chowienczyk PJ, Lawson CP, Lane S, Johnson R, Wilson N, Silverman M, Cochrane GM (1991) A flow interruption device for measurement of airways resistance. Eur Respir J 4:623–628
20. Clausen JL (1982) Pulmonary function testing – Guidelines and controversies. Academic, New York
21. Cockroft DW, Berscheid BA (1983) Measurement of responsiveness to inhaled histamine – comparison of FEV_1 and sG_{aw}. Ann Allergy 51:374–377
22. Cotes JE (1979) Lung function – assessement and application in medicine. Blackwell, Oxford
23. Cotes JE, Peslin R, Yernault JC (1983) Standardized lung function testing – chapter 3 (dynamic lung volumes and forced ventilatory flow rates). Bull Eur Physiopathol Respir 19 [Suppl 5]:22–27
24. Da Silva AMT, Hamosh P (1973) Effect of smoking a single cigarette on the "small airways." J Appl Physiol 34:361–365
25. Desager K, Van Bever H, Làndsér F, Willemen M, De Backer W, Vermeire P (1991) Use of the forced oscillation technique in infants. Eur Respir J 4:248
26. DuBois AB, Botelho SY, Bedell GN, Marshall R, Comroe JH Jr (1956) A rapid plethysmographic method for measuring thoracic gas volume; a comparison with a nitrogen washout method for measuring functional residual capacity. J Clin Invest 35:322–326
27. Dubois AB, Botelho SY, Comroe JH (1956) A new method for measuring airway resistance in man using a body plethysmograph – values in normal subjects and in patients with respiratory diesease. J Clin Inverst 35:327–335
28. DuBois AB, Brody AW, Lewis DH, Burgess DF (1956) Oscillation mechanics

of lungs and chest in man. J Appl Physiol 8:587–594
29. Duvier C, Peslin R, Gallina C (1988) An incremental method to assess linearity of gas flow meters; application to Fleisch pneumotachographs. Eur Respir J 1:661–665
30. Eichenhorn MS, Beauchamp RK, Haper PA, Ward IC (1982) An assessment of three portable peak flow meters. Chest 82:306–309
31. Epstein SW, Fletcher CM, Oppenheimer EA (1969) Daily peak flow measurements in the assessment of steroid therapy for airway obstruction. Br Med J 1:223–228
32. Feldman J, Traver GA, Taussig LM (1979) Maximal expiratory flows after postural drainage. Am Rev Respir Dis 119:239–245
33. Ferris BG (1978) Epidemiology standardization project. Am Rev Respir Dis 118:1–120
34. Ferris BG, Speizer FE, Bishop Y, Prang G, Weener J (1978) Spirometry for an epidemiologic study – deriving optimum summary statistics for each subject. Bull Eur Physiopathol Respir 14:145–166
35. Frank NR, Mead J, Ferris BG (1957) The mechanical behaviour of the lungs in healthy elderly persons. J Clin Invest 36:1680–1687
36. Fry DL, Hyatt RE (1960) Pulmonary mechanics – a unified analysis of the relationship between pressure, volume and gas flow in the lungs in normal and diseased human subjects. Am J Med 29:672–689
37. Gayrard P, Orehek J, Grimaud C (1975) Bronchoconstrictor effects of a deep inspiration in patients with asthma. Am Rev Respir Dis 111:433–439
38. Gelb AF, Molony PA, Klein E, Aronstam PS (1975) Sensitivity of volume of isoflow in the detection of mild airways obstruction. Am Rev Respir Dis 112:401–405
39. Gregg I, Nunn AJ (1973) Peak expiratory flow in normal subjects. Br Med J 3:282–287
40. Guyatt AR, Siddorn JA, Brash HM, Flenley DC (1975) Reproducibility of dynamic compliance and flow-volume curves in normal man. J Appl Physiol 39:341–348
41. Habib MP, Engel AL (1978) Influence of panting technique on the plethysmographic measurement of thoracic gas volume. Am Rev Respir Dis 117:265–271
42. Habib MP, Pare PD, Engel LA (1979) Variability of airways responses to inhaled histamine in normal subjects. J Appl Physiol 47:51–58
43. Hankinson JL, Reger RB, Morgan WKC (1977) Maximal expiratory flows in coal miners. Am Rev Respir Dis 116:175–180
44. Higgins BG, Britton JR, Chinn S, Jones TD, Burney PGI, Tattersfield AE (1988) Relation of methacoline PD20 and peak flow variability measurements to respiratory symptoms in a community population. Am Rev Respir Dis 137 [Suppl 4, 2]:249
45. Hogg JC, Macklem PT, Thurbeck WM (1968) Site and nature of airway obstruction in chronic obstructive lung disease. N Engl J Med 278:1355–1360
46. Hurtado A, Kaltreider NL (1934) Studies of total pulmonary capacity and its subdivisions. VII. Observations during the acute respiratory distress of bronchial asthma and following the administration of epinephrine. J Clin Invest 13:1054–1062
47. Hutcheon M, Griffin P, Levison H, Zamel N (1974) Volume of isoflow. A New test in detection of mild abnormalities of lung mechanics. Am Rev Respir Dis 110:458–465
48. Islam MS (1976) Differential diagnosis of ventilatory disorders with the help of volume/flow diagram. Respiration 33:104–111
49. Jaeger MJ, Otis AB (1964) Measurement of airway resistance with a volume displacement body plethysmograph. J Appl Physiol 19:813–820
50. Jaeger MJ, Bouhuys A (1969) Loop formation in pressure vs. flow diagrams obtained by body plethysmographic techniques. Prog. Respir Res 4:116–130

51. Jansen JM, Peslin R, Bohadana AB, Racineux JL (1980) Usefulness of forced expiration slope ratios for detecting mild airway abnormalities. Am Rev Respir Dis 122:221–230
52. Kelsen SG, Kelsen DP, Fleegler BF, Jones RC, Rodman T (1978) Emergency room assessment and treatment of patients with acute asthma – adequacy of the conventional approach. Am J Med 64:622–628
53. Knudson RJ, Slatin RC, Lebowitz MD, Burrows B (1976) The maximal expiratory flow-volume curve. Normal standards, variability, and effect of age. Am Rev Respir Dis 113:587–600
54. Knudson RJ, Lebowitz MD (1977) Comparison of flow-volume and closing volume variables in a random population. Am Rev Respir Dis 116:1039–1045
55. Knudson RJ, Clark DF, Kennedy TC (1977) Effect of aging alone on mechanical properties of the normal adult human lung. J Appl Physiol 43:1054–1062
56. Knudson RJ, Lebowitz MD (1978) Maximal midexpiratory flow (FEF 25–75%) – normal limits and assessment of sensitivity. Am Rev Respir Dis 117:609–610
57. Làndsér FJ, Nagels J, Demedts M, Billiet L, Van de Woestijne KP (1976) A new method to determine frequency characteristics of the respiratory system. J Appl Physiol 41:101–106
58. Lavelle TF Jr, Rotman HH, Weg JG (1978) Isoflow-volume curves in the diagnosis of upper airway obstruction. Am Rev Respir Dis 117:845–852
59. Leeder SR, Swan AV, Peat JK, Woolcock AJ, Blaclburn CRB (1977) Maximum expiratory flow-volume curves in children – changes with growth and individual variability. Bull Eur Physiopathol Respir 13:249–260
60. Leuallen EC, Fowler WS (1955) Maximal midexpiratory flow. Am Rev Tuberc Pulm Dis 72:783–800
61. Light RW, Conrad SA, Geroge RB (1977) Clinical significance of pulmonary function test. The one best test for evaluating the effects of bronchodilator therapy. Chest 72:512–516
62. Loveland M, Corbin R, Ducis S, Martin RR (1978) Evaluation of the analysis and variability of the helium response. Bull Eur Physiopathol Respir 14:551–560
63. Man PSF, Zamel N (1976) Genetic influence on normal variability of maximum expiratory flow-volume curves. J Appl Physiol 41:874–877
64. Mansell AL, Bryan AC, Levison H (1977) Relationship of lung recoil to lung volume and maximum expiratory flow in normal children. J Appl Physiol 42:817–823
65. Martin J, Powell E, Shore S, Emrich J, Engel LA (1980) The role of the respiratory muscles in the hyperinflation of bronchial asthma. Am Rev Respir Dis 121:441–447
66. McCall CB, Hyatt RE, Nobel FW (1957) Harmonic content of certain respiratory flow phenomena of normal individuals. J Appl Physiol 10:215–218
67. McCarthy DS, Craig DB, Cherniack RM (1975) Intraindividual variability in maximal expiratory flow-volume and closing volume in asymptomatic subjects. Am Rev Respir Dis 112:407–411
68. McCarthy DS, Craig DB, Cherniack RM (1976) The effect of acute, intensive cigarette smoking on maximal expiratory flows and the single-breath nitrogen washout trace. Am Rev Respir Dis 113:301–304
69. McDonald JB, Cole TJ, Seaton A (1975) Forced expiratory time – its reliability as a lung function test. Thorax 30:554–559
70. McMichael J (1939) A rapid method of determining lung capacity. Clin Sci 4:167–173
71. Mead J (1978) Analysis of the configuration of maximum expiratory flow volume curves. J Appl Physiol 44:156–165
72. Mead J, Whittenberger JL (1953) Physical properties of human lungs measured during spontaneous respiration. J Appl Physiol 5:779–796
73. Mead J, Whittenberger JL (1954) Evaluation of airway interruption technique as a method for measuring pulmonary airflow resistance. J Appl Physiol 6:

408–416
74. Melissinos CG, Webster P, Tien YK, Mead J (1979) Time dependence of maximum flow as an index of nonuniform emptying. J Appl Physiol 47:1043–1050
75. Milic-Emili J, Mead J, Turner JM (1964) Topography of oesophageal pressure as a function of posture in man. J Appl Physiol 19:212–216
76. Muller NM, Bryan AC, Zamel N (1981) Tonic inspiratory muscle activity as a cause of hyperinflation in histamine-induced asthma. J Appl Physiol 50:279–282
77. Nagels J, Làndsér FJ, van der Linden L, Clément J, van de Woestijne KP (1980) Mechanical properties of lungs and chest wall during spontaneous breathing. J Appl Physiol 49:408–416
78. Nanchev L (1978) A forced expiration end-segment flow rate to improve diagnosis of reversible bronchial obstruction. Respiration 36:73–77
79. Neuburger N, Levison H, Bryan AC, Kruger K (1976) Transit time analysis of the forced expiratory spirogram in growth. J Appl Physiol 40:329–332
80. Nickerson BG, Lemen RJ, Gerdes CB (1980) Within-subject variability and percent change for significance of spirometry in normal subjects and in patients with cystic fibrosis. Am Rev Respir Dis 122:859–866
81. Orehek J, Gayrard P, Smith AP, Grimaud C, Charpin J (1977) Airways response to carbachol in normal and asthmatic subjects. Distinction between bronchial sensitivity and reactivity. Am Rev Respir Dis 115:937–943
82. Pelzer AM, Thompson ML (1966) Effect of age, sex, stature and smoking habits on human airway conductance. J Appl Physiol 21:469–476
83. Pepys J, Hutchcroft DJ (1975) Bronchial provocation tests in etiologic diagnosis and analysis of asthma. Am Rev Respir Dis 112:829–859
84. Peslin R (1983) Standardized lung function testing chapter 5 (lung mechanics II: resistance measurements). Bull Eur Physiopathol Respir 19 [Suppl 5]:33–38
85. Peslin R, Bohadana A, Hannhart B, Jardin P (1979) Comparison of various methods for reading maximal expiratory flow-volume curves. Am Rev Respir Dis 119:271–278
86. Peslin R, Fredberg JJ (1986) Oscillation mechanics of the respiratory system. In: Macklem J, Mead J (eds) Handbook of Physiology, sect. 3, vol III: mechanics of breathing, part 1. American Physiological Society, Bethesda, pp 145–177
87. Powell Zarins L (1982) Closed circuit helium dilution method of lung volume measurement. In: Clausen JL (ed) Pulmonary function testing – guidelines and controversies. Academic, New York, pp 129–140
88. Prowse K, Cumming G (1973) Effects of lung volume and disease on the lung nitrogen decay curve. J Appl Physiol 34:23–33
89. Quanjer PhH editor (1983) Standardized lung function testing. Bull Eur Physiopathol Respir 19 [Suppl]:5
90. Quanjer PhH, Tammeling GJ (1983) Standardized lung function testing Chapter 1 (Summary of recommendations). Bull Eur Physiopathol Respir 19 [Suppl 5]:7–10
91. Quanjer PhH, Dalhuijsen A, van Zomeren BC (1983) Standardized lung function testing: chapter 10 (appendix b, c and d). Bull Eur Physiopathol Respir 19 [Suppl 5]:67–86
92. Quanjer PhH, Andersen LH, Tammeling GJ (1983) Standardized lung function testing: chapter 2 (static lung volumes and capacities). Bull Eur Physiopathol Respir 19 [Suppl 5]:11–21
93. Ramsdale JW, Tisi GM (1979) Determination of bronchodilatation in the clinical pulmonary function laboratory. Chest 76:622–628
94. Ramsdale EH, Morris MM, Roberts RS, Hargreave FE (1984) Bronchial responsiveness to methacoline in chronic bronchitis – relationship to airflow obstruction and cold air responsiveness. Thorax 39:912–918
95. Rodenstein DO, Stanescu DC, Francis C (1982) Demonstration of failure of body plethysmograph in airway obstruction. J Appl Physiol 52:949–954
96. Rodenstein DO, Stanescu DC (1983) Frequency dependence of plethysmo-

graphic volume in healthy and asthmatic subjects. J Appl Physiol 54:159–169

97. Rossiter CE (1976) Contribution to discussion. Scand J Respir Dis 57:315–316

98. Schanning CG, Gulsvik A (1973) Accuracy and precision of helium dilution technique and body plethysmography in measuring lung volumes. Scand J Clin Lab Invest 32:271–277

99. Stanescu DC, Pattijn J, Clement J, van de Woestjine KP (1972) Glottis opening and airway resistance. J Appl Physiol 32:460–466

100. Stanescu DC, Rodenstein DO, Cauberghs M, van de Woestjine KP (1982) Failure of body plethysmography in bronchial asthma. J Appl Physiol 52:939–948

101. Sterk PJ, Quanjer PhH, van der Maals LLJ, Wise ME, van der Lende R (1980) The validity of the single breath nitrogen determination of residual volume. Bull Eur Physiopat Resp 16:195–213

102. Tager I, Speizer FE, Rosner B, Prang G (1976) A comparison between the three largest and the three last of five forced expiratory maneuvers in a population study. Am Rev Respir Dis 114:1201–1203

103. Tammeling GJ, Quanjer PhH, Visser BF, Lende VD (1976) Airway closure and expiratory flow limitation in relation to smoking habits and symptoms of CNSLD. Scand J Respir Dis 95:73–83

104. Teculescu DB, Pham QT, Hannhart B (1986) Tests of small airway dysfunction – their correlation with the conventional lung function tests. Eur J Respir Dis 69:175–187

105. Tien YK, Elliot EA, Mead J (1979) Variability of the configuration of maximum expiratory flow-volume curves. J Appl Physiol 46:565–570

106. Turner SZ, Blumenfeld W (1973) Heated Fleisch pneumotachometer: a calibration procedure. J Appl Physiol 34:117–121

107. Turner-Warwick M (1977) On observing patterns of airflow obstruction in chronic asthma. Br J Dis Chest 71:73–86

108. Vale JR, Gulsvik A, Kongerud J (1981) Random error with FEV_1. Case for absolute values. Lancet II:313

109. Van Noord JA, Clément J, Cauberghs M, Mertens I, Van de Woestijne KP, Demedts M (1989) Total respiratory resistance and reactance in patients with diffuse interstitial lung disease. Eur Respir J 2:846–852

110. Van Noord JA, Van de Woestijne KP, Demedts M (1991) Clinical applications and modelling of forced oscillation mechanics of the respiratory system. Eur Respir J 4:247–248

111. van Schayck CP, Dompeling E, van Weel C, Folgering H, van den Hoogen HJM (1990) Accuracy and reproducibility of the ASSESS peak flow meter. Eur Respir J 3:338–341

112. Walter S, Nancy NR, Collier CR (1979) Changes in the forced expiratory spirogram in young male smokers. Am Rev Respir Dis 119:717–724

113. Webster PM, Zamel N, Bryan AC, Kruger K (1977) Volume dependence of instantaneous time constant derived from the maximal expiratory flow-volume curve. A new approach to the analysis of forced expiration. Am Rev Respir Dis 115:805–810

114. Woolcock AJ, Read J (1966) Lung volumes in exacerbations of asthma. Am J Med 41:259–273

115. Woolcock AJ, Read J (1968) The static elastic properties of the lungs in asthma. Am Rev Respir Dis 98:788–794

116. Wright BM, McKerrow LB (1959) Maximal forced expiratory flow rate as a measure of ventilatory capacity with a description of a new portable instrument of measuring it. Br Med J 2:1041–1047

117. Zapletal A, Samànek M, Paul P (1987) Lung function in children and adolescent – methods, reference values. Karger, Basel

118. Zapletal A, Samànek M, Paul P (1987) Airway patency. In: Zapletal A (ed) Lung function in children and adolescents – methods, reference values. Karger, Basel, pp 32–67

Distributional Methods and Invasive and Noninvasive Gas Analysis in Asthma

R. Dal Negro[1] and L. Allegra[2]

[1] Department of Lung Pathophysiology, General Hospital, Bussolengo (VR), Italy
[2] Institute of Respiratory Diseases, School of Medicine, University of Milan, Milano, Italy

General Topics in Gas Exchange

The prime function of respiration consists in maintaining alveolar and blood O_2/CO_2 partial pressures at their physiological levels. Under physiological conditions respiration allows an adequate amount of inspired air to contact and arterialize venous blood, thus meeting the body's energy requirements. This is normally achieved by the matched efficiency of alveolar ventilation ($\dot{V}_A$) and pulmonary circulation ($\dot{Q}_C$): the former supplies a sufficient amount of fresh inspired air to the alveolar units, while the latter ensures sufficient blood flow to the terminal sites where gas exchanges take place [1].

Apart from the role of the diffusing capacity, respiratory gas exchanges are influenced by alveolar volume, alveolar ventilation, capillary blood volume, and alveolar blood flow. Alveolar gas volume is the only volume of inspired gas which takes an active part in O_2 and CO_2 exchange. This volume communicates with the ambient air via a system of smaller and larger airways (conducting airways) which constitute the "anatomical dead space," because the air they contain is not involved in gas exchanges. From an anatomical standpoint, alveolar gas volume involves the alveoli, the alveolar ducts, and probably the respiratory bronchioles.

Blood and gas are equally important in respiratory function, though the lung is sometimes seen merely as a pump for moving quantities of air in and out of the chest. Oxygen and carbon dioxide exchange occurs by passive physical diffusion (partial pressure-dependent) when blood and air come into contact at the alveolar interface.

The lung consists of several functional units, each endowed with functional autonomy. The regional distribution of the inspired air depends on local compliance and airflow resistance (i.e., on "time constants"), while blood flow distribution (at the alveolar surface) is mainly influenced by the low-pressure system operating. In other words, this means that all normally perfused lung units require patency of the dependent airways; if this were not the case, significant differences in gas composition would be present in the lung, due to maldistribution of the $\dot{V}_A/\dot{Q}_C$ ratio (R), which, in turn, is related to the dyshomogeneous filling and emptying of the lung units [2].

$\dot{V}_A/\dot{Q}_C$ Unevenness

Uneven ventilation is mainly due to asynchronous ventilation of the lung compartments. When different lung units are characterized by increased resistances (as in obstructive diseases), the units with greater time constants are less efficiently ventilated. They would need more time for inhalation and complete expiration of inhaled air: the shorter the time available (as in rapid shallow breathing), the less efficient will be the regional alveolar ventilation, due in these cases to the particular time dependency of breathing [3].

The lung is sometimes erroneously considered as a uniform structure, in other words, as a magnified reproduction of a simple lung unit. This is not true in practice because, unlike the ideal condition of the "perfect lung," each functional lung unit presents different blood flows and ventilatory supplies, even under absolutely normal conditions. According to the multicompartmental model, even normal lungs show a slight unevenness in the ventilation-perfusion ratio distribution, due to gravitational gradients from the apex to the base, and to postural factors. Blood flow increases down the lung (mainly due to the gradual increase in both perfusion pressure and regional ventilation, though the latter increase is less marked in absolute terms than the former. We can thus assume that, while upper alveolar compartments are characterized by virtual perfusion and excedent ventilation, in lower lung units both perfusion and ventilation are increased in absolute terms, the former to a greater extent than the latter [2].

Regardless of their respective absolute values, inequalities in R distribution (such as blood perfusion and ventilation mismatching) may thus be postulated within the lung and considered as capable of inducing significant changes in respiratory blood gases. Normally, lung perfusion exceeds lung ventilation and the ventilation-perfusion ratio for the lung as a whole is 0.8.

Shunt Effect and Wasted Ventilation

In pathological conditions, namely, in obstructive lung diseases, R distribution is markedly uneven: it is claimed to represent the most important cause by far of arterial hypoxia, much more so than hypoventilation, shunt, and impaired diffusion (Fig. 1). We can therefore imagine and graphically represent by means of the O_2/CO_2 diagram all the situations reflecting the existence of $\dot{V}_A/\dot{Q}_C$ distribution disorders, starting from the extreme condition in which $R = 0$ (that is total absence of ventilation, with unchanged perfusion) to the opposite extreme in which $R = \infty$ (unchanged ventilation, with complete absence of perfusion) (Fig. 2). The line connecting these two extreme functional situations is the R line, the shape of which depends on the O_2 and CO_2 dissociation curves [4].

A marked increase in airway resistance represents the primary cause of R movements towards the venous (v) point of the diagram, i.e., the "shunt effect," due to the prevalence of lung units characterized by a low $\dot{V}_A/\dot{Q}_C$ ratio.

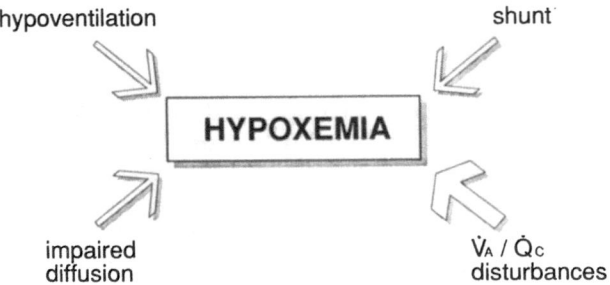

Fig. 1. Factors inducing hypoxemia in diseased lungs

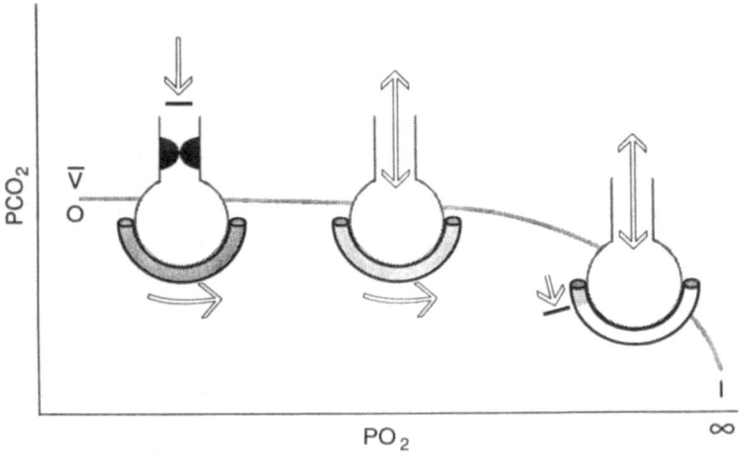

Fig. 2. The O_2-CO_2 diagram. All situations reflecting the existence of $\dot{V}_A/\dot{Q}_C$ disturbances (values from 0 to ∞) are represented

The mechanisms activated to minimize the effects of R inequality on blood gases are: hyperventilation of better ventilated lung units, collateral ventilation and the hypoxic vasoconstriction reflex, in an attempt to increase alveolar ventilation and to reduce the blood flow through the underventilated compartments and shift alveolar blood towards the better ventilated units, respectively. Despite these compensatory mechanisms, the particular shape of the O_2 dissociation curve (sinusoidal) does not allow complete compensation and there will therefore be evident arterial hypoxia, thereby reflecting the increase in the alveolar-arterial PO_2 difference [5]. By contrast, as regards blood CO_2, the particular shape of the CO_2 dissociation curve (practically linear in the physiological range) reflects the fact that the better ventilated lung units (also coexisting within the lung and characterized by higher $\dot{V}_A/\dot{Q}_C$ ratios) are able to compensate for the underventilated ones, the end result frquently being normo- or hypocapnia [5].

The higher the R value, the greater will be the overventilation of the lung units and the closer will be their position to be inspiratory point (I), on the O_2-CO_2 diagram.

Functionally, this situation is indistinguishable from that of the anatomical dead space (namely, ventilated but not perfused) and it is therefore identified as the "dead space effect" or "wasted ventilation," to pinpoint the effect of overventilated units on blood gases.

In conclusion, we can assume an alveolar-arterial CO_2 gradient when the $\dot{V}_A/\dot{Q}_C$ distribution is uneven in the lung, even if the alveolar ventilation volume is normal. Despite the behavior of blood oxygen (invariably decreased in these cases), CO_2 blood levels depend on the compensatory effect of hyperventilation.

$\dot{V}_A/\dot{Q}_C$ Unevenness in Asthma

Most of the pathogenetic findings in bronchial asthma (such as edema of the airway walls, plasma extravasation, mucus hypersecretion, inflammatory cell infiltration, disruption of the epithelial structure, and deranged mucociliary clearance) may represented factors (frequently only peripheral) significantly affecting the normal distributional pattern of ventilation within the lungs, though not always directly related to the clinical evidence of bronchial spasm [6]. These underlying peripheral events may actually operate as factors producing an imbalance in O_2 and CO_2 exchange, even with unchanged overall ventilation. Asymptomatic asthmatics, in fact, frequently show significant gas maldistribution patterns under steady-state conditions (due to preexisting $\dot{V}_A/\dot{Q}_C$ disturbances), particularly when challenged (e.g., following physical exercise) [7]. Furthermore, when symptom-free asthmatics inhale small doses of bronchial challenge (such as histamine or methacholine), some respond with a decreased flow rate with no change in resistance, while in others resistance is impaired without any change in flows, thus denoting the existence of scattered local variations in airway smooth muscle responsiveness [3].

From this point of view, McFadden and Lyons [8] suggested for the first time, in 1968, that maldistribution of inspired gas and frequency dependence of compliance persist after recovery from an acute asthma attack, even when airway resistance has returned to normal and that this might be related to residual long-lasting abnormalities in the small peripheral airways, probably due to their sustained inflammatory involvement.

More recent studies have demonstrated that peripheral airways are the major site of pathological abnormalities in asthma and that the peripheral changes in the mechanical properties of the airways, despite their limited influence on overall pulmonary function, can effectively contribute to increased airway responsiveness in asthmatics, even when asymptomatic [9]. By contrast, even though ventilation-perfusion mismatching has long been claimed to be the main mechanism in respiratory gas exchange abnormalities in bronchial asthma, changes in lung volumes and mechanics during spontaneous and/or induced asthma have undoubtedly attracted the interest of pneumologists and clinical lung physiologists worldwide.

Expiratory volume in 1 s and maximal expiratory flows, along with airway resistance, are the indicators most widely used for assessing spontaneous and induced bronchial obstruction, their major advantage being that they can be used easily, quickly, and inexpensively. By no means negligible drawbacks are the instantaneous nature of the measurements, their dependence on patient collaboration, and the utilization of forced (and/or maximal) maneuvers [6, 10].

It has been proved that the deep inspiration which precedes deep expiration may appreciably minimize the acute response to the bronchial challenge inhalation and that maximal maneuvers may result in measurements which are significantly influenced by extrabronchial factors (such as elastic recoil, changes in lung volumes, and patency of the upper airways). Furthermore, the airway diameter may be affected by the pressure differential across their walls and by mechanical properties, including the air-liquid interphase. Macklem and Wilson [11] have shown that small peripheral airways are stabilized by surfactant in normal conditions, particularly during expiration of low lung volumes. This would mean that in pathological conditions (when the surfactant layer is replaced by fluids with different surface properties) their very small curvature radius may cause airway closure when surface tension is increased.

It is thus likely that the subtler changes in peripheral units remain undetected by this overall functional approach, especially in symptom-free asthmatics. Peripheral gas trapping is particularly liable to occur in such cases, due to forced expiration [12]; the contribution of normal airways to the forced expiration will therefore be overemphasized, while there will be understimation of the role of narrowed or closed airways, which obviously will be measured to a lesser extent or may even pass entirely undetected [12].

In bronchial asthma (spontaneous or induced asthma), functional units characterized by a marked uneven R distribution are obviously predominant and play a leading role in the occurrence of blood gas abnormalities, which are frequently otherwise inexplicable in view of the normality of the spirometric findings.

The main disturbance in patients suffering from bronchial asthma is the increase in $\dot{V}_A/\dot{Q}_C$ mismatching, mainly due to ventilatory unevenness; inspired air is shifted preferentially towards lung units characterized by the lowest flow resistance, determining (in relation to their perfusion) an increase in the $\dot{V}_A/\dot{Q}_C$ ratio, while the remaining units (characterized by the highest regimen of flow resistance) will receive less of the inspired air. The former units will thus induce hypocapnia (i.e., wasted ventilation) and the latter hypoxemia, in agreement with the effects induced by the O_2 and CO_2 dissociation curves respectively [13, 14] (see above).

Also is asymptomatic asthmatics, in spite of their normal (or near normal) volumetric functional pattern, the presence of lung units characterized by a very low $\dot{V}_A/\dot{Q}_C$ ratio has been surprisingly established and their role quantified [6]. These units are estimated as receiving about 20% of the cardiac output, but less that 1% of the ventilation. The bimodal R distribution pattern in lung units has been further related to the markedly reduced patency of distal airways (see above) in the presence of active collateral ventilation [5].

In long-standing chronic asthma, sustained and more severe blood gas abnormalities are obviously to be expected.

Distributional Methods for Measuring Nonuniform Ventilation in Asthma

As we have previously seen, the distribution of inspired gas is markedly unequal in obstructive lung diseases. In bronchial asthma, this has been demonstrated particularly during acute attacks, but also in symptom-free periods and in asymptomatic subjects. Less attention has been paid, however, to the hyperreactive aspects of the problem.

To minimize the influence of maximal expiratory maneuvers on the distributional factors of ventilation, spirometrical measurements taken from partial expiratory flow volume (PEFV) curves have been suggested. Such measurements, in which the forced expiration starts from the functional residual capacity, have proved more sensitive in detecting even mild, peripheral airway narrowing [3].

Generally speaking, the distributional methods available employ gases which undergo practically no exchange with the blood (and are therefore called "inert gases") as tracers. The most commonly used inert gases can be divided into: (1) nonradioactive (nitrogen, N_2; argon, Ar; helium, He) and (2) radioactive (xenon, ^{133}Xe, krypton, ^{81}mKr). They are used as markers and can be traced by serial or continuous expired gas analysis.

The methods for studying uneven distribution of ventilation can be further divided into: (1) single-breath and (2) multiple-breath tests.

O_2 Single Breath Test

This test is very easy to perform and requires a rapid infrared N_2 analyzer. After 100% O_2 inhalation, N_2 is continuously measured during slow expiration. The N_2 expiratory curve is obtained and can be divided into three parts: the first and second portions show the rapid increase in N_2 concentration due to the clearance of the anatomical dead space, while the third corresponds to the alveolar plateau. This phase, during which expiratory gas comes from lung units which are unevenly ventilated and have elevated time constants (as in obstruction), shows an increase in N_2 end-tidal concentration to abnormal levels (Fig. 3); in addition, as compared to normals, a steeper slope of the alveolar plateau is plotted. Although this is the most commonly

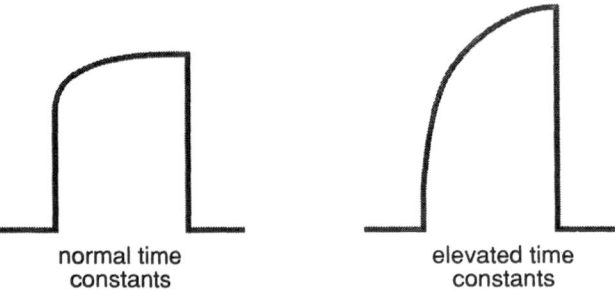

normal time
constants

elevated time
constants

Fig. 3. N_2 expiratory curve. The steeper slope of the third phase (alveolar plateau) identifies the functional role of lung units unevenly ventilated

represented pattern in obstructive disease, some of the severer cases of spontaneous or induced asthma may not be systematically associated with abnormal alveolar plateau slopes.

The curve can be affected by lung volume, flow rates, and posture. Careful interpretation and standardized procedures are required, particularly for assessing the subtler changes, while gross abnormalities are easily discriminated within the curve.

Closing Volume

The term "closing voume" defines the lung volume at which the interruption of ventilation of the lower lung regions occurs due to small airway closure [15]. The method consists of an expiratory manoeuvre up to residual volume (RV), then a low inspiration of the inert gas bolus up to total lung capacity (TLC), and finally a slow expiration to RV, while measuring the inert gas concentration. A second method generally employed for measuring closing volume is to use a gas resistent in the lung, usually N_2 [16]. The curve obtained can be divided into four parts: phases 1 and 2, due to the clearance of the anatomical dead space; phase 3, due to the alveolar plateau, showing a slightly increasing slope; and phase 4, which provides information about the lung volume, as a percentage of vital capacity (VC), at which the peripheral airways of the lower lung units start to make a progressively lower contribution to the expired air. The sudden increase in the inert gas concentration characterizing phase 4 corresponds to the enhanced contribution of the upper lung units (with a higher inert gas concentration) to expiration, when the lower peripheral lung compartments start to close (Fig. 4). This test has been considered particularly suitable in the past for assessing early disturbances, namely, in asymptomatic asthma or in slight increases in bronchomotor tone due to bronchial challenge [6], though with by no means negligible measurement variability. In severer cases, closing volume can be measured only after bronchodilation, when the cut-off between phases 3 and 4 becomes more clearly defined.

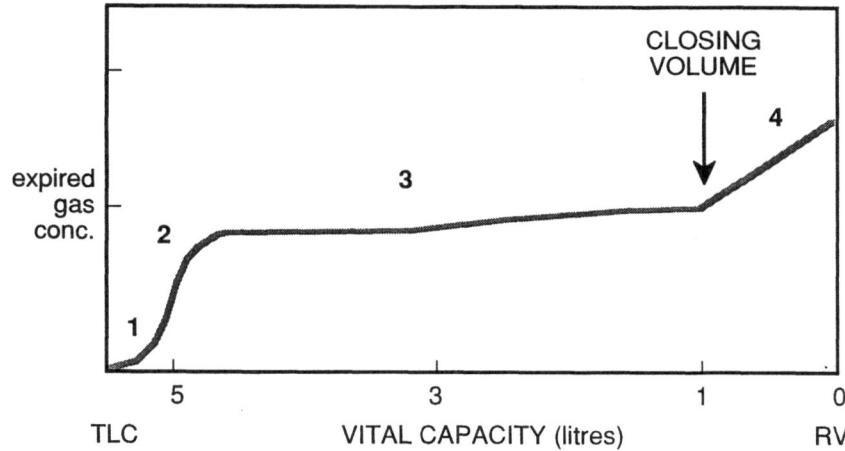

Fig. 4. Closing volume. The four phases of the expired N_2 concentration curve (see text)

Multiple Breath Test

The inert gases most commonly employed in this kind of test are N_2, Ar, and He. When ventilation is equally distributed, an O_2 tidal volume which reaches all lung units in proportion to their respective volumes is expected. In this case, during the subsequent wash-out, the end-tidal alveolar concentrations of the inert gas decrease in all lung units by the same factor, because lung volume and dead space affect its dilution rate according to a linear function. By contrast, when ventilation is uneven (due to increased time constants, such as spontaneous or challenge-induced airway narrowing) the inert gas dilution curve is prolonged and takes on a curvilinear shape, thus denoting the presence of two populations of lung units; fast and slow, according to their emptying pattern during quiet breathing.

Multiple Individual Breath Test

This test is also based on the time constant theory and on thermal conductivity [17, 18]. It consists of a wash-in phase, i.e., quiet breathing of an O_2/He mixture in a closed circuit up to equilibrium, and in a subsequent wash-out phase, which allows measurement of the inert gas (He) emptying pattern and reveals the appearance of air trapping [12].

Measurements with Radioactive Gases

The inhalation of radionuclides detected by means of external scintillation counting or γ-cameras allows topographical study of regional ventilation within the lung and also enables assessment of limited abnormalities, even when pulmonary function shows only mild abnormalities. This kind of measurement was first adopted at the end of the 1950s [19], and a few years later the first study in asthmatics was carried out using ^{133}Xe, which later became the radionuclide of choice (half-life: 5.3 days) [20].

Studies on regional ventilation in asthma have revealed the occurrence of gross, rather than diffuse, abnormalities (with segmental or lobar involvement) in both spontaneous [21] and challenge-induced asthma [22].

Wash-in and wash-out curves have also been determined in bronchial asthma; ^{133}Xe wash-out curves are considered reliable when evaluated over its 70% elimination range and when performed after a wash-in period of less than 2 min [23].

Radionuclides characterized by shorter (^{13}N, 10 min) or much shorter (^{19}Ne, 17 s; ^{81}mKr, 13 s) half-lives have also been employed and high quality images have proved possible. Furthermore, when injected intraveneously, the radionuclide perfusion pattern of distribution allows matching of local blood flow and ventilation.

The intrapulmonary deposition of human albumin minimicrospheres labeled with ^{99}mTc (HAMM) was measured in asymptomatic asthmatics, before and after bronchial challenge (carbachol), to for assess the prevalent site of bronchial constriction in asthma. In bronchial responsiveness thus induced, while central airway involvement was concomitant with increased airway resistance (R_{aw}) values in the early images, there was substantial peripheral airway involvement in the late images, despite R_{aw} normality [24].

Measurement of Continuous Distribution of the $\dot{V}_A/\dot{Q}_C$ Ratio – Multiple Inert Gas Elimination

The technique is based on the simultaneous elimination of six inert (nonradioactive) gases with different solubilities, such as SF6, ethane, cyclopropane, halothane, ether, and acetone, which are first infused intravenously (as saline solution) and then measured in arterial blood and expired gas [5, 9, 14, 25, 27]. Samples are collected only after steady-state levels of inert gas exchange concentrations have been reached. Cardiac output and minute ventilation are also measured. The relationship between blood flow and the $\dot{V}_A/\dot{Q}_C$ ratio and between ventilation and the $\dot{V}_A/\dot{Q}_C$ ratio are obtained by transformation of the "retention-solubility curve" into a distribution of ventilation/perfusion ratios (ratio range from 0.005 to 100, as between real shunt and dead space effect), representing the actual amount of $\dot{V}_A/\dot{Q}_C$ unevenness within the lung units.

Unlike in normal subjects, the distribution of the $\dot{V}_A/\dot{Q}_C$ ratios in asthmatics (with either acute or chronic stable asthma) has been systematically demonstrated as being bimodal and characterized by the presence of a low

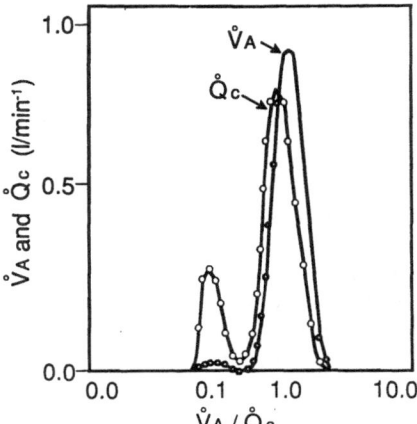

Fig. 5. Multiple inert gas elimination. The distribution of $\dot{V}_A/\dot{Q}_c$ (alveolar ventilation/ blood flow) ratios has been demonstrated as being bimodal, with a substantial amount of blood through poorly ventilated lung units in asthmatics, but not in normals

$\dot{V}_A/\dot{Q}_C$(but not real shunt), suggesting the existence of a substantial amount of blood through poorly ventilated units (about 20% of cardiac output), inducing hypoxia (Fig. 5). This peculiar bimodal pattern of $\dot{V}_A/\dot{Q}_C$ mismatching has often been further verified in asymptomatic asthmatics, in spite of normal spirometer and mechanical function tests.

The poor correlation between the substantial mismatch $\dot{V}_A/\dot{Q}_C$ distribution abnormalities and spirometrical findings [8, 9, 27] provides evidence of the predominant role of peripheral obstructive changes in determining hypoxemia, even in symptom-free patients.

The role of cardiac output and hypoxic vasoconstriction in preventing more severe hyoxemia in asthmatics has been further assessed by this method. A systematic transient increase in the low $\dot{V}_A/\dot{Q}_C$ mode, occurs following $\beta2$-agonist administration, in spite of the improvement in airflow rates [26].

Multiple inert gas elimination has also been used occasionally in asymptomatic asthmatics submitted to bronchial challenge (such as allergen or methacholine) showing different stimulus-specific patterns of $\dot{V}_A/\dot{Q}_C$ disturbances, probably due to the different structural involvement (challenge-related) of the peripheral airways: bimodal distribution was shown with antigen challenge only.

The method is highly reproducible and is much more suitable than the radioactive approach, particularly for repeated measurements and longitudinal studies, though it requires substantial technical capability and is not extensively used for clinical purposes.

Other Tests

Apart from the traditional measurement of RV, other functional tests are based on the time constant theory for the study of distributional ventilation factors [17] and have been described as sensitive indicators for checking small airway dysfunction in asthma:

1. Volume at isoflow is the isovolumetric comparison of maximal expiratory flow rates with air and after the lungs have been filled with a less dense gas mixture (80% He and 20% O_2); a low degree of density dependence indicates that small airways contribute more to flow limitation [6].

2. Frequency dependence of compliance [28] consists of the measurement of pulmonary compliance at different breathing frequencies. It is time-consuming and uncomfortable for the subject [29]. According to the time constant theory, the changes in gas flow observed at different breathing frequencies may reflect bronchial challenge [30].

3. The breathing pattern during exposure to bronchial challenge has also been studied in asthmatics [31]. This functional approach showed a significant increase in mean inspiratory flow (VT/TI) due to bronchial challenge, which was closely related in a dose-dependent manner to the duration of challenge exposure and to the increase in respiratory resistances. This is consistent with the clinical observation that patients with bronchospasm increase alveolar ventilation beyond the level needed to maintain normal $PaCO_2$ [8].

Blood Gas Abnormalities

Invasive Gas Analysis

As previously seen, arterial hypoxemia is common in bronchial asthma and may occur moderately even when airway obstruction is slight. Hypocapnia or normocapnia is usual as well, apart from the most severe cases, in which CO_2 retention mainly reflects the inefficiency of the lung mechanics, i.e., forced expiratory volume in 1 s (FEV_1) about 20% of the predicted value, and hypoxemia is obviously much more severe (Fig. 6).

Lung volumes and mechanics have been extensively studied now for decades in bronchial asthma, but blood gas studies in this disease are considerably fewer in number. Probably the first clinical reports concerning blood gas measurements in asthma were those by Herschfus et al. in 1953 [32] and by Williams and Johman in 1960 [33], carried out in patients with asthma of varying degrees of severity. A systematic decrease in arterial O_2 saturation was found in both studies, and VA/Qc unevenness was suggested as the most likely hypoxemia mechanism.

Only a few years later Tai and Read [27] and McFadden and Lyons [8] obtained the first evidence of more precise changes in O_2 and CO_2 partial pressures in status asthmaticus, in patients with less severe asthma, and during acute asthma attacks. Both of these pioneer studies confirmed the occurrence of consistent hypoxemia, also in many subjects with less severe bronchial obstruction, while the CO_2 behaviour was mainly characterized by nor-

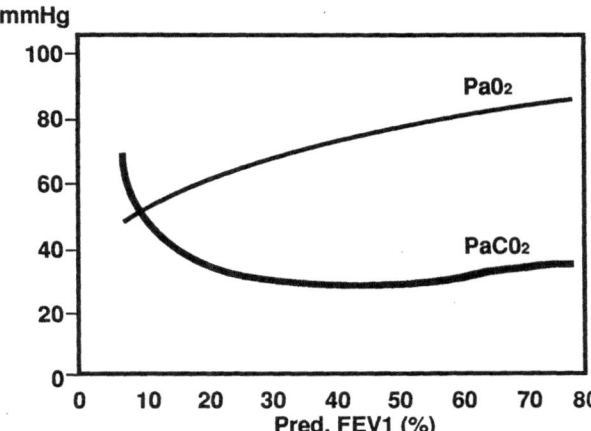

Fig. 6. Effect of airway obstruction on CO_2 and O_2 arterial tensions.

mo- or hypocapnia, with respiratory alkalosis. Despite hypoxemia, which was encountered to some extent in all degrees of airway obstruction, CO_2 retention was in fact related only to particularly severe airway narrowing (FEV_1 about 15% of the predicted value). The explanation provided was that the inspired air is directed preferentially towards the lung units with the lowest flow resistance: as long as the resistance is sufficiently low, these units will tend to hyperventilate (wasted ventilation and hypocapnia; see above), thereby increasing minute and alveolar ventilation. As the bronchial obstruction becomes particularly severe, alveolar ventilation drops and CO_2 retention occurs [13, 27].

Such results stressed, for the first time, that underlying disturbances of blood gas tensions might play a major role in triggering sudden, unexpected, clinical alterations (and sometimes death) in asthmatics. The authors also emphasized that less severe asthmatics should also be considered with particular attention in clinics when the original flow limitation increases (as in infectious exacerbation), because of their "vulnerability" and their liability to rapidly develop severe hypoxemia.

Several further studies have found evidence of hypoxemia and respiratory alkalosis in acute asthma, while a greater tendency towards CO_2 retention has been detected mainly in bronchitic patients [8]. The occasional CO_2 retention sometimes observed in a few patients in the various studies is probably due to the different clinical conditions of the patients included in the same study (such as younger and older subjects, acute and infection-exacerbated asthma, status asthmaticus, and acute bronchospasm in chronic bronchitis) [27, 34, 37].

Frequent measurements of arterial blood gas tensions are clearly of great importance in asthma management and have been described as mandatory to prevent sudden, unexpected, clinical impairment [36]. Similar blood gas abnormalities, together with increases in both O_2 alveolar-arterial difference and in physiological dead space-tidal volume ratio, were also observed in asymptomatic asthmatics despite normal routine pulmonary function by Levine et al. [32]. The authors concluded that, in these symptom-free subjects, obstruction was present in the peripheral airways only (which causes very little increase in resistance) and suggested that, in $\dot{V}_A/\dot{Q}_C$ and gas exchange, abnormalities may occur. These are the only observable irregularities in functional pattern before other lung function defects become apparent. The poor correlation between blood gas abnormalities (particularly CO_2) and spirometry thus obtained further confirmation [34, 37].

Measurements of blood gas tensions are classically performed by arterial puncture. They provide only instantaneous information and several arterial punctures would be required for the monitoring of blood gas changes or longitudinal studies. The reports concerning this kind of study are, in effect, limited, probably also owing to the invasiveness of the measure. Moreover, probably for the same reason, limited information is also available in humans concerning the pattern of response of arterial blood gases to induced bronchoconstriction. Although transient hypoxemia has been reported within a few minutes of challenge inhalation [39–41], CO_2 and O_2 time courses have not been thoroughly examined, particularly as regards asthmatic patients in stable clinical and functional condition. More attention has been paid to the effects of bronchodilators (mainly newer sympathomimetics) on blood gases [5, 9, 26].

It has been emphasized that, despite the improvement in bronchospasm, a transient β-agonist-induced hypoxemia may occur, which may frequently go clinically undetected because of the apparent relief obtained by the patient. The reversal of the compensatory pulmonary hypoxic vasoconstriction due to $\beta2$-mediated stimulation of pulmonary arterial receptors is claimed as being the particular mechanism inducing the transient worsening of $\dot{V}_A/\dot{Q}_C$ (and consequently hypoxemia) in asthmatics. Newer and more selective $\beta2$-bronchodilators are particularly involved, because of their lesser propensity to increase cardiac output, which could act in these cases as a compensatory response to the $\dot{V}_A/\dot{Q}_C$ distributional disturbance [5]. The clinical importance of this kind of transient hypoxemia obviously depends on the patient's preexisting PO_2 level and on the dynamics of its occurrence.

Noninvasive Blood Gas Monitoring

As discussed above, the study of blood gas changes in asthma and/or bronchial hyperreactivity in humans has been mostly approached by invasive (arterial) gas analysis. When the effects of drugs or bronchial challenges are investigated according to this method, several measurements are needed and blood sampling is mostly empirically timed for the patients, following drug or bronchial challenge inhalation. This procedure provides only a sequence of instantaneous information in these cases, but not the precise timing of O_2 and CO_2 changes. The invasiveness of the procedure has probably also contributed to limiting the use of this approach in clinics.

The possibility of performing continuous noninvasive monitoring of blood gas composition may now be achieved by means of electrodes for transcutaneous PO_2 and PCO_2 measurements [42].

The technique of monitoring O_2 and CO_2 partial pressures transcutaneously ($PtcO_2$ and $PtcCO_2$) is based on the assumption that both gases can diffuse through the skin tissues. Although their diffusion rate is low at normal body temperature, it has been proved that the mild heating (42–45 °C) of a localized skin area can increase local blood flow and enhance gas diffusion through the skin, providing a close correlation between transcutaneous and arterial measurements [43].

The principle of the $PtcO_2$ sensor is the reduction of the oxygen which diffuses into the electrolyte (platinum electrode): the electron flow from the silver reference electrode is closely proportional to the O_2 concentration. The $PtcCO_2$ sensor uses the reaction of CO_2 with the water in the electrolyte and the resulting variations in hydrogen ion activity. A glass pH electrode (ion-sensitive) and a silver reference electrode are used to plot CO_2 variations. The most recent devices are equipped with monoelectrodes for the combined measurement of both $PtcO_2$ and $PtcCO_2$. These are characterized by high sensitivity, very short response time, and negligible drift.

The Gasthmatic system is a new technique based on transcutaneous measurements of blood gas changes and has recently been used in the study of both spontaneous asthma and induced bronchoconstriction [43]. It provides an accurate way of monitoring gas exchange variations, with a number of adventages: it is noninvasive; it requires no forced ventilatory maneuvers or active patient cooperation; it is reproducible; it affords the possibility of studying the dynamics of the phenomena measured; it allows a much wider range of ages for investigation. Measurement of the extent and rate of O_2 and CO_2 variations and the precise O_2 and CO_2 time courses throughout all phases of the provocation test, even during challenge inhalation, which was never investigated previously, is possible. This functional approach constitutes a very interesting model for easily assessing, in real time and steady-state breathing conditions, the respiratory gas changes related to the early occurrence of $\dot{V}_A/\dot{Q}_C$ disturbances due to induced bronchoconstriction. The study of the changes in $\dot{V}_A/\dot{Q}_C$ pattern following respiratory drug administration is also possible by this method.

The components of the Gasthmatic system are: (1) a transcutaneous blood gas monitor, with a precise, stabilized heater and electrochemical O_2 and CO_2 sensors; (2) an automatic calibration unit; (3) a personal computer interfaced with both the monitor and the calibration unit; and (4) integrated software for the acquisition, analysis, and calculation of data (namely, parametrization and statistics) and for the real time graphical display of $PtcO_2$ and $PtcCO_2$ time courses. The confidence limits of normal variations are also displayed (Fig. 7).

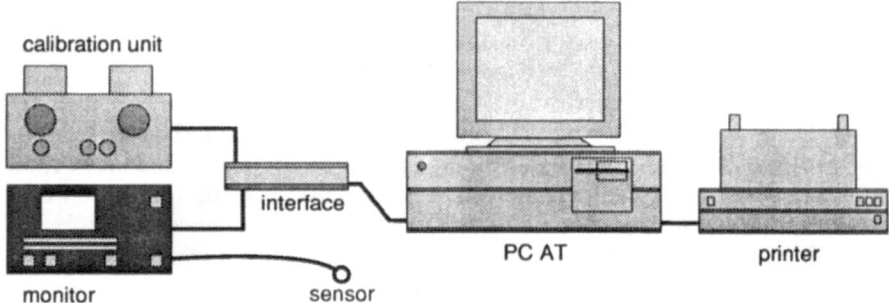

Fig. 7. The Gasthmatic system and its components (see text)

The Gasthmatic System in Induced Bronchoconstriction

Several blood gas response patterns have been assessed according to the bronchial challenge used for the provocation test.

Nonspecific Bronchial Provocation

Methacholine

Methacholine is currently considered the most sensitive challenge for assessing bronchial hyperreactivity in asthma and is, in fact, the most widely employed. Methacholine responsiveness is usually studied by measuring changes in lung mechanics before and after the challenge inhalation (cumulative doses).

FEV_1, 50% maximal expiratory flow (MEF_{50}), peak expiratory flow rate (PEFR) and specific airways conductance (sG_{aw}) are routinely used as functional indicators: the methacholine dose required to cause a "threshold" decrease (provocation dose, PD) from the baseline of these parameters, namely, PD_{20} FEV_1; PD_{30} MEF_{50}; PD_{25} PEFR; PD_{50} sG_{aw}, respectively, is then checked for its ability to identify subjects with enhanced bronchial responsiveness.

This traditional approach provides a sequence of instantaneous measurements, but furnishes no information about the dynamics of functional changes due to the bronchial challenge. When the non invasive monitoring of O_2 and CO_2 time courses is added to this kind of mechanical measurement in the study of asymptomatic asthmatics, two methacholine threshold doses become evident, suggesting that the mechanical response pattern in quite distinct from that of the blood gases, particularly in the case of O_2. The significant reduction in $PtcO_2$ (more than 12% from baseline) due to $\dot{V}_A/\dot{Q}_C$ mismatching systematically precedes the occurrence of significant changes in mechanics: it proved to be much earlier and corresponded to a much lower

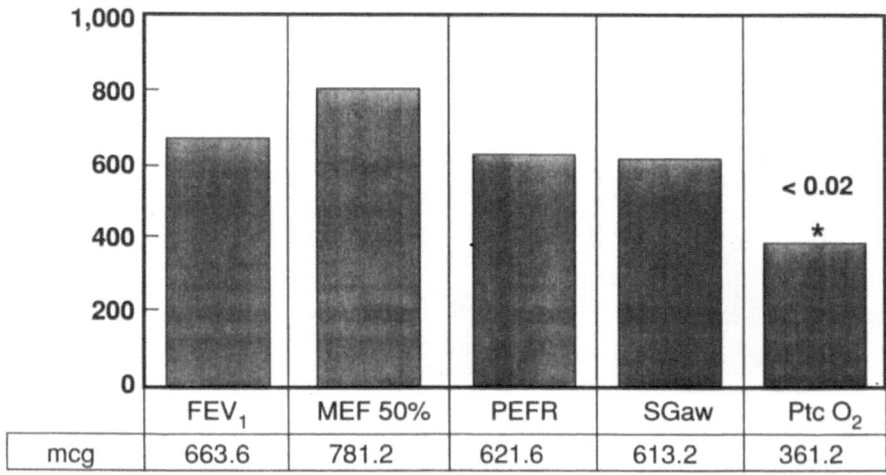

Fig. 8. The significant reduction in $PtcO_2$ systematically precedes the occurrence of significant changes in mechanics during methacholine challenge. FEV_1, forced expiratory volume in 1 s; $MEF_{50\%}$, 50% maximal expiratory flow, $PEFR$, peak expiratory flow rate; sG_{aw}, specific airways conductance; $PtcO_2$, transcutaneous partial oxygen pressure

methacholine threshold dose (about 50%) (Fig. 8) [44]. The existence of both an earlier and a more delayed pattern of methacholine respensiveness can thus be postulated, being chronologically dependent on the particular structural involvement. The earlier pattern is mainly peripheral and detectable by blood gas analysis and the later pattern is more proximal and revealed by mechanical testing.

No significant changes in $PtcCO_2$ time course have been found during methacholine provocation.

Ultrasonic Nebulized Distilled Water

This challenge is known to be an effective bronchoconstrictor in adult asthmatics, when inhaled at a 2 ml/min flow rate for 5 min: the method is simple, reproducible and characterized by a high degree of specificity [45, 46].

Unlike the situation in normals, UNDW induces a particular O_2 and CO_2 response pattern in asthmatics, which is characterized by a sudden but transient hypocapnia (initially concomitant with a transient PO_2 increase) during challenge inhalation followed by a longer-lasting hypoxia (Fig. 9). Hypocapnia becomes evident immediately after the start of UNDW exposure and shows its maximal extent at the third minute of UNDW inhalation. It starts to pick up again immediately after the end of exposure, takes a few more minutes for complete recovery and is undoubtedly linked to an overall increase in alveolar ventilation (hyperventilation). Hypoxia starts to occur at

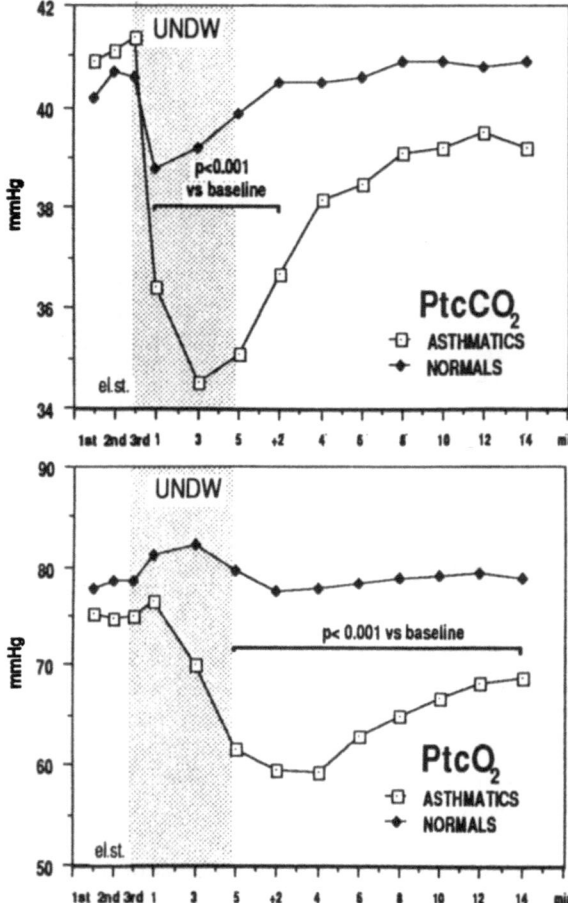

Fig. 9. A sudden but transient hypocapnia during challenge inhalation, followed by a longer lasting hypoxia, characterizes the response to ultrasonic nebulized distilled water (*UNDW*) in asthmatics, but not in normals. *el. st.*, electrode stabilization

the third minute of UNDW inhalation and reaches its lowest value 4 min after the end of exposure (showing a 6 min shift between $PtcO_2$ and $PtcCO_2$ maximal drop), followed by a much slower recovery rate; it reflects a mismatched ventilation/perfusion ratio [43].

In agreement with the principles of uneven ventilation described above, the occurrence of a sequential combination of "wasted ventilation" and "shunt effect" is thus shown to be the distributional pattern of responsiveness to UNDW. There is also a concomitant significant bronchial narrowing (such as a significant flow responsiveness, i.e., a FEV_1 decrease of more than 20% in relation to baseline) in these subjects.

When UNDW is sequentially inhaled for 30, 60 and 120 s at the same flow rate of 2 ml/min, the O_2 and CO_2 time courses show a close dose-response trend. Furthermore, severe hypoxia and sudden hypercapnia can occur simultaneously when the bronchial response to the challenge is characterized by very severe flow limitation; this reflects the occurrence of true alveolar hypoventilation [51].

As stated above, before other lung function defects become apparent, the occurrence of $\dot{V}_A/\dot{Q}_C$ abnormalities, as the only functional pattern suggestive of obstruction confined to the peripheral airways, should be emphasized [34, 37].

The muscular response of the more proximal airways does not constitute the only significant hyperreactive event, though it is certainly the most striking and the most easily detected. Other types of airway response can be expected, particularly responses due to abnormalities within the airway mucosal structures (namely, the epithelial and nervous structures). Some of these events, which have also been described in bronchial biopsy specimens also from mild asthmatics and atopic rhinitics [47], are not necessarily accompanied by notable impairment of routine lung function parameters (such as volumes and flows).

Nevertheless, all these events may act as factors affecting the normal pattern of $\dot{V}_A/\dot{Q}_C$ distribution, even in the early stages of the natural history of bronchial asthma [6]. Furthermore, since recent studies emphasize that bronchial hyperreactivity is distributed according to a unimodal (normal) function in the general population and that traditional flow-responder asthmatics represent only the most sensitive end of the curve [48], the possibility of pinpointing the transition between normality and hyperreactivity becomes a matter of particular importance.

Atopic rhinitics with no history of wheezing when tested to assess their UNDW responsiveness by means of the Gasthmatic system, reproduced the same transcutaneous blood gas response patterns as previously described for asthmatics, even though to a lesser extent and for a shorter duration: a transient hyperventilation during UNDW inhalation (wasted ventilation) and a delayed and persistent hypoxia (shunt effect) (Fig. 10). Regardless of any spirometrical changes, both arterial hypocapnia and hypoxemia were also systematically verified in these subjects, together with respiratory alkalosis [49]. These effects on blood gas time courses strongly suggest the occurrence of significant disturbances in the peripheral distribution of the alveolar ventilation also in subjects with no history of wheezing; the Gasthmatic system proved useful in discriminating "susceptible" individuals of this type (or early stages of hyperreactivity) as an aid to pinpointing the transition between normality and the asthmatic range of hyperreactivity.

When the effects of nature exposure to allergens on blood gas response to UNDW were investigated using the same noninvasive methods in seasonal and nonflow responder atopics, a close correlation was found between the occurrence of significant $\dot{V}_A/\dot{Q}_C$ disturbances and maximal exposure to allergens. The structural involvement leading to appreciable blood gas changes following UNDW proved to be transient and season-dependent, particularly in children, who obviously had a shorter history of exposure to allergens than adults [50] (Fig. 11).

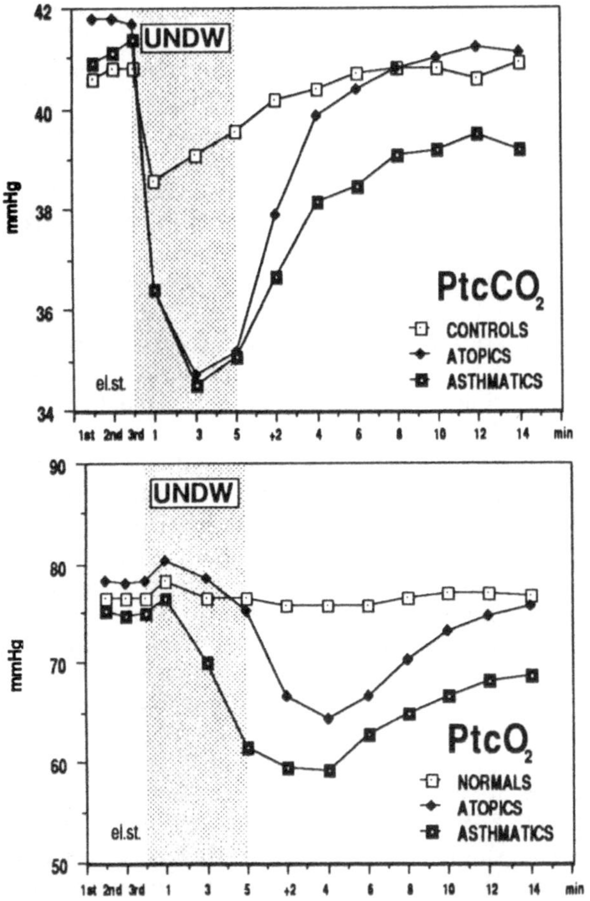

Fig. 10. The PtcCO$_2$ and PtcO$_2$ patterns of response to ultrasonic nebulized distilled water (*UNDW*) in never-wheezy atopic rhinitics reproduce the blood gas response patterns of as described for asthmatics, although to a lesser extent. *el. st.*, electrode stabilization

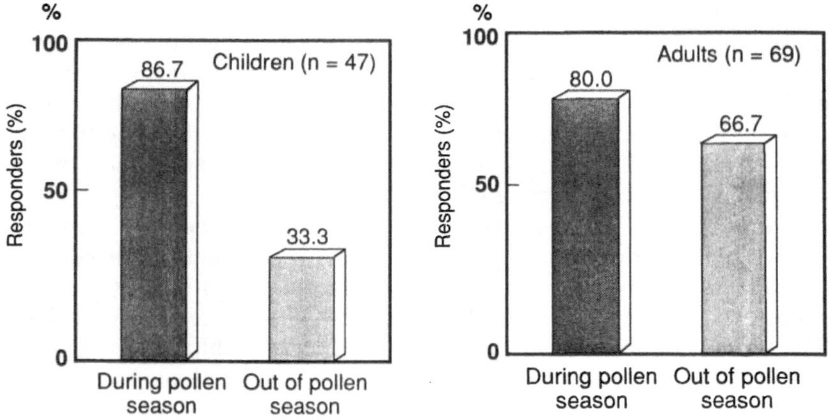

Fig. 11. Appreciable blood gas changes following ultrasonic nebulized distilled water (*UNDW*) inhalation in atopics proved to be season-dependent, particularly in children

Statistical Approach

As previously discussed, a sudden transient hypocapnia and subsequent longer-lasting hypoxia are observed in asthmatics and in never-wheezy rhinitics (though to a lesser extent), but not normals, during UNDW inhalation.

The transcutaneous blood-gas time course (20 min duration) obtained in 104 normal volunteers and 104 atopic rhinitics (FEV_1 nonresponders) [49] were compared (discriminant analysis) in order to establish which monitoring times were the most discriminatory for patterns of response to UNDW in normals and atopics. The Mahalanobis distance (D) was chosen as a measure of discriminatory power. It indicated the third minute of UNDW inhalation as the most predictive time for the $PtcCO_2$ time course ($D = 80.02$, correct discrimination in 81% of cases), while the fourth minute after the end of UNDW challenge proved the most predictive for the $PtcO_2$ time course ($D = 131.17$, correct discrimination in 86% of cases) [52, 53].

The gaussian distributions of the $PtcCO_2$ and $PtcO_2$ values recorded both in normals and in atopic rhinitics at these times were then compared in order to calculate what percentage drop from baseline can be regarded as capable of discriminating between the two response patterns for both gases (i.e., the threshold value). Calculations were performed by equilizing the density functions of the gaussian distributions previously obtained: a 12% drop from baseline was established for both $PtcCO_2$ and $PtcO_2$ [52, 53].

Further Parametric Calculations

A fair amount of parametric information can be derived from both the $PtcCO_2$ and $PtcO_2$ curves, such as the maximal % drop from baseline, the duration of the hypoxic and hyperventilatory (or hypoventilatory) responses, and the time of onset of changes in relation to baseline.

The areas delimited by the $PtcCO_2$ and $PtcO_2$ curves and the steady baseline (i.e., the time line) represent the extent of the functional defect induced; these curves can be measured automatically and their values expressed instantly in screen units (pixels). Each area is approximately triangular in shape (as in the case of the polynomial trend linking the baseline value in the steady-state condition before UNDW inhalation with the value corresponding to the maximal blood gas drop and with the value corresponding to the recovery level towards baseline after challenge). The use of a limited number of trigonometric algorithms leads to a much better interpretation of the monitoring test by adding a number of dynamic parameters to the preexisting static ones, such as drop rate, drop time, recovery rate, recovery time, all of which are important for defining the particular functional patterns in several distinct clinical situations.

A further improvement in parametrization is provided by the simultaneous breath-by-breath recording in graph form of $PtcCO_2$ and $PtcO_2$ in a Cartesian axis system: this furnishes particular planimetric behavior patterns

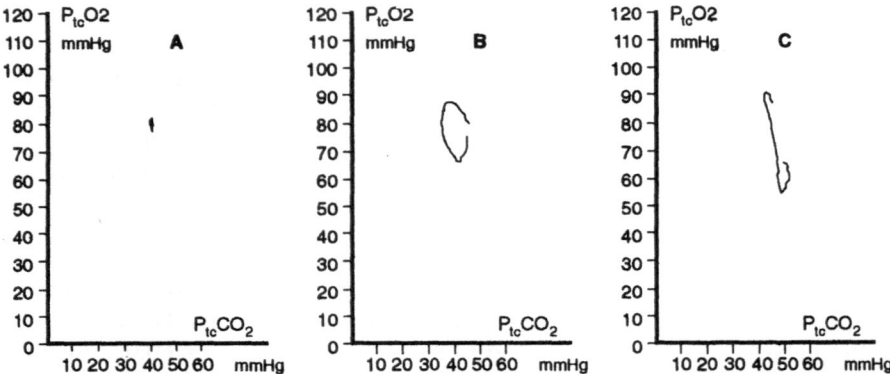

Fig. 12 A–C. Planimetric patterns of response to ultrasonic nebulized distilled water (*UNDW*) in **A** normals ($n=169$); **B** asthmatics ($n=532$), and **C** asthmatics responding with severe flow limitation ($n=52$); 25 min monitoring; values plotted every 30 s. Note the uncomplete $PtcO_2$ recovery in asthmatics

which represent and characterize the patterns of response to UNDW in normals as distinct from those in asymptomatic asthmatics and in asthmatic subjects who respond with a severe flow limitation (Fig. 12).

Specific Provocation

It has been postulated that exposure to allergens may enhance nonspecific bronchial responsiveness in atopic subjects [54].

The transcutaneous blood gas pattern of response to UNDW was assessed before and 60 and 360 min after specific nasal challenge (powdered permato phagoides pteronyssinus, 20 A.U.) in 12 never-wheezy allergic rhinitics and in 12 well matched normal volunteers, together with spirometry and nasal mast cell and eosinophil count.

In rhinitics only, hyperventilation and $\dot{V}_A/\dot{Q}_C$ mismatching gradually increased following UNDW, particularly 360 min after nasal challenge, with no significant change in spirometric parameters. Cell counts also shoped a late (after 360 min) significant ($p < 0.01$) increase, particularly as regards eosinophils.

In rhinitics, despite the negligible involvement of the larger airways, the late blood gas enhanced response emphasizes the occurrence of late functional changes in the peripheral airways, leading to significant $\dot{V}_A/\dot{Q}_C$ disturbances which are concurrent with the inflammatory involvement of the structures [55].

Bronchial Provocation in Pediatric Subjects

In pediatric subjects, the Gasthmatic method has proved to be as effective as in adults in assessing $\dot{V}_A/\dot{Q}_C$ disturbances due to bronchial provocation (UNDW), despite the fact that this challenge is currently considered much less sensitive in small children as regards flow responsiveness.

From a general point of view, the difficulties in performing and measuring traditional lung function parameters (particularly the cooperation-dependent ones) in childhood, together with the earlier occurrence and the longer persistence of $\dot{V}_A/\dot{Q}_C$ distributional disturbances, further enhance the suitability of this functional approach for the early detection and assessment of hyperreactive phenomena in children, and particularly in infants.

In cohort studies carried out in 181 and 116 children, distinguishable $\dot{V}_A/\dot{Q}_C$ patterns of response to UNDW were assessed, showing a close relationship to the clinical situation and disease status (flow responder asthmatics, nonflow responder asthmatics, atopic rhinitics, upper respiratory infection, normal controls). A very high level of specificity was also seen [56] (Table 1).

Furthermore, when FEV_1 and Gasthmatic responsiveness to UNDW were compared double-blind in 62 asthmatic children (ages 4–14 years), the specificity of FEV_1 was found to be poor and closely age-dependent, while the Gasthmatic test specificity was much higher and in no way related to age (Table 2).

Table 1. $\dot{V}_A/\dot{Q}_C$ patterns of response to UNDW show a close relationship to clinical situation and disease status, with a high level of specificity

	n	Spirometry (%)	Gasthmatic system (%)
Asthmatics	62	41.9	96.8
Rhinitics	53	11.3	47.2
URI	32	12.5	43.7
Controls	34	0.0	0.0

UNDW, ultrasonic nebulized distilled water; URI, upper respiratory infection

Table 2. FEV_1 specificity is age-dependent, while Gasthmatic specificity is higher and age-independent

Age (years)	n	Spirometry (%)	Gasthmatic system (%)
4– 6	12	25.0	87.5
6– 8	11	20.0	100.0
8–10	12	25.0	100.0
10–12	17	64.7	100.0
12–14	10	70.0	100.0

Blood Gas Monitoring in Clinical Pharmacology

Not only bronchoconstriction but also bronchodilation can be viewed in terms of changes in $PtcO_2$ and $PtcCO_2$ time courses.

Most respiratory drugs increase both minute and alveolar ventilation, leading to some drop in PCO_2 levels. It has also been known for a number of years that, although airway narrowing is relieved by bronchodilation and alveolar ventilation is increased, there may be some degree of PO_2 impairment, particularly following theophylline and β-agonists [45, 57].

β-Agonists

Though the degree and extent of hypoxemia also depend on preexisting disturbances in $\dot{V}_A/\dot{Q}_C$ pulmonary distribution, the β-agonist-induced stimulation of pulmonary arterial receptors (namely, β_2-receptors) and the subsequent removal of the compensatory pulmonary vasoconstriction are thought to be major mechanisms responsible for the transient increase in hypoxemia in asthma [5, 6, 14].

Due to negligible β_1 stimulation (physiologically leading to a compensatory increase in cardiac output) by the more selective β_2-agonists, a larger decrease in PO_2 levels might thus be expected with these more recent drugs for an equivalent $\dot{V}_A/\dot{Q}_C$ disturbance. In spite of their widespread use, no attempt had been made in clinics to define the precise duration and time course of this phenomenon or the possibility of drug-dependent differences, probably owing to the invasiveness of blood gas measurements.

The transcutaneous PO_2 behavior of 12 asthmatics and 12 normal volunteers has been evaluated according to a cross-over design, following two β_2-agonists with different action kinetics: salbutamol (200 μg), which is a short-acting drug, and bitolterol mesylate (740 μg), which is a "prodrug" and thus takes a longer time (a few minutes) to be active, because of the esterase-dependent release of the active drug (colterol) within the lung [58]. In normal subjects, both drugs induced the same slight increase in $PtcO_2$, probably reflecting the relief of bronchomotor tone in subjects with normal $\dot{V}_A/\dot{Q}_C$ distribution. By contrast, both drugs caused transient hypoxia in asthmatics of the same absolute proportion, though with two distinct kinetic profiles: more abrupt following salbutamol and more delayed with a much more gradual slope following bitolterol mesylate (Fig. 13) [59]. The difference in the time taken (about 6 min) to reach the maximal O_2 decrease strongly indicates appreciable pharmacokinetic differences between the two drugs; the close relationship between $PtcO_2$ and PaO_2 validates the results and also emphasizes the linearity of the variations.

These results obtained with a convenient noninvasive method confirm those of previous studies [5, 14, 26] in asthmatic subjects, showing a marked transient increase in the perfusional pattern within lung units characterized by a low $\dot{V}_A/\dot{Q}_C$ ratio following β-agonists.

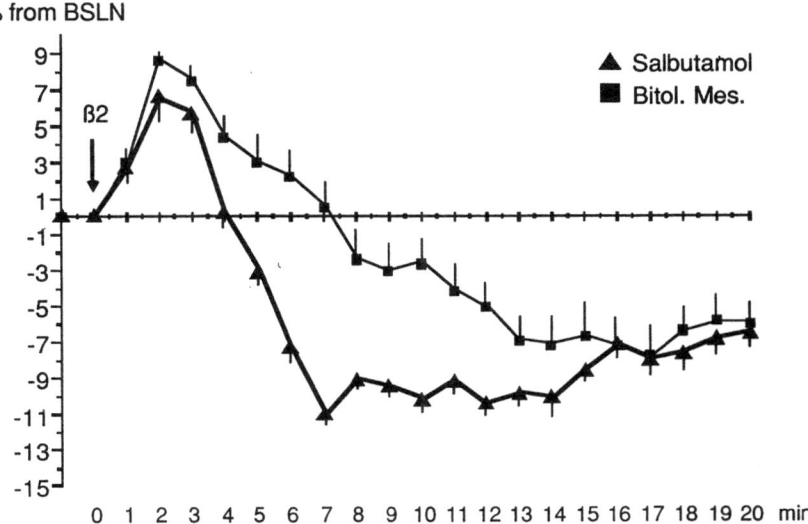

Fig. 13. The onsed of a transient hypoxia has been proved more abrupt following sal-butamol and more gradual following bitolterol mesylate inhalation, thus indicating appreciable pharmacokinetic differences (*BSLN*, baseline)

β-Agonists as Protective Agents

β_2-Bronchodilators are also claimed to be protective agents against airway responsiveness to bronchial challenge, though their protection has never been proved as lasting any longer than their ability to affect airway tone [60, 61].

As previously noted, the $\dot{V}_A/\dot{Q}_C$ disturbances due to UNDW consist in a sequential combination of transient hyperventilation during UNDW inhalation, followed by a longer lasting hypoxia after UNDW, in asthmatics. When UNDW inhalation is repeated in the same subjects 10 min after premedication with salbutamol (200 μg), hypoxia systematically shows prompt complete (or near complete) resolution despite persistence of, or in many cases an increase in, hyperventilation (hypocapnia) (Fig. 14). Arterial blood measurements validate these changes in all cases, even in very mild asthmatics or atopic rhinitics [62, 63].

This dual aspect of PO_2 and PCO_2 time courses is always seen and is systematically reproducible following β_2-agonists. Assuming that the main acute effect of these drugs is airway smooth muscle relaxation, this particular behavior suggests that the $PtcO_2$ time course mainly reflects the dynamics of relief of muscular-dependent events, unlike the $PtcCO_2$ time course, which by contrast, is completely unaffected by β_2-agonists.

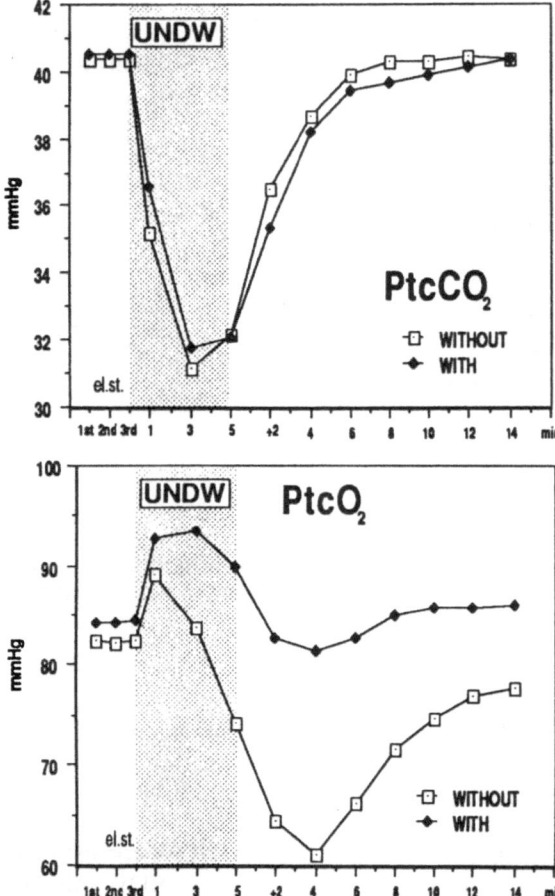

Fig. 14. Short-acting β_2-agonists have been proved to be protective agents only against the occurrence of ultrasonic nebulized distilled water (UNDW)-induced hypoxia. *el. st.*, electrode stabilization

Long-Acting β_2-Agonists

Salmeterol is a new, inhaled, selective β_2-agonist with a much longer bronchodilator activity than other preexisting β_2 agents [64]. The duration of its protective effect against UNDW-induced bronchoconstriction was assessed in eight untreated asthmatics (FEV$_1$ responders to UNDW, PD$_{20\%}$) in a double-blind, cross-over study vs placebo [65]. The spirometric changes to due UNDW and the PtcO$_2$ time course were measured before and 40 min, 8 h, and 12 h after premedication with two puffs of salmeterol (50 µg) and placebo on two separate days. Salmeterol premedication, but not placebo, significantly decreased the FEV$_1$ responsiveness (ANOVA: $p < 0.001$) and minimized the period of UNDW-induced hypoxia (ANOVA: $p < 0.001$) at 40 min, 8 h, and 12 h, thus demonstrating the longer duration of salmeterol activity (up to 12 h) in preventing both the volumetric and the hypoxic patterns of nonspecific bronchial hyperresponsiveness to UNDW.

Drugs Affecting Airway Inflammation

To date, the efficiency of preventive or prophylactic drugs (such as SCG, nedocromile, or ketotifen), and of symptomatic bronchodilators has been assessed by volumetric and mechanical indices of lung function, regardless of their different targets and sites of action. Sometimes, only clinical scores have been employed when negligible spirometrical changes were expected or evoked. Nevertheless, as previously seen, other kinds of measurements (not necessarily correlated with bronchoconstrictional) may be of choice in these cases, particularly to assess earlier or more peripheral airway involvement, which may otherwise be undetectable.

When the efficiency of protective drugs against the challenge-induced $\dot{V}_A/\dot{Q}_C$ disturbances is investigated by means of the Gasthmatic system, the revovery pattern of the $PtcO_2$ and $PtcCO_2$ time courses is completely different as compared with that following symptomatic bronchodilators. First of all, unlike β_2-agonists, these drugs effect both $PtcO_2$ and $PtcCO_2$ time courses, though to a much larger extent in the latter case (Fig. 15).

This effect is not immediate, but gradual and time-dependent during a sufficiently prolonged daily treatment: a few weeks of therapy is required for near complete recovery of O_2 and CO_2 disturbances in mild to moderate asthmatics [66, 67].

Mucosal structures (such as the epithelium and nerve endings) are the main targets for both UNDW [68] and preventive drugs: the sudden and substantial hyperventilation induced by UNDW in conjunction with the particular protection from hyperventilation (afforded by prophylactic agents) lead to the suggestion that the $PtcCO_2$ time course may represent a functional marker for early detection of airway mucosal dysfunction, when CO_2 dependence of ventilatory drive is also considered.

When the effects of inhaled corticosteroids (such as beclomethasone dipropionate) are investigated from this point of view, the only difference worthy of special note is the prompter improvement in $\dot{V}_A/\dot{Q}_C$ disturbances as compared to that induced by preventive drugs, when administered at high doses [62].

Preliminary results, as yet unpublished, indicate that the most recent antihistamines (such as terfenadine, oxatomide, and cyterizine) also show this activity pattern, though to a lesser extent and in atopic subjects only.

Furosemide

It has been shown that inhaled furosemide is effective in preventing bronchoconstriction due to UNDW and osmotic stimuli in asthmatic [69–71].

More recently, significant protection against both UNDW-induced hyperventilation (hypocapnia) and $\dot{V}_A/\dot{Q}_C$ mismatching (hypoxia) has been assessed by the gasthmatic system in 12 stable asthmatics, in whom UNDW was repeated on two different days before and after premedication with

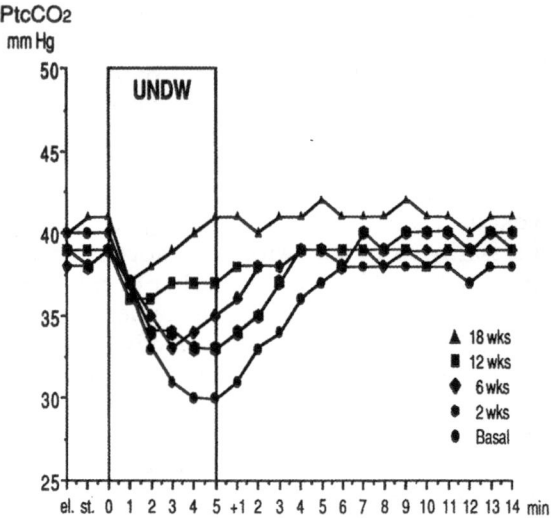

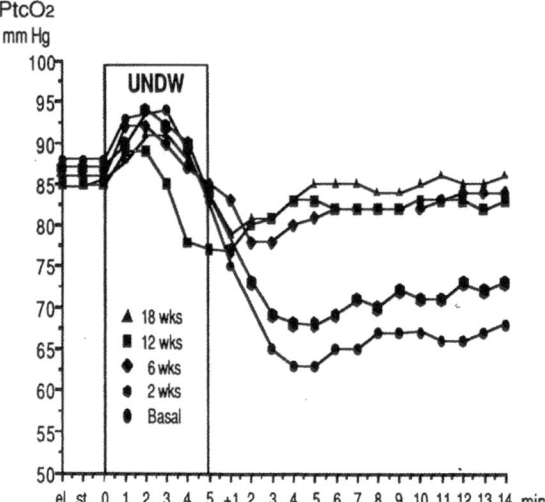

Fig. 15. The influence of protective drugs on PtcCO₂ and PtcO₂ time courses has been shown to be not immediate, but gradual and time-dependent. *el. st.*, electrode stabilization

aerosolized furosemide (40 mg). The same pattern of protection has been previously obtained with sodium cromoglycate (see above): both of these drugs, in fact, are capable of acting on airway sensory nerves [72].

The protection against such gas response patterns is thus probably related to the stabilizing activity of furosemide on bronchial surface triggers.

References

1. Comroe JH (1974) Physiology of respiration. Year Book Medical Publishers, Chicago
2. West JB (1977) Ventilation/blood flow and gas exchange. Blackwell, Oxford
3. Bouhuys A (1977) The physiology of breathing. Grune and Stratton, New York
4. Rahn H, Fenn WO (1956) A graphical analysis of the respiratory gas exchange. American Physiological Society, Washington DC
5. West JB (1980) Pulmonary gas exchange. Academic, New York
6. Macklem PT, Permutt S (1979) The lung in the transition between health and disease. Dekker, New York
7. Friberg S, Bevegard S, Graff-Lonnevig V, Hallback A (1989) Asthma from childhood to adulthood – A follow-up study of 20 subjects with special reference to work capacity and pulmonary gas exchange. J Allergy Clin Immunol. 84: 183–190
8. McFadden ER, Lyons HA (1968) Arterial blood gas tensions in asthma. N Engl J Med 278:1028–1032
9. Ballester E, Roca J, Ramis L, Wagner PD, Rodriguez-Roisin R (1990) Pulmonary gas exchange in severe chronic asthma. Am Rev Respir Dis 141:558–562
10. Orehek J (1982) Measurements of hyperresponsiveness in man. Eur J Respir Dis 63 [Suppl 117]:42–61
11. Macklem PT, Wilson NJ (1965) Measurement of intrabronchial pressure in man. J Appl Physiol 20:653–663
12. Olive JT, Hyatt RE (1972) Maximal expiratory flow and total respiratory resistance during induced bronchoconstriction in asthmatic subjects. Am Rev Respir Dis 106:366–376
13. Udwadia FE (1978) Blood gas studies in bronchial asthma. Indian J Chest Dis Allied Sci 21:10–17
14. Wagner PD, Dantzker DR, Iacovoni VE, Tomlin WC, West JB (1978) Ventilation-perfusion inequality in asymptomatic asthma. Am Rev Respir Dis 118: 511–524
15. Anthonisen NR, Danson J, Robertson PC, Ross WRD (1969) Airway closure as a function of age. Respir Physiol 8:58–65
16. Dolfuss RB, Milic Emili J, Bates DV (1967) Regional ventilation of the lung studied with boluses of 133 Xe. Respir Physiol 2:234–246
17. Otis AB, McKerrow CB, Bartlett RA (1955) Mechanical factors and distribution of pulmonary ventilation. J Appl Physiol 8:427–441
18. Serra R (1967) Courbes expiratoires d'oxygene. PhD thesis, University of Utrecht
19. Martin CJ, Young AC (1956) Lobar ventilation in man. Am Rev Tuberc Pulm Dis 73:330–337
20. Bentivoglio LG, Beerel F, Bryan AC, Stewart PB, Rose B, Bates DW (1963) Regional pulmonary function studies with Xe 133 in patients with bronchial asthma. J Clin Invest 42:1193–1200
21. Fazio F, Palla A, Santolicandro A, Solfanelli S, Fornai E, Giuntini C (1979) Studies of regional ventilation in asthma using 81 mKr. Lung 156:185–194
22. Hughes JMB, Gardiner IG, Ciofetta G (1978) Induced bronchoconstriction. In: Lavander JP (ed) Clinical and Experimental Applications of Krypton-81m. Br J Radiol Spec Rep 15:125–127
23. Ronchetti R, Jones H, Rhodes CG, Herring A, Eiser NM, Renci S, Hughes JMB (1980) Clearance of radioactive nitrogen and xenon from the lungs of anesthetized dogs and human subjects. Bull Eur Physiopathol Respir 16:395–409
24. Santolicandro A, Fornai E, Pulera' N, Giuntini C (1986) Functional aspects of reversible airways obstruction. Respiration 50 [Suppl 2]:65–71
25. Wagner PD, Hedenstierna G, Bylin G (1987) Ventilation perfusion inequality in chronic asthma. Am Rev Respir Dis 136:605–612

26. Rodriguez-Roisin R, Wagner PD (1990) Clinical relevance of pentilation-perfusion inequality determined by inert gas elimination. Eur Respir J 3:469–482
27. Tai E, Read J (1967) Blood gas tensions in bronchial asthma. Lancet 1:644–646
28. Woolcock AJ, Vincent NJ, Macklem PT (1969) Frequency dependence of compliance as a test for obstruction in the small airways. J Clin Invest 48:1097–1106
29. Flenley C, Guyatt AR, Siddorn JA, Brash H (1971) Frequency dependence of compliance. Proc. R Soc Med 64:1234–1238
30. Wanner A, Zarzecki S, Atkins N, Zapata A, Sackner MA (1974) Relationship between frequency dependence of lung compliance and distribution of ventilation. J Clin Invest 54:1200–1213
31. Chada TS, Birch S, Allegra A, Sackner MA (1984) Effects of ultrasonically nebulized distilled water on respiratory resistance and breathing pattern in normals and asthmatics. Bull Eur Physiopathol Respir 20:257–262
32. Herschfus JA, Bresnick E, Segal MS (1953) Am J Med 14:23
33. Williams MH, Johman LR (1960) Cardiopulmonary function in bronchial asthma in comparison with chronic pulmonary emphysema. Am Rev Respir Dis 81:173–177
34. Levine G, Ousley F, Macleod P, Macklem PT (1970) Gas exchange abnormalities in mild bronchitis and asymptomatic asthma. N Engl J Med 282:1277–1281
35. Miyamoto T, Mizuno K, Furuya A (1969) Arterial blood gases in bronchial asthma. J Allergy 4:45–49
36. Palmer KNW, Diament ML (1967) Spirometrical and blood gas tensions in bronchial asthma and chronic bronchitis. Lancet 2:383–384
37. Waddel JA, Emerson PA, Gunstone RF (1967) Hypoxia in bronchial asthma. Br Med J 2:402–404
38. Anonymous (1975) management of acute asthma (leading article). Br Med J iv:65–66
39. Booji-Noord H, DeVries K, Sluiter HJ, Orie NGM (1972) Late bronchial obstructive reaction to experimental inhalation of house dust extract. Clin Allergy 2:43–61
40. Poppius H, Stenius B (1977) Changes in arterial oxygen saturation in patients with hyperreactive airways during histamine inhalation test. Scand. J Respir Dis 58:1–4
41. Stewart IC, Parker A, Catteral JR, Douglas NJ, Flenley DC (1989) Effect of bronchial challenge on breathing patterns and arterial oxygenation in stable asthma Chest 95:65–70
42. Huch R, Huch A, Lubbers DW (1981) Transcutaneous PO_2. Thieme-Stratton, New York
43. Dal Negro R, Allegra L (1989) Blood gas changes during and after non specific airway challenge. J Appl Physiol 67 (6):2627–2630
44. Vocaturo G, Grandi M, Landoni CV et al. (1992) Transcutaneous monitoring of O_2 and CO_2 during bronchial stimulation with methacholine. Am Rev Respir Dis 145:A50
45. Allegra L, Bianco S (1980) Non specific bronchoreactivity obtained with an ultrasonic aerosol of distilled water. Eur J Respir Dis 61 [Suppl 106]:41–49
46. Anderson SD, Schaeffel RE, Finney M (1983) Evaluation of ultrasonically nebulized solutions as a provocation in patients with asthma. Thorax 38:284–291
47. Jeffrey PK, Wardlaw AJ, Nelson FG, Collins JV, Kay AB (1989) Bronchial biopsies in asthma. Am Rev Respir Dis 140:1745–1753
48. Cockcroft DW, Hargreave FE (1990) Airway hyperresponsiveness. Am Rev Respir Dis 142:497–500
49. Dal Negro R, Turco P, Allegra L (1992) Blood gas changes in non asthmatic rhinitics during and after non specific challenge. Am Rev Respir Dis 145:337–339
50. Dal Negro R (1988) Abnormal airways responses in atopy. Triangle 27 (3):87–93
51. Turco P, Dal Negro R, Pomari C et al. (1992) Time course of UNDW-induced hypoventilation in asymptomatic asthmatics. Am Rev Respir Dis 145:A597

52. Dal Negro R, Turco P, Pomari C, Allegra L (1989) Factors discriminating between normals and atopics undergoing bronchial stimulus with UNDW. Eur Respir J 2:777s
53. Dal Negro R, Turco P, Allegra L, Repeto P (1992) Statistical model for discriminating PtcCO$_2$ and PtcO$_2$ time-courses in normals and rhinitics during UNDW inhalation. Am Rev Respir Dis 145:A52
54. Boulet LP, Cartier A, Thomson NC, Roberts RS, Dolovich J, Hargreave FE (1983) Asthma and increases in non allergic bronchial responsiveness form seasonal pollen exposure. J Allergy Clin Immunol 71:399–406
55. Dal Negro R, Perdona' B, Pomari C, Turco P, Allegra L (1990) Non specific bronchial hyperreactivity enhanced by a previous specific nasal challenge. Eur Respir J 3 [Suppl 10]:362
56. Dal Negro R (1989) Studio dei gas respiratori nella patologia asmatica infantile. In: Boschi G, Zanacca C (eds) Nuove tecnologie in pediatria. Bertoni, Reggio Emilia, pp 247–253
57. Palmer KNV (1971) Effects of bronchodilator drugs on arterial blood gas tensions in bronchial asthma. Postgrad Med J 47s:75–77
58. Orgel HA, Kemp JP, Tinkelman DG, Webb DR (1985) Bitolterol and albuterol metered dose aerosols. J Allergy Clin. Immunol 75:55–62
59. Dal Negro R, Cogo A, Turco P, Pomari C, Turati C, Allegra L (1992) Effects of salbutamol and bitolterol mesylate on PO$_2$ levels in asthmatic patients and healthy volunteers. Arzneim.-Forsch 42:959–961
60. Harvey JE, Tattersfield AE (1982) Airways response to salbutamol: therapy on the provocation of asthma by histamine. Thorax 37:280–287
61. McFadden ER (1988) Corticosteroids and cromolyn sodium as modulators of airway inflammation. Chest 94:181–184
62. Dal Negro R, Allegra L (1989) La transizione fra normalita' e risposta iperreattiva. Ital J Chest Dis 43 [Suppl 3]:213–218
63. Turco P, Dal Negro R, Cogo A, Allegra L (1989) Changes in TcO$_2$ and TcCO$_2$ time course due to ultrasonically nebulized distilled water (UNDW) in atopics before and after salbutamol. Eur Respir J 2 [Suppl 8]:866
64. Ullman A, Svedmyr N (1988) Salmeterol, a new long acting inhaled beta-2 adrenoceptor agonist: comparison with salbutamol in adult asthmatic patients. Thorax 43:674–678
65. Cogo A, Turco P, Dal Negro R, Allegra L (1992) Salmeterol: a 12-hour-protection against UNDW-induced hyperreasponsiveness. Am Rev Respir Dis 145:A59
66. Allegra L, Cogo A, Dal Negro R, Pomari C (1990) Bronchial asthma: a new way of assessing the effect of prophylactic drugs. Am Rev Respir Dis 141 (4):754A
67. Allegra L, Turco P, Dal Negro R, Pomari C (1992) P$_{tc}$O$_2$ and P$_{tc}$CO$_2$ monitoring of bronchial responsiveness in FEV$_1$-now-responder asthmatics during ketotifen and placebo treatment. Respiration (to be published)
68. Highenbottam T (1987) The mechanism of aerosol induced bronchoconstriction. Bull Eur Physiopathol Respir 23 [Suppl 10]:77–80
69. Bianco S, Vaghi A, Robuschi M, Pasargiklian M (1988) Prevention of exercise-induced bronchoconstriction by inhaled furosemide. Lancet 2:252–255
70. Robuschi M, Pieroni M, Refini M, Bianco S, Rossoni G, Magni F, Berti F (1990) Prevention of antigen-induced early obstructive reaction by inhaled furosemide in (atopic) subjects with asthma and (actively sensitized) guinea pigs. J Allergy Clin Immunol 85:10–16
71. Barnes P (1990) Frusemide and neural control of airways. Eur Respir J 3 [Suppl 10]:103
72. Wood AM (1990) Effects of frusemide on human airway epithelium. Eur Respir J 3:1234

Part IV

Specific Bronchial Challenges

Skin Tests and Radioimmunological Assays

S. Centanni and G. Piatti

Institute of Respiratory Diseases, School of Medicine, University of Milan, Milano,
Italy

Introduction

Any symptoms of an asthmatic nature must be analyzed from the allergological viewpoint with the aim of evaluating the possible etiological role of an
atopic component in asthma. Furthermore, since asthma is most often characterized by a multifactorial pathogenesis, it is also important to determine
the exact role of the allergic phenomenon in each patient in order to choose
an optimal preventive and therapeutic strategy. Allergy skin tests therefore
represent one of the first investigations which the asthmatic patient must undergo.

Skin Tests

The principle on which these are based is that of recreating artificially, at skin
level, the interaction between the allergen and the IgEs adhering to the surface of mastocytes, in the same way as this reaction occurs spontaneously in
allergic asthmatic subjects at a bronchial level; the skin, in fact, quite accurately reflects the degree of sensitization of airways mucous membranes, while
there are nevertheless some exceptions, as will be seen later [1].

When the subject is sensitive to a certain allergen, the skin responds with
an erythematous-pomphoid type reaction in the space of 10–20 min, since
the reintroduction of the antigen determines local mast cell degranulation
with the rapid release of histamine and other allergy inflammatory agents;
this is therefore an immediate or type I immunopathological reaction,
according to Gell and Coombs' classification. The intensity of the reaction
is influenced by several variables. Of foremost importance, however, is the
degree of sensitization that is produced, i.e., the extent of the overproduction
of specific IgE in response to the allergens. Although it may not always be
linear, this correlation is nevertheless quite evident.

It must be remembered that not all type I reactions are IgE-mediated.
For example, IgG_4, also known as IgG S-TS (short-term sensitizing), can at
times act in a similar manner to IgE and are implicated in some forms of al-

lergic asthma caused by mites and animal dandruff; in these cases, skin tests are positive while RAST is negative [2].

In addition, it is sometimes possible for delayed inflammatory reactions to occur, with odema and erythema and influenced by an immunopathological mechanism of type III (Arthus type), i.e., with an immunocomplex pathogenesis. These reactions may be most frequently observed when carrying out tests with aspergilli in subjects with allergic bronchopulmonary aspergillosis [1, 3, 4]. The same IgE-mediated reactions can, however, determine delayed reactions caused in particular by the release of Histamine Releasing Factor.

The main air contaminants of allergological interest are: pollens, microphytes, dust mites, and animal dandruff. The allergologist will choose the allergens most probably involved to test on the patient on the basis of: (a) the characteristics of the environmental location of each allergen, (b) knowledge drawn from the pollination calender, and (c) the symptoms with which the patient presents.

Skin tests may be carried out according to two methods: (1) "prick tests", which are carried out by means of superficial puncture of the skin through drops of allergenic extract or by the lesser-used scratch tests which are substantially the same; (2) "intradermal reactions". The diagnostic allergens for prick tests are available in concentrated solutions, are usually glycerinated, and are very stable, while those used for intradermal reactions are made up of solutions diluted to differing degrees in a saline-phenycate solution and are therefore less stable.

The concentrations of the allergenic extracts are expressed in terms of weight/volume (w/v) or as protein-nitrogen units (PNU). Extracts with identical w/v or PNU values may, however, vary considerably in the concentration of the allergens since the principal allergens make up only a small and variable percentage of the total protein [5]. It is therefore advisable to use high quality extracts while paying particular attention to the expiration date of the allergens. Titration of the extracts is based on biological tests and immunochemical methods (RAST, cross-over immunoelectrophoresis) from which new biologically based units have been recently derived – AU (allergenic unit), BU (biological unit), etc. Despite numerous attempts, perfect standardization of the allergenic extracts has yet to be reached.

Intradermal injections promote enhanced skin responses in comparison with prick tests; but they are also more likely to cause undesirable side effects, are more painful for the patient, and, without doubt, more invasive. For these reasons, many investigators prefer prick tests to intradermal injections for normal diagnostic routines, while the latter may be used in particular cases, e.g., when the skin response is of dubious interpretation or when it is necessary to establish the threshold dose of skin reactivity. In both cases, the site chosen for the skin tests is the volar surface of the arm and forearm. These are the areas which present greater skin reactivity in relation to the allergens, probably due to differing mast cell concentration or a different skin sensitivity to histamine [1].

Prick Tests

Method of Execution

After disinfecting and carefully cleaning the skin with ether, the investigator places small drops of each allergen, according to a selected order, on the desired area, taking care to maintain sufficient space between allergens (3–4 cm) in order not to superimpose the reactions [6]. Besides the allergenic extracts, a positive (1% histamine chloride) and a negative (glycerinated solution) control are also assayed.

It is important to carry out the test on areas of healthy skin, otherwise skin reactivity may be altered. Furthermore, it is better to avoid placing the drops over the veins since successive puncture with the needle may constitute a potential risk of anaphylactic shock.

Marked dermographism also precludes the possibility of carrying out skin tests, in which case recourse to serological tests is taken.

The second phase is to puncture the skin in order to favour penetration of the allergen and, as a result, reaction with mast cells [7]. For this procedure, lancets are used. They are held at an acute angle (about 60°–70°), with the point inserted at the margin of the drop, just under the epidermis; with a slightly raised movement, the lancet is then rapidly removed.

The dose of extract which penetrates the skin in this way, with concentrated solutions of from 1/20 to 1/100, is 3.10^{-6} ml [2].

If the test has been carried out correctly, no blood will appear at the site of the puncture.

It is advantageous to change lancet for every allergen tested in order to avoid having false positives, linked to the inevitable transport of small quantities of allergens from one site to another on the point of the needle.

After approximately 5 min, the drops are dried individually with cotton wool balls, paying attention once again to avoid transport of any allergenic extract from one area to the other.

Evaluation of the Reactions

A reading of the results is carried out after 15–20 min: if the reaction is negative only a small pink spot is observed where the needle penetrated; when the reaction is positive, an erythematous area is observed and is almost always associated with a wheal of variable size according to the intensity of the allergic reaction. It is advisable to carry out the reading in surroundings well-illuminated by sunlight.

To evaluate the intensity of the reaction, various classifications have been proposed, which on the most part take into consideration the diameter of the wheal, eventual appearance of pseudopodia, and the reaction to histamine for comparison (see Table 1).

It is possible to measure the maximum diameter (D), the diameter perpendicular to this (d) and to express the reaction as $\left(\dfrac{D+d}{2}\right)$, or the dimensions of the wheal and erythema may be transferred onto an acetate and measurements taken successively.

The reaction reaches maximum intensity after 20 min and disappears in the space of a few hours. The areas in which the prick tests have been carried out can be used for further investigations, if necessary, only after several days in order to avoid phenomena of local skin reactivity exhaustion [3].

A correctly carried out skin test yields a high degree of specificity and sensitivity.

Undesired Reactions

Undesired reactions are extremely rare if the test has been carried out correctly. Nevertheless, they may be represented by local reactions such as wheals extending to the surrounding skin, lymphangitis and lymphonodal swelling, by reactions that reproduce the symptoms presented by the patient, or by extremely rare systematic reactions, described in the literature, which may even include the extreme reaction of anaphylactic shock [3]. When such reactions occur, the drops should be dried immediately in order to limit the absorption of the allergens, a tourniquet applied above the interested area, and a 1% solution of adrenaline injected in the reaction area.

Intradermal Reactions

Method of Execution

Intradermal reactions are another method for carrying out allergological skin tests. The solutions used are the same as for the prick test, but, as this is an intradermal test, the allergen dilutions are greater. In particular, concentrations from 10 to 1000 times lower than those used for prick tests are employed. The method consists in introducing about 0.02 ml of test extract into the superficial layers of the skin by means of a 1 ml disposable tuberculin-type plastic syringe [2, 8]. After disinfection, the patient's skin is stretched with one hand and with the other the needle is introduced almost parallel to the skin surface, with the smooth part of the needle point facing the skin. Once the extract has been injected, a thin epidermal layer remains raised, forming a small wheal. Attention must be payed not to inject air, to avoid the reflux of liquid when the needle is extracted, and to not inject the allergen subcutaneously in order to avoid false negatives.

Distances of 4–5 cm must be maintained between each intradermal reaction in order to avoid superimposition which causes difficulties in reading the

Table 1. Suggested classifications for assessing skin reactions

Serafini [3]
-     No difference from negative control
- +   Erythema and wheal just noticeable
- + +   Wheal (10 mm in diameter) with pseudopodia and slight erythema
- + + +   Wheal (15 mm in diameter) with pseudopodia and marked erythema
- + + + +   Wheal (20 mm in diameter) with pseudopodia and marked erythema

D'Amato [1]
- + + +   Wheal of same dimensions as histamine control
- + + + +   Intermediate-type reaction
-     Reaction equal to that of negative control

Muiesan [19]
-     No wheal or erythema
- +   Erythema <20 mm in diameter
- + +   Erythema >20 mm in diameter
- + + +   Wheal and erythema
- + + + +   Wheal, erythema, and pseudopodia

results. As for the prick tests, a negative control with 0.02 ml of physiological solution and a positive control with a 0.1 mg/ml concentration of histamine are included.

Evaluation of the Reactions

Readings of the reactions are carried out after 5–15 min and the diameter of every positive reaction is measured (see Table 1). In this case too the diameter is represented by an erythema-pomphoid reaction.

A vast number of allergens may be assayed with this method. The main advantage of intradermal reaction tests compared to prick tests lies in the possibility of varying the concentration of the solutions employed, beginning with the lowest, and in this way evaluating the skin reaction threshold.

The intradermal reaction is more exact and more constant than the prick test and reveals a state of sensitization with particularly low concentrations of allergen. Furthermore, the determination of the threshold of sensitization to an allergen may be useful for the eventual beginning of desensitization treatment. Nonetheless, intradermal reactions are more likely to cause undesirable reactions, and it is for this reason that the use of prick tests, also without doubt easier to carry out, is becoming more and more widespread.

Conclusions

Findings of skin positivity do not necessarily mean that sensitization towards that particular allergen is responsible for the symptoms presented in the patient. Skin positivity exists which is not accompanied by any symptoms and which may be the warning sign of future development of atopic symptoms, the after-effects of a preceding allergic diathesis, or symptoms which are totally or partially independent of any allergic etiopathogenesis, even if positivity was highlighted in the skin tests (false positivity).

Latent or "potential" allergy is mainly observed for pollens in children with a positive family history of allergic disorders who have not yet developed evident clinical symptoms. In these cases, the positivity of the skin tests may precede the clinically detectable allergic signs by several years.

It must also be considered that some subjects, e.g., those treated with a specific desensitization treatment, may retain persistent positivity of skin reaction without presenting any symptoms on exposure to the specific allergen [3, 5] and that 6%–10% of the asymptomatic population presents unexplainable positive skin reactions [6].

Furthermore, the correlation between skin positivity and the symptoms induced by the allergen is good for inhaled allergens but less so for alimentary allergens. It is also possible that an individual has allergy-type clinical signs but that these are not expressed in an evident skin positivity; that is to say, false negatives exist. Often, these are patients in whom clinical symptoms have only recently appeared and, as a consequence, antibodies have been produced mainly locally, at the site of the allergic phlogosis but are still scarce at skin level. On other occasions the lack of a skin response may be attributable to the variability and low sensitivity of the extracts used. In these cases, if the clinical symptoms suggest an atopic etiopathogenesis, the immunoserological RAST test (see below) is of help.

The pomphoid reaction diminishes with age, but even individuals of the same age may have different cutaneous reactivity.

Prick tests are not normally carried out in children below 3–5 years of age due to the weak skin reactivity present at this age. According to age, the skin tests which first give positive results are those for dust, followed by those for animal fur and only later, towards the age of five, those for pollens [6, 9–11]. It is particularly important to emphasize that certain drugs are capable of inhibiting skin reactivity. It is, in fact, good practice to inquire about any treatment which the patient may have undergone in the recent past before carrying out a prick test, since antihistamines and ketotifen have an inhibitory action on skin tests. The period of inhibition varies according to the molecule involved; for terfenadine the inhibitory effect on the allergic wheal stops within 48 h of the last administration, while for asthemizol this effect is still present 13 days after the last administration. Theophyllines, β_2-stimulants, cromoglycate, and corticosteroids, at the commonly used doses, do not interfere with immediate IgE mediated responses. Moreover, corticosteroids have an inhibitory action on the late component of the allergic reaction and, as has been recently discovered, also seem to have an effect on the immediate reaction, thus determining a certain reduction of the pomphoid reaction. Systemic β_2-stimulants also have a slight depressant effect.

It is therefore necessary to suspend all treatment with antihistamines and ketotifen at least 1 week before carrying out allergy tests. It is possible to check the state of conservation of the skin reactivity with a 1:100 solution of histamine. Specific immunotherapy also causes a reduction in pomphoid skin reactivity.

The circadian cycle influences skin reactivity, as the response to the tests improves at night. Furthermore, skin responses are maximal on the first day of the menstrual cycle.

We can thus conclude that it is always important to evaluate the results of prick tests with respect to the clinical symptoms presented by the patient and by considering the diverse factors which play a part in depressing or enhancing skin reactivity.

In Vitro Tests: RAST and ELISA

In order to evaluate the atopic diathesis of an asthmatic subject, the allergologist also has recourse to laboratory tests, which will generally be employed after a primary screening with skin tests. The most important and most widely used allergological in vitro tests is the RAST followed by the ELISA.

The RAST (radioallergosorbent test) is a laboratory test used to determine the quality and quantity of specific IgE antibodies produced in allergic subjects against certain allergens, with a sensitivity in nanograms.

The allergen is fixed with a stable bond to an insoluble support (solid phase) which may be a cellulose disk or a polystyrene spherule. The allergen plus the support are incubated for 3 h together with a small quantity of the serum under examination (50 µl): if specific IgE antibodies are present, these will bind to the allergen. The successive washing of the support ensures removal of those IgE which do not react. Following this, the support is incubated with anti-IgE antibodies and labelled with a radioactive isotope tracer (^{125}I) or with an enzyme in the case of ELISA.

Excess anti-IgE antibodies which do not bind are removed and the radioactivity of the support is then counted by means of a γ-camera. The quantity of specific IgE is expressed in RAST units or as class 0, 1, 2, 3, 4, which begins to have clinical significance with positivity between 1 and 2, and, more directly, as a percentage of specific bound radioactivity [12]. However, owing to the low level of allergen purification, not all the specific IgE present in the serum bind to the support and as a result the RAST does not reveal specific IgE in a truly quantitative manner [14, 15]. There is usually a good correlation between the prick test and the RAST, especially in the presence of high degrees of sensibilization. The relation is less good for low degrees of sensibilization, as is also the case between the RAST and the intradermal reaction tests, since the latter also highlight all slight cases of allergy. It is difficult to have negative skin tests and positive RAST [12], while the contrary is possible. It is thought that 15% of patients with positive skin tests have a negative RAST [13].

The RAST is not as sensitive as the skin test. In fact, the serum ratio of IgE is influenced by the extent of their synthesis and therefore by allergenic stimulation [12, 16] and by their fixing to mast cells and basophils [13]. Moreover, since the level of IgE in the serum varies with exposure to the allergen, it is theoretically possible to find negative RAST which become positive only after the pollination season, as, in the same way, the RAST may be negative in the presence of a high number of mast cells available to bind the IgE. Furthermore, the RAST does not reveal the specific IgE adhering to the mast cells of the skin mantle as the skin tests do, but rather the circulating IgEs in the serum, that is, that quota which is not fixed to mast cells and which is only a portion of the total amount of IgE in the organism. False negatives are possible when high levels of IgG with the same allergenic specificity as IgE, as, for example, are produced during desensitization treatment, can bind the allergen to the support, so impeding their recognition by IgE.

Investigation by RAST involves minimum discomfort for the patient: only a few milliliters of blood are required. Moreover, unlike the PRICK test, the RAST test can be carried out in a manner which is completely independent of drugs, which is a great advantage.

Despite these facts, the RAST remains a test which is only carried out, in most cases, after the skin tests and when these give dubious responses. For this reason, requests for RAST are usually restricted to one or two allergens, in order to settle diagnostic uncertainties, and are always founded on accurate anamnesis.

Nevertheless, it must be pointed out that the RAST may be positive even in the absence of allergic symptoms: these are usually cases of recently occurring sensitization which is not yet clinically evident [12, 13].

The RAST is preferred to the skin test only when the latter cannot be carried out due to existing treatment, when the skin is altered because of a common disease or presents marked dermographism, or in the case of children.

Many allergens are used in the RAST technique but are, however, less numerous than those employed in skin tests, due to the difficulty, in some cases, of fixing them to the support.

Concerning the interpretation of the results, there is usually a good correlation between the clinical data and the RAST data in cases of pollens and mites, but the same cannot be said for food. The reason for this may be found in the poor purity of the allergens and in the probable involvement, in food allergies, of other immunopathological mechanisms which are not IgE-mediated. The same problem arises in regard to drugs.

With the same technical principle employed for the RAST, it is possible to dose the total serum IgE (paper radioimmunosorbent test, PRIST), the levels of which are usually increased in the allergic asthmatic subject (200 IU/ml in the adult, 1 IU = 2.4 ng). Nevertheless, at a clinical level, the quantity and the quality of the specific IgE assumes major importance rather than the absolute value of the total ratio of IgE [14] (Fig. 1).

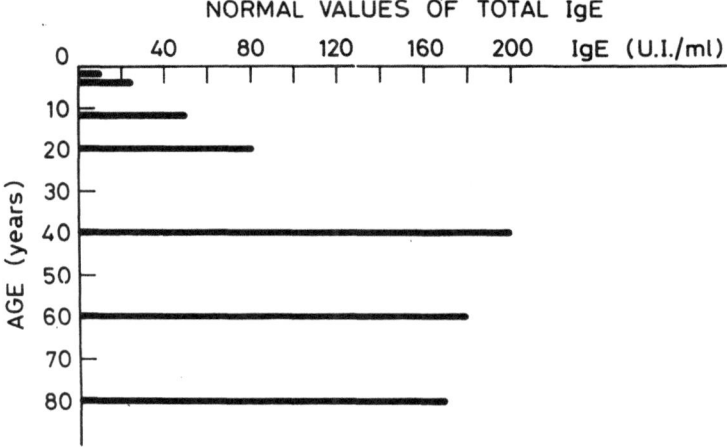

Fig. 1. IgE values in the various periods of life

References

1. D'Amato G (1981) Allergie respiratorie de pollini e da miceti. Lombardo, Roma, pp 231–237
2. Pigatto P, Riva F (1984) Diagnostica allergologica: tests cutanei "in vivo". In: Tassi GC, Sertoli A (eds) Allergologia applicata e immunologia. Pensiero Scientifico, pp 232–247
3. Serafini U (1982) Immunologia ed allergologia clinica. USES 425–435
4. Pepys J, Turner-Warwick M, Dawson PL, Hinson KF (1968) Arthus (type III) skin test reactions in man. Clinical and immunopathological features. Allergology, Excepta Medica, New York, pp 221–235
5. Aas K, Backmann A, Berlin L, Weeke B (1978) Standardization of allergen extracts with appropriate methods. The combined use of skin prick testing and radio-allergosorbent test. Allergy 33:130–137
6. Charpin J (1980) Tests cutanés d'allergie. Allergologie, Flammarion, Paris, pp 288–295
7. Brown HM (1985) Allergologia clinica. Practitioner 82:99–102
8. Norman PS (1978) In vivo methods of study of allergy. In: Middleton E, Reed CE, Ellis EF (eds) Allergy principles and practice, Vol 1. pp 256–264
9. Hannaway P, Hyde JS (1970) Scratch and intradermal skin testing: a comparative study in 250 atopic children. Ann Allergy 28:413–419
10. Voorhorst R, VanKrieken M (1973) Atopic skin test revaluated. II. Variability in results of skin testing done in octuplicate. Ann Allergy 31:195–202
11. Whitcomb N (1971) Incidence of positive skin tests among medical students. Ann Allergy 29:67–70
12. Sorzini MR (1984) Presupposti teorici e applicazioni pratiche del RAST e del PRIST. In: Tassi GC, Sertoli A (eds) Allergologia applicata e immunologia. Pensiero Scientifico, pp 209–231
13. Guerin N, Didierlaurent A, Derer M, Stadler B (1985) Seuil de positivité. Interpretation des résultats du RAST. Rev Franc Allerg 25:189–195
14. Charpin J (1980) Tests biologiques in vitro. Allergologie, Flammarion, Paris, pp 296–307
15. Gleich GJ, Jacob GL (1975) Immunoglobin E antibodies to pollen allergen ac-

count for high percentages of total immunoglobulin E protein. Science 190: 1106–1108
16. Mygind N (1986) Malattie allergiche, vol 1. Momento Medico, Salerno, pp 123–128
17. Aas K (1980) Some variables in skin prick testing. Allergy 35:250–256
18. Lundkvist U (1975) Research and development of the RAST technology. In: Eans R (ed) Advances in diagnosis of allergy: RAST. Medical Book Publisher, Miami, pp 85–99
19. Muiesan P (1982) Pneumologia, UTET, Turin

Allergen Administration in Bronchial Provocation Tests

B. J. O. WONG and F. E. HARGREAVE

Firestone Regional Chest and Allergy Unit, St. Joseph's Hospital, Hamilton, Ontario, Canada

Introduction

Allergen inhalation tests measure the respiratory response to inhaled allergen. The response can be localised to the airways, to the peripheral respiratory tissues or both. In this chapter we will deal only with airway (asthmatic) responses. The materials and methods described in this chapter are those used in our laboratory, however, the principles are generally applicable. Alternative methods are considered in the Discussion.

The first thorough description of the response to inhaled allergen was made by Herxheimer [17] in the 1950s with a description of both early and late asthmatic responses. Altounyan [1] subsequently described that natural exposure to grass pollen during the grass pollen season could also increase airway responsiveness to inhaled histamine in sensitized subjects. This allergen-induced increase in airway responsiveness was subsequently found to occur particularly in people who also had a late asthmatic response (LAR) [3, 6].

The importance of allergens as a cause of asthma and exacerbations was highlighted by their effect on heightening histamine (or methacholine) airway responsiveness. The presence of hyperresponsiveness is a sensitive indicator of abnormal airway function since it is present even when spirometry is normal [30]. The degree of hyperresponsiveness correlates closely with the degree of diurnal variation of peak flow rate (PFR) [30] and less closely with symptoms and treatment requirements [19]. When methacholine hyperresponsiveness is reduced by treatment with inhaled corticosteroid the symptoms of asthma, PFR variability and the need for β_2-agonist becomes less [20, 31].

Allergen inhalation tests have been a valuable research method to investigate the mechanisms and treatment of allergen-induced asthma. However, they are usually not of clinical value today because the diagnosis of allergy can be made from skin tests [16], airway responsiveness to allergen can be predicted from the results of skin tests plus histamine inhalation tests [8], allergen extracts are not standardized, and the tests are time-consuming and can be dangerous if not carefully performed.

Allergen inhalation tests are performed in a dose/response way. Many aspects of the procedure are similar to other inhalation provocation tests to nonsensitizing (nonallergic) stimuli described in this book. Differences include problems with standardization of test extracts, the dependence of the early asthmatic response (EAR) on the severity of the allergic reaction and airway responsiveness to the released mediators like histamine, the different time course of the allergen-stimulated EAR which peaks later, and the frequent occurrence of LAR with the associated prolonged increase in histamine airway responsiveness.

Materials and Methods

The components of allergen inhalation tests include subject selection, identification and selection of the allergen, preparation and storage of the allergen extract, prediction of the dose to cause a fall in FEV_1 of 20% (allergen PC_{20}) and the starting dose of inhaled allergen, confounding factors to be avoided, allergen inhalation, measurement of the response and aspects of safety. While administration of the allergen is central to the test, the other steps are crucial to its success and safety.

Subject Selection

Subjects must be hypersensitive to the allergen as determined by skin tests and should have a history of asthma.

The asthma should be stable and mild. Subjects should not require current treatment with corticosteroid. At the time of testing spirometry should be normal, or near normal (FEV_1 >70% predicted and FEV_1/VC >70%).

Subjects should be able to understand the nature of the test and appreciate that asthma symptoms might become worse for several days after the test.

Identification and Selection of the Allergen

Relevant allergens are identified by a history of symptoms related to exposure and by skin tests with a number of common allergen extracts. The symptoms, which can include cough, chest tightness, wheezing and shortness of breath, can onset soon after exposure or can recur or begin hours after exposure has ceased. They can be prolonged. The description of a late onset or of prolonged symptoms suggests the occurrence of a LAR. An increase in the ease with which symptoms are triggered by nonsensitizing stimuli such as exercise suggests that airway responsiveness to these stimuli has been heightened and airway inflammation has resulted from the allergen exposure [6, 12].

Preparation and Storage of the Allergen Extracts

The term "allergen" refers to an immunologically pure compound that specifically reacts with IgE. The term allergen extract refers to a complex antigenic mixture from a common source and with the same properties as allergens [24]. The potency of allergen extracts can be compared to an international standard (IS) developed by the International Union of Immunological Societies [23]. Different preparations of the same allergen extract contain different concentrations of antigenic proteins and different ratios of individual allergens. If several inhalation tests are to be performed for comparison then a sufficient quantity of the preparation must be available for each test at the time of the first test. Potentially different preparations of the same allergen extract could be used with reference to the IS to ensure the same potency of allergen is administered. However, this allows for increased error in administration and interpretation of results and is not recommended. Highly purified allergen is available for a number of allergens, e.g. Dac g 1, Amb a 1, Der P 1 for grass, ragweed and house dust mite allergen, respectively. When these are available the difficulty with variation in potency of crude extracts can be avoided.

Crude allergen extracts and purified allergen degrade with time. The degradation can be reduced by storage at $4\,^\circ C$ or $-20\,^\circ C$. One approach to storage when several inhalation tests with the same allergen extract are to be performed in the same person is to divide the extract into several aliquots of appropriate volume and to store them at $-20\,^\circ C$. Each aliquot can then be thawed separately and prepared for each test to avoid repeated thawing of extracts.

Doubling dilutions of the allergen extract are made using a sterile technique for both skin and inhalation tests. For skin tests we use serial doubling dilutions to 1:8196. For allergen inhalation, five serial doubling dilutions are made available initially, with the most dilute preparation being the predicted starting dose for inhalation (see below).

The diluent we use is phosphate buffered saline. The dilutions are used immediately or stored at $4\,^\circ C$ for up to an arbitrary maximum of 24 h before use.

Prediction of Allergen PC_{20} and Starting Dose

The method we use to predict the allergen PC_{20} has been investigated and described by Cockcroft et al. [8], and is supported by other studies [2, 9]. Prediction of the dose of allergen to cause an early fall in FEV_1 of 20% is made from skin tests using serial dilutions of allergen extract and from the histamine PC_{20} using a previously determined regression equation [8]. These tests should be performed on the day before, or a few days before, the allergen inhalation test. The histamine PC_{20} is measured by the method described by Cockcroft et al. [5] and brought up to date by Juniper et al. [21]. The skin prick tests are performed with serial dilutions of allergen to determine the allergen concentration which causes a mean wheal of 2 mm diameter. Our technique is as follows:

1. On the clean anterior surface of the forearm two rows of skin prick tests are performed with the serial dilutions of allergen extract and diluent control.

2. The direction of increasing dilutions for the two rows of prick tests are performed in opposite directions, to minimise the effect of arm location of the test on wheal size.

3. A drop of each dilution is placed and the keratinous layer of the skin is lifted using a fresh sterile 25 gauge needle. A new needle is used for each dilution.

4. After 10 min each wheal is measured in two perpendicular directions. Therefore, for each dilution, four measurements are made. The mean wheal size produced by the saline control is subtracted from the mean wheal produced by allergen diluent to give the wheal produced by allergen alone.

5. The most dilute extract to cause a 2 mm wheal is then used to calculate the allergen PC_{20} from the equation:

$$\log \text{allergen } PC_{20} = 0.68 \times \log (SS_{2 \text{ mm}} \times \text{histamine } PC_{20})$$

where $SS_{2 \text{ mm}}$ is the allergen concentration causing a 2 mm skin wheal and PC_{20} is the provocative concentration causing a 20% fall in FEV_1 (Table 1).

The calculation provides a rough guide. *To be safe the usual starting concentration for inhalation should be three doubling dilutions below the predicted allergen PC_{20}*, e.g. in the example of Table 1, a starting dilution of 1:64 would be used.

Table 1. Sample calculation of allergen PC_{20}

Dilution causing mean wheal of 2 mm	$= 1 : 128$
Histamine PC_{20}	$= 4.0$ mg/ml
Log allergen PC_{20} $= 0.68 \times \log (1/128 \times 4.0)$	
$= 0.68 \times \log (0.03125)$	
$= 0.68 \times (-3.4657)$	
$= -2.3567$	
Allergen PC_{20} $= $ antilog (-2.3567)	
$= 0.094732$	
or allergen dilution factor $1/0.094732 = 10.556$	

An allergen dilution of 1:120 or 1:8 could be expected to produce a 20% fall in FEV_1 immediately after administration.

Confounding Factors

Before commencing the inhalation test, subjects should be told to avoid factors which can cause either bronchodilatation or bronchoconstriction which are extraneous to the study. Certain asthma and hayfever medications affect the responses to allergen and therefore should be withheld for their duration of action before the test [15]. Some examples of recommended times are as follows: Inhaled short-acting β_2-agonists 8 h, ingested short acting β_2-agonists 12 h, inhaled anticholinergics 12 h, theophylline 24 h, slow release theophylline 48 h, antihistamines (except astemizole) 4 days, astemizole 6 weeks.

Bronchoconstricting stimuli to avoid include cold air and strenuous exercise. Patients should be told not to rush to the laboratory before the test and, if it is cold outside, to wrap a scarf over the nose and mouth and to limit any time outside to a minimum.

Patients should not be currently exposed to allergens to which they are allergic (except the dust mite) since this will interfere with the interpretation of results. For example, allergen inhalation tests should not be performed during the pollen season in pollen sensitive subjects.

Factors which stimulate pulmonary inflammation such as smoking, should be avoided for the entire testing period. Tests should not be performed within 4 weeks of a respiratory infection.

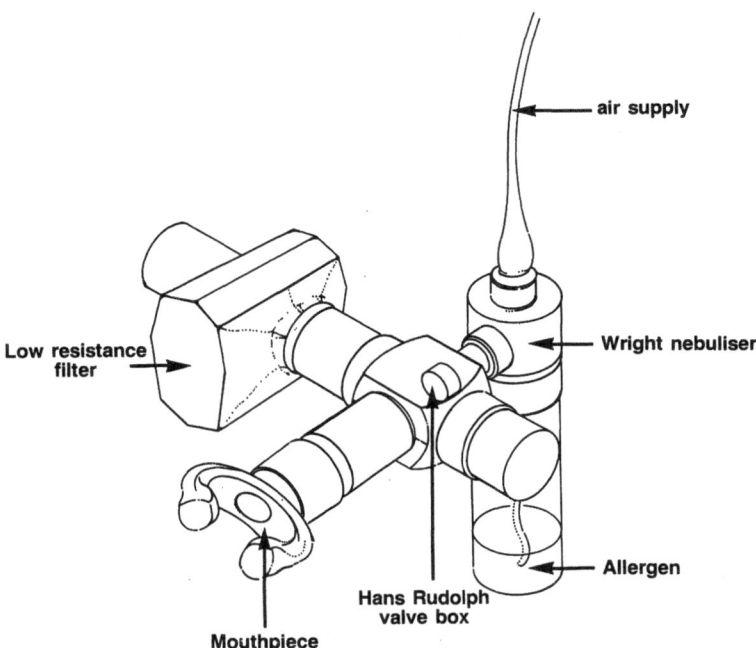

Fig. 1. Apparatus for allergen inhalation

Allergen Inhalation

The methods of aerosol generation and inhalation are described elsewhere in this volume. The crucial aspects are the accurate and reliable delivery of each allergen concentration in a reproducible manner.

The equipment used in our laboratory is for a tidal breathing technique [13, 21]. Nebulisation of the allergen extract is achieved with an English Wright nebuliser connected to a Hans Rudolph inspiratory/expiratory valve box plus mouthpiece (Fig. 1). A low resistance absorption filter is attached to the expiratory port of the valve box. A minimum of 3 ml of solution is added to the nebuliser to ensure that a consistent output is achieved over 2 min. The nebulizer is operated with dry air or oxygen at the flow rate required to give an output of 0.13 ml/min. The patient sits inside a chamber equipped with an exhaust system vented outside. The filter and exhaust chamber prevent others in the laboratory from exposure.

Inhalation Test Procedure

The procedure is shown in Fig. 2.

1. On arrival in the laboratory the subject rests for at least 15 min. During this time a questionnaire is completed concerning confounding factors and the severity and stability of the asthma.

2. Baseline VC is measured at intervals of 1 min, three times or until it is reproducible within 5%. Then the FEV_1 is measured, similarly. The best, mean or lowest value can be used for analysis, as long as this is decided before the start of the study. In addition, PFR is measured three times for comparison with further measurements after going home after the test; this is further discussed below.

3. On the first day, a control inhalation of the diluent of the allergen extract, usually phosphate buffered saline, is inhaled for 2 min, three times at intervals of 10 min. The control inhalation is required to investigate the possibility of any nonspecific airway constriction in the first hour and to document any diurnal variation of FEV_1, giving information which is required to interpret allergen-stimulated EAR and LAR.

4. Allergen inhalation is performed on the next day, or within a few days, beginning with three twofold dilutions below the concentration predicted to give a fall in FEV_1 of 20%. The extract is discarded after use. The subject is instructed to remove the mouthpiece if symptoms (e.g. cough, chest tightness, dyspnea) occur and is kept under continuous observation, to ensure that aerosol generation and inhalation are optimum and to detect and act on any adverse event.

5. The effect of each inhalation is measured by FEV_1 after 10 min. The FEV_1 is performed only once, unless it is technically poor when the best of the two measurements is used for analysis.

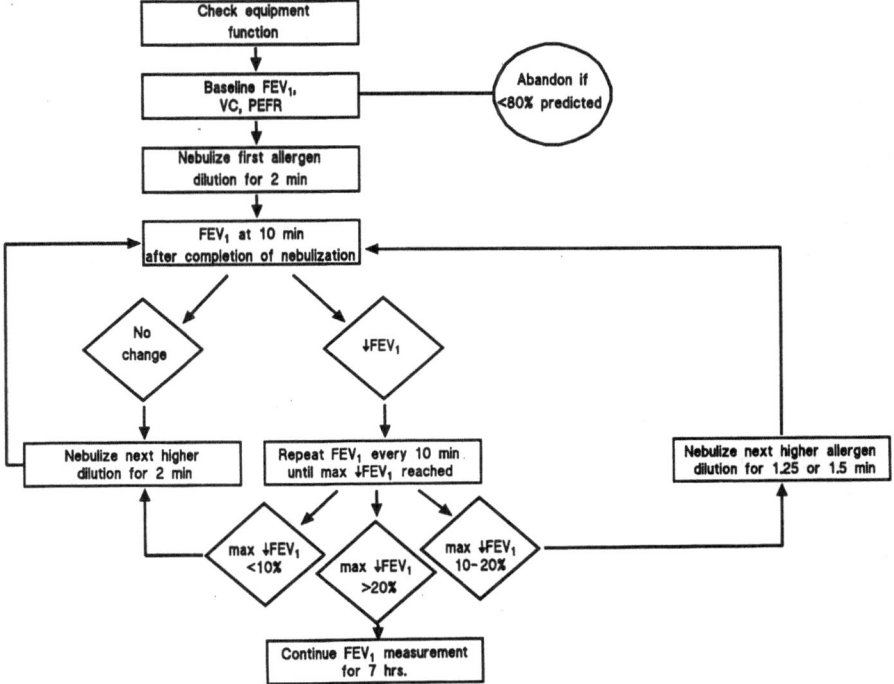

Fig. 2. Allergen administration procedure

- If there is no change in the FEV_1, the allergen concentration is increased twofold and inhaled for 2 min.
- If the FEV_1 falls by $\geq 5\%$, the measurement is repeated at intervals of 10 min until it is no longer falling. If the maximum fall is less than 10% the next twofold increase in allergen concentration is inhaled for 2 min.
- If the maximum fall in FEV_1 is between 10% and 20% then administering the next higher allergen concentration for 2 min could cause an exaggerated EAR. For safety, the next higher concentration is therefore inhaled for 1 min 15 s or 1 min 30 s.
- Once the fall in FEV_1 is $\geq 20\%$ below baseline, no further inhalations are given.

6. Subsequent measurements of FEV_1, are made at 10, 20, 30, 45 and 60 min then at hourly intervals for 7 or 8 h.

7. At 7 or 8 h, any reduction in FEV_1 is treated with inhaled β_2-agonist and the measurement is repeated after 10 min. If this value is $\geq 80\%$ of baseline, the subject can be sent home. If the value is $<80\%$, consideration should be given to keeping the subject under supervision and/or starting treatment with inhaled or ingested corticosteroid according to severity.

Treatment with inhaled corticosteroid can also be considered to reverse mild late effects more quickly if it will not interfere with subsequent studies.

8. When the subject goes home, instructions must be given as to when, who and where to call for advice based on PFR and need for β_2-agonist use.

9. Other tests will depend on the aims of the study, e.g., histamine PC_{20} can be measured 24 h or more after allergen inhalation.

10. The results are best illustrated by a graphical plot of percentage change in FEV_1, compared to baseline, with a plot of the effects of the control inhalation on the same graph (Fig. 3).

Repeat Allergen Inhalation Tests

If more than one allergen inhalation test is to be performed on the same subject during the course of a study, care must be taken to ensure the measurements have returned to baseline before repeat tests are performed. Specifically, the FEV_1, should be within 10 % and histamine PC_{20} should be within one doubling concentration of baseline of the first test. Often 2 weeks or longer are necessary for these to occur if the patient is untreated.

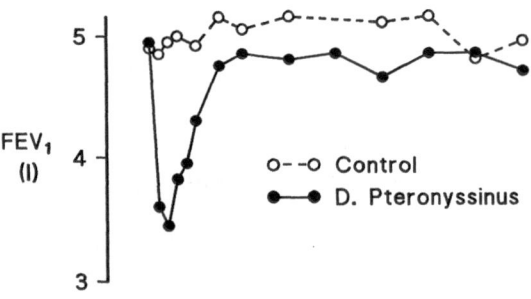

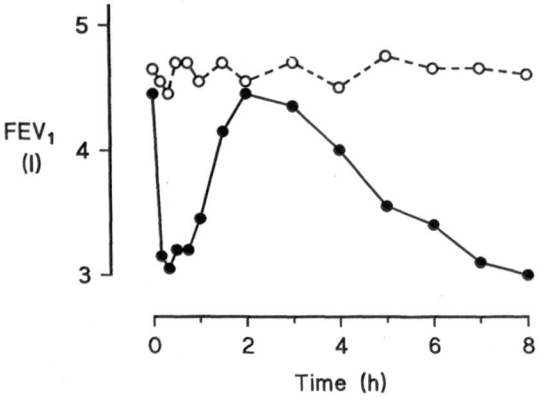

Fig. 3. An isolated early asthmatic response after inhalation of dust mite extract (*D. pteronyssinus*) (*upper panel*). An early followed by a late asthmatic response after inhalation of house dust mite (*lower panel*). The control mesurements (*open circles*) are made after inhalation of the diluent alone. The measurements made after allergen inhalation (*closed circles*) are made at the same time points as the control measurements. (From [27])

At each repeat challenge only the final three allergen dilutions used in the initial test are required. The test is performed by sequentially administering these three dilutions as described above. The test is terminated if a 20% fall in FEV_1 is achieved or the final dose determined previously has been given, whichever occurs first.

If a higher final concentration of allergen than previously determined is required to cause an EAR then there is the possibility of a more severe late response [14, 22]. This situation might arise when investigating the effect of medications on allergen PC_{20}.

Safety Aspects

Allergen challenge tests are safe if care is taken to ensure the amount of allergen inhaled is carefully titrated. The potential exists for creating a dramatic EAR and/or an unexpectedly severe LAR. A physician who understands the test procedure and is skilled in resuscitation should therefore always be in attendance during allergen inhalation and the EAR, and readily available during the LAR. Appropriate resuscitation equipment should be available including a fully equipped "crash cart" with a loaded syringe of 1 ml 1:1000 epinephrine and β_2-agonist inhalers.

Care must be taken to avoid contact with the allergen by laboratory personnel, particularly if they are known to be sensitive to the allergen. Allergen inhalation in a chamber vented to the outside and an absorption filter on the expiratory port of the Hans Rudolph valve minimises this problem. Allergen should not contaminate of the outside of the nebuliser as this can cause superficial reactions in the subject. Disposal of allergen extract should be performed carefully to eliminate accidental exposure of either laboratory personnel or test subjects [18].

Results

Allergen inhalation can elicit three types of response, an EAR, a LAR and an increase in airway responsiveness to histamine (or other nonsensitizing stimuli) [27].

The EAR begins within 10 min after allergen inhalation, reaches a maximum within 30 min, and generally resolves spontaneously within 1–3 h (Fig. 3 upper panel).

The LAR begins 3–4 h after allergen inhalation, reaches a maximum during the next few hours (Fig. 3 lower panel), and reverses over 24–48 h or so depending upon its severity. The LAR is considered to be definite if there is a fall in FEV_1 of $\geq 15\%$, and possible if the fall in FEV_1 is between 5%–15% [3]. Approximately 50% of randomly selected subjects who have an EAR go on to develop a LAR. Occasionally, the LAR is not preceded by a clinically evident EAR, this is called an isolated LAR.

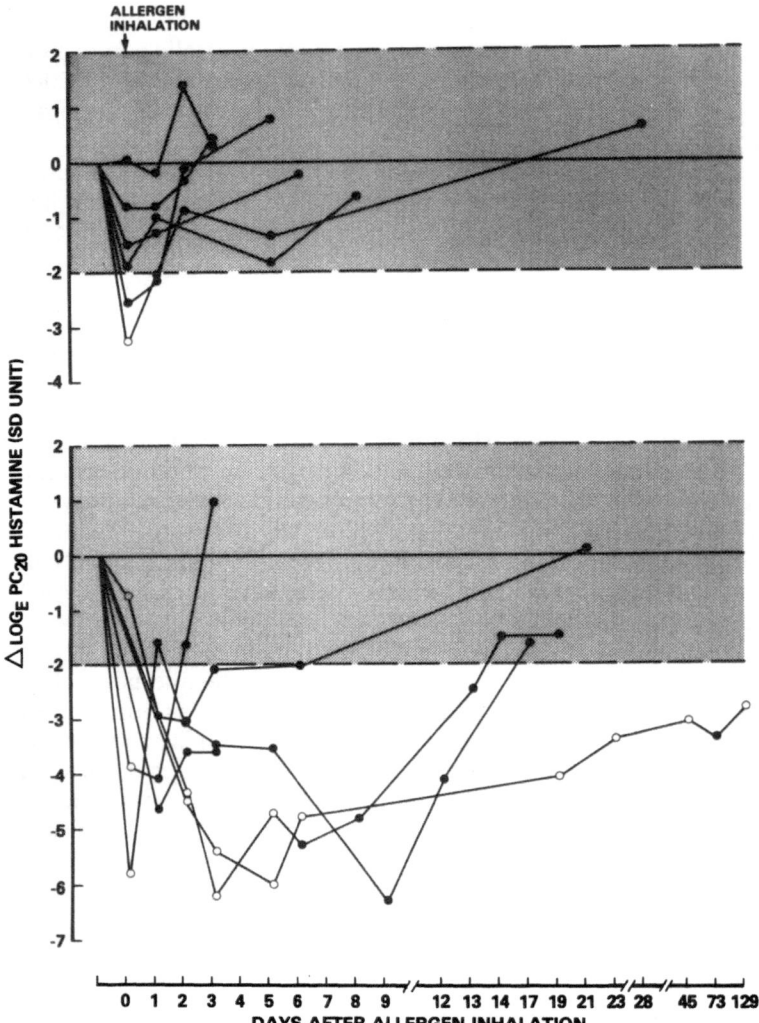

Fig. 4. Changes in the provocation concentration of histamine causing a 20% fall in FEV_1 (PC_{20} histamine) after allergen inhalation tests (expressed as the mean preallergen PC_{20}/postallergen PC_{20}). *Upper panel* gives values for subjects with an equivocal allergen-induced late asthmatic response, i.e., a fall in FEV_1 of less than 14% between 3 and 8 h. Lower panel gives values for subjects with a definite allergen-induced late asthmatic response, i.e., a fall in FEV_1 of greater than 14% between 3 and 8 h. Shaded areas indicate the normal range of variability in PC_{20} histamine in the control period, expressed as log units of the pooled within-subject standard deviation. Open circles are measurements when FEV_1 was more than 10% below preallergen inhalation baseline values. Closed circles are measurements when FEV_1 was within 10% of preallergen inhalation baseline values. (From [3])

The increase in histamine (or methacholine) airway responsiveness after allergen challenge starts as early as 2–3 h after the last dose of allergen [7, 10] and can, unless treated, last for several days or weeks (Fig. 4). It can be conveniently measured 24 h or more after allergen inhalation. It is usually associated with a LAR; however, the LAR and increase in airway responsiveness can occur independently after allergen inhalation [3, 6, 22]. Both the LAR and prolonged increase in airway responsiveness are a result of airway inflammation [25, 27]. However, the LAR has other determinants and the prolonged increase in airway responsiveness is probably a more sensitive indicator of the inflammation [12].

Discussion

The subject selection, methods and study design can be modified according to the objectives of the study. A control inhalation test is essential for the accurate interpretation of the different responses. Good reproducibility of allergen responses is possible providing that confounding factors are regulated, baseline subject characteristics are similar and technical aspects of aerosol generation and inhalation are standardized between tests [11, 28, 29]. Ideally, the reproducibility should be investigated in the study.

A commonly used method to determine the starting dose of allergen extract for inhalation is to start allergen inhalation with a suitably low concentration of allergen. This can be determined from prick tests with dilutions of the allergen to be used for inhalation; the starting concentration being the weakest to cause a wheal of 2 mm [15].

Other methods of aerosol generation and inhalation of allergen extract than continuous generation and tidal breathing can be used, such as the dosimeter method [4], providing that the technical factors required to give a reproducible dose are regulated. Allergen extract can also be inhaled as a powder with a spinhaler [26].

Acknowledgement. We would like to acknowledge Mrs. Laurie Whitely for her excellent secretarial assistance.

References

1. Altounyan REC (1970) Changes in histamine and atropine responsiveness as a guide to diagnosis and evaluation of therapy in obstructive airways disease. In: Pepys J, Frandland AW (eds) Disodium cromoglycate in allergic airways disease. Butterworth, London, pp 47–53
2. Bryant DH, Burns MW (1976) Bronchial histamine reactivity: its relationship to reactivity of the bronchi to allergens. Clin Allergy 6:523–532.
3. Cartier A, Thomson NC, Frith PA, Roberts R, Hargreave FE (1982) Allergen-induced increase in bronchial responsiveness to histamine: relationship to the late

asthmatic response and change in airway caliber. J Allergy Clin Immunol 70: 170–177
4. Chai H, Farr RS, Froehlich LA, Mathison DA, McLean JA, Rosenthal RR, Sheffer AL, Spector SI, Townley RG (1975) Standardization of bronchial inhalation challenge procedures. J Allergy Clin Immunol 56:323–327
5. Cockcroft DW, Killian DN, Mellon JJA, Hargreave FE (1977) Bronchial reactivity to inhaled histamine: a method and clinical survey. Clin Allergy 7:235–243
6. Cockcroft DW, Ruffin RE, Dolovich J, Hargreave FE (1977) Allergen-induced increase in non-allergic bronchial reactivity. Clin Allergy 7:503–513
7. Cockcroft DW, Murdock KY (1987) Changes in bronchial responsiveness to histamine at intervals after allergen challenge. Thorax 42:302–308
8. Cockcroft DW, Murdock KY, Kirby J, Hargreave F (1987) Prediction of airway responsiveness to allergen from skin sensitivity to allergen and airway responsiveness to histamine. Am Rev Respir Dis 135:264–267
9. Crimi E, Brusasco V, Losurdo E, Crimi P (1986) Predictive accuracy of late asthmatic reaction to dermatophagoides pteronyssinus. J Allergy Clin Immunol 78: 908–913
10. Durham SR, Craddock CF, Cookson WO, Benson MK (1988) Increases in airway responsiveness to histamine precede allergen-induced late asthmatic responses. J Allergy Clin Immunol 82:764–770
11. Frith PA, Ruffin RE, Juniper EF, Dolovich J, Hargreave FE (1981) Inhibition of allergen-induced asthma by three forms of sodium cromoglycate. Clin Allergy 11:67–77
12. Gibson PG, Manning PJ, O'Byrne PM, Girgis-Gabardo A, Dolovich J, Denburg JA, Hargreave FE (1991) Allergen induced asthmatic responses: relationship between increases in airway responsiveness and increases in circulating eosinophils, basophils and their progenitors. Am Rev Respir Dis 1991; 143:331–335
13. Hargreave FE (1987) Inhalation provocation tests. In: Lessof MH, Lee TH, Kemeny DM (eds) Allergy: an international textbook. Wiley, Chichester, pp 289–303
14. Hargreave FE, Dolovich J, Robertson DG, Kerigan AT (1974) II. The late asthmatic responses. Can Med Assoc J 110:415–424
15. Hargreave FE, Fink JN, Cockcroft DW, Fish JE, Holgate ST, Ramsdale EH, Roberts RS, Shapiro GG, Sheppard D (1986) Workshop 4: the role of bronchoprovocation. J Allergy Clin Immunol 78:517–524
16. Hargreave FE, Marone G, Platts-Mills T (1989) Diagnostic procedures. In: Holgate ST (ed) The role of inflammatory processes in airway hyperresponsiveness. Blackwell, Oxford, pp 80–107
17. Herxheimer H (1952) The late bronchial reaction in induced asthma. Int Arch Allergy 3:323–328
18. Hoeppner VH, Murdock KY, Kooner S, Cockcroft DW (1985) Severe acute occupational asthma: caused by accidental allergen exposure in an allergen challenge laboratory. Ann Allergy 55 (1):36–37
19. Juniper EF, Frith PA, Hargreave FE (1981) Airway responsiveness to histamine and methacholine: relationship to minimum treatment to control symptoms of asthma. Thorax 36:575–579
20. Juniper EF, Kline PA, Vanzieleghem MA, Ramsdale EH, O'Byrne PM, Hargreave FE (1990) Effect of long-term treatment with an inhaled corticosteroid (budesonide) on airway hyperresponsiveness and clinical asthma in nonsteroid-dependent asthmatics. Am Rev Respir Dis 142:832–836
21. Juniper EF, Cockcroft DW, Hargreave FE (1991) Histamine and methacholine inhalation tests: a laboratory tidal breathing protocol. AB DRACO (subsidiary of ABASTRA) Lund, Sweden 1991
22. Lai CKW, Twentyman OP, Holgate ST (1989) The effect of an increase in inhaled allergen dose after rimiterol hydrobromide on the occurrence and magnitude of the late asthmatic response and associated change in nonspecific bronchial responsiveness. Am Rev Respir Dis 140:917–923

23. Lowenstein H (1983) Report on behalf of the International Union Standardization Subcommittee. Arb Paul Ehrlich Inst 78:41–48
24. Lowenstein H, Ipsen H, Lind P, Matthiesen F (1987) The physicochemical and biological characteristics of allergens. In: Lessof MH, Lee TH, Kemeny DM (eds) Allergy: an international textbook. Wiley, Chichester, pp 87–104
25. Machado L, Stalenheim G (1990) Factors influencing the occurrence of late bronchial reactions after allergen challenge. Allergy 45 (4):268–274
26. Melillo G (1986) Bronchial Challenge with a micronized, freeze-dried allergen extract administered as a powder by a special turboinhaler. In: Melillo G, Cocco G, Centanni G (eds) XIIIth congress on of the European academy of allergology and clinical immunology – workshop on "The use of allergen in powder form for provocation tests and for immunotherapy in allergic asthma", pp 3–14
27. O'Byrne PM, Dolovich J, Hargreave FE (1987) Late asthmatic responses. Am Rev Respir Dis 136:740–751
28. Pepys J, Hargreave FE, Chan M, McCarthy DS (1968) Inhibitory effects of disodium cromoglycate (Intal) on allergen inhalation tests. Lancet ii:134
29. Ruffin RE, Cockcroft DW, Hargreave FE (1978) A comparison of the protective effect of fenoterol and Sch1000 on allergen-induced asthma. J Allergy Clin Immunol 61:42–47
30. Ryan G, Latimer KM, Dolovich J, Hargreave FE (1982) Bronchial responsiveness to histamine: relationship to diurnal variation of peak flow rate, improvement after bronchodilator and airway calibre. Thorax 37:423–429
31. Woolcock AJ, Yan K, Salome CM (1988) Effect of therapy on bronchial hyperresponsiveness in the long-term management of asthma. Clin Allergy 18:165–176

Part V

Nonspecific Bronchial Challenges

Radiogas and Radioaerosol Production, Imaging, and Dosimetry in Asthmology

P. Gerundini, R. Benti, and A. Bruno

Department of Nuclear Medicine, IRCCS, Ospedale Maggiore, Milan, Italy

Introduction

Using imaging techniques nuclear medicine studies the function of different organs and systems. When introduced in to a live organism, a radioactive chemical species with specific biological properties has a metabolic fate similar or identical to the same "cold" (nonradioactive) chemical agent. For example, the radioisotope of iodine, iodine-131 (^{131}I), when administered orally in humans, is extracted from the intestine with the same efficiency as the cold iodine contained in food. Like dietary iodine, the radioactive ^{131}I, after being concentrated from the blood in the thyroid and conjugated with thyroxine, also enters into the synthetic pathways of thyroid hormones. Due to these characteristics, a picomolar quantity of administered radioiodine allows "tracing" of the metabolic behavior of the total cold iodine contained in the thyroid. Therefore, it may be considered a tracer of thyroid metabolism of iodine.

In a biopsy specimen of the thyroid, it is possible to measure the absolute content of ^{131}I and correlate it with the efficiency of metabolism of the cold iodine in thyrocytes. This invasive sampling of an organ to measure a certain metabolic activity may be substituted by measuring, with external detectors, the radioactive decay of the tracer, obtaining a reliable estimate of several functions of the organ under investigation.

This simplification leads from quantitative or absolute estimates of a certain function to relative ones. The absence of invasiveness, though, and the possibility of serial measurements has favored the practical introduction of these imaging procedures in clinical nuclear medicine.

This approach to functional imaging also offers definite advantages in the evaluation of many lung diseases. Pulmonary functions can be studied separately by using different tracers. For example, lung perfusion and ventilation can be separately evaluated in the same clinical situation using two different radioactive tracers. Similarly, the activity of bronchial ciliated cells and the permeability of the alveolar epithelium can be assessed noninvasively before and after therapeutic interventions. The physiopathology of several pulmonary diseases can also be clarified by measuring the volumes of the vascular and extravascular lung spaces or the alveolar surfactant production-related uptake in the lung of lipophilic substances.

The selection of the proper radioactive tracer is of crucial importance in the clinical applications of nuclear medicine. The characteristics of an ideal tracer can be summarized as follows:

1. Metabolic behavior (i.e., chemical properties) identical or similar to that of the cold (nonradioactive) species in the organism.

2. Use of the smallest amount of radioactive substance administered to avoid interference with the selected metabolic pathway being studied and unnecessary irradiation of the patient.

3. No toxicity or pharmacologic activity.

4. Easy and stable conjugation with a proper radioactive isotope, if the selected substance does not have a natural radioactive decay. These cold substances suitable for labeling with a proper radioactive element are also called radiopharmaceuticals.

5. Easy measurement of the radioactive decay in the target organ with external detectors (imaging) for its morphofunctional assessment.

Many of these properties can be found in the first radioactive species used in diagnostic pulmonary nuclear medicine. In 1955 the inhalation of the noble radiogas, xenon-133 (^{133}Xe), was suggested in the early diagnosis of bronchial carcinoma to evaluate the impairment of regional ventilation, caused by bronchial stenosis or pleural thickening, by measuring ^{133}Xe radioactive decay over the chest wall by detectors. An insoluble radiogas such as ^{133}Xe, if administered intravenously, can be used to assess pulmonary blood flow because its low solubility allows the passage of more than 95% of the tracer from the blood into the alveolar spaces, thus being distributed proportionally to the capillary blood flow. Regional perfusion can be assessed diagnostically by measurement of its distribution in the lungs by detectors (Fig. 1).

Other soluble radiogases such as oxygen-15 (^{15}O), carbon-11 (^{11}C) dioxide, and carbon (^{11}C) monoxide have been used to determine regional venti-

Fig. 1. A–F. Radiopharmaceuticals for diagnostic lung imaging: Time-activity curves ▶ (TAC) after administration. **A** TAC from normoperfused (A) and hypoperfused (B) lung regions after i.v. injection of ^{99m}Tc-labeled particles. The distribution of the tracer is reduced in hypoperfused areas. **B** TAC from normal (A) and pathological lung regions with impaired Q and/or V (B, C and D) after i.v. administration of ^{133}Xe. **C** TAC from normoventilated (A) and hypoventilated (B) regions after ^{133}Xe inhalation. Radiogas penetration and clearance rate are both reduced in hypoventilated areas. **D** TAC from normoventilated (A) and hypoventilated (B) regions after ^{81m}Kr inhalation. Radiogas penetration only is reduced in hypoventilated areas. **E** TAC from regions with normal (A) and abnormal (B) lung epithelial permeability (LEP) after inhalation of small sized (MMAD <1.5 μm) idrosoluble DTPA radioaerosols. The alveolar damage increases the lung clearance rate of the inhaled radioaerosols (shorter half-life). **F** TAC from regions with normal (A) and reduced (B) muco-ciliary clearance (MCC) after inhalation of small sized (MMAD 4–8 μm) nonidrosoluble particulated radioaerosols. The reduced clearance rate of bronchial secretions proportionally decreases the lung clearance rate of the inhaled radioaerosols (longer half-life)

lation after inhalation. The subsequent rate of removal of soluble radiogases from the alveoli (wash out) can reflect the entity of regional pulmonary blood flow, because a soluble gas rapidly diffuses through the alveolo-capillary membrane and is dissolved in the blood. Unfortunately these ideal soluble gases have very short half-lives (very rapid decay) and are impractical for diagnostic purposes, requiring an in-house cyclotron unit for their produc-

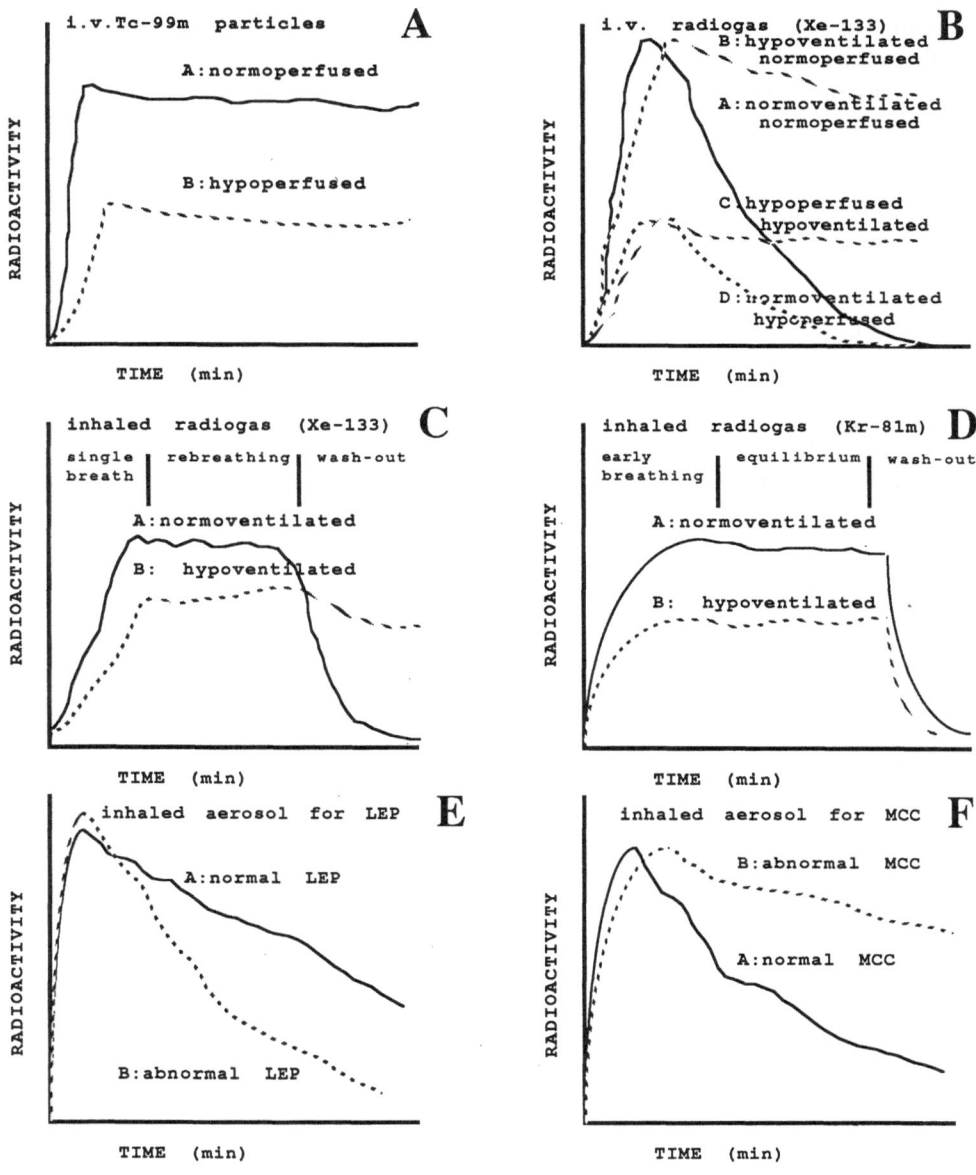

tion and a dedicated camera for the detection of positron emission. In spite of this, these soluble radiogases can be used in quantifying several lung functions for research purposes.

There have been striking improvements in the performance of nuclear medicine detectors and computers, and the use of nuclear imaging in many pulmonary diseases has largely benefited from those made to the γ-camera. This device allows one not only to detect (measure) with good approximation the regional distribution of a tracer in the lungs, as in earlier scanning with probe detectors, but also to assess both perfusion and ventilation in single pulmonary segments. Thus, if not otherwise specified, the clinical applications described below should be considered as being obtained with a γ-camera.

The principal element of a γ-camera is a large sodium iodine (NaI) crystal with thallium impurities in the crystalline reticule (Fig. 2). When a γ-ray emitted from the studied organ is absorbed in a region of the crystal, these impurities allow conversion of the high energy incident photon to a low energy visible photon (scintillation phenomenon) that is recorded and amplified by a group of photomultipliers positioned close to the crystal. This way the resultant photon energy from each scintillation is converted into a discrete electron flux (electronic signal) proportional to the original energy of the incident photon. The electric signals of the photomultipliers are then collected into the electronic components of the γ-camera, measured, and stored in a computer and/or displayed in a persistence video screen. The entire procedure takes less than 20 ns and allows, with the crystal of the γ-camera, lo-

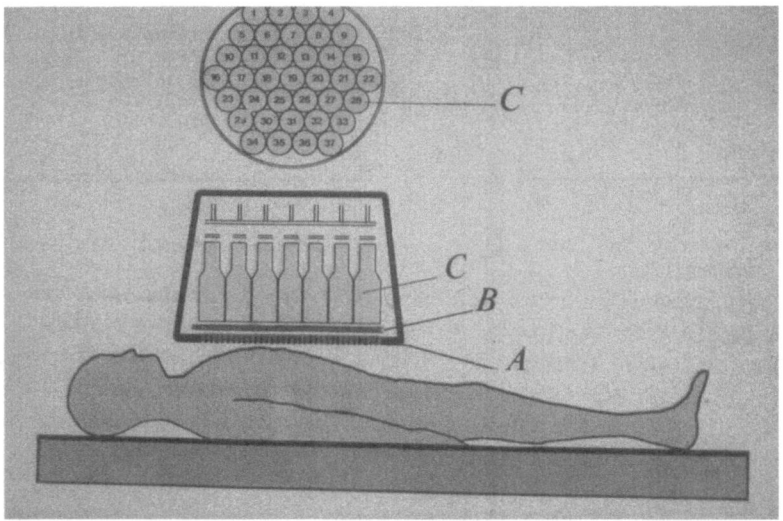

Fig. 2. The γ-camera. *A*, the collimator; *B*, the crystal (NaI detector); and *C*, the photomultipliers

calization of the spatial coordinates and measurement of the energy of each incident photon. For each projection, the measurement of a large number of photons from a radioactive source organ takes a few minutes to obtain an image of the regional distribution of the tracer. For example the entire pulmonary system can be imaged in less than 30 min with minimal discomfort to the patient.

Physical Properties of Radionuclide Decay

The majority of the chemical elements of a living organism, such as carbon, oxygen, nitrogen, calcium, phosphorus and hydrogen, have a stable nuclear configuration because of a balance between nuclear protons and neutrons. This nuclear energetic balance is stabilized by the electron cloud surrounding the nucleus, which determines the chemical properties of each atom and its electric charge. The changes in energetic state of the whole stable atom depend almost completely on the changes in the charge of the electronic cloud. The rare exceptions to this situation are the "unstable" atoms, quite similar in external charge and chemical properties to the stable element, but different in atomic weight (lower or higher).

The atomic weight is assumed to be the weight of the nucleus, i.e., proportional to the total number of protons and neutrons. The number of protons is the same for each atom of an element. For example, all the isotopes of iodine have 53 protons. However, the number of neutrons in the nucleus can vary, changing the nuclear weight, either higher than the stable isotope weight in "neutron rich" atoms or lower in "neutron poor" unstable atoms. This neutron imbalance, in these very few atoms with an unstable energetic status of the nucleus, causes the atom to try and lose (or gain) neutrons and thus convert to a stable isotope. This result can be obtained through two main pathways: by an isobaric or an isomeric transition of nuclear energy (Table 1). An isobaric transition implies a small change of nuclear mass following the decay; the result is a change of the chemical properties of the element and the emission of a large amount of energy during the decay. An iso-

Table 1. Physical properties of radionuclides

Radioactive atom	Energetic transitions	Type of decay	Type of emitted radiation
Unstable nucleus	Isobaric transitions Neutron "poor" nucleus Neutron "rich" nucleus	Positron emission or electron capture Electron emission	β^+ (positron) X-rays (photons) β^- (electron)
	Isomeric Transitions Neutron "balanced" nucleus	Internal conversion or metastable conversion	X-rays (photons) γ-rays (photons)

meric transition of nuclear energy is obtained by photonic emissions only, without changing the chemical properties of the element following the radioactive decay. If the unstable nucleus is "neutron poor" a proton can be converted into the lacking neutron. This phenomenon releases energy with the resulting emission of a positron, a particle with the same mass as an electron. The positron is an antimatter positively charged particle that is attracted after a variable pathway by the negative charge of an electron. The contact of the two particles results in their annihilation, which is the complete conversion of their mass into two highly energetic photons (511 keV) that originate from the annihilation site and leave it at 180° from each other. The annihilation site of a positron with the electron can be determined exactly in living organisms by measuring the two photonic emissions with a positron emission tomograph.

The conversion of a proton in a neutron into a neutron poor nucleus is also possible by the nuclear capture of an orbiting electron. This situation implies the release of an amount of energy smaller than that in positron emission. The new stable nuclear configuration of the element induces a rearrangement of the electronic cloud with the emission of measurable X-rays of different energies whose total amount equals the excess of energy of the unstable parent nucleus. Conversely, a neutron rich element reaches a stable nuclear status emitting a negatively charged electron with the conversion of a nuclear neutron into a proton.

Another type of unstable atom can convert the excess nuclear energy in a single photonic emission by the nucleus (a γ-ray), whereas the emission of a X-ray is produced by electronic cloud rearrangement. The latter energetic transition transfers the excess of nuclear energy from the inner to the outer electrons which produces the emission of X-rays. All these nuclear phenomena are called "nuclear disintegrations" because a small part of the nuclear mass is converted into irradiated energy. The original unstable element is called the "father" radionuclide and the product of the nuclear disintegration is called a "daughter" element, with different chemical properties but a more stable nuclear configuration.

The first relevant characteristic of a radionuclide is the type of energy emitted during each nuclear disintegration (particulate or photonic) that selects its utility for diagnostic (γ-ray emitters) or therapeutic (particulate emitters) purposes. The radioactive decay is measured in disintegrations per second; the unit is the becquerel (Bq), one disintegration per second. Another unit in which the radioactivity of a source can be practically expressed is the curie (Ci): 1 Ci is the disintegration rate per second of a gram of radium: 3.7×10^{10} disintegrations per second.

The second relevant characteristic of radioactive decay is its half-life, that is the time required for a radioactive source to halve its energetic emission. This ranges from seconds to a few days for the radionuclides suited for clinical applications. Similarly, the rate of decay (λ) of a radioactive isotope (expressed as min^{-1}) is peculiar to each radiotracer and allows assessment of the amount of radioactivity to be administered for imaging.

A group of radioactive γ-emitters, "metastable isotopes," has peculiar diagnostic applications because the disintegration does not change the chemical properties of the father isotope and results in the emission of an unique γ-ray with characteristic energy. One of these metastable tracers is technetium 99m (^{99m}Tc), currently the radioactive element most widely used in clinical nuclear medicine. This radionuclide is easily produced by a generator containing the father isotope molybdenum-99 (^{99}Mo) absorbed in an ionic resin. The ^{99m}Tc obtained by ^{99}Mo disintegration can be periodically washed out by a sterile solution introduced in the generator. The daily "milking" of the generator allows ready availability of ^{99m}Tc with low costs and no shipping problems unlike the majority of the other radioisotopes used in clinical nuclear medicine. Furthermore, the short half-life of ^{99m}Tc ($t_{1/2}$ 6.02 h) and its γ-ray emission (140 keV) are almost ideal for γ-camera measurement.

The preferential use in human studies of radiotracers with photonic emission reduces radiation exposure because only a small fraction of the emitted photon flux is absorbed by vital tissues. By contrast, radiotracers with particulate nuclear emission (electrons) produce maximal irradiation because almost all the energy released from nuclear disintegration is absorbed by vital tissue, with resulting poor detection of the radioactivity by currently used γ-cameras. The administration of a particulate emitter radioisotope is instead suitable for therapy, being the maximal amount of irradiation delivered to the pathologic tissues.

The diagnostic use of a γ-emitter is also conditioned by the energy of its photonic emission. The standard γ-cameras offer the best performance in detecting photons with energies ranging between 80 and 400 keV, and this limits the number of radionuclides for diagnostic nuclear medicine to less than 20 elements. Another limiting factor that precludes the clinical use of a great variety of radionuclides is the cost of production, which is particularly relevant for positron emitters and other cyclotron-produced γ-emitters with especially shelf-lives.

Radiopharmaceuticals in Pulmonary Nuclear Medicine

The major efforts in radiochemistry are being directed to the synthesis of molecules suitable for labeling with selected radionuclides to assess specific pulmonary functions by measurement of their regional distribution and metabolic fate in normal or pathologic lungs. Though none of the current imaging procedures allows precise quantification using γ-cameras, the measurements obtained with these radiopharmaceuticals offer the advantage of low invasiveness, feasibility of repeated evaluations, and possibility to study different pulmonary functions in the same clinical setting, thus providing a clinically useful alternative to other invasive procedures Table 2 lists the principal radionuclide and radiopharmaceuticals used for the assessment of lung function by nuclear imaging techniques.

Table 2. Radiopharmaceuticals and radiation doses in pulmonary imaging

Radio-nuclide	Gamma Emission (keV)	Dose (mCi)	Agent	Administration	SPET imaging	Clinical applications	Radiation dose (mrad/mCi) Lungs	Radiation dose (mrad/mCi) Whole body
99mTc	140	3–5	Particles	i.v. (10–50 μm)	Yes	Perfusion studies	230	<15
99mTc	140	0.3–0.5	DTPA aerosols	Inhalation (<1 μm)	Yes	Ventilation studies	48	<20
					No	LEP measurements		
99mTc	140	0.5–0.8	Graphite aerosols	Inhalation (0.05 μm)	Yes	Ventilation studies	450	<10
99mTc	140	0.5–1	HM-PAO aerosols	Inhalation (<1 μm)	No	LEP measurements	85	<20
99mTc	140	0.5–1	Particulate aerosols	Inhalation (4–10 μm)	No	MC measurements	190	<8
99mTc	140	0.5–0.8	Autologous RBC aerosols	Inhalation (5–6 μm)	No	MC measurements	180	<8
99mTc	140	0.5–2	Pertechnetate aerosols	Inhalation (<1 μm)	No	LEP measurements	25	<20
113mIn	392	0.8–2	Particulate aerosols	Inhalation (<1 μm)	No	Ventilation studies	250	<2
123I	159	4–5	HIPDM	i.v.	No	Alveolar damage	85	<20
133Xe	81	5–10	Gas in saline solution	i.v.	No	Perfusion/ventilation	10	<1
133Xe	81	5–10	Gas single breath	Inhalation	No	Ventilation studies	10	<1
133Xe	81	5–10	Gas rebreath/min	Inhalation	No	Ventilation studies	50	<2
127Xe	170–203	5–10	Gas in saline solution	i.v.	No	Perfusion/ventilation	4	<1
127Xe	170–203	5–10	Gas single breath	Inhalation	No	Ventilation studies	5	<1
127Xe	170–203	5–10	Gas rebreath/min	Inhalation	No	Ventilation studies	20	<2
81mKr	190	5–10	Gas continuous breath/min	Inhalation	Yes	Ventilation studies	2.5	<1
81mKr	190	5–10	Gas in glucose solution/min	i.v.	Yes	Perfusion studies	2	<1

SPET, single photon emission tomography; DTPA, diethylenetriamine pentaacetic acid; HM-PAO, hexa-methyl-propilene-amine-oxime; HIPDM, N,N,N-trimethyl-N´-(2-hydroxy-3-methyl-5[123I]-iodobenzyl)-1,3-propanediamine; RBC, red blood cell; LEP, permeability of alveolar epithelium; MC, mucociliary clearance

Particulate Tracers

The standard technique in clinical applications for the assessment of regional perfusion of the lungs is the i.v. injection of macroaggregates (diameter 10–50 µm) or microspheres (10–30 µm) of heat denatured human albumin labeled with ^{99m}Tc. This type of particle mixes uniformly with the venous blood while passing through the right heart and distributes into the lungs in proportion to the blood flow, being trapped by the pulmonary arteriocapillary bed.

The preferential use of ^{99m}Tc for labeling these particles is due to its availability, short half-life, stable labeling, and low dose for the patient. The ideal number of particles to be injected for perfusion imaging in an adult ranges from 100 000 to 300 000. Since adult lungs contain $200–300 \times 10^6$ precapillary vessels and 280×10^9 capillaries, the intravenous injection of 10 µg of ^{99m}Tc particles results in a variable embolization of 0.15 %–0.30 % of the total pulmonary arteriocapillary bed without patient discomfort. The minimal toxic dose is 20 µg/kg. However a smaller number of particles must be used in patients with pulmonary hypertension and in pediatric imaging, especially in newborns and infants; the optimal number of injected particles in these cases ranges from 60 000 to 120 000. This caution in pediatric applications is conditioned by the incomplete maturation of the arteriolar tree at birth. The number of arterioles ranging in diameter from 20 to 50 µm increases about three fold, particularly in the first 3 years. In older children the increased vessel number per volume unit of lung parenchyma is less relevant because the alveolar spaces are more inflated and the ratio between alveolar and capillary volumes grows slightly more slowly. The injection of less than 50 000 labeled particles can frequently result in poor diagnostic quality images, with a patchy distribution of the activity in the lungs, even in normal subjects.

Radiogases

The measurement of lung ventilation by an imaging procedure requires an inert radiogas which does not interfere with lung metabolism, has suitable radiation energy, and is readily available. The most widely used radiogas for diagnostic nuclear imaging is xenon-133 (^{133}Xe). However, its low energy photons (81 keV) are suboptimal for the γ-camera and result in high absoption of the activity in the deeper segments of the lungs; furthermore ^{133}Xe single photon emission tomography (SPET) studies of lung ventilation are not feasible. ^{133}Xe is available in different forms for administration: as a saline solution for i.v. injection in the serial evaluation of regional perfusion and segmental ventilation (wash-out phase) of the lungs, or as a free radiogas in a closed delivery circuit, mixed with air or oxygen, for the evaluation of bronchial patency and convection ventilation (early inspiration phase) and regional diffusive ventilation (equilibrium of activity in the lungs during tidal ventilation of xenon in the delivery system and regional wash-out of the lung activity during expiration).

The use of other radioisotopes of xenon is unusual. Only xenon-127 (^{127}Xe) ventilation studies are practically feasible. The advantages of ^{127}Xe are its shelf-life ($t_{1/2} = 36.4$ days), which makes it always available, and its γ-emission (172 and 203 keV), which is higher than ^{99m}Tc, allowing execution of ventilation studies immediately after perfusion scintigraphy of the lungs with ^{99m}Tc macroaggregates. The disadvantages are the greater cost and higher radiation dose than ^{133}Xe. All these problems result in limited utilization of xenon radioisotopes in most cases, even if ^{133}Xe imaging remains a proper diagnostic approach in the assessment of regional ventilation of the lungs by nuclear medicine imaging.

Another inert radiogas suitable for lung ventilation imaging is krypton-81m (^{81m}Kr). ^{81m}Kr is produced by a generator containing the father rubidium-81 (^{81}Rb), has a very short shelf-life ($t_{1/2}$ 13 s), and a characteristic γ-ray of 190 keV. The principal advantage of ^{81m}Kr is the possibility of obtaining images of ventilatory spaces of the lungs in different planar projection or, with a SPECT study, that are easily comparable with the corresponding perfusion images previously obtained with ^{99m}Tc macroaggregates or during continuous i.v. injection of the same ^{81m}Kr dissolved in saline solution. The disadvantages are the high cost of the cyclotron-produced ^{81}Rb/^{81m}Kr generator and the necessity of its daily shipment. Also the dose of an entire ventilation study with ^{81m}Kr (six projections) exceeds that of ^{133}Xe ventilation scintigraphy.

Radioaerosols

The inhalation of a labeled aerosol allows the separate assessment of bronchial patency, activity of ciliated cells of the bronchial tree, and permeability of alveolar epithelium in different pulmonary diseases. While inhalation scintigraphy offers definite advantages over other scintigraphic techniques in lung imaging, only recently has it achieved widespread use in routine clinical applications.

The biological behavior of an inhaled radioaerosol can widely vary, even in normal subjects, mainly by two parameters: the mass median aerodynamic diameter (MMAD) and its geometrical standard deviation (GSD). The latter provides an indication of the distribution of particulate diameters and differentiates the monodisperse aerosols with GSD >1.2 μm from the heterodisperse aerosols having GSD >1.2 μm. Therefore, the measurable accumulation of a labeled aerosol in the lungs depends mainly on the latter two factors, the mode of inhalation (low or high flow rate), and the anatomy of the target airways. All the aerosols that can be inhaled have MMADs less than 10 μm. When the diameter decreases, the accumulation in the nonciliated airways (distal to terminal bronchioles) increases.

The optimal aerodynamic diameter to selectively measure the mucociliary clearance (MC) of an insoluble monodisperse aerosol from ciliated airways is nearly 8 μm with a small GSD. The tussive clearance (TC) can also be measured during the same scintigraphic study. However, the scintigraphic data obtained have to be corrected for the distal retention of the aerosol in nonciliated airways via the measurement of lung retention of the activity at 24 h, when the MC of the activity from ciliated bronchi is completed. The evaluation of the clearance from distal nonciliated airways is possible with insoluble monodisperse aerosols with MMADs less than 2 μm, but it is impractical for clinical purposes due to the necessary prolonged measurements – over days or weeks – of the activity retained in the lungs.

The measurement of the permeability of the alveolar epithelium (LEP) requires an aerosol size less than 1 μm to minimize central airways deposition and reduce the interference of mucociliary transport of the aerosol. These particles are mainly deposited in respiratory bronchioles and more distal alveolar surfaces.

These considerations regarding size and composition of the droplets of an inhaled aerosol limit the choice of the substance to be aerosolized to obtain an inhalation scintigraphy. Some inert nontoxic substances that have been used as monodispersed or heterodispersed radioaerosols for MC or LEP measurements are listed in Table 3.

Monodispersed particulate (insoluble) aerosols for MC measurement are usually obtained in a spinning disk generator by centrifugal dispersion.

Table 3. Aerosols for nuclear imaging

Insoluble (for ventilation studies)
Graphite
Albumin microspheres
Insoluble (for mucociliary clearance measurements)
Solids
Albumin macroaggregates
Lucite
Teflon
Polystyrene latex
Fluorocarbon
Iron oxide
Colloids
Sulfur
Albumin
Others
Autologous red blood cells
Soluble (for measurements of alveolar epithelium permeability)
DTPA (also ventilation studies)
Pertechnetate
Albumin
HM-PAO

Abbreviations, see Table 2.

The liquid solution, once dripped on to the spinning disk, collapses to form droplets of 1–10 μm MMAD. Droplets with the same MMAD can also be generated by vaporization of organic or inorganic substances with subsequent condensation of the vapor onto small solid nuclei. All the particles produced can be labeled with various radionuclides during production or prior to resuspension and inhalation.

Heterodispersed solid aerosols for MC measurements can be produced by fluorocarbon-propelled canisters or dry powder inhalers. The main advantage of these products is the possibility to incorporate a pharmaceutical into the suspension, allowing the measurement of MC prior to and after deposition of the drug on the airways to be studied.

Heterodispersed aqueous aerosols for LEP measurements are produced by jet atomization of the labeled solution using compressed air or ultrasonic nebulizers. These devices are quite similar to those utilized for aerosol therapy, with various sizes (0.5–0.8 μm) and delivery rates (< 1 ml/min) of the generated aerosols. A wet aerosol with MMAD < 1 μm has to be obtained for LEP evaluation. This implies the sedimentation of the nebulized product in a separator or a settling bag for a few minutes before inhalation, because most standard nebulizers also produce a certain amount of radioaerosols with MMAD > 2 μm.

Although a large number of radioisotopes were used to label monodispersed and heterodispersed aerosols, the isotope of choice in human measurements of MC and LEP is ^{99m}Tc. Technetium is easily and steadily bound to diethylenetriaminepentacetate (DTPA), albumin particles, colloids, or autologous erythrocytes. In addition, their nebulization does not change the labeling efficiency of the final inhaled substance. Indium-113m (^{113m}In) labeled aerosols can also be used for LEP measurement in humans, even if their major clinical application remains the study of lung ventilation soon after a perfusion scintigraphy with ^{99m}Tc macroaggregates.

Other Radiopharmaceuticals

The assessment of diffuse alveolar damage can be obtained measuring the distribution in the lungs of a neutral lipophilic complex such as iodine-123-HIPDM. The presence of diffuse interstitial or epithelial damage reduces the production of a lipid fraction contained in the alveolar surfactant, resulting in lower pulmonary uptake of the lipophilic ^{123}I-HIPDM injected intravenously. The lung/whole body uptake ratio of ^{123}I-HIPDM will be proportionally reduced and will offer a noninvasive means to grade the impairment of alveolar functions.

The clinical application of the short-lived positron emitters is limited by their costly production and by the necessity of a dedicated PET camera for their detection. However PET technology offers a series of advantages in the characterization of structure-function relationships of the normal and pathological lung. A quantitative measurement of ventilation-perfusion (V/Q) is feasible by unique i.v. injection of nitrogen-13 (^{13}N), or separately with i.v. administration of oxygen-15 (^{15}O) water for perfusion measurements, followed by neon-19 (^{19}Ne) inhalation for ventilation determination. In addition, lung vascular volume and extravascular lung water can be measured with inhaled [^{11}C] carbon monoxide and [^{11}C] carbon dioxide, respectively. Measurements of glucose consumption and endothelial cell metabolism in the lung are feasible with [^{18}F] fluorodeoxyglucose (^{18}FDG) and [^{11}C] imipramine, which allow quantification of cellular damage in various pathologies of the lung, such as sarcoidosis, pulmonary edema, or chronic airflow obstruction. Another limiting factor for PET quantitative assessment of the pathologic lung is the necessity to have a normal reference distribution for each parameter to be obtained based on a large control group. Furthermore, PET technolgy is not as sophisticated as for the γ-cameras, frequently resulting in a cumbersome comparison of the same functional parameter values between different PET utilizers.

Imaging Techniques

Lung Perfusion Studies

Perfusion scintigraphy is currently performed utilizing ^{99m}Tc-labeled particles and γ-cameras. Usually 74–148 mBq (2–4 mCi) of macroaggregates are injected slowly in a cubital vein. The ultimate distribution of these particles is determined by lung perfusion at the time of injection, reflecting accurately regional pulmonary blood flow. The distribution of the radioactivity can vary according to the gravity effects over the blood mass in the lung. If the patient is injected in an erect position the perfusion is greater at the lung bases and decreased toward the apices. This perfusion gradient is almost abolished when the patient lies supine. Therefore, the radiopharmaceutical has to be injected with the patient in supine decubitus to obtain the most uniform perfusion to the lungs. Imaging can be then performed in other projections, as there is no change in particle position after initial fixation occurs. If imaging is postponed for more than an hour, the lung metabolization of labeled particles becomes relevant, and image quality becomes impaired by the extrapulmonary radioactivity due to free ^{99m}Tc released from aggregates. The best imaging results are obtained with a large field of view γ-camera (diameter >40 cm) and acquired in at least four projections: anterior, posterior, left, and right oblique posterior images. In most cases lateral images do not offer relevant adjunctive diagnostic information.

A normal four view perfusion scintigraphy is presented in Fig. 3. The anatomy of the lungs, which are asymmetric and nonuniform organs, is reflected by these images. The cardiac area is prominently seen in anterior projection. The hilar structures are normally seen mainly in the right posterior oblique projection, where they appear as a central area of decreased radioactivity; the left hilum is generally less prominent. A tomographic assess-

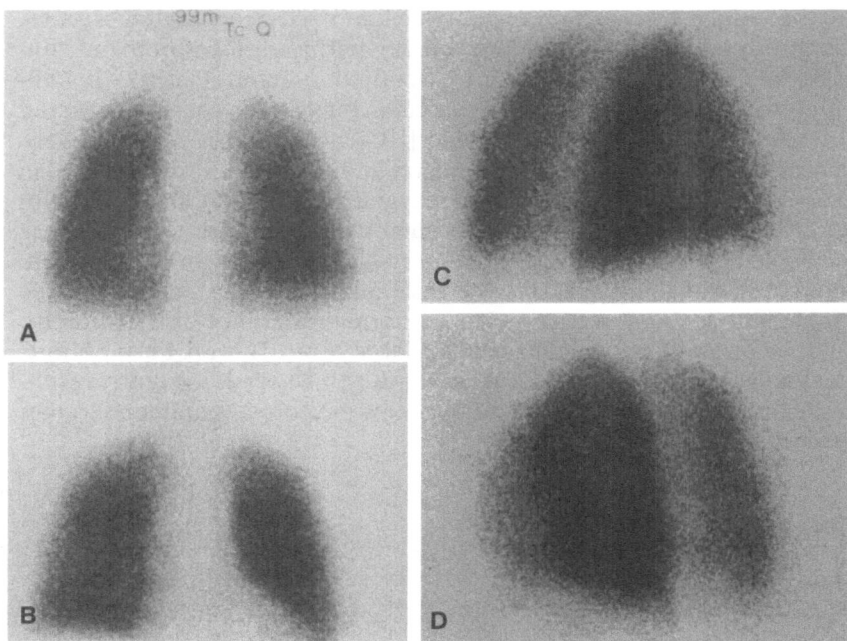

Fig. 3 A–D. Perfusion scintigraphy with ⁹⁹ᵐTc particles in a normal subject. **A** posterior; **B** anterior; **C** right oblique posterior images and **D** left oblique

ment of lung perfusion can also be performed. The reconstructed slices can show, in more detail than planar images, the anatomic features of the lungs and their relationships with contiguous structures.

More than 90% of perfusion studies are performed for the detection of suspected pulmonary embolism. The typical scintigraphic pattern of pulmonary embolism is the presence of segmental or lobar defects in the distribution of ⁹⁹ᵐTc aggregates, whereas the ventilation appears normal in a scintigraphic study with radiogases or radioareosols (Fig. 4).

The most common technical artifacts in perfusion images are caused by adhesion of ⁹⁹ᵐTc aggregates to fibrin clots occurring in the syringe when venipuncture is difficult or when the administration is made via a venous catheter that sometimes contains small clots. These iatrogenic emboli can be appreciated as hot spots in the perfusion images and do not cause discomfort to the patient.

Another technique to assess lung perfusion is the i.v. administration of an insoluble radiogas such as ¹³³Xe or ⁸¹ᵐKr. Perfusion studies with ⁸¹ᵐKr can offer some advantages versus ⁹⁹ᵐTc aggregates only when a combined SPET evaluation of perfusion and ventilation with krypton is to be obtained. During the continuous i.v. administration of ⁸¹ᵐKr the right heart, central veins, and pulmonary vessels are always visualized, but not the left ventricle be-

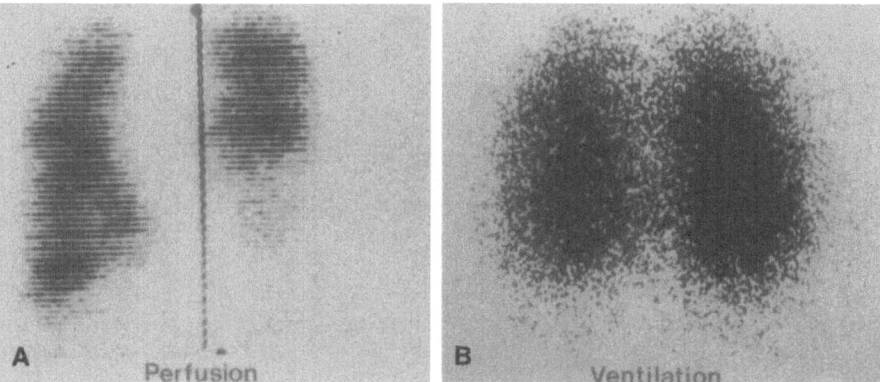

Fig. 4A, B. Pulmonary embolism: **A** perfusive defect in the lower right lobe (posterior view); **B** normal pattern during ^{133}Xe early ventilation in the same area

cause the krypton decay is quite complete in the lung circulation. This uncommon technique makes feasible the calculation of the regional distribution of V/Q ratios in normal and pathological lungs as in PET studies.

Lung Ventilation with Long-Lived Radiogases

The most widely used agent for ventilation scintigraphy is ^{133}Xe ($t_{1/2} = 5.3$ days). It is added to the reservoir of a closed circuit shielded spirometer to produce a concentration of 370 mBq (10 mCi)/liter. The entire imaging procedure is done with the γ-camera positioned behind the patient. In the posterior view the distribution of the activity is homogeneous and almost symmetrical in the lungs, allowing evaluation of a pulmonary surface that is greater than with other projections and more easily comparable with a standard radiogram of the chest.

The patient inhales the mixture of radioxenon and air from a face mask or a mouthpiece, in this case the nostrils should be closed with a nose clip. Exhaled ^{133}Xe is captured in a lead-shielded gas trap. Despite adequate precautions, up to 20% of the radiogas utilized leaks into the room during ventilation, resulting in significant irradiation of the personnel.

The first part of the study consists in the "single breath" phase (Fig. 5B). After a maximal expiration, the patient performs a first maximal inspiration of the xenon/air mixture, than holds his breath for 10–20 s. The outcome of the single breath maneuver is mainly conditioned by the cooperation of the patient; thus results of this phase may be misleading in compromised subjects or in infants and children.

During the second, "equilibrium," phase the patient quietly breathes the xenon mixture from the spirometer for 4–6 min. In this period the xenon dis-

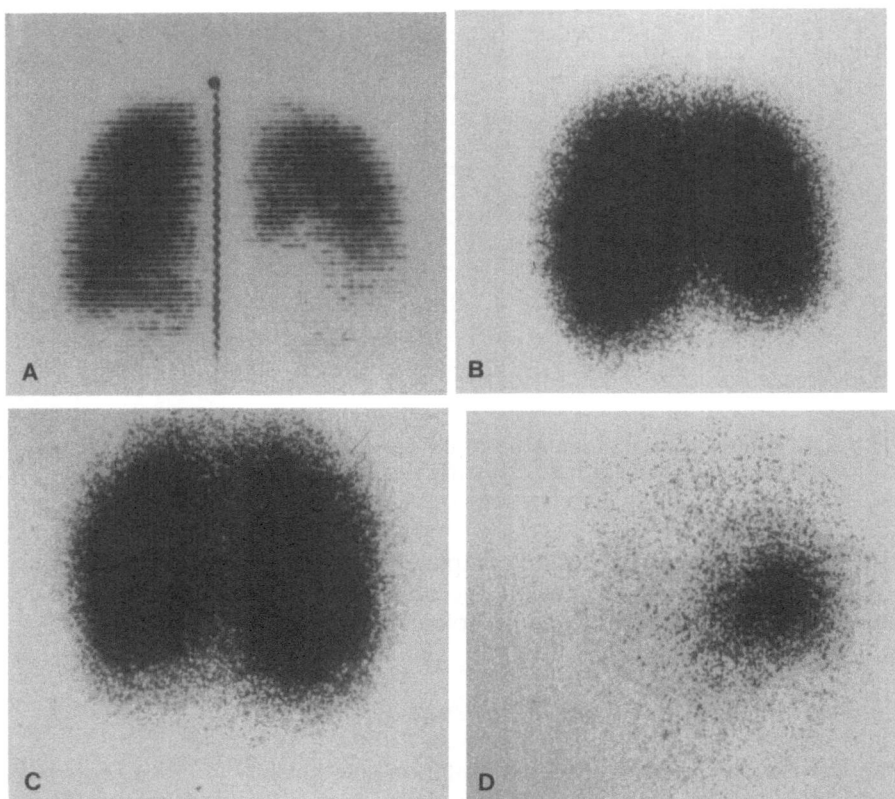

Fig. 5 A-D Stable asthma: **A** Perfusive defect in the inferior right lobe; **B–D** sequential ^{133}Xe ventilation images show a retention of activity in the last image consistent with lobar bronchial stenosis in the same area

tributes in areas with impaired but not abolished ventilation (Fig. 5C). After this equilibrium is obtained, the radioactivity is not detectable in nonventilated areas of the lung, thus appearing as "cold" areas.

In the last phase (wash-out phase) the spirometer is deconnected and the patient slowly breathes room air while expiring through the gas trap. The areas of impaired ventilation will reduce their xenon content more slowly than normally ventilated areas and are visualized in the wash-out phase images as regions of increased radioactivity caused by ^{133}Xe retention (Fig. 5D).

The typical pattern of the hypoventilated lung areas is thus a "cold defect" in early images which turns into a "hot spot" during the wash-out phase. Usually the single breath images alone visualize only 65% of the abnormalities observed in the entire study, while the wash-out phase alone reveals about 95% of the hypoventilated areas. In the equilibrium and wash-out images some artifacts due to xenon swallowing may be seen in the gastric area or under the right pulmonary base due to hepatic steatosis, with liver uptake of the highly lipophilic xenon (2%–8% of inhaled gas).

[127]Xe ventilation is identically performed and offers the additional possibility to follow a perfusion study with ^{99m}Tc particles. In this situation the entire study can be performed in the projection more consistent for perfusion defects and not necessarily in the posterior projection as for ^{133}Xe ventilation studies.

Lung Ventilation with Short-Lived Radiogases

[81m]Kr is the short-lived radiogas of choice for lung ventilation studies. Imaging is performed differently than with xenon. The selection of a [81m]Kr ventilation study implies its comparison with perfusion scintigraphy and its main application is the detection of normally ventilated segments with impaired perfusion, consistent with pulmonary embolism. After the patient has been injected with ^{99m}Tc particles and the first perfusion image is obtained, the krypton ventilation study is performed (Fig. 6).

After the ventilation image is obtained, [81m]Kr flow is stopped and the patient is positioned for the next perfusion image. The execution of a complete

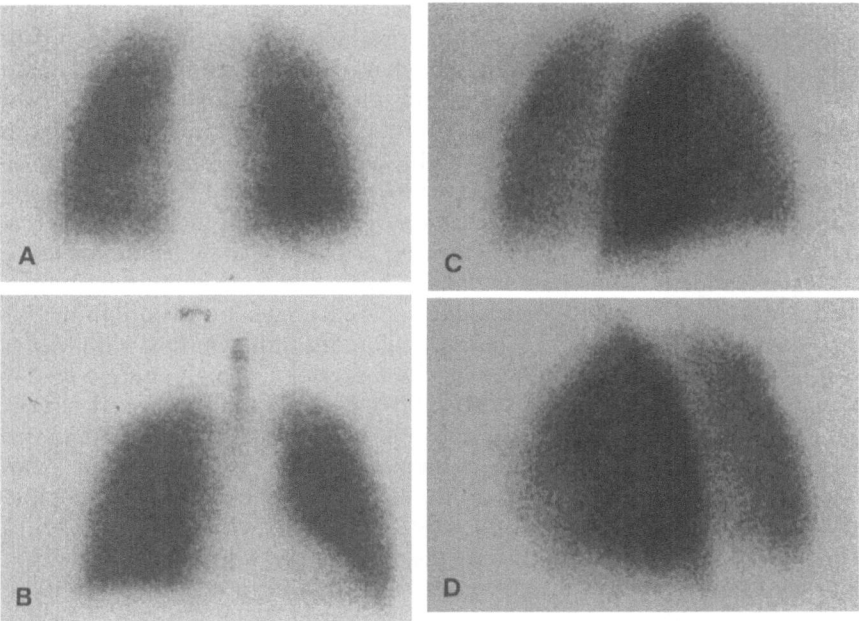

Fig. 6 A–D. Normal ventilation scintigraphy during [81m]Kr inhalation (same subject and projections as in Fig. 3)

^{99m}Tc perfusion/^{81m}Kr ventilation imaging session requires about 40 min. Planar acquisitions can be substituted with SPET studies, improving the diagnostic assessment of pulmonary embolism or other pathologies with V/Q mismatches.

Due to the short (13 s) half-life of this radiogas, there is no problem of storage and room contamination. The patient can breathe the krypton/air mixture, produced by passing compressed air through the ^{81}Rb/^{81m}Kr generator, by a simple face-mask. A stable distribution of the activity in the ventilatory spaces is obtained by the continuous inhalation of the mixture without patient effort and no need for gas recovery, ^{81m}Kr decay being completed in the exhaled air mixture. This rapid decay precludes the imaging of equilibrium and wash-out phases as in xenon studies (Fig. 1D). Krypton and xenon images can show different patterns of a mildly hypoventilated area of the lung. ^{81m}Kr steady-state images may show areas of normally distributed radioactivity, whereas xenon wash-out images frequently manifest a discrete retention of radioactivity. However, SPET imaging with krypton ventilation studies improves the detection of abnormal scintigraphic patterns in these mildly ventilated areas of the lung.

Lung Inhalation with Radioaerosols

The selection of a system for the production and administration of radioactive aerosols for nuclear imaging of the lung is mainly conditioned by the possibility of obtaining a final inhaled product with specific characteristics. Size, chemical composition, electrical charge, and dissolution rate must be suitable for tracing the functions of the selected anatomic structures of the lungs where the inhaled substances preferentially distribute. In the proximal ciliated airways, deposition is caused by the impact of relatively larger droplets due to convection ventilation, whereas in the distal nonciliated airways deposition is obtained by sedimentation of smaller droplets. The preferential deposition in distal nonciliated airways of certain small insoluble aerosols allows assessment of the patency of the bronchial tree, being distributed in the respiratory spaces proportional to regional convection ventilation.

The production of this type of particulate insoluble aerosol with MMAD < 1.5 μm requires a jet nebulizer in which is added a small volume (1–2 ml) of solution containing 400–1500 MBq (10–40 mCi) of labeled particles, commonly the macroaggregates or microspheres of human serum albumin used also for perfusion studies. The nebulized product is collected in a large shielded settling bag (10–20 liters) for 10–15 min allowing almost complete sedimentation of the fraction of produced droplets with MMAD > 1.5 μm. The patient is then connected with the settling bag and inhales the suspension by a mouthpiece after closing the nostrils with a noseclip. The patient cooperation required is minimal, but in compromised or mechanically ventilated subjects the use of a rubber balloon for aspiration and inflation of the radioaerosol to the patient is feasible without technical complications. The exhaled suspension is then collected by a filter resulting in a limited dispersion of the radioactivity in the environment. The administered radioactive dose is low because only a small fraction (1%–3%) of the nebulized aerosol is distributed in the distal airways, a negligible amount is deposited in the ciliated airways, and most of the tracer remains in the exhaled air.

Aerosol labeling with ^{113m}In ($t_{1/2} = 100$ min), produced by a ^{113}Sn/^{113m}In generator, allows execution of a ventilation scintigraphy soon after a complete perfusion study with ^{99m}Tc particles to assess pulmonary embolism, since its energetic γ-rays (392 keV) permit the ventilation images to be obtained without the interference of ^{99m}Tc emission. Ventilation images with ^{113m}In radioaerosols are obtained with a γ-camera in the same projections used in perfusion scintigraphy to assess ventilation/perfusion mismatches (Fig. 4B). The quality of ^{113m}In inhalation images is less satisfying than that of ^{99m}Tc, but ^{113m}In inhalation remains one of the most important techniques to obtain a ventilation/perfusion study in a single clinical setting, if the more costly ^{127}Xe and ^{81m}Kr are not available. If only ^{99m}Tc is available for aerosol labeling, the inhalation study must be delayed for at least 24 h, until the ^{99m}Tc, aggregates injected have been cleared from the lung capillary bed (Fig. 7).

An alternative system for production and delivery of ^{99m}Tc-labeled monodispersed insoluble aerosols for convection ventilation assessment requires the heating of a free ^{99m}Tc concentrated solution (110–140 mBq in less

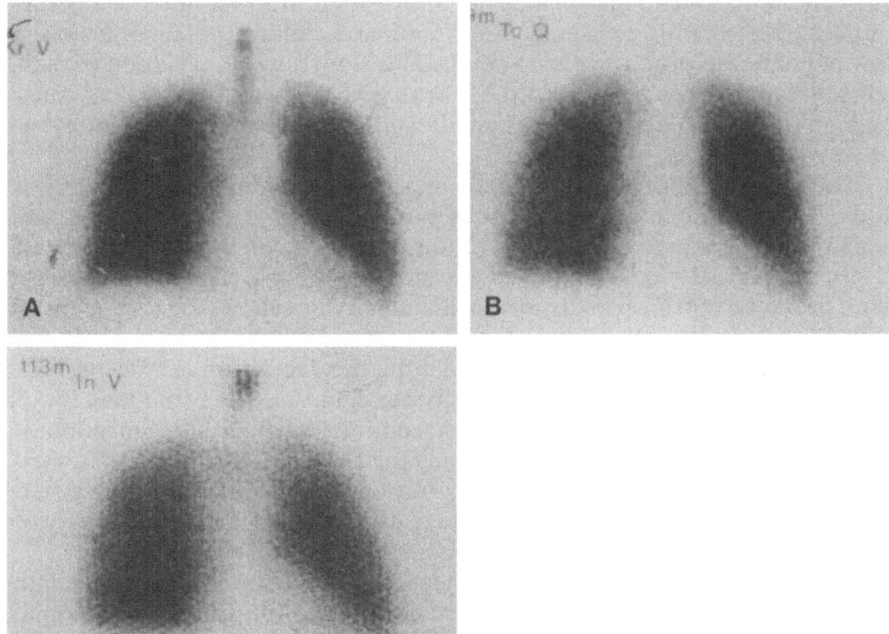

Fig. 7A–C. Ventilation images obtained in a normal subject (same as in Fig. 5) with ^{81m}Kr (**A**), ^{133}Xe (**B**) and ^{113m}In radioaerosol (MMAD <1.5 μm) inhalation (**C**)

than 0.05 ml) deposited over a small stick of pure graphite to 2500 °C in argon atmosphere. The ultrafine carbon dispersion (MMAD < 0.05 μm) obtained is collected in a 2–3 liter reservoir and inhaled by a mouthpiece for two or three tidal breaths. The exhaled airborne activity is trapped by a filter. The administration procedure is rapid, requires little collaboration from the patient, and can immediately precede a ^{99m}Tc perfusion study. The limited activity deposited in the lungs (8–12 MBq) interferes only marginally with the interpretation of perfusion images obtained after i.v. injection of a 20-fold greater amount (160–240 MBq) of ^{99m}Tc-radiolabeled particles. However, ^{99m}Tc radioaerosol images should be obtained, for optimal comparison of ventilation and perfusion, postponing the ventilation study for 24 h.

The most relevant clinical application of these "pseudogas" particles is the diagnostic assessment of pulmonary embolism. However, it is also possible to use them for the assessment of other lung diseases with V/Q mismatch. The main disadvantage of the device for pseudogas production is its high cost and the impossibility to produce soluble gas-like radioaerosols for the optimal assessment of LEP. By contrast, the production of small monodisperse soluble radioaerosols (MMAD < 1.5 μm, GSD < 1.2 μm) is feasible with the same jet nebulizer/settling bag systems employed for small particulate insoluble radioaerosols production. These systems allow proper delivery even in pediatric patients. The nebulizers without settling bag or reservoir and with continuous high-flow air administration are less suitable for this purpose. The small lung capacity of infants and children requires a slower flow of nebulized product than in adults. This slow-flow nebulization of radioaerosols can result in a larger MMAD or GSD of the inhaled droplets, causing high bronchial deposition of the radioactivity and cumbersome interpretation of the images.

The radiopharmaceutical currently most commonly employed for clinical studies is diethylenetriamine-pentaacetic acid (DTPA), which is readily available, inexpensive, and easily produced and labeled with technetium (^{99m}Tc-DTPA). The scintigraphic assessment of ^{99m}Tc-DTPA monodisperse small droplet deposition in distal nonciliated airways allows measurement of LEP. Before starting the inhalation, the camera is positioned close to the back of the sitting patient. During inhalation, the deposition of ^{99m}Tc-DTPA is measured for a few minutes until a proper count/rate over the lung is obtained; the aerosol inhalation is then discontinued, while the acquisition of scintigraphic images (2–4/min) continues for at least 2 h (Fig. 1E). Toward the end of the acquisition, a small amount of ^{99m}Tc-DTPA can be injected intravenously to define and subtract the contribution to lung radioactivity of the reabsorbed DTPA circulating through the pulmonary vessels.

The scintigraphic technique to measure the clearance of particulate monodispersed aerosols with larger size (MMAD 8–10 μm) from proximal ciliated airways for MC and TC measurements is similar to that described for LEP measurement but usually does not require additional injection of tracer because lung reabsorption of the radioactivity is negligible. The measurement of MC requires acquisition of a 24 h delayed image to measure the small fraction of inhaled aerosol in the distal airways retained in the lungs, and it is possible to subtract from the initial images the contribution of the radioactivity distally penetrated to avoid underestimation of MC from pericentral bronchi.

Data Processing and Analysis

The relative measurement of pulmonary function obtained by imaging requires processing of the acquired images. Many of these measurements imply the calculation of the residence time of the administered tracer in the lungs as a whole or in specific regions. Image processing is usually semiautomated, requires less than 30 min, and the demands on the operator's are reasonable. Mathematical analysis of static, dynamic, and SPET images is currently feasible with a computer connected to the γ-camera. The software configuration is usually well enough suited for the compilation of original processing programs; dedicated array processors for the time-consuming reconstruction of SPET acquisitions are advantageous.

Perfusion Images

The instrumental information on pulmonary perfusion is mostly evaluated by comparing scintigraphic perfusion/ventilation images with other imaging procedures, such as spot radiograms of the thorax, and/or other morphological imaging procedures, such as computed tomography or magnetic resonance. When a SPET study of the lung is performed after i.v. injection of ^{99m}Tc aggregates or ^{81m}Kr, a series of projections (64–128 images) are acquired by rotating the γ-camera in a circular or elliptical orbit around the patient. The multiple images are then processed and the measured activity in each part of the field of view is mathematically analyzed by applying a back-projection interpolating algorithm to obtain, as in CT studies, a variable number of transaxial slices of the thorax which represent the distribution of the labeled particles or radiogas in the vascular bed of the lungs.

SPET techniques are achievable in most nuclear medicine departments using many currently available radionuclides and with limited additional cost for the instrumentation and dedicated software programs. Despite its utility in the separation of overlying structures of the thorax and in the assessment of small perfusion defects, the absolute quantification of lung perfusion by SPET with particulate tracers is far from clinical application. The percent distribution of the labeled particles can, though, be assessed for each pulmonary lobe and segment in many pulmonary diseases, such as in the diagnosis of pulmonary embolism. A precise definition of perfusion improvement during therapy is possible with serial studies and the V/Q SPET ratios can be calculated with ^{81m}Kr in discrete segments of the lungs by comparison with a ventilation SPET study.

Xenon Ventilation Images

The sequential images obtained during a typical three-phase ventilation study with ^{133}Xe or ^{127}Xe allow regional quantification of regional ventilation by different methods. The use of a computer simplifies the mathematical analysis. The calculation of regional and whole lung clearance rates that express the diffusive ventilation efficiency per unit time of the alveolar volume requires only a few minutes (Fig. 8).

A practical way to express regional ventilation clearance is the area/height ratio (A/H) over the time/activity curve of the lungs. The area (A) is the count rate (counts/minute) at equilibrium multiplied for the average clearance time τ that is 1.44 times the clearance half-time in wash-out phase. A can be expressed as counts eq $\times$ τ, and H is espressed as counts $\times$ Δt, where Δt is the chosen interval of 1 min. Thus the clearance time τ is $A \times \Delta t/H$. The regional distribution of A/H ratios can also be represented in a single parametric image obtained by subtracting the image acquired in the first minute of the wash-out phase from the image obtained in the last minute of the equilibrium phase, that is a distribution of $(A/H)^{-1}$ parameter. A is low in poorly ventilated areas, with resulting low $(A/H)^{-1}$ ratios and cold areas in subtracted images. In normally ventilated areas, A is high and the $(A/H)^{-1}$ ratios are higher, being represented on subtracted image as hot areas.

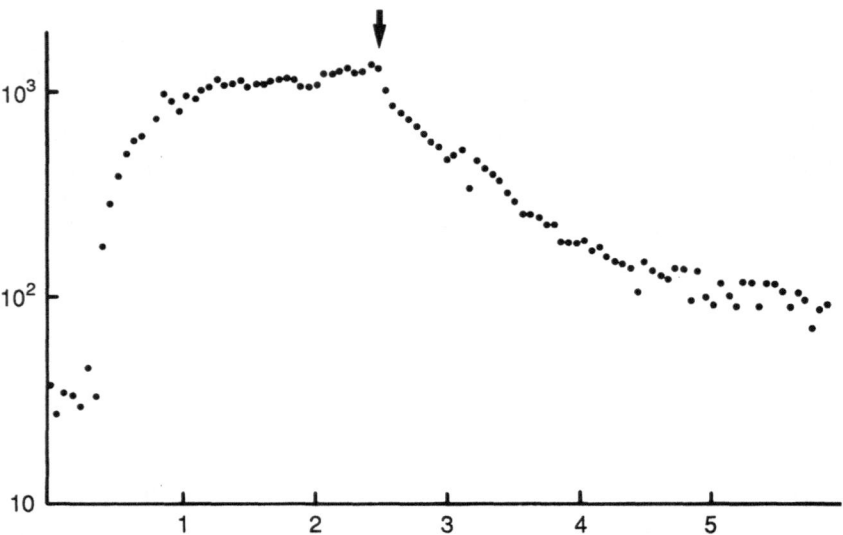

Fig. 8. Time/activity curve representing lung distribution of inhaled ^{133}Xe in a normal subject (wash-out phase start is at the *arrow*)

Krypton Ventilation Images

Typically, ^{81m}Kr images represent the effectiveness of the regional ventilation when equilibrium is obtained, the gas decaying almost completely after entering the alveoli. The distribution in the lungs of ^{81m}Kr at equilibrium is similar to that of ^{133}Xe or ^{127}Xe during the inhalation phase (Fig. 1D). The ^{81m}Kr count rate in the lungs is expressed as $V/(V/\text{volume}) + \lambda$, where V is the ventilation rate of the krypton/air mixture (near 2.5 liters per min in adult normal subjects) and λ is the constant decay of ^{81m}Kr (3.2 min^{-1}). Thus a direct relationship between activity and volume of inflated lung regions can be obtained, the measured decay of ^{81m}Kr expressing lung inflation efficiency. This behavior can explain the observed Kr/Xe mismatches in ventilation images, due mainly to ^{81m}Kr decay before it reaches the hypoventilated areas.

The feasibility of SPET tudies has recently renewed the interest in ^{81m}Kr ventilation. The reconstruction algorithms allow the calculation of V/Q ratios of combined SPET ^{81m}Kr perfusion and ventilation in small segments of the lungs. These V/Q ratios are reproducible within 10%–15%, allowing serial V/Q measurements in different clinical settings prior to and after therapeutic intervention.

Radioaerosol Images

The analysis of radioaerosol studies is usually applied to inhalation scintigraphy obtained with small monodisperse ^{99m}Tc-DTPA aerosols (MMAD <0.8 μm) for LEP measurements or with insoluble (particulate) larger aerosols (MAD 5–8 μm, GSD <3 μm) for the measurement of MC and TC. A sequence of images is acquired after inhalation for periods ranging from 0.5 to 3 h for LEP assessment and from 1 to 2 h in MC and TC measurements.

The initial penetration of the radioaerosol in the lungs is conditioned by bronchial patency and is calculated as a penetration index, expressed as the percent of whole lung activity distributed in peripheral lung airways in the first image acquired after inhalation. This parameter can be used to asses the broncodilatation or bronchoconstriction obtained with various pharmaceutical agents (Fig. 9).

The retention of activity in the lungs, also defined as regions of interest (ROIs), at each particular point of the study is expressed in counts/min. In most cases rough counts in the lung ROIs, obtained from hilar and peripheral areas, are corrected for tracer decay and/or for background (intravascular) activity (Fig. 1F). The levels of the radioactivity in lung areas can be plotted as the logarithm of counts vs time.

The pulmonary time/activity curve plotted for MC and TC determination presents several exponential components; each component is easily expressed with its $t_{1/2}$ and represents the clearance rate of the tracer in airway, portions of different size. MC of radioaerosols in ROIs of the lungs (hilar,

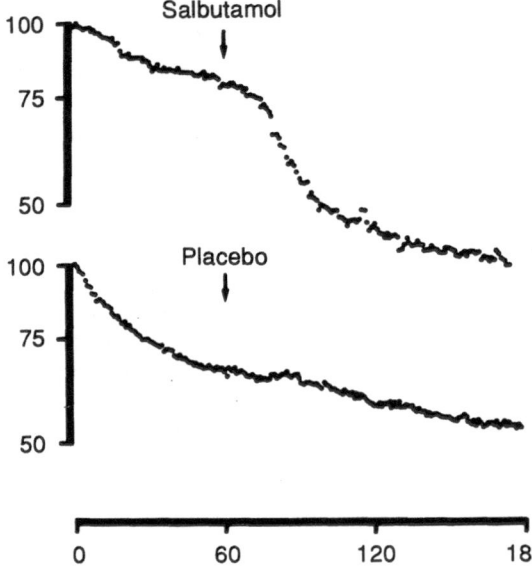

Fig. 9. Effects of salbutamol and placebo administration (*arrows*) on mucociliary clearance in stable asthma. Time/activity curvbes obtained in two asthmatic patients after ^{99m}Tc particulate aerosol (MMAD 5–6 μm) inhalation

pericentral, and peripherical areas) can also be expressed as percent of maximal activity cleared per hour in the selected areas or in whole lungs (Fig. 10). Normal clearances values vary from 200% to 300% in central areas of the lungs, after correction of the data for the contribution of distally sedimented radioactivity, and less in peripheral regions. The TC rate is usually obtained in the last minutes of the acquisition of a study performed for MC measurements. The values of TC in normal subjects, which can be expressed as percent of activity in the pericentral bronchi released after a minute of active coughing, ranges from 0.5% to 1%, but becomes more relevant in obstructive bronchial diseases.

The separation of each component of the total lung clearance curve in central areas of the lungs is mathematically possible by sequential graphical extrapolation of each component from the original multiexponential curve or by fitting the data with a multiexponential regression equation or a polynomial function. The time/activity curves obtained for LEP measurements are similarly analyzed. The pattern of the total curve is monoexponential in normal nonsmoker subjects and becomes biexponential in the presence of lung damage. When this second component of the curve is considerably increased, the presence of vascular intrapulmonary radioactivity caused by DTPA reabsorption and recirculation in the lungs often overestimates the true pulmonary half-time of this component extrapolated from the rough time/activity curve. In these cases, data correction is feasible by monitoring the activify in the lungs and in other background regions after i.v. injection of a small dose (4–8 mBq) of ^{99m}Tc-DTPA in order to subtract from the original curve the activity present in the pulmonary circulation.

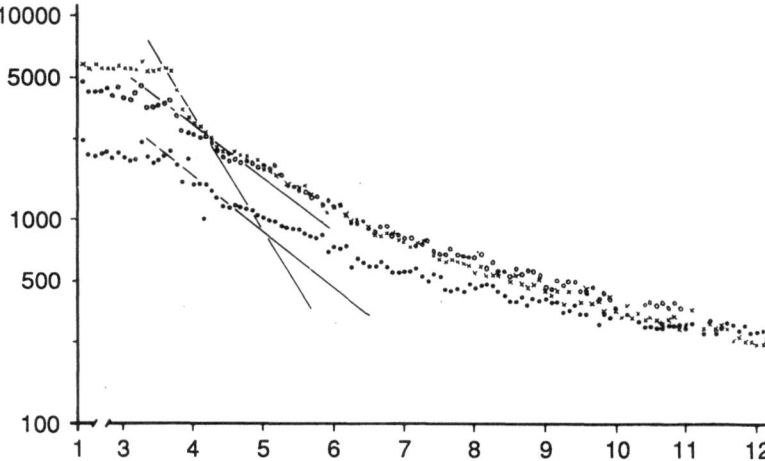

Fig. 10. Regional time/activity curves from apical (○○), basal (●●), and central (× ×) areas of the lungs for regional mucociliary clearance assessment in a control subject after ^{99m}Tc aerosol inhalation

The functional measurement of LEP is expressed for clinical purposes either as the half-time of the clearance of the activity from lungs to blood ($t_{1/2L/B}$) or as the downslope (k) of the retention curve in the first 20 min of acquisition. The distribution of LEP values in normal nonsmokers has not been definitively assessed. This situation is mainly due to the combination of various factors affecting the distribution of DTPA in the alveolar spaces such as DTPA instability in vivo, normal variability of convection ventilation between apices and bases, flow rates of inflation, variability and effective size of the aerosol sedimented in the alveoli, and mathematical procedures employed for the fitting of each component of the rough retention curve. A normal reference distribution of $t_{1/2L/B}$ or k values is to be obtained in each center if LEP measurements are used for clinical purposes. The mean $t_{1/2L/B}$ values obtained in various centers in normal controls vary widely, from 40 to 250 min. However, the reproducibility of an LEP measurement in the same normal subject is usually good. The alveolar clearances of other nebulized radiopharmaceuticals, such as ^{99m}Tc pertechnetate or ^{99m}Tc-HM-PAO, a neutral lipophilic oxime complex, are measureable for diagnostic purposes. The inhaled pertechnetate shows a short mean $t_{1/2}$ (10 min) in normals and is slightly affected by alveolar damage. The clearance rate of ^{99m}Tc-HM-PAO from the lungs is slower than ^{99m}Tc-DTPA clearance; mean HM-PAO $t_{1/2}$ from the lungs is 53 min and is significantly prolonged in various interstitial pathologies of the lungs.

Nuclear Medicine Applications in Asthma

The main changes of regional pulmonary perfusion and ventilation occur in asthmatic patients at the onset of an acute episode. These are the result of bronchospasm and the change in secretion rheology which is followed by blood shunting from the hypoventilated lungs areas. As an extreme consequence of the loss of gas exchange capability, these patients develop hypoxemia. The clinical resolution of an acute episode implies recovery of normal lung perfusion, while regional ventilation remains defective in a large number of patients in remission.

The role of nuclear medicine in the instrumental assessment of asthma is to demonstrate the functional impairment of regional ventilation and perfusion in stable asthma, acute episodes and remission. The extension of the ventilatory deficit, as assessed by spirometry, is closely related to the severity of airways obstruction. By contrast, ventilation and perfusion mismatches assessed by nuclear imaging can be related to the development of hypoxemia independently of the degree of chronic airflow limitation observed during remission or stable asthma.

Both the tracheobronchial clearance, that is, the clearance of bronchial secretions from the first sixteen generations of the airways, and the TC, obtained by coughing from the first six generations of the airways, can be mildly or severely decreased in asthmatic patients. When severe symptoms occur, the measurement of tracheobronchial clearance rates is redundant; conversely, the assessment of long-dated alterations of airways diameter and/or rheology of bronchial secretions by nuclear imaging plays an important role in the adjustment of pharmacologic therapy. The improvement of convection ventilation and mucus rheology, obtained with a proper physical or pharmacological therapy, can be measured non invasively by nuclear imaging techniques.

Perfusion and Ventilation Imaging in Acute Asthma

In 1963 the first report of nuclear imaging in a patient with an asthmatic attack documented the impairment of regional lung perfusion by i.v. injection of labeled macroaggregates. During acute episodes, a standard perfusion study demonstrates, in 95%–100% of the patients) multiple bilateral defects in the deposition of ^{99m}Tc labeled particles (cold spots). The distribution pattern of these perfusion defects is generally segmental or lobar and is attributed to the functional shunting of blood from the regions of the lung developing hypoxia as a consequence of neurogenic or biochemical bronchospasm. The localization of these defects may actually change from one episode to another. The typical lobar or segmental perfusion defect observed in early acute episodes is quite similar to that observed in pulmonary embolism, but the pattern may change if the study is performed soon after the onset of therapy. The distribution of the cold areas becomes more patchy, due to partial resolution of regional hypoxia with rearrangement of vascular resistances and progressive reflow of blood in shunted areas. However, a deficient distribution of particulate tracer is usually observed in lung areas where bronchospasm persists. A perfusion study repeated after 12–24 h, when wheezing has abated, is normal in 75%–90% of these subjects. This rapid change in the perfusion pattern is typical of asthmatic patients. The lung perfusion defects observed in patients with pulmonary embolism show a slower return to a normal perfusion pattern, 4–10 days after the onset of therapy. Therefore, when the clinical presentation suggests an unusual acute asthmatic component in a lung perfusion impairment primarily related to pulmonary embolism and a scintigraphic ventilation study is not readily feasible, a perfusion scintigraphy should be repeated 24 h after resolution of the symptoms to avoid an overestimation of the severity of pulmonary embolism.

A certain degree of cooperation is required from the patient for breath holding during injection and wash-out breathing maneuvers when a combined assessment of lung perfusion and ventilation can be practically performed by i.v. administration of ^{133}Xe or ^{127}Xe. The typical scintigraphic pattern observed after i.v. administration of radioxenon is a diffuse reduction of perfusion in both lungs. Retention of radioxenon can be demonstrated in 10%–20% of the normoperfused or mildly hypoperfused segments. This association of perfusion defects with V/Q mismatches is commonly observed in asthmatic patients with FEV_1 <30% and in acute episodes. Combined ventilation and perfusion studies with ^{133}Xe inhalation and ^{99m}Tc particles injection can, conversely, show the association of perfusion defects matched with ventilation reduction and/or ventilation defects with conserved regional perfusion.

The combined V/Q assessment of acute asthma with ^{99m}Tc particle injection and ^{81m}Kr inhalation is less commonly employed due to the high cost and limited availability of krypton. However, ^{81m}Kr images are qualitatively better than xenon images, and a regional assessment of ventilation by comparison with perfusion images is easily obtained by inspection only. Multiple ventilation defects can be observed in ^{81m}Kr images in all patients during acute asthma. These are usually matched with the perfusion defects seen in ^{99m}Tc images. However, up to 30%–40% of hypoventilated areas show also a less relevant decrease of perfusion without a constant apex/base distribution of these areas in the lungs.

When bronchodilation is obtained by therapeutical interventions, a certain degree of hypoventilation may persist in areas where the rheologic changes of secretion and the edema of the bronchial mucosa are still significant. In this phase the symptoms improve but the ^{81m}Kr penetration is still reduced in areas at the periphery of the lungs, with a more patchy distribution of radioactivity. Most perfusion defects also improve significantly in repeated ^{99m}Tc particles scintigraphic studies.

Quantification of ^{81m}Kr ventilation is possibly obtained by an underventilation score, which expresses the total degree of lung hypoventilation by comparison with a normal reference range for ^{81m}Kr ventilation into each lung's region. This parameter is positively correlated with the presence of airway obstruction as assessed by spirometric tests.

The evaluation of V/Q match or mismatch in $^{81m}Kr/^{99m}Tc$ studies is improved by automated analysis of the lung distribution of the tracers. The processing of the data results in a regional distribution of V/Q ratios which can be compared with the normal V/Q ratios distribution in the same lung regions or with other V/Q studies obtained in the same patient.

In addition, the presence and severity in acute episodes of hypoxiemia, as assessed by arterial PO_2 saturation, is positively correlated with the extension of V/Q mismatch in the lungs, as assessed by $^{81m}Kr/^{99m}Tc$ imaging.

The inhalation of small sized insoluble aerosols labeled with ^{99m}Tc is an alternative scintigraphic technique to radiogases in the assessment of ventilation during acute asthma. Unfortunately, the comparative evaluation of perfusion and ventilation images must be postponed since the inhaled ^{99m}Tc can interfere significantly with the interpretation of perfusion images when the ^{99m}Tc articles are injected too soon after the ventilation study. Obviously, the comparison of V/Q images for diagnostic purpose over a 8–12 h timespan is heavily affected by the environment and the effects of physical or pharmacological treatment performed during this interval.

In acute asthma, nuclear imaging techniques allow precise assessment of the degree of airflow limitation and perfusion impairment caused by bronchospasm and the consequent vasoconstriction in discrete areas of the lungs. Perfusion images are an excellent alternative to monitor the response to therapy in uncooperative or pediatric patients in which the use of spirometric tests is problematic. The high cost of radiogases and their radiation burden makes these techniques impractical for monitoring the development of symptoms in acute episodes. The use of less expensive radioaerosols for ventilation assessment does not offer advantages in acute episodes because a higher deposition of radioaerosol in proximal airways negatively affects the diagnostic quality and interpretation of the images. Perfusion/ventilation studies can also be employed to evaluate asthmatic patients before and during the acute administration of acetylcholine or during other provocative tests.

Perfusion and Ventilation Imaging in Stable Asthma and Remission

The abnormalities of ventilation and perfusion observed during acute asthma improve during remission and the values of the standard spirometric tests may return to within normal range. During remission, a number of sophisticated inhalation tests, using mixtures of nonradioactive noble gases with different solubilities in the lungs, can be used to demonstrate abnormal persistence of narrowing in the small airways. In other cases the normalization of spirometric test values is incomplete and the extent of airways obstruction can be assessed and clinically graded according to the percent reduction of predicted FEV_1%, FEV_1/FCV ratio, or other spirometric parameters. The primary clinical information obtained by nuclear imaging in these subjects is the extent and degree of lung hypoventilation. The qualitative comparison between [81m]Kr ventilation images and ^{99m}Tc particles perfusion images in the asthmatic patient reveals a variable degree of regional hypoventilation in 15%–20% of asymptomatic patients with FEV_1 >75%. A usually matched reduction of perfusion is observed in these areas (Fig. 5). When severe or discrete impairment of spirometric tests is observed, the ventilation images show reduced radioactive content in multiple areas of the lungs in 100% and 83% of the patients, respectively. A variable percent of these ventilation defects, 20% and 8% respectively, show relatively preserved perfusion (V/Q mismatch).

The scintigraphic assessment of ventilation in asthmatic patients, as obtained by accurate analysis of [81m]Kr images, has been found to be more sensitive than chest radiogram analysis. Indeed, large ventilation defects can be observed in asthmatics with normal chest radiograms. The administration of bronchodilators improves both ventilation and perfusion on scintigraphic images with [81m]Kr and [99m]Tc. The degree of improvement is related to both the clinical resolution of symptoms and the spirometric deficit. However, ventilation and/or perfusion can be persistently reduced in patients with an increase of more than 24% of FEV_1 induced by therapy.

The quantification of regional hypoventilation for diagnostic purposes is feasible in asthmatics with radiogas inhalation only, but still remains an uncommon procedure. Quantitative analysis of V/Q ratios in asthmatic patients has been recently obtained by combining SPET perfusion studies during continuous i.v. infusion of [81m]Kr with SPET ventilation during continuous breathing of [81m]Kr in air. Tomographic sections of the lungs in control subjects in supine position have demonstrated increased perfusion along the gravity axis, from anterior to dorsal regions. In normals, ventilation follows the same distribution, but with an alveolar distribution of [81m]Kr in the anterior areas that is better than the one in the vascular compartment. The V/Q gradient observed in supine controls showed higher V/Q values in dorsal and central areas than in anterior areas.

Asthmatic subjects, asymptomatic and with normal spirometric tests, show, when studied supine, a perfusion distribution gradient within the normal range. By contrast, the ventilatory gradient appears abnormal in SPET sections, with significantly lower ventilation in dorsal areas and higher in anterior areas. The V/Q ratio gradient is more significantly altered in asthma than the gradient of ventilation. In asthma the V/Q ratios are higher in the anterior regions and lower in the dorsal ones than in control subjects.

The inhalation of salbutamol significantly improves ventilation in the anterior regions with a consequent increase in perfusion and fall of V/Q ratios. This impairment of V/Q SPET ratios observed in the anterior areas after bronchodilation may explain in part the reduction of oxygen saturation in arterial blood samples observed after salbutamol inhalation. Thus the automated quantification of V/Q scintigraphic studies improves the instrumental assessment obtained in asthmatic patients by other quantitative tests of lung function, even if the well known fluctuations of arterial oxygen saturation and FEV_1 values in asthmatic patients confine the quantitative analysis of scintigraphic images to same-day data. The need for repeated SPET studies and the high cost of ^{81m}Kr generators makes this technique impractical for routine use even if it may clarify the acute or chronic response to pharmacological interventions or the results of therapeutic bronchial drainage in severe asthma.

The quantitative assessment of the clearance rates of inhaled radioxenons (^{133}Xe or ^{127}Xe) also shows the regional distribution of airflow impairment and can accurately define the improvement of regional ventilation obtained by pharmacologic and/or physical therapy. Unfortunately, only a limited number of centers perform ventilation or perfusion studies with noble radiogases, while most currently perform routinely radioaerosol imaging for the assessment of lung ventilation.

For ventilation imaging an aerosol should be either insoluble (particulate) or slowly absorbed (DTPA) in the distal nonciliate airways and have the lowest amount of deposition in the proximal ciliate airways and maximal deposition in small distal bronchi (MMAD >1.5 μm, GSD >1.2 μm). The peripheral penetration (penetration index) of this type of aerosols has been found to be positively correlated to FEV_1 and RV in controls and mild asthmatics. However, the inhalation of this optimal radioaerosol in patients with severely diminished lung ventilation, as in severe asthma or status asthmaticus, often gives a poorer peripheral penetration than that obtained with radiogas inhalation, resulting in poorer quality and sometimes misleading diagnostic interpretation of the scintigraphic images. The diffuse bronchial narrowing generates high airflow velocities in these structures, possibly enhancing the probability of particles deposition by inertial impact, is probably responsible for this phenomenon. Therefore, in severe asthma ventilation assessment is better performed with radiogas administration rather than with radioaerosol inhalation.

The comparison of ^{81m}Kr ventilation images and ^{99m}Tc radioaerosol inhalation images in normal nonsmokers shows no significant differences in the semiquantitative scores obtained from inspection of the images or by comparing the distribution of the two tracers in the peripheral, central, and hilar regions of the lungs. The variability in the distribution of ^{99m}Tc between the ventilatory spaces and the distal ciliate airways in radioaerosol images appears to be greater than in ^{81m}Kr images. In asymptomatic asthma (mean FEV_1 102%), more ventilation abnormalities have been observed in radioaerosol images than in krypton images (respectively, 60% and 40% of the patients show peripheral defects of ventilation). However, the presence and extent of these abnormalities, assessed with either of the two tracers, is positively correlated with the spirometric values distribution in both asthmatics and controls. The apparent overestimation of the ventilation abnormalities observed with radioaerosol inhalation vs krypton inhalation can be partly related to the different pulmonary distribution volume of the two tracers.

If stable narrowing of the small airways is present in asthmatics patients, the peripheral deposition of inhaled aerosols is more affected than the penetration of ^{81m}Kr in alveolar spaces. Moreover, the high airflow velocity in stenotic bronchi during ventilation results in an extensive deposition of aerosols by impact, while krypton retention in proximal ciliate airways during equilibrium is not significantly conditioned by airways diameters but only by their total volume.

In conclusion, ventilation images obtained with ^{81m}Kr and ^{133}Xe are potentially useful in the assessment of the response of regional bronchospasm to bronchodilation, even when spirometric tests return to normal values. ^{81m}Kr quantification is particularly useful in assessing ventilation in pediatric patients and in exercise-induced asthma. In situations in which the regional ventilation widely varies within minutes or hours and patient cooperation is problematic, ^{81m}Kr inhalation allows precise assessment of the ventilatory response to therapy or exercise, which is performed poorly by spirometry.

The assessment of ventilation by radioaerosol inhalation is feasible in the instrumental approach to mild and asymptomatic asthma. However, the quantitative analysis of ventilation, achievable with radiogas imaging, is still negatively conditioned in this technique by the lack of an ideal "gas-like" radioaerosol. Radioaerosol ventilation imaging is helpful in assessment of optimal breathing maneuvers to obtain the maximal effect of nebulized drugs in asthmatics. The pharmaceutical is mixed with the radioaerosol before inhalation, and the measured distribution of the aerosol in the lung obtained with either breathing maneuver is compared with the intrinsic effects of the nebulized drug. Therefore, the role of radioaerosol techniques for ventilation studies in asthma is still debated from a methodological point of view and offers some advantages over radiogases only in selected clinical and experimental situations.

Tracheobronchial Clearance Measurements by Radioaerosol Imaging in Asthma

The measurement of MC and TC by nuclear imaging is relatively easy to perform, inexpensive, and results in low radiation exposure for the patients. This allows repeat studies in the same subjects to assess the effects of physical maneuvers or therapy on the tracheobronchial transport velocity of inert colloids. To trace surface transport on ciliate airways, an inhaled radioaerosol must be insoluble in lung secretions (i.e., particulate), chemically stable, easily bound with ^{99m}Tc, have no intrinsic pharmacologic activity, and should have a diameter larger (MMAD 4–8 μm, GSD < 1.2 μm) than the radioaerosols described for the study of regional ventilation or alveolar permeability of the lung. With this type of radioaerosol, maximal deposition in small ciliate airways and minimal penetration in alveolated lung spaces beyond the terminal bronchioles is achieved.

The standard maneuver to obtain preferential impact of the radioaerosol on the distal bronchi is the slow vital capacity inspiration. This inhalation procedure results in constant deposition of the tracer in the lungs that is mandatory for the interpretation of MC and TC measurements, especially when repeated studies are performed in the same patient. In addition, the lack of deposition in trachea and main bronchi improves the measurement of mucus transport velocity from the central bronchi and makes the measurement of TC more reproducible. The clearance rate of radioaerosols in the ciliate airways of normal subjects increases from 0.02 mm/min in the 16th bronchial generation to 13 mm/min in the trachea. High inspiration flow rates, large particle inhalation (>8 μm), or airways stenosis result in an improperly large deposition of radioactivity in the proximal airways, in which the intrinsic rate of transport of mucus is faster, and reduced impact within the smaller bronchi, in which the clearance rates of particles are slower. This leads to an overestimation of the clearance rates from central and hilar bronchi when the initial deposition of the inhaled aerosol is prevalent in proximal airways. Tracheobronchial clearance is thus evaluated by several mechanisms, such as mucociliary transport, cough, gas/liquid layer movements, phagocytos, and liquid solutes reabsorption by bronchial capillaries and lymphatics.

In asthmatics and normal subjects only MC, TC, and two-phase gas/liquid layer movements in the bronchi can be improved by drug administration. Measurements of MC and TC following the administration of substances with intrinsic activity on the bronchial structures are conditioned by ultimate bronchial clearing effects, that is, the result of bronchodilation, rheology, and secretion composition changes obtained. Radioaerosol image quantification is currently performed in pharmacologic studies of asthmatic subjects to assess the response of MC to therapeutic or provocative administration of various substances. MC measurements are frequently associated with inhalation studies using noble radiogases to assess diffusive ventilation. Unfortunately, radioaerosol production and delivery are often designed only for single administrations, resulting in a difficult comparison of MC quantitative measurements obtained by different groups even with the same administered substance.

The pharmacological effects of many chemical compounds on tracheobronchial clearance have been extensively studied in asthmatics, the most widely studied being bronchodilators and mucolytics in single or associated administration. The effects of these substances on mucus transport and on airways resistance are easily quantified in clinical practice by spirometry and by measurement of the sputum viscoelastic properties and volume of the expectorated. A comparison between scintigraphic measurements of MC and TC with spirometric data is particularly relevant if the pharmaceutical tested has specific effects on the lungs and if it has been administered in association with other substances with synergic or opposite activity. For example, the association of two or three bronchodilators improves the ultimate effects on airways patency, mucus rheology, and secretion and allows the use of submaximal doses of the single pharmaceuticals, with a consequent reduction of side effects and toxicity during chronic therapy. The effects on MC, TC, and convection ventilation of single substances used in chronic and acute therapy of asthma are briefly reported on below.

Parasympathicolytics. Bronchodilation with these substances is obtained in asthma by inhalation of quaternary ammonium compounds such as ipratropium or oxitropium bromide. There are substantial differences between the effects of tertiary (atropine and its derivatives) and quaternary ammonium compounds. The tertiary ammonium compounds reduce mucociliary transport up to 24 h after acute administration. This reduction is probably related to an impairment of ciliary activity and decreased mucus secretion and viscoelasticity in patients with bronchorrhea. Quaternary ammonium compounds do not affect MC or TC rates after single or chronic administration in asthmatics. Sputum rheology and volume are also not affected.

β-2-Sympathicomimetics. These substances are included in chronic and acute therapeutical protocols in treating almost all asthmatics. The positive effects of inhaled salbutamol on MC and TC observed in stable symptomatic asthma is mainly due to an increase in ciliary movement and secretion volume (Fig. 9). The administration of salbutamol results in an increase in the peripheral distribution of the radioaerosol as compared with the baseline scintigraphic pattern. The penetration index in small airways and the alveolar distribution of inhaled tracers is increased from baseline values, also in nonatopic asthma during remission. This response is conditioned by bronchodilation which significantly improves spirometric tests. However, the measured clearance rates of radioaerosols are not significantly improved by salbutamol or other different β_2-agonists in asymptomatic asthma. This "surprising" bronchodilatative effect of salbutamol in asymptomatic asthma, as assessed by spirometry, results in better airways patency and less coughing, a better penetration of the radioaerosol, and selective faster clearance rates in the small distal bronchi that are more consistently visualized in scintigraphic images after treatment. However, the total amount of radioaerosol cleared per hour from the lungs is not significantly increased by salbutamol, also in association with theophylline, in asthmatic patients during remission.

Methylxanthines. Theophylline increases MC with a dose-dependent mechanism in acute and stable asthma. This increase is inversely related to primary bronchial damage and is directly affected by theophylline's stimulation of bronchial epithelium. Other methylxanthines do not show effects on bronchial clearance in asthmatics.

Mucolytics. MC measurements are not significantly improved by the administration of secretolytics such as cysteine, carbocysteine, and ambroxol. No differences in the transport of radioaerosols toward the bronchial tree have been observed after administration of these substances. However, an individual positive response of MC in asthmatics, possibly dependent on baseline

MC values, has been substantiated by radioaerosol imaging. This positive effect on mucus transport is possible only if a normalization of sputum rheology is obtained with the secretolytics.

In conclusion, the applications of nuclear medicine in tracheobronchial clearance measurements allows noninvasive assessment of the response of the bronchial tree to provocative tests, therapeutic intervention, and environmental factors in asthmatics. However, the clinical relevance of these quantitative measurements in asthmatics seems ancillary for the management of the single patient. Further progress in radioaerosol production and labeling will possibly result in more standardized nebulized products suitable for quantitative measurement of MC and TC, also in the clinical setting of asthma, in addition to conventional spirometric quantification of lung ventilation.

Measurement of Lung Epithelial Damage by Radioaerosols in Asthma

The clearance of nebulized radioaerosol of ^{99m}Tc-DTPA sedimented in the alveolar spaces has been studied in a variety of clinical conditions including allergic alveolitis and exposure to toxic substances that can produce bronchospasm in asthmatics. The major environmental cause of lung epithelial damage is cigarette smoke. This is substantiated by an increased permeability of the alveolar surfaces to inhaled DTPA and by an increased lung clearance rate of the tracer. Usually the effects of smoke and other combustion products on airway diameters and tracheobronchial clearance are mediated via both nonspecific and specific reactivity of the ciliate epithelium. However, inhaled smoke also damages directly the alveolar epithelium. In addition, alveolar release of inflammatory mediators may possibly enhance the response of the epithelium to chronic exposure to these substances.

The clinical relevance of LEP measurement in asthma is limited, even if the presence of an abnormal permeability of the alveoli can be observed in persistently hypoperfused areas of the lungs, such as in status asthmaticus and allergic alveolitis. An increase from baseline values of DTPA clearance has been observed in control subjects up to 24 h after inhalation of histamine. This observation suggests a use for LEP measurement to assess the delayed response of the alveolar surface to provocative testing in asthmatics after resolution of bronchospasm.

References

Freeman LM (1984) Freeman and Johnson's clinical radionuclide imaging, vol 2. Grune and Stratton, Orlando
Clarke SW, Pavia D (1984) Aerosols and the lung: clinical and experimental aspects. Butterworths, London
Moren F, Newhouse MT, Dolovich MB (1985) Aerosols in medicine: principles, diagnosis and therapy. Elsevier, Amsterdam

Physical Agents in Bronchial Provocation Tests: Nebulized Hypoosmolar Aerosol

L. Allegra[1] and R. Dal Negro[2]

[1] Institute of Respiratory Diseases, School of Medicine, University of Milan, Milano, Italy
[2] Clinical Respiratory Physiology Department, Bussolengo General Hospital, Verona, Italy

Introduction

The bronchial challenge consisting in getting subjects to inhale ultrasonically nebulized distilled water (UNDW) has for some time now been adopted as an economical "physiological" method for documenting bronchial hyperreactivity [1, 2].

Evidence for the bronchospasmogenic effect of aerosols of nonisotonic solutions in asthmatics was not reported until 1974 [1, 3], though prior to that a number of investigators had observed a generic hazard in chronic bronchitis [4, 5]. In 1980, Allegra and Bianco [2] described a technique whereby, after ultrasonic inhalation of distilled water, adult asthmatics, unlike normal subjects, exhibited a bronchoconstrictor response which could be easily documented (Fig. 1).

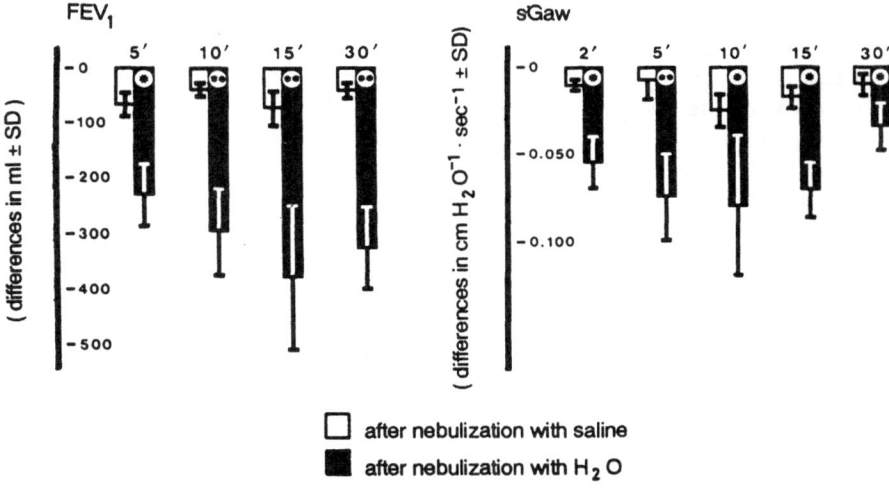

Fig. 1. The first published observation on the spirographic and mechanical behavior of asthmatics submitted to 5 min inhalation of isoosmotic (*white bars*) or hypoosmotic ultrasonic nebulization. * $p \leq 0.05$, ** $p \leq 0.01$

The basic reason for investigating this type of challenge was the clinical observation of the frequent attacks of bronchial constriction experienced by asthmatics on foggy days, which are a common feature of the northern Italian winter. This phenomenon, moreover, was observable not only in patients living in cities or in highly polluted areas and therefore exposed to smog, but also in populations from rural areas breathing uncontaminated fog, which prompted the authors to reproduce exposure to pure distilled water in the laboratory by means of aerosol nebulization [2].

Later it was demonstrated that in asthmatics, unlike normal subjects, FEV_1 is reduced as a result of exposure both to hypotonic and hypertonic ultrasonically nebulized solutions [6]. The bronchial response was standardized not so much as a function of exposure time (which, in their protocol, varied from case to case) or ventilation (the sensitivity of which was inadequate), but rather as a function of the aerosol volume inhaled to obtain a 20% FEV_1 reduction (PD_{20} FEV_1) [7].

The fog test, which has been increasingly used over the past 10 years, may require further studies for standardization of nebulization techniques [8, 9], nebulizer characteristics [8, 10], and aerosol retention [7] and possibly through comparative investigations vs other tests [7], but can now unquestionably be regarded as an already established, though recent, technique for provoking airway obstruction.

Many observations have been possible in recent years thanks to this challenge technique, and new interpretative hypotheses have been proposed regarding bronchial hyperreactivity phenomena on the basis of fog test findings.

Characteristics of the Test

The test is easy to use and is very well tolerated, probably more so than the other provocation tests commonly used [5]. Its reproducibility is good, even when repeated after several months [8, 9], but not when repeated after only a few minutes [2, 3].

Its specificity is excellent (100%) [9, 18], inasmuch as normal subjects invariably test negatively.

As regards the sensitivity of the test, in our own experience, in adults evaluated spirometrically, 91% of subjects testing positively in other specific or nonspecific provocation tests yield positive fog test findings. In reports by other investigators, the sensitivity ranges from 67% [19] to 100% [20]. The test, however, proves much less sensitive in children (Fig. 2), and its sensitivity increases progressively with age (Table 1).

Very recently, however, it has been observed that, using a different measurement technique consisting in the transcutaneous measurement of PO_2 and PCO_2 ($PtcO_2$ and $PtcCO_2$), i.e., by noninvasive transcutaneous monitoring of blood gases (Gasthmatic® method), the fog test proves capable of providing more detailed information on bronchial hyperreactivity (Fig. 3) in

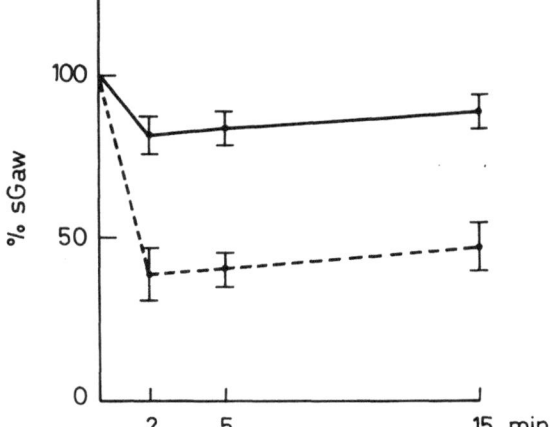

Fig. 2. Average values and standard errors of the changes in specific conductances (sGaw) 2, 5 and 15 min following a challenge with 5 min nebulization of ultrasonically nebulized distilled water in 62 asthmatic children (*solid line*) and 91 asthmatic adults (*dashed line*)

Table 1. Bronchial challenge in asthmatic patients with ultrasonically nebulized distilled water (UNDW)

Patients	Number[a]	Positive challenge	Negative challenge	UNDW challenge positive (%)	negative (%)
5– 8 years old	16	2	14	14	86
9–12 years old	25	11	14	43	57
Adults	114	104	10	91	9

[a] Patients positive to another challenge (such as: exercise, $PGF_{2\alpha}$, metacholine, allergen extracts)

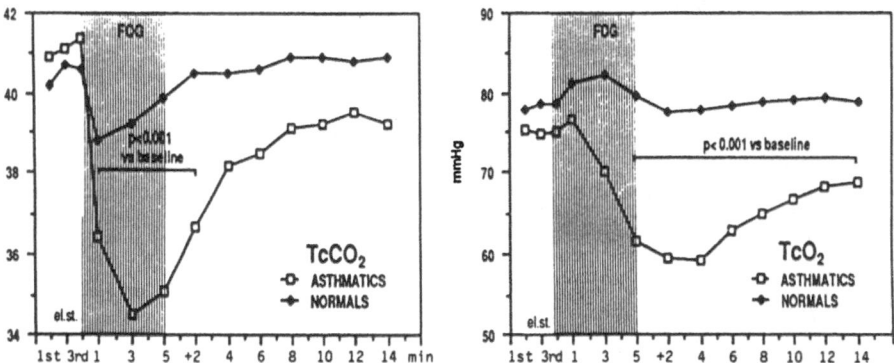

Fig. 3. Transcutaneous CO_2 and O_2 ($TcCO_2$ and TcO_2) monitoring before, during (*shaded area*), and after a challenge with ultrasonically nebulized distilled water ("FOG") inhalation in 28 asthmatics and 28 normal subjects. *El. st.,* electrode stabilization

Table 2. $\dot{V}_A/\dot{Q}_C$ patterns of response to UNDW showed a close relationship to clinical situation and disease status, with a high level of specificity

Patients	Number	Spirometry (%)	Gasthmatic (%)
Asthmatics	62	41.9	96.8
Rhinitics	53	11.3	47.2
Upper respiratory infections	32	12.5	43.7
Controls	34	0.0	0.0

adult asthmatics than traditional spirometry [12]; this is true not merely in adults but also in children (Table 2) who, as mentioned above, are very often FEV_1 nonresponders (our own observations). What is more, even nonasthmatic rhinitics exposed to challenge with ultrasonically nebulized distilled water, though not responding spirometrically, show changes in $PtcO_2$ and $PtcCO_2$ similar to those observed in asthmatics (albeit of shorter duration). Thus, the combination of the UNDW fog test and this new method of evaluating bronchial hyperreactivity by blood gas monitoring presents the distinct advantages of revealing a hitherto neglected pattern of hyperreactivity and of discriminating "predisposed" individuals or early stages of airways disease (it is not yet clear which). The combination allows us to pinpoint the transition from normality to the asthmatic range of bronchial reactivity and permits identification of a borderline area between normal subjects and subjects who are hyperreactive according to classic criteria, i.e., spirometric responders [13].

Applications of the Test

Alongside mechanical changes, moreover, changes in breathing pattern have also been detected depending upon exposure time to ultrasonic nebulized distilled water, which has allowed dose-effect correlations to be constructed (dose meaning exposure time) in asthmatics undergoing the fog test [14].

The test has proved ideal for evaluating the bronchospasm preventive properties of molecules such as disodium cromoglycate [2], nedocromile [15], ketotifen [16], furosemide [11], salbutamol [2], and salmeterol [17]. A drug for which no such activity has been found appears to be ipratropium bromide, at least not at the dose of 80 μg [2].

Mechanisms

There are important differences between challenges with nonisotonic aerosols and the more usual forms of challenge such as histamine and methacholine [18–20]. Unlike the latter, nonisotonic aerosols do not act directly on the bronchial smooth muscle receptors to induce contraction [11], but probably act indirectly by stimulating the release of histamine and other mediators by the mast cells [2, 22, 23]. Since the release of mediators by mast cells more closely resembles what happens following bronchoconstrictor stimulation caused by phenomena occurring naturally in asthmatics, such as the effect of muscular exercise or of air-borne allergens, bronchial challenge with nonisotonic aerosols, and in particular the very simple challenge with ultrasonically nebulized distilled water, would appear preferable for the diagnosis of asthma and for the choice of treatment to be implemented. This, we feel, is all the more true if the Gasthmatic method of monitoring blood gas patterns is used before, during, and after the fog test, since only the transcutaneous measurement of PO_2 and PCO_2 has enabled us to study the very early short-lasting phenomena associated with bronchial hyperreactivity but not with bronchospasm, such as hyperventilation and consequent hypocapnia which are detected only if the subject is monitored during the challenge. This information, in addition to data on the intensity and duration of the $\dot{V}_A/\dot{Q}_C$ mismatch and consequent hypoxia following the challenge, is proving to be of great importance with a view to clarifying the bronchial reactivity phenomenon, detecting hidden hyperreactivities, and perhaps discovering subjects "susceptible" to asthma [12, 13].

As regards the mechanism whereby the fog test induces bronchoconstriction, a limited number of in vivo studies are now available which suggest that mast-cell mediators are at least partly responsible for triggering the bronchoconstrictor response to the nonisotonicity in the airways, the mast cells being situated on the wall, superficially between the epithelial cells and even more superficially in the airway lumen [23] and thus being ideally placed to mediate the response to the changes in osmolarity occurring in the lumen and in the epithelium [19, 25, 26]. Contrary to the opinion of other investigators, we believe that it has only been demonstrated that the fog test is "associated" with the synthesis and release of inflammatory mediators and that these phenomena are related only in a chronologically sequential, and not a causative, manner with the events occurring early in the airways of hyperreactive subjects. We take this view in the light of the results of the only studies considering the time courses of the functional changes induced by exposure to fog challenge not only in asthmatics but also in nonasthmatic rhinitics (in whom clear-cut inflammation of the bronchial airways is inconceivable, insofar as these subjects are unmistakeable FEV_1 nonresponders to provocation testing). These studies show that hyperventilation with a decrease in PCO_2 occurs immediately, from the very first few breaths following inhalation of UNDW, and that a ventilation-perfusion mismatch begins to manifest itself after 60–100 breaths [12, 13]. We therefore believe that the fog test immediately induces an osmolar alteration on the surface of the bronchial epithelium and on the intercellular receptor sites of the irritant receptors, with an instantaneous hyperventilatory response independent of bronchoconstrictor phenomena (it also occurs, in fact, in FEV_1 nonresponders). We are convinced that $PtcCO_2$ monitoring enables us to split this "epithelial" and "neuroreceptor" effect off from the "muscular" effect (bronchial and perhaps also vascular) revealed by the $PtcO_2$ trend, which may possibly be associated with release of inflammatory mediators (though, in this case, too, we cannot be sure that it is a direct, not to mention an exclusive, result of such release). We believe that inflammation is not the factor responsible for the initial phases of bronchoconstriction, but is responsible for chronologically less immediate stages, and that, on the contrary, physical "distorsions" related to osmolarity are directly responsible for the early phenomena, particularly the hyperventilation.

References

1. Allegra L, Bianco S, Petrigni C, Robuschi M (1974) Lo sforzo muscolare e la nebulizzazione ultrasonica di H_2O come test di provocazione aspecifica del broncospasmo. In: Pasargiklian M, Bocca E (eds) Progressi in medicina respiratoria '74, Terme Sirmione, pp 81–86
2. Allegra L, Bianco S (1980) Non-specific bronchoreactivity obtained with ultrasonic aerosol of distilled water. Eur J Respir Dis 61 [Suppl 106]:41–49
3. Allegra L, Robuschi M, Bianco S (1975) Tests di provocazione bronchiale aspecifica. In: Melillo G, Pisaneschi M (ed.) Atti I Congr. Naz. Assoc. Ital. Aerosols in Med. Salsomaggiore, pp 107–112
4. Cheney FW Jr, Butler J (1968) The effects of ultrasonically produced aerosols on airway resistance in man. Anesthesiology 29:1099–1106
5. Pflug AE, Cheney FW Jr, Butler J (1970) The effects of an ultrasonic aerosol on pulmonary mechanics and arterial blood gases in patients with chronic bronchitis. Am Rev Respir Dis 101:710–714
6. Schoeffel RE, Anderson SD, Altounyan RCE (1981) Bronchial hyperreactivity in response to inhalation of ultrasonically nebulized solutions of distilled water and saline. Br Med J 283:1285–1287
7. Anderson SD, Schoeffel RE (1985) The inhalation of ultrasonically nebulized aerosols as a provocation test for asthma. In: Hargreave FE, Woolcock AS (eds) Airway responsiveness: measurements and interpretation. Astra Pharmac Canada, Mont St. Marie, pp 39–48
8. Anderson SD, Schoeffel RE, Finney M (1983) Evaluation of ultrasonically nebulised solutions for provocation testing in patients with asthma. Thorax 38:284–291
9. Goddard RF, Mercer TT, O'Neill PX, Flores PL, Sandez R (1968) Output characteristics and clinical efficacy of ultrasonic nebulizers. J Asthma Res 5:355–358
10. Bianco S, Robuschi M, Damonte C (1983) Drug effect on bronchial response to $PGF_{2\alpha}$ and water inhalation. Eur J Respir Dis 64 [Suppl 128]:213–221
11. Robuschi M, Gambaro G, Spagnotto S, Vaghi A, Bianco S (1989) Inhaled furosemide is highly effective in preventing ultrasonically nebulized water bronchoconstriction. Pulm Pharmacol 1:187–191
12. Dal Negro R, Allegra L (1989) Blood gas changes during and after nonspecific airway challenge in asthmatic and normal subjects. J Appl Physiol 67(6): 2627–2630
13. Dal Negro RW, Turco PA, Allegra L (1992) Blood gas changes in nonasthmatic rhinitis during and after nonspecific airway challenge. Am Rev Respir Dis 145: 337–339
14. Chadha TS, Birch S, Allegra L, Sackner MA (1984) Effects of ultrasonically nebulized distilled water on respiratory resistance and breathing pattern in normals and asthmatics. Bull Eur Physiopathol Respir 20:257–262
15. Robuschi M, Vaghi A, Simone P, Bianco S (1987) Prevention of fog-induced bronchospasm by nedocromil sodium. Clin Allergy 17:69

16. Allegra L, Turco P, Dal Negro R, Pomari C (1992) $P_{tc}O_2$ and $P_{tc}CO_2$ monitoring of bronchial responsiveness in FEV_1-now-responder asthmatics during ketotifen and placebo treatment. Respiration (to be published)
17. Cogo A, Turco P, Dal Negro R, Allegra L (1992) Salmeterol: a 12-hour-protection against UNDW-induced hyperreasponsiveness. Am Rev Respir Dis 145: A59
18. Smith CM, Anderson SD (1990) Bronchial hyperresponsiveness as assessed by non isotonic aerosols. In: Olivieri D, Bianco S (eds) Airway obstruction and inflammation. Prog Resp Res 24:105–116
19. Rosati G, Mormile F, Ciappi G (1983) Bronchial challenges with ultrasonic mist histamine and carbachol: a comparison in 87 asthmatic subjects. Eur J Respir Dis 64 [Suppl 128]:417–420
20. Magyar P, Dervaderics M, Toth A, Lantos A (1983) Inhalation of hypertonic potassium chloride solution: a specific bronchial challenge for asthma. Giorn It Mal Tor 37:29–34
21. Finney MJB, Anderson SD, Black JL (1987) The effect of non isotonic solutions on human isolated airway smooth muscle. Respir Physiol 69:277–286
22. Shaw RJ, Anderson SD, Durham SR, Taylor KM, Schoeffel RE, Green W, Torgillo P, Kay AB (1985) Mediators of hypersensitivity and "fog"-induced asthma. Allergy 40:48–57
23. Eggleston PA, Kagey-Sobotka A, Lichtenstein LM (1987) A comparison of the osmotic activation of basophils and human lung mast cells. Am Rev Respir Dis 135:1043–1048
24. Tomioka M, Ida S, Shimdoh Y, Ishihara T, Takishima T (1984) Mast cells in bronchoalveolar lumen of patients with bronchial asthma. Am Rev Respir Dis 129: 1000–1005
25. Silber G, Proud D, Warner J et al. (1988) In vivo release of inflammatory mediators by hyperosmolar solutions. Am Rev Respir Dis 137:602–612
26. Eschenbacher WL, Grovelyn TR (1988) Mediator release after local asmolar challenge to the airways. In: Armour C, Black JL (eds) Mechanisms in asthma: pharmacology, physiology and management. Liss, New York, pp 355–363

Physical Agents in Bronchial Provocation Tests: Nebulized Hyperosmolar Aerosol

C. M. SMITH

Department of Allergy and Allied Respiratory Disorders.
Guy's Hospital, London, UK

Introduction

Probably the most important development leading to the recognition that abnormal osmolarity of the respiratory tract is a potent stimulus that can provoke airway narrowing was the introduction of ultrasonic nebulizers in the 1960s. Since these nebulizers produce dense aerosols (usually in excess of 3 ml of aerosol per minute), with a large proportion of respirable droplets [31], they were considered superior to the nebulizers and humidifiers available at that time [18–20]. However, it became apparent that inhalation of ultrasonically nebulized aerosols could be associated both with an increase in airway resistance [11, 22, 23, 30] and a decrease in arterial oxygen tension [23, 29] in patients with chronic bronchitis [11, 23], chronic obstructive airways disease [22, 29] and asthma [6, 11]. The use of ultrasonically nebulized aerosols specifically for the purpose of diagnosis and assessment of bronchial hyperresponsiveness was investigated in the 1970s by Allegra et al. [1, 3] and Allegra and Bianco [2], who used ultrasonically nebulized water to challenge patients with asthma. In 1981, Schoeffel et al. [25] extended these findings by demonstrating that the response to ultrasonically nebulized aerosols is largely determined by the osmolarity of the aerosol and that hyperosmolar aerosols are also potent agents for provoking airway narrowing in asthmatic subjects.

Why challenge with ultrasonically nebulized hyperosmolar aerosols?

To date, challenge with hyperosmolar aerosols has been used largely for research purposes. However, it is now apparent that here may be some advantages to using this form of challenge in the routine assessment of bronchial hyperresponsiveness. The challenge is simple, inexpensive and requires little effort from the patient. Unlike challenge with more conventional pharmacological agents, such as histamine and methacholine, it is a highly specific test, in that normal subjects do not respond even at high doses [4, 21, 27, 28]. However, the test is not as sensitive as the pharmacological challenges, and subjects with intermittent or past symptoms of asthma are unlikely to respond to hyperosmolar aerosol challenge [4, 27, 28]. The fact that it is mostly patients with asthma of clinical significance who respond to challenge with hyperosmolar saline may relate to the mechanism whereby hyperosmolarity induces a response. Unlike histamine and methacholine, hyperosmolarity does not act directly on smooth muscle receptors to cause bronchoconstriction [16]. Rather, it is believed to act indirectly, by stimulating the release of inflammatory mediators from cells found in the lumen and submucosa of the bronchi [7, 12, 13, 15]. Thus the challenge may reflect more closely the extent of inflammation and/or the degree of activation of inflammatory cells within the airways.

Methods

Here, a technique for challenge with ultrasonically nebulized hyperosmolar (4.5%) saline is described. It was used to challenge 41 adults and 18 children with a clinical diagnosis of asthma and 10 normal subjects

Subjects

Normal Subjects. Ten healthy nonsmoking subjects (9 female, 1 male) were used as normal controls. All had a normal FEV_1 [22] at rest (mean ± 1 SD, 117 ± 10), and none had a history of wheeze or chronic cough, or had ever required the use of a bronchodilator.

Subjects with Asthma. The technique was used to challenge 60 subjects (29 male and 31 female) aged between 6 and 57 years, all of whom had a clinical diagnosis of asthma made by specialist physicians. A summary of their prescribed medication is given in Table 1.

Table 1. Summary of medications used by the 60 patients with asthma

Medications	Number (%)
β-Adrenocepter agonist	
Regularly	38 (63%)
As required	15 (25%)
Glucocorticosteroids	
Inhaled	24 (40%)
Oral	4 (7%)
Theophylline	17 (28%)
Disodium cromoglycate	19 (31%)
None	7 (12%)

Equipment

The equipment used and the manufacturers' names and addresses are given in Table 2.

Table 2. Equipment used for challenge with ultrasonically nebulized hyperosmolar saline, together with the manufacturer and place of manufacture

Equipment	Manufacturer and address
Ultrasonic nebulizer: Mist-O_2-Gen EN 143A	Mistogen Equipment Co Lancaster, Pa USA Oakland, California USA
Two-way valve: Hans Rudolph	Hans Rudolph Inc, Kansas City, MO USA
Autospirometer: Minato AS-500 or AS-800	Minato Medical Science Co Ltd, Osaka Japan
Gasometer: Tissot gasometer (350 L)	W.E. Collins, Braintree, MA USA
Recorder: Devices M19	Electromed, Jersey UK
Balance: Sartorius 1216MP	Sartorius GmbH, Göttingen, Germany

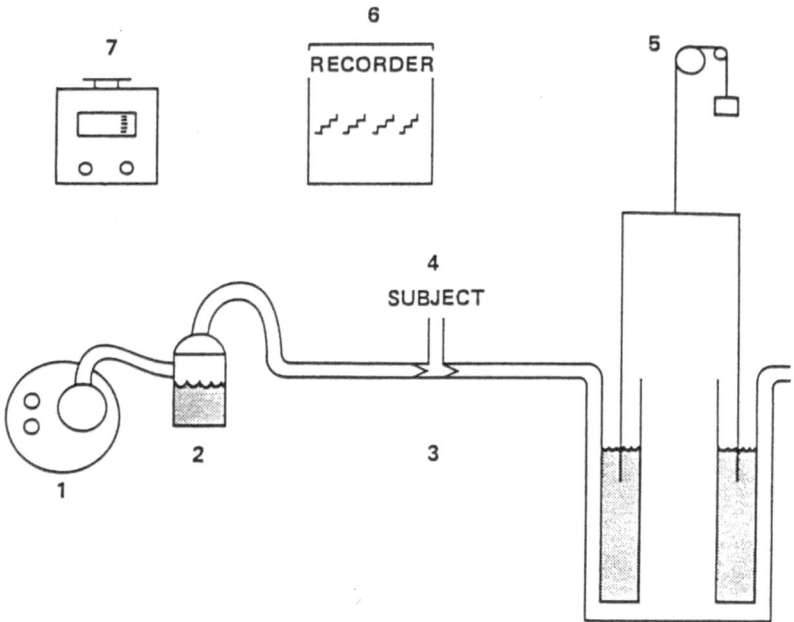

Fig. 1. Apparatus used to challenge subjects with hyperosmolar saline. Details of the equipment used are given in Table 2. 1, ultrasonic nebulizer; 2, nebulizer canister with 4.5% NaCl; 3, low resistance 2-way valve; 4, subject; 5, 350 liter Tissot gasometer; 6, chart recorder for ventilation; 7, balance

A Mist-O_2-gen EN143A ultrasonic nebulizer was used to generate an aerosol of 4.5% saline. The aerosol was delivered to the subject via a large two-way valve that was connected to the nebulizer by flexible noncorrugated tubing (68 cm in length and 20 mm in diameter). A schematic diagram of the circuit is shown in Fig. 1. The droplet size distribution of the aerosol was measured with a seven-stage cascade impactor using the method described by Phipps et al. [24], both with and without the valve and connecting tube. The mass median aerodynamic diameter (MMAD) of the aerosol at the port of the nebulizer (i.e without the valve and tubing) was 5.7 μm (geometric standard deviation 1.2 μm). Placing the tubing and respiratory valve in the circuit produced major modifications to the droplet size distribution. The MMAD was reduced to 3.6 μm and was almost monodisperse. Presumably, the large droplets impacted on the tubing and the inspiratory valve. The output of the nebulizer was also modified when the circuit was included. With the patient breathing at rest, the output of the nebulizer to the inspiratory port of the valve was reduced from 3.0 ml/min to about 1.2 ml/min, again because of deposition of the larger droplets.

Challenge Procedure

Initially the subjects were instructed to inhale 30 liters of room air through the valve at a comfortable resting rate of ventilation. A nose clip was used to ensure mouth breathing. The FEV_1 was measured before and after this procedure to determine whether there was any change in airway calibre in response to breathing through the apparatus. The subjects were then instructed to breathe 10 liters of aerosol, again at tidal volume. Following this, the FEV_1 was again measured, this time at 0.5, 1.5, and 3 min and, if necessary, at further 2 min intervals until the values had reached a plateau or had begun to rise. If the reduction in FEV_1 was less than 10%, the volume of aerosol inhaled during the next challenge period was doubled. If it was between 10% and 20% the previous dose was repeated rather than doubled. The challenge continued in this fashion until the FEV_1 had been reduced by more than 20% or until a total of 250 liters of aerosol had been inhaled. The most usual progression of the challenge was 10, then 20, 40, 80 and 100 liters. However, for some subjects with a history of severe asthmatic responses, the initial dose given was 5 rather than 10 liters.

The ventilation (L BTPS) was determined by collecting the expired air in a 350 liter chain-compensated gasometer. The signal from a potentiometer attached to the gasometer was displayed on a chart recorder.

The doses administered were reported in terms of the cumulative volume of 4.5% saline delivered to the inspiratory port of the valve. This was determined by weighing the nebulizer canister and tubing up to the inspiratory port of the valve before and after challenge.

Stimulus-response plots were drawn relating the cumulative dose of 4.5% saline delivered to the inspiratory port of the valve (ml) on a logarithmic scale, to the percent fall in FEV$_1$ on an arithmetic scale. The dose that provoked a 20% fall in FEV$_1$ (PD$_{20}$) was obtained from these plots by linear interpolation and used as an index of sensitivity.

Results

Distribution of PD$_{20}$ Values

The mean maximum percent fall in FEV$_1$ (± 1 SD) in normal subjects was 6% (± 2%). This reduction, though small, was significant. The subjects also experienced a moist and sometimes productive cough both during and following challenge, although this was not systematically documented.

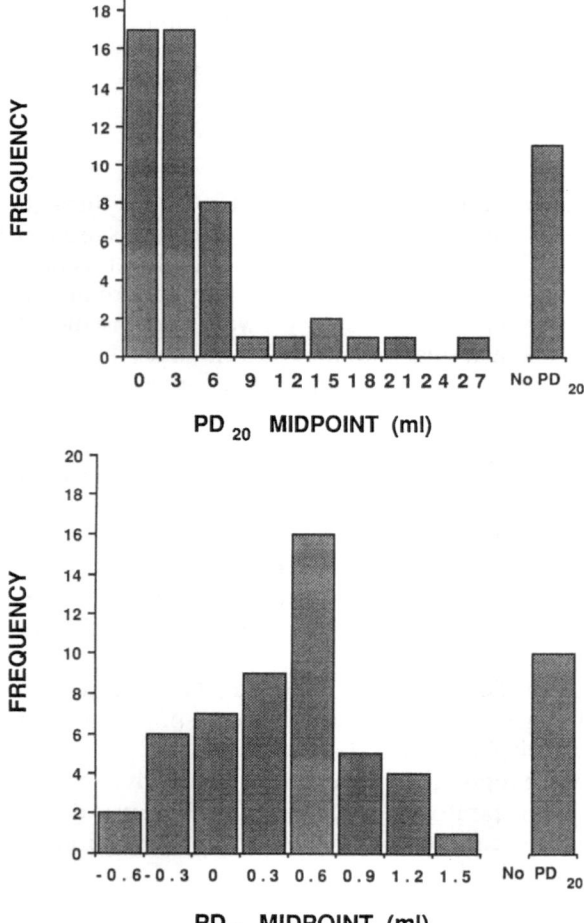

Fig. 2. Frequency histogram of the volume of a aerosol required to induce a 20% fall in FEV$_1$ (PD$_{20}$) in 60 subjects with asthma (top panel). In those subjects with a PD$_{20}$ value, the distribution is normalized by logarithmic transformation (bottom panel) of the PD$_{20}$ values

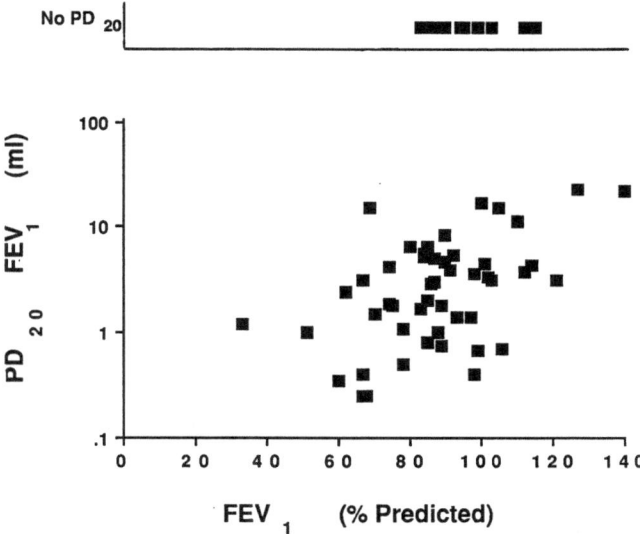

Fig. 3. Relationship between baseline FEV_1 (expressed as a percentage of the predicted normal value) and PD_{20}

Of the 60 asthmatic subjects studied, 49 (82%) responded with at least a 20% fall in FEV_1 in response to inhaling up to 210 liters of 4.5% saline aerosol. Of the 49 subjects who did respond, 34 (70%) did so after inhaling less than 5 ml. With our nebulizer and delivery circuit, this volume would be delivered after a total of about 40–60 liters had been inhaled. Thus, the distribution of PD_{20} values was highly skewed. In those subjects who did respond, logarithmic transformation of the PD_{20} values, however, produced a normal distribution (Fig. 2).

Relationship Between Response and Baseline FEV_1

There was a significant relationship between baseline FEV_1 and PD_{20} values (Spearman's correlation coefficient = 0.46, $p < 0.001$). Despite this significant trend, however, it would not be possible to confidently predict the outcome of challenge based on baseline FEV_1 (Fig. 3).

Repeatability of Challenge

Eight of the asthmatic subjects also underwent a second challenge with 4.5% saline within 37 days of the initial challenge. During this period there had been no change in medication or in severity of symptoms. The geometric

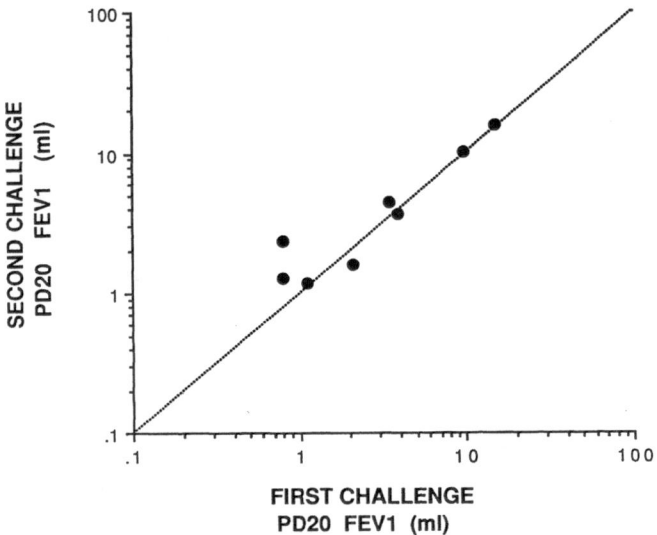

Fig. 4. PD_{20} values measured in eight subjects after two separate challenges performed within 37 days

mean PD_{20} (and 95% confidence limits) for the first challenge was 2.69 ml (1.06–6.85) and for the second challenge 3.36 ml (1.52–7.43). The coefficient of variation was 14%, and the correlation coefficient for these values was 0.92 ($p < 0.001$) (Fig. 4).

Discussion

Equipment

There are a number of different models of ultrasonic nebulizers now on the market. The droplet size varies as a function of the frequency of the nebulizer, but is fairly constant at operating frequencies between 0.5–4 MHz [9]. However, it is important to realise that although the manufacturers usually specify both the droplet size distribution and nebulizer output, these specifications will be modified considerably by the circuit used to deliver the aerosol to the patient. For this reason, it is preferable, if facilities exist, to determine droplet size distribution and output with the delivery circuit attached. If a respiratory valve is used, it is possible to report the volume of nebulized solution delivered to the inspiratory port of the valve. This is because the inspiratory valve closes during expiration, and thus the aerosol in the tubing is either inhaled during the following breath or is deposited. If a mask is used, it is more difficult to assess the dose delivered to the patient, because the aerosol is dissipated during expiration.

Technique

Three observations arising from these studies suggest that the protocol could be improved. First, when the dose is measured in terms of ventilation, it does not take into account the different rates at which people breathe. Since the output of the nebulizer is constant with time, more aerosol is delivered to those subjects with a slower rate of ventilation than is delivered to those with a faster rate of ventilation. To some extent, this problem is overcome by reporting the doses in terms of ml of 4.5% saline delivered to the valve. However, to standardize the delivered dose, it is probably better to time the doses rather than measure the ventilation. Second, the response was either fully developed or almost fully developed within 90 s of each challenge interval. Thus it is not necessary to continue to measure FEV_1 for more than 90 s after each dose. Third, of those subjects who did respond, 93% had done so by the time 15 ml or less had been delivered to the inspiratory port of the valve. With our nebulizer and delivery circuit, the output is 1.2 ml/min (± 0.2). Thus the time taken to deliver 15 ml is about 12.5 min.

The challenge procedure has therefore been modified so that the doses are timed, spirometry is measured 90 s after each dose and a total of 15–20 ml is delivered to the subject. The first exposure is for 30 s, and subsequent doses are progressed by doubling the time as follows; 1 min, 2 min, 4 min and 8 min. Again, if the subject responds with a greater than 10% fall in FEV_1 from that measured before the previous dose, then the dose is repeated rather than doubled. Since the nebulizer output is constant with time, the dose can either be reported in terms of ml of aerosol delivered to the valve or number of minutes of nebulization. However, the output of ultrasonic nebulizers can decrease with use, and for this reason it is probably better to continue to determine the dose delivered gravimetrically, by weighing the nebulizer and tubing before and after challenge.

The response to challenge with hyperosmolar aerosols can be brisk in some patients, and, as for all forms of bronchial challenge, nebulized bronchodilator should be readily available, preferably prepared before challenge has begun. Facilities for cardiopulmonary resuscitation should also be available.

Comparison with Other Forms of Challenge

When challenge with hyperosmolar saline is performed using techniques identical or similar to those described in the Methods section, responsiveness to hyperosmolar saline correlates with responsiveness to methacholine [28], histamine [8], exercise [8, 28] and eucapnic hyperventilation [28]. Surprisingly, responsiveness to ultrasonically nebulized hyperosmolar aerosols is not correlated with responsiveness to ultrasonically nebulized water [21, 28], and although both challenges have been considered as "osmotic" challenges [4], they should in fact be considered as being two quite distinct forms of challenge.

Specificity of the Response to Saline

The response to 4.5% saline is specific for the detection of abnormal bronchial hyperresponsiveness; normal subjects do not respond. However, the challenge is not specific for asthma and will detect bronchial hyperresponsiveness in subjects with chronic obstructive airways disease (COAD). In a group of 16 current smokers with COAD who demonstrated hyperresponsiveness to histamine, nine also demonstrated abnormal responsiveness to ultrasonically nebulized 4,5% saline aerosol. In those smokers who did respond, the distribution of PD_{20} values was not different from that seen in asthmatic controls. Thus, on the basis of PD_{20} values it was not possible to differentiate the subjects with COAD from those with asthma.

Standardization

A number of different techniques for challenge with ultrasonically nebulized aerosols have been described. Although most describe a technique in which a single concentration of aerosol is delivered in incremental doses [5, 7, 21], it is also possible to increase the stimulus by increasing the output of the nebulizer [26] or the concentration of the aerosol [10, 17].

As yet there has been no study examining the comparability of these various techniques. However, for theoretical reasons, it is possible that different outcomes may be expected. Unlike the pharmacological agents that act directly on receptors, challenges with hyperosmolar aerosols act by changing the physical environment within the airways. This will depend on a combination of how much aerosol is delivered and the rate at which it is able to increase osmolarity. For example, it is possible for a subject to show very little responsiveness to 2.7% saline, regardless of how long it is delivered for and yet to respond very briskly to 4.5% and 5.4% saline, even when delivered for a relatively short time. This may occur despite the fact that the number of moles of NaCl delivered during the 2.7% saline challenge are considerably more than that delivered over a shorter period during the 4.5% and 5.4% saline challenges (Fig. 5). Thus, this form of challenge does not display a simple relationship between the cumulative moles of NaCl delivered and the response. Changing the rate at which osmolarity is increased by changing the nebulizer output or concentration of aerosol may alter sensitivity considerably.

The type of solution used may also influence the outcome of challenge. Eschenbacher et al. [14] reported that the response was slightly enhanced if the solution contained ions, but concluded that osmolarity was the most important determinant of the response. However, Magyar et al. [21] reported that the response was more brisk if 10% KCl was used in place of 10% NaCl, despite the fact, that the solutions were of almost identical osmolarity, and suggested that this may be due to the ability of potassium to directly depolarize the membranes of mast cell and smooth muscle.

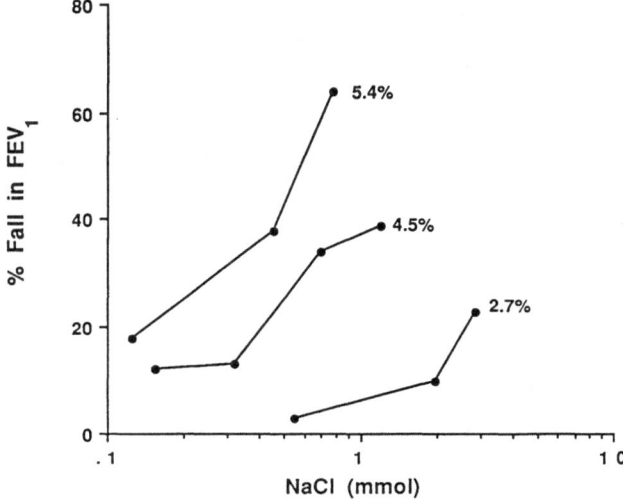

Fig. 5. Relationship between the percent fall in FEV_1 and the number of millimoles of NaCl delivered during challenge with 2.7%, 4.5% and 5.4% saline in a patient with asthma

The permeance of the ion may also be important, since less permeant ions are able to maintain a greater osmotic gradient across cell membranes than are more permeant ions [15].

Conclusions

Challenge with ultrasonically nebulized 4.5% saline is a repeatable, cheap and simple test of bronchial hyperresponsiveness that can be completed within 25 min. It is therefore suitable for use in both the research and routine laboratory. It is able to detect bronchial hyperresponsiveness of clinical significance, but is unlikely to detect mild or borderline hyperresponsiveness. Since this form of challenge is associated with the release and synthesis of mediators of inflammation, it is an appropriate test to use to assess the effectiveness of pharmacological agents, both acutely and after long-term therapy.

References

1. Allegra L, Bianco S, Petrigini G, Robuschi M (1974) Lo Sforzo muscolare e la nebulizzazione ultrasonica die H_2O come tests di provocazione aspecifica del broncospasmo. In: Pasargiklian, Bocca (eds) Progressi in medicina respiratoria '74. Edizioni scientifiche terme e grandi alberghi di Sirmione, Sirmione, p 81
2. Allegra L, Bianco S (1980) Non-specific bronchoreactivity obtained with an ultrasonic aerosol of distilled water. Eur J Respir Dis 61:41–49

3. Allegra L, Robuschi M, Bianco S (1975) Tests di provocazione bronchiale aspecifica. In: Mellillo, Pisaneschi (eds) Attidel 10 Congresso Nazionale dell'Associazione Italiani Aerosol in Medicina. Terme di Tabiano, Salsomaggiore, pp 107–121
4. Anderson SD, Smith CM (1989) The use of non-isotonic aerosols for evaluating bronchial hyperresponsiveness. In: Spector S (ed) Provocative challenge procedures: background and methodology. Futura, Mount Kisco, pp 227–252
5. Anderson SD, Schoeffel RE, Finney MJB (1983) Evaluation of ultrasonically nebulised solutions for provocation testing in patients with asthma. Thorax 28: 284–291
6. Barker R, Levison H (1972) Effects of ultrasonically nebulized distilled water on airway dynamics in children with cystic fibrosis and asthma. J Pediatr 80:396–400
7. Belcher NG, Murdoch RD, Dalton N, House FR, Clark TJH, Rees PJ, Lee TH (1988) A comparison of mediator and catecholamine release between exercise- and hypertonic saline-induced asthma. Am Rev Respir Dis 137:1026–1032
8. Belcher NG, Lee TH, Rees PJ (1989) Airway responsiveness to hypertonic saline, exercise and histamine challenges in bronchial asthma. Eur J Respir Dis 2:44–48
9. Boucher RMG, Kreuter J (1968) The fundamentals of ultrasonic atomization of medical solutions. Ann Allergy 26:591–600
10. Boulet L-P, Legris C, Thibault L, Turcotte H (1987) Comparative bronchial responses to hyperosmolar saline and methacholine in asthma. Thorax 42:953–958
11. Cheney F, Butler J (1968) The effects of ultrasonically-produced aerosols on airway resistance in man. Anesthesiology 29:1099–1106
12. Eggleston PA, Kagey-Sobotka A, Lichtenstein LM (1987) A comparison of the osmotic activation of basophils and human lung mast cells. Am Rev Respir Dis 135:1043–1048
13. Eggleston PA, Kagey-Sobotka A, Schleimer RP, Lichtenstein LM (1984) Interaction between hyperosmolar and IgE-mediated histamine release from basophils and mast cells. Am Rev Respir Dis 130:86–91
14. Eschenbacher WL, Boushey HA, Sheppard D (1984) Alterations in osmolarity of inhaled aerosols cause bronchoconstriction and cough, but absence of a permeant anion causes cough alone. Am Rev Respir Dis 129:211–215
15. Eschenbacher WL, Gravelyn TR (1988) Mediator release after local osmolar challenge to the airways. In: Armour CL, Black JL (eds) Mechanisms in asthma: pharmacology, physiology and management. Liss, New York, pp 355–363
16. Finney MJB, Anderson SD, Black JL (1987) The effect of non-isotonic solutions on human isolated airway smooth muscle. Respir Physiol 69:227–286
17. Finney MJB, Anderson SD, Black JL (1989) Terfenadine modifies airway narrowing induced by the inhalation of non-isotonic aerosols in subjects with asthma. Am Rev Respir Dis (in press)
18. Goddard RF, Mercer TT, O'Neill PXF, Flores RL, Sanchez R (1968) Output characteristics and clinical efficacy of ultrasonic nebulizers. J Asthma Res 5: 355–368
19. Harris RL, Riley HD (1967) Reactions to aerosol medication in infants and children. J A M A 201:953–955
20. Herzog P, Norlander OP, Engstrom C-G (1964) Ultrasonic generation of aerosol for the humidification of inspired gas during volume-controlled ventilation. Acta Anaesthesiol Scand 8:79–95
21. Magyar P, Dervaderics M, Toth A (1984) Bronchial challenge with hypertonic KCl solution in the diagnosis of bronchial asthma. Schweiz Med Wochenschr 114:910–913
22. Malik SK, Jenkins DE (1972) Alterations in airway dynamics following inhalation of ultrasonic mist. Chest 62:660–664
23. Pflug AE, Cheney FW, Butler J (1970) The effects of an ultrasonic aerosol on pulmonary mechanics and arterial blood gases in patients with chronic bronchitis. Am Rev Respir Dis 101:710–714
24. Phipps P, Borham P, Gonda I, Baily D, Bautovich G, Anderson S (1987) A rapid

method for the evaluation of diagnostic radioaerosol delivery systems. Eur J Nucl Med 13:183–186

25. Schoeffel RE, Anderson SD, Altounyan REC (1981) Bronchial hyperreactivity in response to inhalation of ultrasonically nebulized solutions of distilled water and saline (Br Med J 283:1285–1287

26. Sheppard D, Rizk NW, Boushey HA, Bethel RA (1983) Mechanism of cough and bronchoconstriction induced by distilled water aerosol. Am Rev Respir Dis 127: 691–694

27. Smith CM, Anderson SD (1990) Provocation tests for asthma using non-isotonic aerosols. J Allergy Clin Immunol (in press)

28. Smith CM, Anderson SD (1989) Inhalation challenge using hypertonic (4.5%) saline in asthmatic subjects: a comparison with responses to hyperpnoea, methacholine and water. Eur Respir J (in press)

29. Taguchi JT (1971) Effect of ultrasonic nebulization on blood gas tensions in chronic obstructive lung disease. Chest 60:356–361

30. Waltemath CL, Bergman N (1973) Increased respiratory resistance provoked by endotracheal administration of aerosols. Am Rev Respir Dis 108:520–535

31. Wolfsdorf J, Swift DL, Avery ME (1969) Mist therapy reconsidered; an evaluation of the respiratory deposition of labelled water aerosols produced by jet and ultrasonic nebulizers. Paediatrics 43:799–808

Chemical Agents in Bronchial Provocation Tests

P. MAGYAR

Department of Pulmunology, Semmelweis Medical University, Budapest, Hungary

Introduction

In addition to bronchoconstriction mediators, various pharmacological agents, and hypo- and hyperosmolar solutions, several other chemical agents can provoke bronchospasm if they are inhaled. With few exceptions these are occupational agents or air pollutants and are discussed as such in the approporiate chapters of this book. However, they are also used for bronchial provocation tests (BPTs) in order to clarify the etiological or stimulating factors of bronchospasm, especially in patients with asthma, or for research purposes.

Among the chemical agents used for BPTs, potassium chloride (KCl), as a nonoccupational and nonpollutant agent seems to have particular importance in the differential diagnosis of asthma [21]. Inhalation of nebulized KCl solution was found to cause significant bronchospasm in patients with asthma [20] but does not do so in healthy subjects and in patients with chronic bronchitis [21] and "wheezy bronchitis" [24]. Although KCl BPTs are performed with hyperosmolar (10%) solutions,, its bronchospastic activity is mainly due not to its osmotic properties but to a specific ionic action of potassium [20]. In vitro studies on mast cells demonstrated that potassium surplus causes a very fast and significant release of histamine, with the highest rate at isomolar concentrations [25].

Potassium was found to contract human bronchial smooth muscle preparations in a dose-dependent way [8], in contrast to hyperosmolar solutions [8, 13]. These observations strongly suggest an essential difference in the mechanism of action of KCl BPTs and tests using inhalation of hyperosmolar solutions, such as NaCl [27], which has a much weaker bronchospastic effect at the same concentration [20]. Several drugs used in the prevention and therapy of asthma were found to inhibit KCl-induced bronchospasm [20]. The latter could also be inhibited by a previously performed exercise test, even if it did not provoke bronchospasm [29, 30].

Inhaled KCl produces no change in serum K^+ levels [9, 22] or cardiovascular function [9]. Bronchoconstriction induced by KCl is usually easely reversed with inhaled bronchodilator drugs [20]; thus KCl-induced bronchoconstriction is safe [9]. The nonsignificant and dose-independent bronchial response to KCl of nonasthmatic subjects [21] has allowed a new method of estimation of positive criteria regarding differentiation between asthmatics and nonasthmatics [23]. This method is described here along with that of the KCl BPT used for differential diagnostic purposes in our laboratory in patients suspected of having asthma.

Methods

Subjects

Healthy subjects ($n = 55$; 23 males, 32 females; age: 32 ± 12 years) and patients with chronic bronchitis ($n = 209$; 116 males, 93 females; age: 42 ± 12 years), allergic rhinitis ($n = 71$; 38 males, 33 females; age: 33 ± 11 years), and asthma ($n = 329$; 148 males, 181 females; age: 36 ± 14 years) were challenged with nebulized KCl solution.

Inclusion criteria for the group of healthy subjects were: no history of wheeze or chronic cough and normal airway resistance (R_{aw}) and FEV_1 according to the reference values recommended by the European Community for Coal and Steel [26]. For the diagnosis of chronic bronchitis and asthma, criteria recommended by the American Thoracic Society [3] were used. The diagnosis was based primarily on the history and clinical and lung function data observed during a long-term (2–8 yerar) follow-up period in our in- and outpatient departments. Only patients who had asthma attacks that were observed by us during the follow-up period were included in the group of patients with asthma.

Most of the patients with allergic rhinitis were sensitive to grass and/or ragweed pollens (86%) and showed regular seasonal nasal symptoms. At the time of BPT 19% of them had mild nasal symptoms. Patients who also had a history of wheeze were not included in this group.

The inhalation challenge test was performed only in subjects with R_{aw} below 0.6 kPa s l^{-1}. They were asked not to take any medicine affecting the bronchial system and not to drink coffee, tea, or cola in the day prior to the test. Regular steroid, disodium cromoglycate, and ketotifen treatment was ceased 1 week before testing. In the 4 day period prior to BPT with KCl, other BPT or exercise tests were not allowed. The BPT was carried out between 9 and 11 a.m.

Patients were informed about the test procedure and gave their consent.

Nebulization and Challenge Test Procedure

Nebulization of a 10% KCl solution (potassium chloride 10% ampule, 10 ml; Chinoin, Budapest, Hungary) was performed with an ultrasonic nebulizer (TUR-USI-50, Dresden, FRG). The ultrasound frequency was 2.6 MHz. The rate of nebulizer delivery was 3 ± 0.25 ml/min at setting position no. 5; in position no. 4 of the ventilator flow scale, the air flow was 12 l/min. The nebulizer and its heater were switched on at least 5 min before starting inhalation of the aerosol in order to have sufficient time to heat both the system and the fluid to be nebulized. The temperature of the aerosol measured at the port of the mouthpiece was 34°–37°C at room temperature of 18°–22°C.

The nebulized KCl solution was delivered to the subject via a mouthpiece attached to a two-way valve system that was connected to the nebulizer by flexible corrugated plastic tubing (63 cm in length and 24 cm in diameter).

Inhalation was carried out through a mouthpiece during tidal breathing, controlling the inhaled dose by counting the number of inhalations while the nose was closed with a noseclip. The distinctly visible high aerosol density of air leaving the exhalation ort of the nebulizer mouthpiece made it possible to easily count the number of breaths.

Lung function parameters, namely, airway resistance (R_{aw}), specific airway conductance (sG_{aw}) and FEV_1 were measured by a constant volume body plethysmograph (Bodytest, Erich Jäger; Würzburg, FRG) before and after KCl inhalations. In the majority of cases R_{aw} was used to assess the bronchial response to inhaled KCl.

Dose–response curves were determined in healthy persons and in patients with asthma, chronic bronchitis, and allergic rhinitis by increasing the inhaled dose (number of inhalations) at constant concentrations (1.16%, 2.5%, 5%, or 10%) of KCl solution. For nonasthmatic subjects only 10% KCl was used. Physiologic saline solution was inhalaed as a control. Inhalation was interrupted at given doses in order to measure bronchial response (Figs. 1–3). The time intervals needed for lung function measurements (i.e., for R_{aw} and/or FEV_1) were 2–3 min.

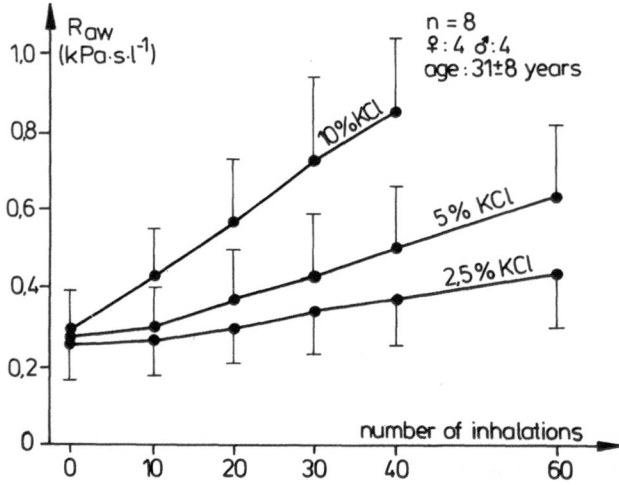

Fig. 1. The effect on R_{aw} of inhaled KCl solutions in patients with asthma

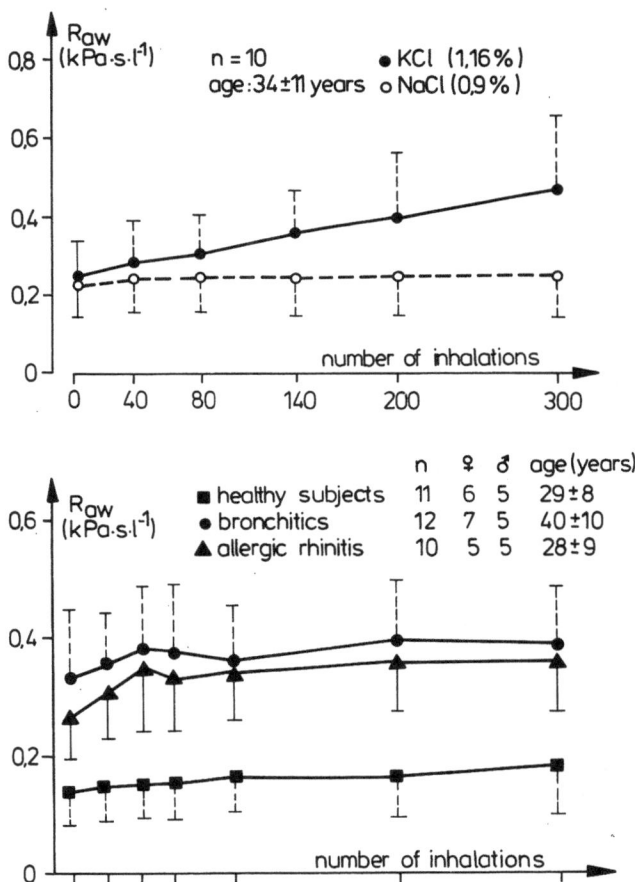

Fig. 2. The effect on R_{aw} of inhaled isotonic saline and KCl solution in patients with asthma

Fig. 3. Inhaled KCl (10%) dose–bronchial response curves in healthy subjects and in patients with chronic bronchitis and allergic rhinitis

Inhalation of KCl aerosol was ceased if the increase of R_{aw} was equal to or more than 100% of baseline value and at the same time exceeded 0.6 kPa s l^{-1}. If no significant change in R_{aw} could be detected, KCl inhalation was continued to a maximum of 300 inhalations.

Estimation of Limit Values for Asthma

Determination of the upper limit values of bronchial response to KCl was based on the dose-independent and nonsignificant bronchospastic action of KCl in nonasthmatics (Fig. 3). Upper limits of postchallenge changes of R_{aw}, sG_{aw}, and FEV_1 were estimated in the following way: values of these parameters, after large or even extreme doses of KCl solution (120–140 or 300 inhalations), were plotted against prechallenge values; limit lines were then

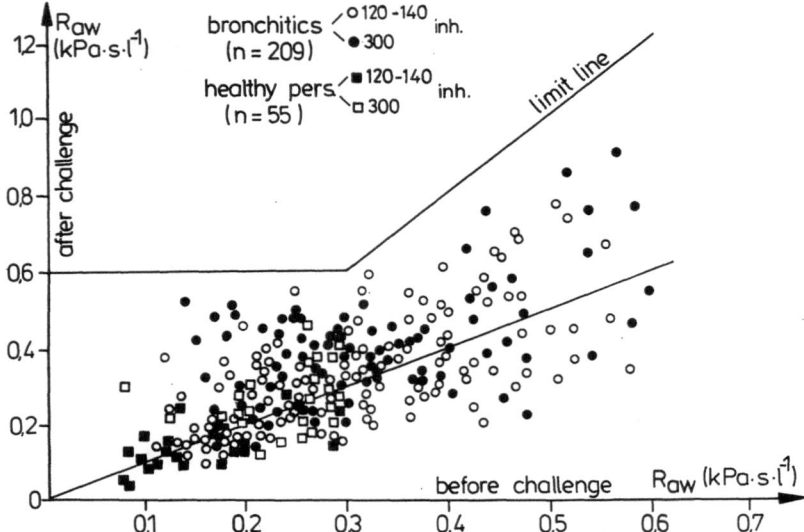

Fig. 4. Change of individual R_{aw} values in healthy persons and patients with chronic bronchitis after 120–300 inhalations of a 10% KCl solution. Values below and above the *straight line* starting from zero point indicate R_{aw} decrease and increase, respectively. *Line* drawn from 0.6 kPa s l^{-1} R_{aw} value on the *ordinate* represents the chosen limit values. At baseline R_{aw} values which are less than 0.3 kPa s l^{-1}, the postchallenge limit value is 0.6 kPa s l^{-1}; at R_{aw} baselines of more than 0.3 kPa s l^{-1}, the limit value is twice that of the baseline

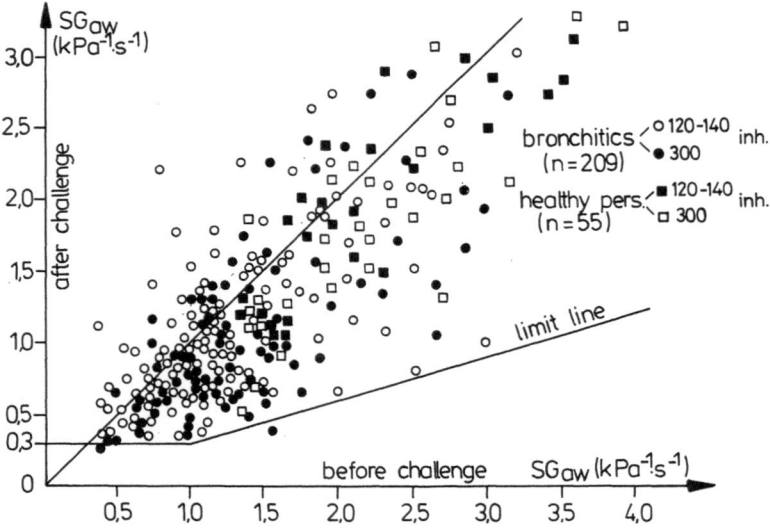

Fig. 5. Pre- and postchallenge sG_{aw} values in the same groups as in Fig. 1. Line starting from 0.3 kPa^{-1} s^{-1} sG_{aw} value of ordinate represents limit values for sG_{aw}. At baseline, sG_{aw} value below 1.0 kPa^{-1} s^{-1} postchallenge limit value is 0.3 kPa^{-1} s^{-1}; at baseline values above 1.0 kPa^{-1} s^{-1}, the limit value is 70% less than the baseline

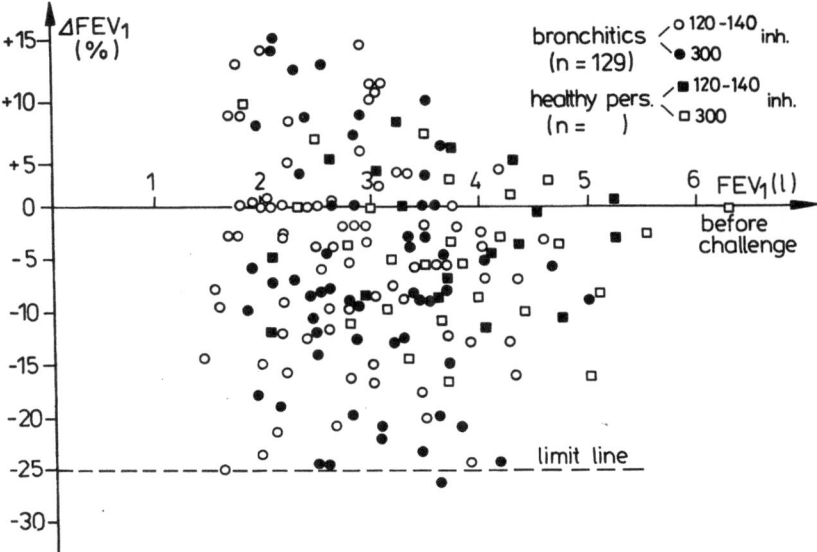

Fig. 6. Percentage change of FEV_1 values after 120–300 inhalations from KCl solution taken as a function of FEV_1 baseline. *Broken line* represents limit value (−25%)

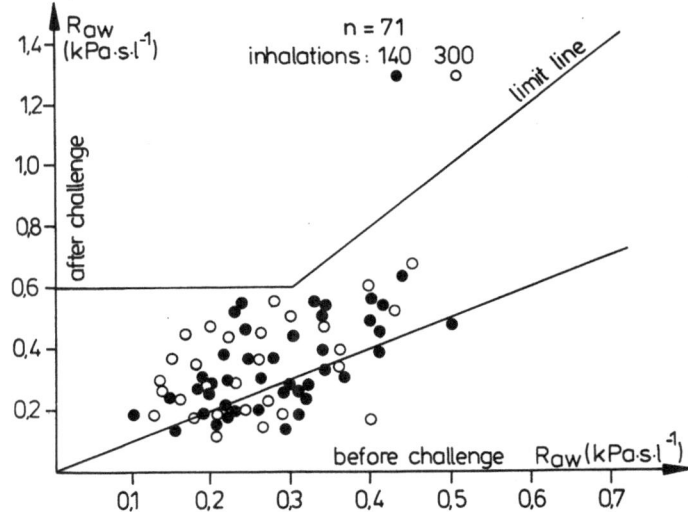

Fig. 7. Pre- and postchallenge value of R_{aw} of patients with allergic rhinitis. Lines are identical with those of Fig. 4

drawn empirically such that they would not be exceeded by postchallenge values of ≤1% of the nonasthmatics (Figs. 4–7). Limit values of postchallenge changes represented by the limit lines could be accepted as cut-off values (positive criteria) for differentiating between asthmatics and nonasthmatics,

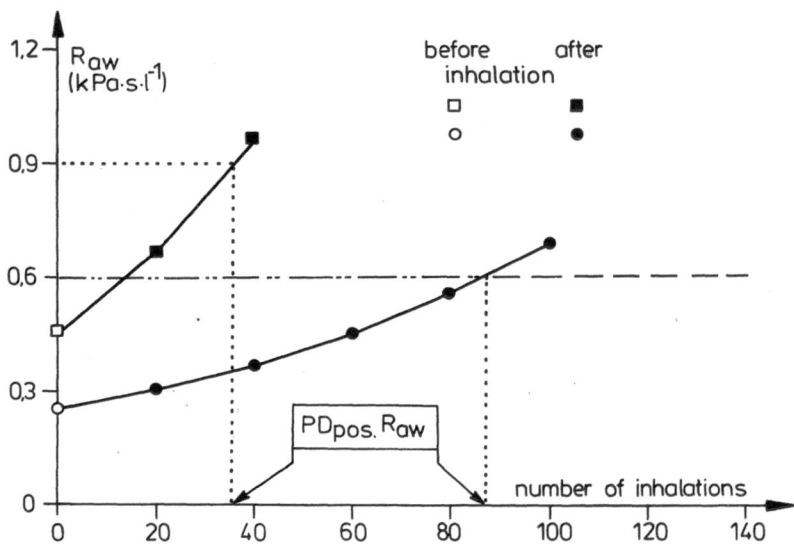

Fig. 8. Estimation of inhalation dose required for achieving a positive test for R_{aw} (PD$_{pos}$ R_{aw}) of two representative patients. At a baseline below 0.3 kPa s l^{-1}, the lowest postchallenge R_{aw} value which can just fit positive criteria has to be 0.6 kPa s l^{-1}. In patients with a baseline between 0.3–0.6 kPa s l^{-1}, the minimum postchallenge value has to be twice that of baseline in order to fit criteria for a positive test

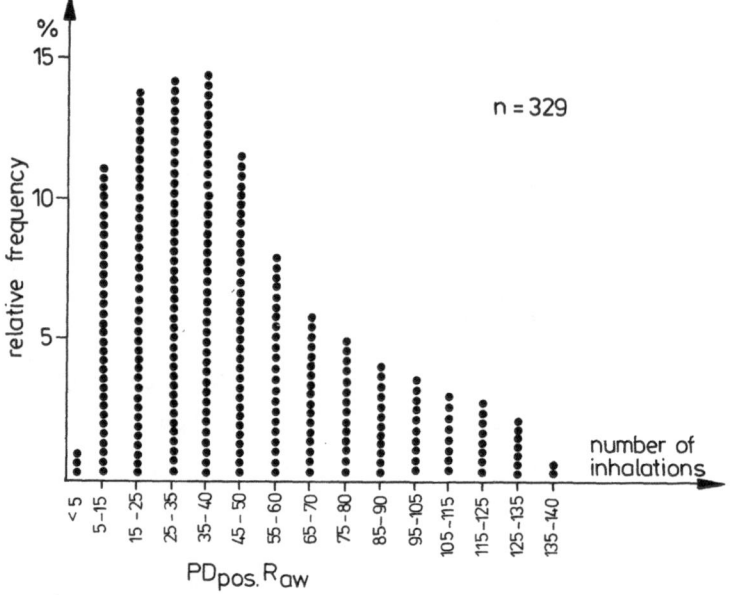

Fig. 9. Frequency distribution of PD$_{pos}$ R_{aw} values in the group of patients with asthma

because a bronchial response exceeding these values at any dose could be expected only in patients with asthma.

The method of estimation of dose which is needed for provoking an increase of R_{aw} positive for asthma (PD_{pos} R_{aw} value) is demonstrated in Fig. 8. Using the positive criteria for R_{aw}, the PD_{pos} R_{aw} value can be estimated by linear extrapolation. The frequency distribution of these doses was studied in 329 patients with symptom-free asthma (Fig. 9) and the highest PD_{pos} R_{aw} value (the dose at the right end of the distribution "curve") was taken as the threshold dose for excluding the possibility of asthma with great probability if the bronchial response in a given patient did not reach the level of limit values for R_{aw} changes.

Results

Inhalation of nebulized KCl solution caused significant bronchospasm in a just linear or slightly curvilinear dose-dependent way (Figs. 1, 2). Healthy subjects and patients with chronic bronchitis [21] and allergic rhinitis did not show significant airway narrowing even after high doses of KCl (Fig. 3). Some mild changes in airways caliber, however, could be provoked in these groups but the individual changes did not exceed values represented by the limit lines shown in Figs. 4–7. These limit values of postchallenge changes of R_{aw}, sG_{aw}, and FEV_1 in nonasthmatics were considered as positive criteria for asthma (postchallenge $R_{aw} \geq 2 \times$ prechallenge $R_{aw} \geq 0.6$ kPa s l^{-1}; postchallenge $sG_{aw} \leq 0.3$ kPa s^{-1} or $\leq 30\%$ of prechallenge sG_{aw}; postchallenge decraease of FEV_1 $\geq 25\%$). A more or less remarkable postchallenge improvement in R_{aw}, sG_{aw}, and FEV_1 values was found in about one fourth to one third of nonasthmatics (Figs. 4–7).

As was expected on the basis of the dose-response curves, each patient with asthma exceeded the limit values (positive criteria) of R_{aw} at a certain number of inhalations of 10% KCl solution. In some patients, less than ten inhalations were needed to reach limit values for R_{aw}, while in others much higher doses were necessary. Each patient with asthma had a positive reaction for R_{aw} at doses between 2 and 140 inhalations. The PD_{pos} R_{aw} value was found to be greater than 100 inhalations in only 10% of asthmatics.

In asthmatics in whom BPTs were ceased at KCl doses which induced R_{aw} increases corresponding to the positive criteria, 14.2% and 22.3% were nonetheless negative according to the positive criteria for sG_{aw} and FEV_1, respectively. A relatively low percentage (1.5% and 3.9%) of patients had a positive reaction for R_{aw} and at the same time were still negative to sG_{aw} and FEV_1 at doses between 100 and 140 inhalations.

PD_{pos} R_{aw} values of asthmatics did not show any dependence on baseline R_{aw} values, age, sex, season, type of asthma [18], or the current condition of this illness. Patients in a long-lasting (more than a half year) symptom-free period that had not been taking any antiasthmatic drug could also exhibit a positive reaction, even at low KCl doses in some cases.

KCl-induced bronchospasm reached its peak within 2 min after cessation of inhalation in more than 95% of patients. A complete reversal of bronchospasm could be achieved within a few minutes after inhalation of β-2 agonists [20].

A long-lasting relative refractory period could be demonstrated after KCl BPTs in asthmatics. Repeated challenges 1 or 2 days after the first ones – performed under the same conditions – induced a significantly smaller increase in R_{aw} than was previously abserved. Bronchial responsiveness to KCl returned to the original level 3 days after the first challenge [22]. The coefficient of variation of repeated tests carried out in 4 day intervals in 16 patients with asthma was found to be 17.6%.

Side effects of KCl inhalation in decreasing order to their frequency of occurrence were: increased salivary secretion, tickling in the throat, cough, mild burning sensation in the upper airways [20], nausea, and stridulous inspiration.

Tickling in the throat or laryngeal irritation and cough occurred in one third of healthy persons and patients with allergic rhinitis and asthma, while more than half of patients with chronic bronchitis noticed these complaints. In about one fifth of patients in the latter group, cough was hardly tolerable during the first 20–30 inhalations. By further increasing the inhaled KCl dose, the coughing stimulus decreased and after 40–50 inhalations cough rarely was observed.

A burning sensation in the upper airways was not frequent in healthy persons and patients with allergic rhinitis but in patients with asthma and chronic bronchitis it appeared in 11% and 19% of patients, respectively. This complaint appeared mostly at higher doses of inhaled KCl, disappeared 1–2 min after cessation of inhalation, and returned again after 10–20 additional inhalations of 10% KCl solution.

Stridulous inspiration (37 out of 1043 patients), which was due to temporary laryngospasm at the very beginning of KCl inhalation, could be abolished after instructing the patients to inhale slowly. Most of these patients identified this dyspnea of laryngeal origin with their former complaint; only one of them had asthma.

All the above mentioned complaints disappeared some minutes after the challenge.

Discussion

Standardization

The KCl inhalation test used for diagnostic purposes does not need a precise measurement of inhaled dose due to a qualitative rather than a quantitative difference in response to KCl between asthmatics and nonasthmatics. An overdose of inhaled KCl does not cause a false positive response but an underdose may result in a false negative test. Thus the most important requirement is to inhale a sufficient quantity of KCl such that a positive bronchial response in patients having asthma is provoked.

The inhaled dose is characterized by the KCl concentration, the delivery rate of nebulization, and the number of inhalations. If KCl concentration and delivery are constant, the inhaled dose during tidal breathing is determined by the duration of aerosol inhalation or by the number of breaths. Using a 10% KCl solution, the highest PD_{pos} R_{aw} value found in a large group of asthmatics was 140 inhalations (about 10 min) at a delivery of 3 ml/min of fluid particles. KCl solutions of lower concentrations (e.g., 5% or 2.5%) or nebulization with lower delivery rates either would significantly increase the number of inhalations (i.e., the time) needed for performing the test or might result in a false negative test in patients with asthma less sensitive to KCl. Thus it is advisable to use a 10% KCl solution nebulized at high delivery rate, although the side effects are less at lower concentrations and aerosol densities.

KCl BPTs can also be standardized for timing the inhaled doses, but theoretically no substantial difference exists between dose measurement based on timing and counting the number of breaths during regular breathing.

In repeated BPTs carried out for research purposes, the same amount of KCl inhaled in the same concentration is required. In order to decrease the possible differences in inhaled doses at the same number of inhalations, only patients without any side effects during the first BPT were selected for repeated challenges.

Test Positivity, Specificity, and Sensitivity

The upper limit values of bronchial response of nonasthmatics have been considered as positive criteria for asthma, because a greater response can be achieved with great probability only in patients with asthma. Thus the high specificity for asthma of the KCl BPT is determined by the method of estimating positive criteria.

The postchallenge decrease in airway caliber in each subject with asthma exceeds the limit values at individually different KCl doses, ranging between 2 and 140 inhalations for R_{aw}. This means that the KCl BPT is highly sensitive for detecting asthma. Premedication with antiasthmatic drugs [20, 22], drinking coffee or tea, and exercise [29, 30] may at least partially protect the bronchial response to KCl and may lead to decreased sensitivity by causing a false negative test result in some asthmatics.

There was a relatively large number of patients positive for R_{aw} but still negative for FEV_1 at given KCl doses. On the basis of the asthmatics' dose-response curves, by continuing the KCl inhalations a positive reaction for both FEV_1 and sG_{aw} would have eventually resulted. The relatively low percentage of patients with asthma that were positive for R_{aw} between 100 and

140 inhalations and at the same time were still negative for sG_{aw} and FEV_1 suggests that less than 5% of patients with asthma had a positive reaction in terms of these parameters but only at a KCl dose of over 140 inhalations. This is nonetheless of importance in case of measurement of FEV_1 alone, e.g., if R_{aw} cannot be measured due to lack of adequate equipment. In a subject suspected of having asthma, if the FEV_1 change is close to the positive level (e.g., between 20% and 25%) after 140 inhalations, it is advisable to increase the number of inhalations to over 140 in order to include – as far as possible – false negative cases of bronchial asthma.

It should be mentioned that positive criteria determined for KCl BPTs in adults are not necessarily suitable for children. Filtsev et al. [11] found less sensitivity and specificity of the test in children; but the method of estimating positive criteria was different from that used by us (personal communication).

Simplifying Possibilities of the Method

In bronchitics and partly in healthy persons as well, after increasing the inhalation dose of KCl, the R_{aw} irregularly fluctuated to a certain extent but not with a great amplitude. However, it is not characteristic in asthma for the values of parameters detecting obstruction to show stagnation or improvement before reaching the positive level when the 10% KCl inhalation dose is increased considerably, e.g., by 40 inhalations. That is why, e.g., if R_{aw} of FEV_1 values improve or do not change after 100 inhalations compared to baseline or values at 60 inhalations, asthma can be excluded with great probability; for this purpose it is not necessary to continue KCl inhalations to 140 or more breaths. If the R_{aw} increase or FEV_1 decrease does not exceed even half of the limit values after 100 inhalations, challenge can be stopped since practically it cannot be expected to reach positive reaction with further increases of the inhalation dose. It is advisable to use this method especially when KCl inhalation is not well tolerated because of possible laryngotracheal irritation and coughing.

Determination of PD_{pos} values (PD_{25} FEV_1 or PD_{pos} R_{aw}) for diagnostic purposes in a given patient is not necesssary because more than 99% of non-asthmatics did not reach a 25% decrease in FEV_1 or a positive reaction in terms of R_{aw} at any dose below 140 or even at more inhalations of a 10% KCl solution. Thus the differentiation of symptom-free asthmatics using the KCl BPT is based solely on a positive bronchial reaction, independent of the exact dose at which they reach positivity.

Therefore a simplified method of KCl BPT for differential diagnosis of asthma can be used without determination of dose-response curves and PD_{pos} values in a particular patient. This method has been used recently in our practice in patients suspected of having asthma. After informing the subject about the test procedure, the baseline R_{aw} (or FEV_1) value was measured and the jugular region was auscultated by using a phonendoscope. Inhalation of the 10% KCl solution was then started. If the patient indicated dyspnea or if wheezing could be detected by auscultation during the challenge, inhalation was interrupted and R_{aw} (or FEV_1) was measured. If the R_{aw} increase reached or exceeded both 100% and the value of 0.6 kPa s l^{-1} (or the decrease of FEV_1 was found to be 25% or more), inhalation was discontinued. If the R_{aw} (or FEV_1) change did not fit these criteria, inhalation was continued until a possible positive bronchial reaction was reached or, in case of negativity, to 140 inhalations.

Comparison with Other Tests

It is well known that in BPTs performed by inhalation of acetylcholine (methacholine) or histamine, a significant bronchospasm can be provoked by increasing the dose of inhaled material in any group of patients and in healthy persons too. Reaching any accepted limit value indicating a positive bronchial reaction is thus a question of inhaled dose. There is a great overlap between asthma and other respiratory diseases [7, 16, 17] as regards inhalation doses needed to reach a positive bronchial reaction, e.g., 20% decrease in FEV_1 (PD_{20} FEV_1). Thus the differential diagnostic value of these tests is rather limited [6, 10, 16, 17].

Results obtained by KCl BPT reflect entirely different conditions. The essential difference derives from the finding that, while in a few but nonetheless significant number of nonasthmatics, KCl does not decrease the caliber of airways (and may even increase it), the decreased airway caliber observed in the majority of nonasthmatics is not dose-dependent and does not reach or exceed the level of the positive criteria, in contrast to asthmatics. Thus bronchial hyperreactivity to KCl inhalation is characteristic of bronchial asthma only.

The positivity of the challenge test performed with inhalation of ultrasonically nebulized distilled water (UNDW) [2] also seems to be specific for asthma [19]. Comparing the KCl BTP with the UNDW inhalation test under the same conditions, a 10% KCl solution had a stronger bronchospastic action than distilled water [20], i.e., more inhalations of UNDW than of 10% KCl solution are needed to provoke a positive bronchial reaction. Using the same positive criteria regarding postchallenge R_{aw} changes as applied to the KCl test, UNDW did not induce positive bronchial reaction in five out of 24 patients with asthma, even after 300 inhalations, due to a plateau-like character of their dose-response curve [21]. Thus, the negativity of the UNDW test – in contrast to the KCl test – does not exclude the diagnosis of asthma.

The vice versa protection found between KCl and exercise-induced bronchospasm [29, 30] suggests, at least in part, a common pathway. Evaporative water loss from bronchi is thought to be one of the main factors in the mechanism of exercise-induced asthma [4, 5], which leads to an increase in osmolarity [4] and thus to an increased potassium concentration in the airway surface liquid. This may also be a causal factor in exercise-induced bronchospasm in patients with asthma most reactive to KCl.

Mechanism of Action of Inhaled KCl

The dose-response curve of 0.9% saline solution suggests the negligible effect of water as a solvent in bronchospasm induced by KCl. The observation that a 10% KCl solution (molarity 1.34) induced a much higher increase in R_{aw} than did a 10% NaCl solution (molarity 1.73) at the same inhalation doses in the same patients with asthma [20] and that an isomolar (1.16%) KCl solution caused a dose-related increase in R_{aw} (Fig. 2) suggests that hypertonic KCl-induced bronchospasm is due not only to an osmotic effect but also to a specific ionic action of potassium [20].

KCl challenge was found to increase serum histamine levels in patients with athma [14]. This effect of inhaled KCl may primarily be due to a direct action, because even a mild excess of KCl in the incubation fluid degranulated mast cells [25]. This action is not an osmotic one because the highest degranulation rate (71%) was observed at isomolar concentration of KCl.

In human smooth muscle preparations a significant KCl dose-related increase in tension was demonstrated [8]. This direct effect on smooth muscle can be another possible action of inhaled KCl. An extracellular surplus of potassium produced locally by inhalation in the mucosa of the bronchi may influence not only mast cells and smooth muscle but also sensory (irritant) receptors probably by depolarization [21]. Thus KCl may induce bronchospasm also through a reflex pathway. It is still not clear why an inhaled KCl solution failed to provoke significant bronchospasm either in healthy persons or in patients with chronic bronchitis and allergic rhinitis, even after extreme doses. Differences in releasability of mast cells and/or basophils [12, 13] of asthmatics and nonasthmatics or an increased sensitivity to KCl of the above mentioned structures (mast cells, bronchial smooth muscle and irritant receptors) may play a role in the increased bronchial responsiveness of asthmatics. Another possibility may be a markedly slower resorption of KCl in nonasthmatics than in asthmatics due to differences in bronchial mucosal permeability [15] and disturbances in electrolyte transport functions of the bronchial mucosa in the latter group of patients [1].

In patients with wheezy bronchitis KCl inhalation was found to cause a short-term slight worsening in airway obstruction which was followed by a significant decrease in R_{aw} persisting for more than 5 h [24]. The reason why KCl inhalation induced a decrease rather than an increase in R_{aw} in these patients and in about one third of nonasthmatics also remains to be answered in further studies. One of the explanations may be that potassium-induced selective prostaglandin E_2 production in the bronchi [28[, which overcomes the bronchospastic action of KCl, is weak in these patients. This may also, at least partly, be responsible for the protective effect of the KCl BPT on exercise-induced bronchospasm, since indomethacin decreased or abolished such protection [30].

Conclusions

A BTP with 10% KCl inhalation is simple and safe. In using the test for diagnostic purposes, precise standardization is not needed, because an overdose, i.e., more KCl than that getting into the bronchi during regular tidal breathing after 140 inhalations, does not increase the possibility of obtaining false positive reaction due to the dose-independent bronchial response of nonasthmatics. Applying the positive criteria determined in the above described way BPTs performed with 10% KCl solution proved, in a large number of patients, to be not only highly sensitive but also highly specific for asthma. Its sensitivity and specificity for detecting asthma in adults are close to 100%. Thus a patient with a positive test, asthma can be diagnosed, while a negative test excludes the diagnosis of asthma with great probability in patients suspected of having asthma.

References

1. Agrawal CT, Reed CE, Hyatt RE, Imber WE, Krell WS (1986) Airway responses to inhaled oubain in subjects with an without asthma. Mayo Clin Proc 61: 778–784
2. Allegra L, Bianco S (1980) Non-specific bronchoreactivity obtained with ultrasonic aerosol of distilled water. Eur J Respir Dis 61 [S106]:41–49
3. American Thoracic Society, Committee on Diagnostic Standards for Nontuberculous Diseases (1962) Definitions and classification of chronic bronchitis, asthma and pulmonary emphysema. Am Rev Respir Dis 85:762–768
4. Anderson SD (1984) Is there a unifying hypothesis for exercise induce asthma? J Allergy Clin Immunol 73:660–665
5. Chan JY, Horton DJ (1977) Heat and water loss from airways and exercise-induced asthma. Respiration 34:305–313
6. Cocroft DW, Killian DN, Mellon JJA, Hargreave PE (1977) Bronchial reactivity to inhaled histamine: a method and clinical survey. Clin Allergy 7:235–243
7. Curry JJ (1946) The action of histamine on the respiratory tract in normal and in asthmatic subjects. J Clin Invest 25:785–799
8. Debreczeni L, Magyar P (1988) Effect of hypo- or hyperosmotic solutions on the tone of isolated human bronchial smooth muscle. Eur Respir J 1 [S2]:212S
9. Dixon CMS, Williams AJ, Ind PW (1989) Inhaled potassium chloride (KCl) induced bronchoconstriction is safe. Thorax 44:333–334
10. Emarson DA, Vedal S, Schulzer M, Dybuncio A, Chan-Young M (1987) Asthma, asthmalike symptoms, chronic bronchitis, and the degree of bronchial hyperresponsiveness in epidemiologic surveys. Am Rev Respir Dis 136:613–617
11. Filtschev SI, Haluszka J, Werys R (1989) The usefullness of the challenge with 10% KCl for diagnosing asthma in children. Eur Respir J 2 [S5]:303s
12. Findlay SR, Lichtenstein LM (1980) Basophyl releasibility in patients with asthma. Am Rev Respir Dis 122:53–59
13. Finney MJB, Anderson SWD, Black JT (1987) The effect of non-isotonic solutions on human isolated airway smooth muscle. Respir Physiol 69:227–286

14. Herceg R, Magyar P, Németh A, Huszti Z (1986) Non-osmotic degranulation of mast cells induced by KCl solution. In: Allegra L, Rizzato G (eds) Bronchitis and Emphysema. Eur J Respir Dis 60 Suppl 146: A74
15. Hogg JC (1981) Bronchial mucosal permeability and its relationship to airways hyperreactivity. J Allergy Clin Immunol 67: 421–425
16. Klein RC, Salvaggio JE (1966) Nonspecificity of the bronchoconstricting effect of histamine and acethyl-beta-metacholine in patients with obstructive airway disease. J Allergy 37: 158–168
17. Laitinen LA (1974) Histamine and metacholine challenge in testing bronchial hyperreactivity. Thesis, University of Helsinki
18. Lantos A, Magyar P (1988) Independence of bronchial sensitivity to KCl inhalation from baseline R_{aw} values, age, sex, season and type of asthma. Eur Respir J 1 [S2]: 315S
19. Lilker ES (1982) Letter to the editor: bronchial reactivity in response to inhalation of ultrasonically nebulised distilled water and saline. Br Med J 284: 417
20. Magyar P, Dervaderics M, Tóth A, Lantos A (1983) Inhalation of hypertonic potassium chloride solution: a specific bronchial challenge for asthma. Ital J Chest Dis 37: 29–34
21. Magyar P, Dervaderics M, Tóth A (1984) Bronchial challenge with hypertonic KCl solution in the diagnosis of bronchial asthma. A comparison with the challenge performed by inhalation of distilled water. Schweiz Med Wochenschr 214: 910–913
22. Magyar P, Dervaderics M, Tóth A, Wollák A, Zsámboki G (1984) The specificity of bronchial provocation test with 10% KCl solution in the differential diagnosis of asthma. Respiration 46 [S1]: 32
23. Magyar P, Miskovits G, Dervaderics M, Herceg R, Tóth A (1986) KCl bronchial provocation test: positivity criteria for differentiation between asthmatics and nonasthmatics. Bull Eur Phyiosopathol Respir 22 [S8]: 106S
24. Mészáros L, Magyar P (1986) Types of bronchial reaction of challenge test with KCl inhalation in patients with asthma, chronic bronchitis, allergic rhinitis and in healthy persons. Eur Respir J 1 [S1]: 173
25. Németh A, Magyar P, Herceg R, Huszti Z (1987) Potassium-induced histamine release from mast cells and its inhibition by ketotifen. Agents Actions 20: 149–152
26. Quanjer PH (1983) Standardized lung function testing. Report working party standardization of lug function tests. Recommendations of the European Community for Coal and Steel. Bull Eur Physiopathol Respir 19 [S5]: 1–95
27. Schoeffel RE, Anderson SD, Altounian REC (1981) Bronchial hyperreactivity in response to inhalation of ultrasonically nebulised solutions of distilled water and saline. Br Med J 283: 1285–1287
28. Steel L, Platson L, Kaliner M (1979) Prostaglandin generation by human and guinea pig lung tissue: comparison of parenchymal and airway responses. J Allergy Clin Immunol 64: 287–293
29. Tóth A, Magyar P (1989) Refractory period after exercise and hypertonic (10%) KCl challenge. Eur Respir J 2 [S8]: 776S
30. Tóth A, Magyar P, Wollák A (1990) Refractory period between exercise and hypertonic KCl challenge after indomethacin pretreatment. Clin Exp Allergy 20 [S1]: 89

Pharmacological Agents in Bronchial Provocation Tests

A. SZCZEKLIK and E. NIZANKOWSKA

Department of Medicine, Copernicus Academy of Medicine, Kraców, Poland

Introduction

In about 10% of adults with asthma, but rarely in asthmatic children, aspirin and other nonsteroidal antiinflammatory drugs (NSAIDS) precipitate asthma attacks. This distinct clinical syndrome is called aspirin-induced asthma (AIA) [12, 16–18, 22].

The course of the disease and its clinical picture are very characteristic [12, 17]. The intolerance presents itself as a unique picture: within 1 h following ingestion of aspirin, acute asthmatic attacks develop, often accompanied by rhinorrhea, conjunctival irritation, and scarlet flush of the head and neck. These reactions are dangerous; indeed, a single therapeutic dose of aspirin or other anticyclooxygenase agent can provoke violent bronchospasm, shock, unconsciousness, and respiratory arrest [9]. Asthma runs a protracted course, despite the avoidance of aspirin and other NSAIDS. The eosinophil count is elevated. Skin tests with common aeroallergens are often negative, and those with aspirin are always negative.

While the clinical history might raise the suspicion of aspirin-induced asthma, the diagnosis can be established with certainty only by aspirin challenge. There are no in vitro tests suitable for routine clinical diagnosis.

Methods and Materials

Preconditions for Carrying Out the Aspirin Challenge Tests

Patients are challenged when their asthma is in remission and their FEV_1 is greater than 1.5 l or FEV_1/VC >60% of predicted values. They continue regular medication, including corticosteroids, but stop sympathomimetics and methylxanthines for 10 h and antihistamines for at least 48 h prior to the challenge. Regular intake of sodium cromoglycate and ketotifen should be interrupted at least 72 h before the challenge. Aspirin reactions can be blocked by ketotifen [4, 19, 23], and modified by H_1-antihistamines [21]. Sodium cromoglycate can alleviate aspirin reactions [1, 6], though this has not been a uniform experience [3, 5]. Glucocorticosteroids attenuate aspirin-precipitated reactions [7].

Oral Challenge Tests

Oral challenges with aspirin can be carried out either on an outpatient basis or during short hospitalization, usually 3–5 consecutive days. The challenges consist of administration of increasing doses of aspirin (see below) and placebo, according to a single-blind procedure and careful monitoring of clinical symptoms, pulmonary function tests, and parameters reflecting nasal patency during 6–12 h following administration of the drug. All doses of aspirin and placebo are prepared by the hospital pharmacy in identical gelatin capsules.

Within the frame of clinical observation particular attention is paid to the following symptoms and signs: sensation of warmth over the face, neck and upper part of the body, accompanied usually by erythema; appearance of cough, dyspnea and chest tightness with signs of airways obstructions: wheezes, prolongation of the expiration; nasal symptoms, i.e., rhinorrhea and diminished nasal patency. Quite frequently lacrimation with conjunctival irritation occurs. Patients seldom report pruritus of the eyes, ears, nose, gingiva, or skin.

It is particularly important to look for "preliminary" symptoms: cough, rash over the upper part of the body, and discrete nasal signs. They usually precede more definitive bronchial symptoms; their appearance affects the decision whether the next dose of aspirin should be administered.

The characteristics of the symptoms, the time of their appearance, and their intensity is recorded in 30 min intervals following aspirin administration (see Results). For example, the intensity of nasal symptoms: rhinorrhea and nasal obstruction (blockade, diminished patency) are rated by the patients themselves using a 4-pointgrading scale (0, none; 1, small intensity; 2, moderate; 3, severe). These subjective recordings are accompanied by measurements of peak nasal inspiratory flow (PNIF) with the Youlten peak nasal inspiratory flow meter (Airmed Ltd., UK).

For the objective assessment of the bronchopulmonary effects of aspirin, pulmonary function tests are performed every 30 min over a period of 6–12 h. Usually we measure spirometric parameters (FEV_1 and FVC) and maximal expiratory flows ($MEF_{25,50,75}$) on a flow-integrated computerized pneumotachograph (Master Lab, E. Jaeger, Germany) for 6 h on every test day. If longer monitoring of pulmonary function tests is required, we measure peak expiratory flow rate (PEFR) with Wright's peak flow meter (Airmed Ltd., UK). These simple measurements could be done the entire day following the challenge, even after discharge of the patient from the pulmonary function test laboratory. We do not perform oral challenges when baseline FEV_1 is smaller than 1300–1500 ml or $FEV_1/FVC < 60\%$.

Scheme of the Challenge

The aspirin challenge test is as follows:

Day 1: placebo
Day 2:   20 mg aspirin +   40 mg aspirin
Day 3:   80 mg aspirin + 150 mg aspirin
Day 4: 300 mg + 300 mg of aspirin

On the first day placebo is administered twice, separated by a 3 h interval. Careful monitoring of clinical symptoms and pulmonary function tests is carried out. This procedure identify patients with unstable pulmonary function parameters and allows the patients to familiarize themselves with the pulmonary function tests methodology. The patients with marked variations in FEV_1, especially those in whom FEV_1 falls below 15% of baseline following placebo, are not fit for further testing but may be tested later when their disease becomes more stable.

On the second day the challenge is begun with the smallest dose of aspirin. In our department this is usually 20 mg of aspirin (only rarely, in patients who have a history of anaphylactic shock and/or severe dyspnea necessitating mechanical ventilation following ingestion of analgesic, do we start with 10 mg of aspirin). The reaction is considered positive if a fall in $FEV_1 > 15\%$ of baseline and/or intense (grade 3) nasal symptoms and a decrease in PNIF $> 50\%$ of baseline occur. In case of negative reaction, the second dose, i.e., 40 mg of aspirin, is administered 3 h following the first dose. If no response occurs, the doses are gradually increased during the next 2 days in the following way: day 3: 80 mg and 150 mg 3 h later; day 4: 300 and 300 mg of aspirin. If at the end of the 3 h observation period following the first dose, the untoward reaction only begins (for example gradual fall in FEV_1, intensification of symptoms), the second dose of that day is postponed (not administered). The higher dose is administered the next day if the symptoms provoked by the previous dose were inconclusive. This procedure allows for safe challenge and avoids precipitation of severe bronchial and systemic reactions.

Questionable responses to aspirin challenge are unusual, but if present may require rechallenge with a particular dose of aspirin and once again placebo some days later. If during the 4 day study period the reactions are of very mild intensity, despite augmentation of the aspirin dose, "desensitization" to aspirin should be taken into account. In this case, the challenge should be repeated 10 days later, starting usually with higher dose (e.g., 80 mg).

The adverse reaction following aspirin administration usually starts 1–2 h following ingestion of the drug; in some patients it may appear 3–5 h later. We have seen patients in whom moderate bronchial and nasal symptoms appeared in the afternoon. These "late" reactions could be recorded by monitoring PEFR and PNIF every hour for 12 h.

In majority of patients pulmonary function tests are done every 30 min but if a prompt decrease in FEV_1 is observed, FEV_1 should be followed every 10 min. When the fall reaches values below 20% of baseline, the reaction should be stopped immediately. In a majority of patients quick relief of adverse symptoms can be achieved by administration of 1–2 puffs of fenoterol (Berotec) or salbutamol. If the reaction is more severe (tendency to progressing fall in FEV_1 despite β-mimetics) we administer aminophylline slowly i.v. (or in perfusion) with 40–80 mg of Solumedrol (Upjohn, USA). Antihistaminic drugs (Teldane, Zyrtec) and nasal corticosteroids (Syntans, Rhinocort) usually stop nasal symptoms. Most patients recover from acute reactions within 1–2 h. In rare cases, following severe reactions a general feeling of malaise and excessive bronchial and nasal secreation might persist for a day or two.

We start oral challenges usually in the morning between 8:30 and 9:30 A.M. The challenges are performed in the pulmonary function tests laboratory in our department by very experienced nurses, closely supervised by the physician. The physician is always present when the reaction occurs and decides each time whether the next dose should be administered. All severe reactions could be followed in the intensive care unit located in the same building.

Inhalation Challenge Tests with Aspirin

A modification of the challenge test has been developed, in which, instead of giving aspirin orally an aerosol of lysine acetylsalicylate is administered by inhalation [2, 11, 13, 14]. Here we present the method described by Phillips et al. [8].*

All patients should fulfill the preconditions described above.

Lysine-aspirin (Laboratorios Andromaca S.A., Spain), as a powder containing 1800 mg of lysine-acetylsalicylate with 200 mg of glycine, is made up freshly on each challenge day with 5 ml of sterile water to produce a lysine-aspirin solution containing 360 mg/ml (1.1 mol/liter), which is equivalent to 200 mg/ml of acetylsalicylic acid. This solution, which has a pH of 4.55 and an osmolality of 3100 mosmol/kg, is diluted in 0.9% (wt/vol) of sodium chloride to produce a range of increasing doubling concentrations, 11.25–360 mg/ml (34.5–1100 mmol/liter). A placebo solution consisting of 1200 mg of lysine with 300 mg of glycine (BDH Chemicals) is reconstituted with 5 ml of water for injection to produce an identical osmolality and pH to the lysine- aspirin solution. This is diluted with 0.9% (wt/vol) sodium chloride in a similar fashion to the active agent to produce a range of increasing doubling concentrations.

---

* For the further developement of this method see: Dahlen B., Zetterström O. Comparison of bronchial and per oral provocation with ASA in ASA-sensitive asthmatics. Eur. Resp. J., 1990, 3:527–534

These solutions are administered as aerosols generated from a starting volume of 3 ml in a disposable Inspiron mininebulizer (C. R. Bard International Ltd., UK) driven by compressed air at 8 liters/min. Under these conditions, the nebulizer has an output of 0.48 ml/min and generates an aerosol with a mass-median particle diameter of 4.7 μm. Wearing a noseclip, subjects inhale the aerosolized solution via a mouthpiece in five breaths from end tidal volume to full inspiratory capacity.

All the provocations are carried out at the same time of day, and challenges with lysine-aspirin or matched placebo are performed at least 7 days apart.

On the study day, after a 15 min rest, three baseline measurements of FEV_1 are made at intervals of 3 min, followed by inhalation of 0.9% (wt/vol) sodium chloride and repeat FEV_1 measurements at 1 and 3 min. Provided FEV_1 does not change by >10% of the baseline value, the proper provocation is started. This consists of concentration-response studies with lysine-aspirin or matched placebo. Measurements of FEV_1 are made at 5 min intervals for 45 min after inhalation of each concentration. If FEV_1 decreased by <15% of the postsaline baseline value, the next lysine-aspirin concentration is administered. Increasing doubling concentrations of lysine-aspirin are inhaled in this manner until FEV_1 has fallen by >20% of the postsaline baseline value or the highest concentration has been administered. If the decrease in FEV_1 from baseline with the highest concentration of lysine-aspirin failed to achieve the value of 20%, then one additional dose of this agonist consisting of ten breaths of the highest concentration is administered. Subjects who fail to respond to this last dose are termed "unresponsive."

The percentage decrease in FEV_1 from postsaline baseline is plotted against the cumulative concentration of lysine-aspirin on a logarithmic scale and the PC_{20} value derived by linear extrapolation.

Results

Oral Provocation Tests

Since 1973 we have carried out oral aspirin challenges in about 800 patients with histories suggestive of intolerance to aspirin and other NSAIDSs. As a result of oral challenges, performed according to the procedure described above, not only hypersensitivity to aspirin could be confirmed or excluded, but also on individual "threshold dose" of aspirin could be established for each individual patient. In our patients the threshold doses varied between 20 and 300 mg; most of patients reacted to 40–80 mg of aspirin. This dose of aspirin is fairly stable in the individual patient, providing their treatment and clinical status has not changed significantly.

Some typical examples of oral challenges performed in our department and standard recordings of the parameters measured are described below. A male patient, age 43 years, has suffered from mild bronchial asthma since age

35. In the past, he had two severe attacks of dyspnea and rhinorrhea following administration of an analgesic probably containing aspirin. The results of
oral challenges are as follows: day 1 (placebo) no symptoms, stable pulmonary function tests; day 2 (20 mg aspirin + 40 mg aspirin 3 h later), a 10% fall
in FEV_1 and mild rhinorrhea (30% decrease in PNIF); day 3 (80 mg aspirin),
typical bronchial and nasal reaction with gradual fall of FEV_1, MEF_{50},
PEFR, and complete nasal obstruction (Table 1).

A female patient, 40 years old, has suffered from chronic rhinosinusitis
since 1979 and bronchial asthma since 1983. She had four polypectomies in
the past and described an attack of dyspnea following ingestion of an unknown drug for relief of severe headache. The results of aspirin challenge are
as follows: day 1 (placebo), stable pulmonary function tests: day 2, no symptoms following 20 mg of aspirin but significant fall in FEV_1 after 40 mg of the
drug; dyspnea was quickly relieved by fenoterol (Fig. 1).

A female patient, 37 years old, has suffered from bronchial asthma and
chronic rhinitis since age 34. She once had a very severe attack of dyspnea,

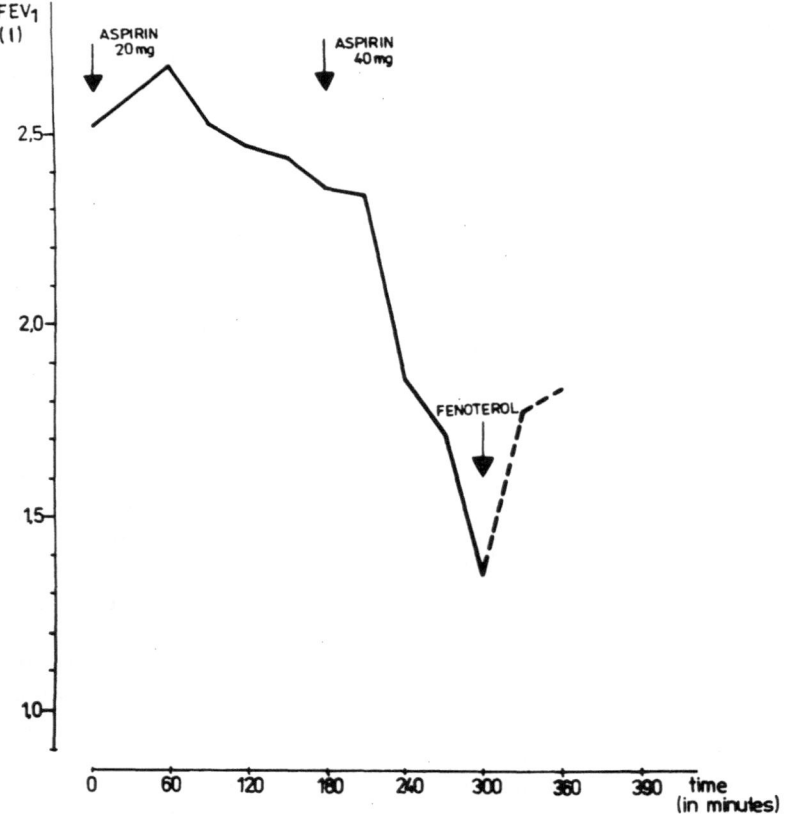

Fig. 1. Oral aspirin challenge of a female patient, age 40 years old; second test day

Table 1. Oral aspirin challenge (third test day) of a 43 year old male patient

Parameter	Baseline (8.30 A.M.)	Response to 80 mg aspirin					Subsequent response to fenoterol	
		30 min	60 min	90 min	120 min	150 min	15 min	60 min
FVC (l)	4.90	4.78	4.70	4.76	4.47	4.37	4.30	4.51
FEV$_1$ (l)	3.19	3.10	3.00	3.05	2.75	2.30	2.61	2.91
MEF$_{25}$	1.3	1.3	1.2	1.2	1.0	1.1	1.0	1.1
MEF$_{50}$	2.5	2.5	2.4	2.6	2.2	1.6	2.0	2.4
MEF$_{75}$	4.2	4.3	4.3	4.2	3.5	2.8	3.2	4.4
PEFR (l/min)	400	390	390	380	360	230	340	390
PNIF[a]	120	100	100	90	50	–	–	50
Dyspnea	–	–	–	–	+	+ +	+	–
Rhinorrhea	–	–	–	+	+ +	+ +	+	+
Nasal obstruction	–	–	–	+	+ +	+ + +	+ + +	+ +
Others	–	–	–	Face rash	Face rash; throat irritation; cough	Face rash; lacrimation; cough		

[a] In arbitrary units (Youlten peak nasal inspiratory flow).

during an influenza infection, when she took two tablets of aspirin (1000 mg). Some weeks later she was admitted to our department for diagnostic challenge with aspirin. Her physician supposed that not aspirin but acute viral infection could have precipitated such as severe exacerbation of asthma. The results of aspirin challenge were as follows: day 1, stable pulmonary function tests following placebo. Day 2, she received 20 mg aspirin and another 20 mg 3 h later. The second dose of aspirin was not doubled because after the first dose she developed rash, rhinorrhea, and moderate nasal obstruction. Dyspnea, which appeared 90 min following the second dose of aspirin, resolved spontaneously; nasal symptoms were recorded during the next 6 h (Table 2).

A female patient, 54 years old, has suffered from chronic severe rhinorrhea for at least 15 years. For the past 7 months she has had mild sporadic asthma attacks and 4 months ago she had mild dyspnea after ingestion of analgesic, probably containing aspirin. Oral challenge with aspirin was per-

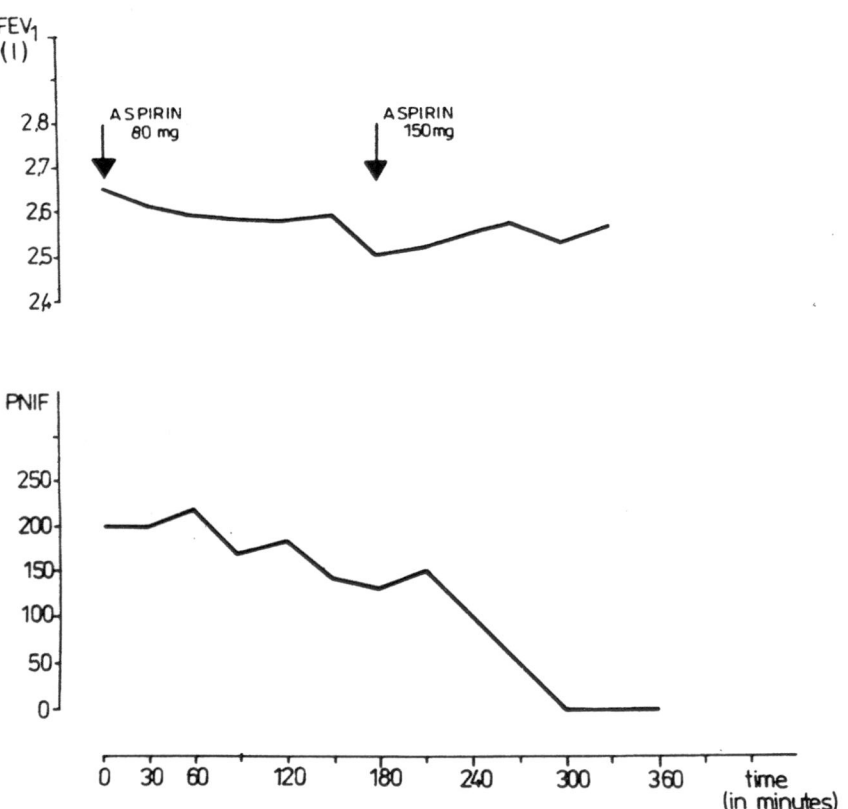

Fig. 2. Oral aspirin challenge of a female patient, age 52 years old; third test day

Table 2. Oral aspirin challenge (second test day) of a 37 year old female patient

Parameter	Baseline (9 A.M.)	Response to first dose of 20 mg aspirin								Response to second dose of 20 mg aspirin					
		30 min	60 min	90 min	120 min	150 min	180 min	210 min	240 min	270 min	300 min	360 min	420 min	480 min	540 min
FVC (1)	3.40	3.30	3.29	3.37	3.30	3.20	3.28	3.11	3.10	2.90	2.91				
FEV_1 (1)	2.74	2.64	2.70	2.67	2.69	2.50	2.56	2.30	2.25	2.07	2.10				
MEF_{25} (1/s)	1.5	1.4	1.4	1.6	1.4	1.5	1.4	1.3	1.2	1.1	1.2				
MEF_{50}	5.2	4.8	5.3	4.3	4.2	4.0	3.9	3.9	3.8	3.7	3.7				
PEFR (1/min)	400	390	390	400	370	360	350	340	300	230	230	300	280	330	360
$PNIF^a$	120	120	120	100	80	80	70	60	–	–	–	40	50	60	80
Dyspnea	–	–	–	–	–	–	–	–	+	++	++	+	–	–	+
Rhinorrhea	–	–	–	+	+	++	++	++	+++	++	++	+	+	+	–
Nasal obstruction	–	–	–	–	–	+	++	++	+++	+++	+++	++	++	++	+
Others	–	–	–	Face rash	Face and upper trunk rash	As at 120 min	Rash, rhinorrhea, moderate nasal obstruction	Cough	Cough, small dyspnea	Moderate dyspnea complete nasal blockade	As at 270 min				

^{a} In arbitrary units (Youlten peak nasal inspiratory flow).

formed; she had only nasal symptoms following administration of $80 + 150$ mg of aspirin during the third day of the challenge (Fig. 2).

Inhalation Provocation Tests

The PC_{20} lysine aspirin values determined in 11 aspirin-intolerant asthmatics varied between 30 and 220 mg/ml [8] with a geometric mean of 65 mg/ml. After inhalation of lysine-aspirin, bronchoconstriction (FEV_1 fall by about 20%) developed from 20 min to 2 h after the challenge. Recovery from induced bronchoconstriction varied from 20 min up to 6 h. The response was confined to the respiratory tract and was not accompanied by any symptoms of rhinitis, conjunctivitis, or flushing.

In seven of another nine subjects [8] the lysine-aspirin bronchoprovocation procedure was repeatable to within a single doubling concentration difference. The 95% confidence interval for the difference in results between the two lysine-aspirin challenges was 0.3- to 2.9-fold.

Discussion

Oral challenge tests are commonly performed. In inhalation provocation tests the increase in aspirin dose is achieved every 30–45 min, and the test is completed in one morning. It is, therefore faster than oral challenge which often takes 2–3 days. However, in oral tests there is no need for special equipment and the chances that aspirin will evoke other than bronchial symptoms are much higher.

In a few patients only naso-ocular responses are provoked by orally administered aspirin. These patients usually exhibit bronchial asthma at other times. Pleskow et al. [10] recorded this type of reaction in three of 50 patients with documented aspirin idiosyncrasy and chronic respiratory tract disease.

In a majority of patients, aspirin intolerance, once developed, remains for the rest of their life. Repeated aspirin challenges are therefore positive, though some variability in intensity and spectrum of symptoms occurs. Nonetheless, we and others [15] have observed an occasional patient in whom a positive aspirin challenge became negative after a period of a few years.

Provocation tests are the only way of diagnosing aspirin intolerance and should be performed in any suspected case in order to avoid unexpected and serious reactions in the future. If performed by an experienced team, they are quite safe. However, since they do carry a potential risk, they must not be carried out by a general practitioner, and their use, though important, should be limited to specialized centers.

In patients with aspirin-induced asthma, not only aspirin but several other anti-inflammatory drugs precipitate bronchoconstriction. Major offenders and safe alternatives are listed in Table 3. Not all of the offending drugs produce adverse symptoms with the same frequency. This depends on a drug's

Table 3. Tolerance of anti-inflammatory drugs in aspirin-induced asthma

Precipitate attacks of asthma	Well tolerated (caused no bronchoconstriction)
Salicylates	Sodium salicylate
Aspirin	Choline salicylate
Diflunisal	Choline magnesium trisalicylate
Salasate (salicylsalicylic acid)	Salicylamide
Polycyclic acids	Dextropropoxyphene
Acetic acids	Azapropazone
Indomethacin	Benzydamine
Sulindac	Chloroquine
Tolmetin	Paracetamol[a]
Aryl aliphatic acids	Azapropazone
Naproxen	
Diclophenac	
Fenoprofen	
Ibuprofen	
Ketoprofen	
Tiaprofenic acid	
Enolic acids	
Piroxicam	
Fenamates	
Mefenamic acid	
Flufenamic acid	
Cyclofenamic acid	
Pyrazolones	
Aminopyrine	
Noramidopyrine	
Sulfinpyrazone	
Phenylbutazone	
Steroids	
Hydrocortisone hemisuccinate	

[a] When beginning therapy, give half a tablet of paracetamol and observe patient 2–3 h for symptoms, which occur in no more than 5% of patients.

anticyclooxygenase potency and dose and on the individual sensitivity of the patient.

Many other drugs can also cause transient obstruction to the airflow. Such reactions are rarely a subject for clinical diagnostic testing. The reader is referred to a recent review on this topic [20].

References

1. Basomba A, Romar A, Pelaez A, Villamanzo IG, Campos A (1976) The effect of sodium cromoglycate in preventing aspirin-induced bronchospasm. Clin Allergy 6:269–275
2. Bianco S, Robuschi M, Petrigni G (1977) Aspirin-induced tolerance in aspirin-asthma detected by a new challenge technique. IRCS J Med Sci 5:129–130

264   A. Szczeklik and E. Nizankowska: Pharmacological Agents

3. Dahl R (1981) Oral and inhaled sodium cromoglycate in challenge test with food allergens or acetylsalicylic acid. Allergy 36:161–165
4. Delaney JC (1982) The effect of ketotifen on aspirin-induced asthmatic reactions. Clin Allergy 13:247–251
5. Hollingsworth HM, Downin ET, Braman SS, Glassroth J, Binder R, Center DM (1984) Identification and characterization of neutrophil chemotactic activity in aspirin-induced asthma. Am Rev Respir Dis 130:377–379
6. Martelli NA, Usandivaras G (1977) Inhibition of aspirin-induced bronchoconstriction by sodium cromoglycate inhalation. Thorax 32:684–690
7. Nizankowska E, Szczeklik A (1989) Glucocorticosteroids attenuate aspirin-precipitated adverse reactions in aspirin-intolerant patients with asthma. Ann Allergy 63:159–164
8. Phillips GD, Foord R, Holgate ST (1989) Inhaled lysine-aspirin as a bronchoprovocation procedure in aspirin-sensitive asthma: its repeatability, absence of a late phase reaction, and the role of histamine. J Allergy Clin Immunol 84:232–241
9. Picado C, Castillo JA, Monserrat JM, Augusti-Vidal A (1989) Aspirin-intolerance as a precipitating factor of life-threatening attacks of asthma requiring mechanical ventilation. Eur Respir J 2:127–129
10. Pleskow WW, Stevenson DD, Simon RA, Mathison DA, Schatz M, Zeiger RS (1983) Aspirin-sensitive rhino-sinusitis/asthma: spectrum of adverse reactions to aspirin. J Allergy Clin Immunol 71:574–580
11. Sakakibara H, Tsuda M, Suzuki M, Handa M, Saga T, Umeda H, Suetsugu SD, Konishi Y (1988) A new method for diagnosis of aspirin-induced asthma by inhalation test with water soluble aspirin (aspirine-D,L,-lysine, Venopirine). J Jpn Thor Soc 26:275–283
12. Samter M, Beers RF Jr (1968) Intolerance to aspirin. Clinical studies and consideration of its pathogenesis. Ann Intern Med 68:975–983
13. Schmitz-Schumann M, Schaub E, Virchow C (1982) Inhalative Provokation mit Lysin-Azetylsalicylsäure bei Analgetika-Asthma-Syndrom. Prax Klin Pneumol 36:17–21
14. Schmitz-Schumann M, Juhl E, Costabel U, Ruehle K-H, Menz G, Virchow C, Matthys H (1985) Analgetikaprovokationsproben bei Analgetika-Asthma Syndrom. Atemwegs Lungenkrankh 11:479–486
15. Simon RA, Pleskow WW, Stevenson DD, Mathison DA (1984) Aspirin sensitivity: description of aspirin (ASA) respiratory sensitivity. In: Kornblat J, Wedner C (eds) Allergy, theory and practice, Grune and Stratton, New York, pp 435–452
16. Stevenson DD (1984) Diagnosis, prevention and treatment of adverse reactions to aspirin and nonsteroidal anti-inflammatory drugs. J Allergy Clin Immunol 74:617–622
17. Szczeklik A (1986) Analgesics, allergy and asthma. Drugs 32 [Suppl 4]:148–163
18. Szczeklik A, Nizankowska E (1992) Asthme bronchique et médicaments anti-inflammatoires non stéroïdiens. In: Charpin J, Vervloet D. Allergologie, 3e édition, Flammarion, Paris, pp 762–779.
19. Szczeklik A, Czerniawska-Mysik G, Serwonska M, Kuklinski P (1980) Inhibition by ketotifen of idiosyncratic reactions to aspirin. Allergy 35:421–424
20. Szczeklik A, Nizankowska E (1989) Drug-induced asthma and bronchospasm. In: Akoun GM, White JP (eds) Treatment-induced respiratory disorders. Elsevier, Amsterdam, pp 189–209
21. Szczeklik A, Serwonska M (1979) Inhibition of idiosyncratic reactions to aspirin in asthmatic patients by clemastine. Thorax 34:654–657
22. Virchow C (1976) Analgetika-Intoleranz bei Asthmatikern (Analgetika-Asthma-Syndrom) vor laufige Mittelung. Prax Pneumol 30:684–692
23. Wuetrich B, Fabro L (1981) Azetylsalicylicsäure und Lebensmittel additiva-Intoleranz bei Urtikaria, Asthma bronchiale und chronischer Rhinopathie. Schweiz Med Wochenschr, 111:1445–1449

Occupational Agents in Bronchial Provocation Tests

L. M. FABBRI[1], A. PAPI[1], C. E. MAPP[2] and A. CIACCIA[1]

[1] Institute of Infections and Respiratory Diseases, University of Ferrara, Ferrara, Italy
[2] Institute of Occupational Medicine, University of Padova, Padova, Italy

Introduction

In 1700 Bernardino Ramazzini, Professor of Medicine at the University of Padova, Italy, firstly described grain dust asthma and baker's asthma [1]. Some 200 years later, in 1911, Karasek and Karasek [2] described asthma caused by exposure to platinum salts in photographic workers. This interest in occupation as a cause of asthma was continued in the late 1960s, mainly through the work of Jack Pepys, in London, England, who conducted routine bronchoprovocation tests with occupational agents and established their importance in the diagnosis of the disease [3]. Around the same time, the problem of occupational asthma was noted by several investigators, including Massimo Crepet, Professor of Occupational medicine at the University of Padova from 1954 until 1980, who organized a pioneering meeting in Padova on "Le allergie professionali" in 1963 [4].

Definition

Occupational asthma may be defined as a respiratory disease characterized by variable airway obstruction and variable airway hyperresponsiveness caused by a specific, as opposed to an irritant, agent present in the workplace [5].

Asthma-like symptoms, variable airway obstruction, and a persistent increase of nonspecific airway responsiveness may be caused by acute exposure to strong respiratory irritant gases at work ("reactive airway disfunction syndrome") [6]. Some investigators would call this syndrome "occupational asthma;" however, while this syndrome is undoubtedly an occupational respiratory disease, it should be differentiated from classic occupational asthma induced at work by a specific sensitizing agent. Indeed, both syndromes represent clear examples of an acute inflammatory process in the airways "switching on" nonspecific airway hyperresponsiveness, but occupational asthma is a classic example of an acquired hypersensitivity response, that is, it occurs only in a proportion of the subjects exposed to the specific agent, develops after an initial disease-free period of exposure (weeks, months, or years), and asthmatic reactions in the sensitized subjects are provoked by exposure to concentrations of the specific agent which were previously tolerated and which do not cause airway responses in subjects similarly exposed.

Byssinosis should not be considered occupational asthma because it is not associated with airway hyperresponsiveness, the hallmark of asthma. Patients with preexisting asthma may develop bronchoconstriction at work after exercise or exposure to low levels of irritants. This form of variable airway obstruction should also not be regarded as occupational asthma [5].

Epidemiology

Occupational asthma is becoming the most frequent occupational pulmonary disease in industrialized countries, and its incidence and prevalence are increasing. The overall prevalence of occupational asthma is difficult to determine, since, in many instances, there is a "self-selection" by workers who leave the workplace once they become affected and a lack of an exact definition of asthma; a lack of specific questionnaires; and the use, in previous studies, of nonstandardized lung function tests all of which represent confounding factors that bias prevalence studies.

Prevalence and Incidence

Although the true prevalence of work-related asthma is unknown, it is clear that this disorder has been reported with increasing frequency. Surveys suggest that 2%–6% of the general adult population has asthma. It is estimated that 2%–15% of this asthma may be of occupational origin. This figure varies depending on the country, the type of industry, the potency of the agent to which workers are exposed, and the working environment. Figures may vary from 2% to 90% [7]. Some prevalence rates of occupational asthma reported in the literature are listed in Table 1 [8]. As mentioned, accurate epidemiological data on occupational asthma are not easily obtained [7–9]. Almost all the epidemiological studies performed so far have been cross-sectional. These surveys may underestimate the prevalence of occupational asthma; however, they can give a quick estimate of asthma frequency. The best approach would be to perform cross-sectional studies followed by longitudinal studies [10–12].

Occupational asthma is becoming the most frequently claimed respiratory disease of occupational origin. Statistics provided by the Quebec Ministere or by the Comite' local des Maladies Pulmonaires Professionnelles show that, while the number of claims for pneumoconiosis and other occupational lung diseases was stable or decreased comparing the data of 1984 with the data of 1987, in the same period the number of claims for occupational asthma sharply increased (personal communication of J. L. Malo).

Table 1. Prevalence of occupational asthma according to job and sensitizing agent (from [8])

Occupation	Agent	Prevalence (%)
Bakery, mill	Grain, flours	21
Detergent industry	Bacillus subtilis	21
Laboratory	Small animals	30
Laboratory	Small animals	27
Food industry	Prawn	36
Laboratory	Locust	28
Electronics	Colophony	22
Solder manufacturing	Colophony	21
Chemical processing	Platinum salts	60
Isocyanates	TDI	5
Chemical industry	Piperazine	8

TDI, toluene diisocyanate

Sensitizing Agents

The number of agents reported to induce occupational asthma will increase with the continuing introduction of new agents in the workplace. An extensive list of these agents has been published in several review articles (e.g., [5]). For convenience we summarize the three major groups of agents in Table 2. Isocyanates are small molecular weight potent sensitizers widely produced and used in industrialized countries [10]. In some places, e.g., the UK, isocyanates are the most frequently recognized cause of occupational asthma, as shown by the number of cases of occupational asthma diagnosed in the period March 1982–1984 in the UK for each of the agents listed (personal communication of F. G. Ward).

Table 2. Principal agents causing occupational asthma

Substances of animal origin
  Mammalian allergens
  Arthropod debris
Substances of vegetable origin
  Flowers, leaves, roots, seeds
  Flours
  Wood and byproducts
Substances of chemical origin
  Plastic industries
  Pharmaceutical industry
  Metal industry
  Other chemicals

Predisposing Factors

Host factors may be important for a proportion of workers exposed to a sensitizing agent. While age, race, sex, genetic predisposition, airway hyperresponsiveness, and previous asthma have not yet been demonstrated to be predisposing factors for the development of occupational asthma, there is some evidence that atopy, viral infections, and smoking may indeed predispose exposed subjects to the development of occupational asthma. For example, atopy has been considered a predisposing factor for exposures to high molecular weight agents, and cigarette smoking has been demonstrated to have a permissive effect on IgE antibody production and development of asthma (one example is occupational asthma induced by the acid anhydride TCPA). The role of cigarette smoking is far from being clear, and in fact it exerts opposing effects in other diseases such as extrinsic allergic alveolitis, in which it reduces the risk of specific IgG antibody and the development of the disease. Environmental factors such as the intensity of exposure, the potency of the sensitizer, and the length of exposure seem to be of greater importance for the development of occupational asthma [5].

Diagnosis of Occupational Asthma

The diagnosis of occupational asthma is based on patient history and lung function measurements at work and in the laboratory [5, 13]. Objective confirmation of the diagnosis of occupational asthma may be obtained with specific inhalation challenge [14].

History

A correct collection of the patient's history is the most important step for the diagnosis of occupational asthma. In the history of subjects with suspected occupational asthma, it is important to recognize symptoms of occupational asthma; dry cough, particularly nocturnal cough, breathlessness, wheezing, and chest tightness are the most frequently reported. Symptoms may develop at work, but in many cases they develop after cessation of work, during evenings and nights. Symptoms of occupational asthma usually improve during the weekends, but in some cases they may require weeks to improve. This latency should be considered in the so-called stop/resume work test, which is otherwise useful. History may help in the identification of triggering factors, and in the definition of the relationship between the first exposure and the onset of the disease.

Immunologic Tests

Immunologic evaluation of the subject suspected of having occupational asthma may be important to confirm sensitization, particularly to high molecular weight substances which are believed to act through an IgE-mediated mechanism. However, immunologic tests, and especially skin tests, are not, at the present time, required to establish the diagnosis [5, 13–15], because the demonstration of a specific immunological response to an inhaled allergen is not in itself sufficient evidence that the allergen is the cause of occupational asthma, and a negative test does not exclude occupational asthma [5].

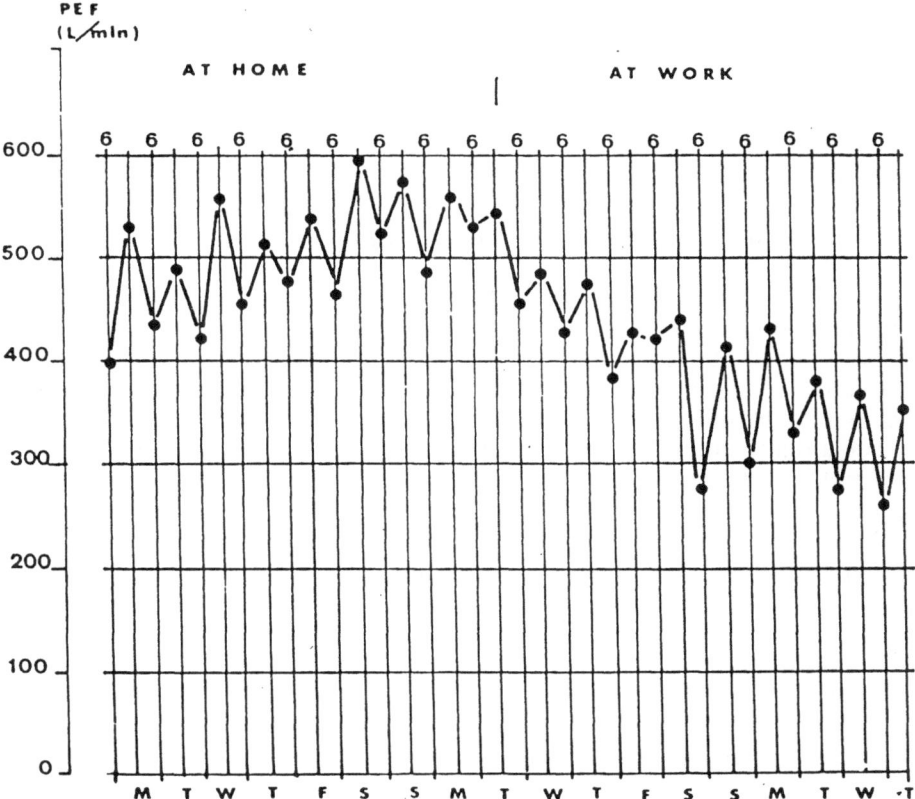

Fig. 1. Peak expiratory flow records (PEFRs), obtained from a furniture worker with a history of job-related asthma, show lower and more variable values of PEFRs during the week he was at work compared to the week he was not working

Peak Flow Records

The measurement of peak expiratory flow rates (PEFR) is the most widely used and probably the best method of assessing asthma. Simple, inexpensive devices (e.g., the popular Mini-Wright) are available. Measurement of lung function, and particularly PEFR, before and after a workshift has been used to evaluate the acute bronchoconstrictive effect of exposure to a noxious agent at work. This method, used in the past for the diagnosis of byssinosis, has never been properly tested for its sensitivity and specificity in the diagnosis of occupational asthma. Actually, the absence of changes in lung function at the end of the work shift may not exclude the presence of occupational asthma, because in many subjects exposure to the sensitizing agent causes a late asthmatic reaction rather than an immediate reaction. In addition, the exposure may be transient and not present during each working day. This method should not be used for the diagnosis of occupational asthma. By contrast, repeated measurements of peak expiratory flow rate performed at home and at work over several weeks may provide objective confirmation of occupational asthma (Fig. 1) [16].

Airway Hyperresponsiveness to Methacholine or Histamine

Airway hyperresponsiveness to methacholine or histamine is the hallmark of asthma both of occupational and nonoccupational origin, and thus repeated measurements of the nonspecific airway responsiveness to methacholine or histamine should be included in the diagnostic procedure of occupational asthma [5]. Normal airway responsiveness does not exclude the presence of occupational asthma, because when the subject is examined after a period of nonexposure to the sensitizing agent, airway responsiveness may be in the normal range. The measurement of nonspecific airway responsiveness to methacholine or histamine should be performed with standardized methods, either with the dosimeter or with the continuous inhalation method, both being properly standardized and providing reproducible results [17]. The results of the dose-response curves to inhalation challenge should be plotted in a semi-log scale and the results expressed in term of PC_{20}-FEV_1 or PD_{20}-FEV_1 [17].

In subjects with occupational asthma the degree of airway responsiveness to methacholine or histamine is usually increased, but it may be normal. Figure 2 shows the variability of PEFRs and PC_{20}-FEV_1 in a subject sensitized to toluene diisocyanate (TDI) and the relationship with exposure [18]. Also, at the time of diagnosis of occupational asthma in the laboratory, airway responsiveness to methacholine or histamine may be normal, but it usually increases (i.e., PD_{20}-FEV_1 decreases) in the asthmatic range after an inhalation challenge with the sensitizing agent [19]. The increase in airway responsiveness to methacholine may last for days or even longer [20, 21].

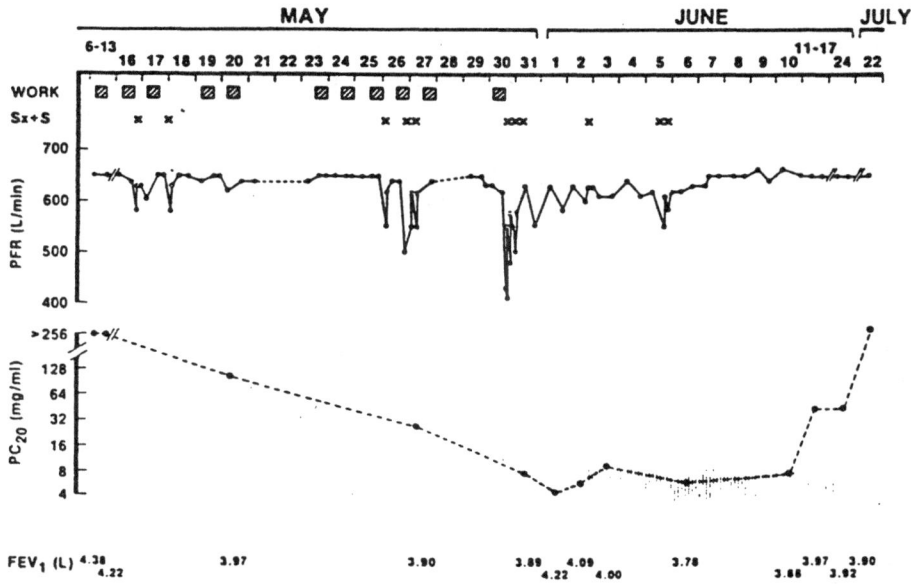

Fig. 2. Decreased peak expiratory flows and increased airway responsiveness during exposure which recovered when the subject, a worker sensitized to toluene diisocyanate (*TDI*), was away from work. Serial measurements before, during (May 9 to 30), and after periods at work. Days at work (XX), symptoms (*Sx*), and use of salbutamol (200 μg) (*S*), PFR (L/min) (● = after salbutamol), PC$_{20}$ methacholine (mg/ml), and baseline FEV$_1$ (L) at the time of methacholine tests. *Shaded area* indicates bronchial hyperresponsiveness (From Ref. 18).

Specific Inhalation Challenges

Specific inhalation challenges remain the "gold standard" for the confirmation of occupational asthma [13, 14]. Recommendations for specific inhalation challenges were recently provided by a committee of the American Academy of Allergy and Clinical Immunology, and the reader is referred to those guidelines for further information [14]. Unfortunately there is no gold standard for an exposure chamber for specific inhalation challenge with occupational agents. Most centers performing these tests developed their own, usually simple, exposure chamber, but more sophisticated exposure chambers have been designed and built [22]. In the past, specific inhalation challenges were performed in the laboratory simulating the exposure to the suspected sensitizing agent present at work, mostly without monitoring the concentration of the occupational sensitizer [4], such as simply exposing bakers to flour, electronic workers to soldering fumes, or painters to paint vapors. Since specific inhalation challenges may be dangerous if the exposure is not properly monitored and controlled, these tests should be performed only in specialized centers where careful measurement of the concentration of the occupational sensitizing agent and resuscitating facilities are available.

Cloutier and coworkers recently developed a new method for specific inhalation challenges with occupational agents in powder form [23], and the same group developed a similar device for specific inhalation challenges with isocyanates. An accurate description of the device may be obtained directly from the authors (Prof. J. L. Malo, MD, personal communication).

Inhalation challenges with occupational agents may cause early, progressive, dual, or late asthmatic reactions, and thus lung function should be monitored for at least 8 h after exposure [4, 14, 24] (Fig. 3). FEV_1 is the most reliable lung function test to assess the response, and an asthmatic response is considered to occur when FEV_1 decreases more than 20% from baseline. Since some asthmatic subjects may have increased diurnal variability of lung volumes, either spontaneously or due to the withdrawal of medications, it has been recommended to include a sham-exposure study day, and to exclude subjects with a daily variability of FEV_1 larger than 10%. Asthmatic reactions induced by occupational agents may be associated with increased airway responsiveness to methacholine or histamine, particularly dual and late asthmatic reactions, which are associated with pulmonary inflammation [25, 26]. When the level of exposure is properly monitored and a control day is included in the protocol, false positive reactions are not very likely to occur [24]. By contrast, a large number of false negative reactors (convincing history of occupational asthma, negative inhalation challenge) has to be expected, probably because of the low level or too short duration of exposure during the challenge or because the agent used for the challenge is not the one which caused asthma. Also, a test may become negative when a sensitized subject has not been exposed at work for a long enough time. Thus, even a negative inhalation challenge does not exclude the presence of occupational asthma. However it certainly excludes a severe sensitivity to the agent tested.

Inhalation challenges with low molecular weight sensitizers, e.g. TDI and plicatic acid, may cause early (10%–20%), dual (30%–50%), or late (30%–50%) asthmatic reactions in about 40% of the subjects with a history of asthma induced by these agents [5, 24]. The challenge is highly specific, because no reaction is induced in normal subjects or in asthmatics not sensitized to TDI [24]. By contrast, a larger proportion of early or dual asthmatic reactions has been recorded after inhalation challenges with high molecular weight sensitizers. Dual and late, but not early, asthmatic reactions induced by TDI are associated with an increased responsiveness to methacholine. Such an increase of bronchial responsiveness is specific because it is not observed in normal subjects or in asthmatics not sensitized to TDI [24].

In conclusion, inhalation challenges with occupational agents remain the gold standard for confirming a diagnosis of occupational asthma in an individual worker, but they may be risky, and thus informed consent from the subject should be obtained before they are performed. They should be performed in specialized centers with all the safety measures recommended by

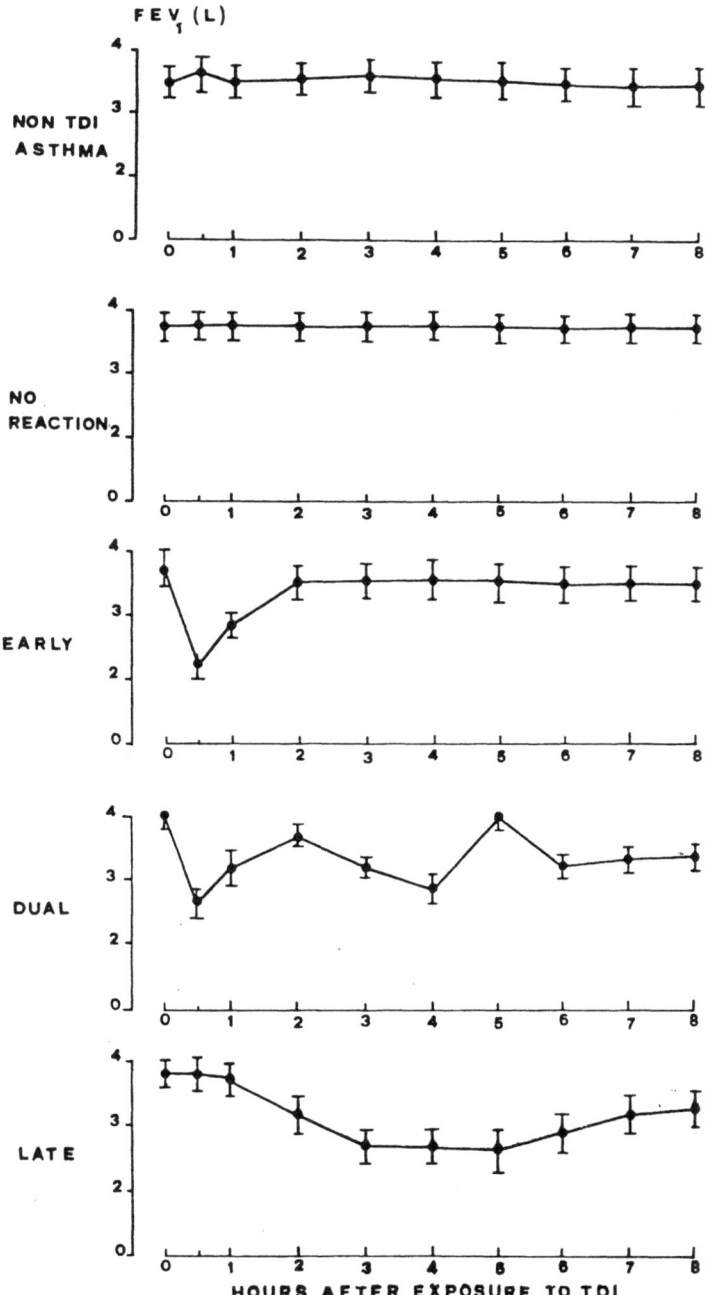

Fig. 3. FEV$_1$ before and after exposure to toluene diisocyanate (*TDI*) in asthmatic subjects nonsensitized to TDI (**a**), normal controls (**b**), subjects sensitized to TDI who developed an early asthmatic reaction (**c**), a late asthmatic reaction (**d**), and a dual asthmatic reaction (**e**). (From [24])

the guidelines provided by international committees [14]. Inhalation challenges with occupational agents are highly specific but poorly sensitive, and thus a negative inhalation challenge with an occupational agent does not exclude the presence of occupational asthma.

Other Approaches to Diagnosis

Other approaches have been recently recommended for the diagnosis of occupational asthma. Measurements of airway responsiveness combined with peak flow records for a week at home and a week at work may be helpful, but they have been shown to be neither more sensitive nor as specific as a simple combination of history and peak flow records [27]. A reproducible increase of airway responsiveness after a negative inhalation challenge may be considered in some cases as objective evidence of occupational asthma [21]. Nonetheless, it may be helpful to confirm occupational asthma in individuals who refuse, or are not eligible, to undergo specific inhalation challenges. At the present time, bronchoalveolar lavage, a useful tool for clinical research, has no practical use in the diagnosis of asthma and particulary of occupational asthma [28].

Comparing the different approaches to the diagnosis of occupational asthma, the patient's history seems to be the most sensitive but the least specific test, whereas the subjective evaluation of repeated PEFRs is almost as sensitive as history, but by far a more specific test in the diagnosis of occupational asthma, for example, induced by red cedar [7]. In subjects with a positive inhalation challenge with plicatic acid (the sensitizing agent responsible for red cedar induced-asthma), 93% had a positive history and 86% had evidence of work-related changes of PEFR, whereas in subjects with a negative inhalation challenge with plicatic acid, only 45% had a negative history (true negative) but as many as 89% did not have evidence of work-related changes of PEFR. Changes of FEV_1 or PC_{20}-FEV_1 methacholine were less sensitive and less specific. In the same study, Cote' and colleagues showed that the combination of changes of PEFR and/or PC_{20}-FEV_1 methacholine, and the combination of history and/or changes of PEFR further improved the sensitivity of each test, but only slightly increased the specificity [27].

In subjects with suspected occupational asthma induced by high molecular weight sensitizers, the diagnosis may be established with the history; evidence of exposure, determined either through the history or in the work place; evidence of sensitization to the suspected causative agent in an immunologic tests, and particularly skin tests. Nonetheless, the diagnosis needs to be confirmed by physiological measurements either at work or in the laboratory [5, 29]. In subjects with suspected occupational asthma induced by low molecular weight sensitizers, the diagnosis may be established with the history, evidence of exposure, and physiological measurements either at work or in the laboratory, whereas skin tests and other immunologic tests are available for a limited number of substances. Moreover the role of IgE against protein-apten conjugatès remains to be established. Skin tests with common allergens may still be useful to identify atopic subjects [5, 30]. In conclusion, the diagnosis of occupational asthma can be reliably established with the combination of history and repeated measurements of lung function, and particularly of PEFR. However, inhalation challenges with occupational agents may be required to confirm the diagnosis in some patients. Skin tests, serologic tests, and tests of cell immunity are useful to demonstrate a response to exposure (sensitization), but these tests may be positive also in exposed asymptomatic workers. Although evidence of an occupational sensitization may be helpful in evaluating a subject with work-related respiratory symptoms, it is not required to establish the diagnosis of occupational asthma. Chest X-rays, blood tests, ECG, and other clinical tests may be helpful for the differential diagnosis of asthma from other pulmonary and nonpulmonary diseases, but they are not required for the diagnosis [5, 13].

Prognosis of Occupational Asthma

Factors Influencing Prognosis

If exposure continues after diagnosis, occupational asthma does not recover, but often persists or may even deteriorate [5, 31–33]. Fatal attacks may be triggered at work in sensitized subjects [34]. The majority of patients with occupational asthma do not even recover after several years of cessation of exposure both to low and high molecular weight sensitizers [5, 31–33, 35]. The prognosis of occupational asthma is better in subjects who, at the time of diagnosis and cessation of exposure, have better lung function, a milder degree of nonspecific airway hyperresponsiveness, a shorter duration of exposure and of symptoms, and who develop an early (compared with a late or dual) asthmatic reaction at the diagnostic inhalation challenge with the occupational sensitizer. Prognosis is not influenced by race, sex, atopy, smoking habits, and is not always improved by relocation to working areas with lower exposure [36, 37].

Persistence after Cessation of Exposure

Percentages of persistence of asthma symptoms and airway hyperresponsiveness in subjects with occupational asthma after cessation of exposure are reported in Table 3. The data clearly show that, when sensitized, most subjects remain asthmatic even after cessation of exposure.

Table 3. Persistence of symptoms and airway hyperresponsiveness in subjects with occupational asthma after leaving work (from [37])

Agent	Number of subjects	Duration of follow-up (years)	Persistence of symptoms (%)	Persistence of hyperresponsiveness (%)
Red cedar	75	1–9	49	25/33 (76)
Colophony	20	1.3–3.8	90	7/20 (35)
Snow-crab	31	0.5–2	61	28/31 (90)
Snow-crab	31	4.8–6	100	26/31 (84)
Isocyanates	50	>4	82	12/19 (63)
Isocyanates	20	0.5–4	50	9/12 (75)
Isocyanates	22	1	77	17/22 (77)
Isocyanates	12	1.3	66	7/12 (58)
Various	32	0.5–4	93	31/32 (97)

Management of Occupational Asthma

Short- and Long-Term Management

When the causal relationship between occupational sensitizers and asthma has been confirmed, the worker should be entitled to paid sick leave, particularly if she/he needs medical treatment, relocation of her/his job to areas of no exposure, and/or to use protective devices that guarantee total avoidance of exposure. In addition the worker should receive compensation for temporary disability. Management of occupational asthma on a long-term basis requires more fundamental interventions. Employers should develop all the possible preventive measures, i.e., an efficient environmental control of processes involving sensitizing agents, a change in product formulation or industrial process whenever possible, and, finally, substitution of harmful material. Sensitized workers should be entitled to removal from exposure, either by job relocation or by compensated retirement and/or change of their job, and to compensation for disability. Symptomatic patients should be treated the same as patients with active asthma.

Therapy

Drug treatment of occupational asthma is identical to that of non-occupational asthma. Several treatment protocols have been recently published or are presently in press. The guidelines for asthma treatment have been summarized in an article produced by a group of several investigators interested in and experienced in the assessment and treatment of asthma [38].

Pharmacologic Prophylaxis

Since it is often difficult for a sensitized subject to completely avoid exposure to the sensitizing agent, it may be helpful to know the most effective pharmacologic treatment which prevents late asthmatic reactions induced by specific exposure. For example, for subjects sensitized to TDI, the most effective prophylactic treatment (i.e., prevention of asthma attacks induced by TDI) is a high dose of inhaled steroids [39], whereas theophylline is effective only at very high blood concentrations, and cromolyn, verapamil, and ketotifen are not effective [39, 40]. Whether this applies to other sensitizers is not known. β-2 Agonists may be used to prevent or reverse acute, early asthmatic reactions [4], but more severe attacks of asthma induced by occupational agents should be treated as any attack of asthma, i.e., with high dose inhaled β-2-agonists and high dose systemic steroids [38]. In conclusion, the management of occupational asthma is identical to the management of nonoccupational asthma, i.e., avoidance is preferable to medical treatment, and medical treatment is identical in occupational and nonoccupational asthma.

Evaluation of Impairment and Compensation

Subjects with occupational asthma should be awarded compensation for permanent disability whenever permanent disability is proven to exist. Unfortunately, there are no definite guidelines for the evaluation of impairment in asthma, and the guidelines for evaluation of impairment of subjects with other pulmonary diseases are not adequate for asthma, particularly for occupational asthma [41]. Evaluation of impairment might be based on history, lung function tests including spirometry and measurement of airway responsiveness, and on the amount of medication required to keep asthma under control [41]. Symptomatic subjects with nonspecific airway hyperresponsiveness should be considered impaired even if they have normal lung volumes. Tentative guidelines derived from the literature are the following: lung function tests should be performed before and after the administration of a bronchodilator, it should include the measurement of the degree of airway responsiveness either to histamine or methacholine, and the minimum amount of medication required to keep asthma under control (i.e., normal lifestyle, absence of symptoms, normal or "best" lung function) should be taken into account. Finally, each worker who receives compensation should undergo periodic reevaluation of lung function, degree of airway responsiveness to methacholine, and history to check for asthmatic symptoms and amount of medication [5, 41]. Recently the Canadian Thoracic Society proposed tentative criteria for rating the severity of asthma and impairment from the degree of obstruction (determined by FEV_1, % predicted), airway responsiveness, and current medications [42].

Conclusions

In conclusion, occupational asthma is the most frequent occupational pulmonary disease in industrialized countries, and its incidence and prevalence are increasing. The diagnosis of occupational asthma is based on history, repeated measurements of lung function, and repeated measurements of airway responsiveness. However, inhalation challenges with occupational agents may be necessary to confirm the diagnosis. These challenges are risky, and thus they should be performed only in specialized centers and after informed consent is obtained by the patient. The mechanisms, pathology, pathophysiology, and treatment are similar in occupational and nonoccupational asthma. Occupational asthma may become more severe; it does not recover and may even be fatal on continuation of exposure. It also often persists after several years of cessation of exposure. Evaluation of impairment and disability caused by occupational asthma should include measurements of lung function, of airway responsiveness, and of the amount of medication required to maintain asthma under control.

References

1. Ramazzini B (1713) Be morbis artificum. Diatriba. Edition Novissima. Ex typographya Caroli Columbi Romae MCMLIII (A reprint of the edition published in Padova in 1713)
2. Karasek Sr, Karasek M (1911) Preliminary report on the injurious effects of metal platinum, chromates, cyanides, hydrofluoridric acid, and of material used by silver miners. Report of the Illinois State Commission on occupational diseases, p 97
3. Pepys J, Hutchroft BJ (1975) Bronchial provocation tests in etiologic diagnosis and analysis of asthma. Am Rev Respir Dis 112:829–859
4. Crepet M, Gaffuri E, Vallerani G (1966) Aspetti Clinici e diagnostici dell' asma allergico professionale. In: Le allergie professionali. Atti del XXVI Congresso Nazionale di Medicina del Lavoro tenutosi a Padova dal 11 al 13 Ottobre 1963. Cedam Editrice, Padova
5. Chan-Yeung M, Lam S (1986) Occupational asthma. Am Rev Respir Dis 133: 686–803
6. Brooks SM, Weiss MA, Bernstein IL (1985) Reactive Airways Disfunction Syndrome (RADS). Persistent asthma syndrome after high level irritant exposures. Chest 86:376–384
7. Venable KM (1987) Epidemiology and the prevention of occupational asthma. Br J Ind Med 44:73–75
8. Keskinen H (1983) Epidemiology of occupational lung diseases: asthma and allergic alveolitis. In: Kerr JW and Gandertone MA (eds). Proceedings of XI International Congress of Allergology and Clinical Immunology. McMillan, London, pp 403–407
9. Sears M (1990) Epidemiology of asthma. In: O'Byrne PM (ed). Asthma as an inflammatory disease. Dekker, New York, chap 2
10. Mapp CE, Boschetto P, Dal Vecchio L, Maestrelli P, Fabbri LM (1988) Occupational asthma due to isocyanates. Eur Respir J 1:273–279
11. Burge PS, Perks WH, O'Brien IM et al. (1979) Occupational asthma in an electronic factory: a case-control study to evaluate aetiological factors. Thorax 34: 300–307

12. Thiel H (1983) Baker's asthma. Epidemiological and clinical findings – need for prospective studies. In: Kerr JW, Gandertone MA (eds) Proceedings of the XIth international congress of allergology and clinical immunology. McMillan, London, pp 429–433
13. Bernstein DI (ed) (1989) Guidelines for the diagnosis and evaluation of occupational lung diseases. J Allergy Clin Immunol 84:5 (part 2)
14. Cartier A, Bernstein IL, Burge PS et al. (1989) Guidelines for bronchoprovocation on the investigation of occupational asthma. J Allergy Clin Immunol 84: 823–828
15. Cockcroft AE (1988) Occupational asthma and alveolitis – unanswered questions. J R Soc Med 81:255–257
16. Burge PS, O'Brien IM, Harries MG (1979) Peak flow rate records in the diagnosis of occupational asthma due to colophony. Thorax 34:308–316
17. Hargreave FE, Woolcock AJ (eds) (1985) Airway responsiveness. Measurement and interpretation. Astra Pharmaceutical Canada
18. Hargreave FE, Ramsdale EH, Pugsly SO (1984) Occupational asthma without bronchial hyperresponsiveness. Am Rev Respir Dis 130:513–515
19. Mapp CE, Dal Vecchio L, Boschetto P, De Marzo N, Fabbri LM (1986) Toluene diisocyanate-induced asthma without airway hyperresponsiveness. Eur J Respir Dis 68:89–95
20. Mapp C, Polato R, Maestrelli P, Hendrick DJ, Fabbri LM (1985) Time course of the increase of airway responsiveness associated with delayed asthmatic reactions to toluene diisocyanate in sensitized subjects. J Allergy Clin Immunol 75:568–572
21. Cartier A, L'Archeveque J, Malo' JL (1986) Exposure to a sensitizing occupational agent can cause a long lasting increase in bronchial responsiveness to histamine in the absence of significant changes of airway caliber. J Allergy Clin Immunol 78:1185–1190
22. Hammad YY, Rando RJ, Abdel-Kader H (1985) Considerations in the design and use of human inhalation challenge delivery system. Folia Allergol Immunol Clin 32:37–44
23. Cloutier Y, Lagier F, Lemieux R et al. (1989) New methodology for specific inhalation challenges with occupational agents in powder form. Eur Respir J 2: 769–777
24. Mapp CE, Di Giacomo R, Broseghini C et al. (1986) Late, but not early, asthmatic reactions induced by toluene diisocyanate (TDI) are associated with increased airway responsiveness. Eur J Respir Dis 68:276–284
25. Chan-Yeung M, Lam S (1990) Evidence for mucosal inflammation in occupational asthma. Clin Exp Allergy 20:1–5
26. Fabbri LM, Mapp CE, Saetta M, Allegra L (1990) Occupational asthma. In: O'Byrne PM (ed) Asthma as an inflammatory disease. Dekker, New York, chap 6
27. Cote' J, Kennedy S, Chan-Yeung M (1990) Sensitivity and specificity of PC20 and peak expiratory flow rate in cedar asthma. J Allergy Clin Immunol 85: 592–598
28. Fabbri LM, De Rose V, Godard Ph, Boschetto P, Rossi GA (1992) Guidelines and recommendations for the clinical use of bronchoalveolar lavage in asthma. Eur Respir Rev 2:116–123
29. Novey HS, Bernstein IL, Mihalas LS, Terr AI, Yunginger JW (1989) Guidelines for the clinical evaluation of occupational asthma due to high molecular weight (HMW) allergens. J Allergy Clin Immunol 84:829–833
30. Butcher BT, Bernstein IL, Schwartz HJ (1989) Guidelines for the clinical evaluation of occupational asthma due to low molecular weight (LMW) chemicals. J Allergy Clin Immunol 84:834–838
31. Yeung M, Grzybowski S (1985) Prognosis of occupational asthma. Thorax 40: 241–243
32. Cote' J, Kennedy S, Chan Yeung M (1990) Outcome of patients with cedar asthma with continuous exposure. Am Rev Respir Dis 141:373–376

33. Mapp CE, Chiesura-Corona P, De Marzo N, Fabbri LM (1988) Persistent asthma due to isocyanates. A follow-up study of subjects with occupational asthma due to toluene diisocyanate. Am Rev Respir Dis 137:1326–1329
34. Fabbri LM, Danieli D, Crescioli S, Bevilacqua P, Meli S, Saetta M, Mapp CE (1988) Fatal asthma in a toluene diisocyanate sensitized subject. Am Rev Respir Dis 137:1494–1498
35. Paggiaro PL, Paoletti P, Bacci E et al. (1990) Eosinophils in bronchoalveolar lavage (BAL) of patients with toluene diisocyanate (TDI) asthma after cessation of work. Chest 98:536–542
36. Banks DE, Rando RJ, Barkman HW (1990) Persistence of toluene diisocyanate induced asthma despite negligible workplace exposures. Chest 97:121–125
37. Allard C, Cartier A, Ghezzo H, Malo JL (1989) Occupational asthma due to various agents. Absence of clinical and functional improvement at an interval of four or more years after cessation of exposure. Chest 96:1046–1049
38. Hargreave FE, Dolovich J, Newhouse MT (eds) (1990) The assessment and treatment of asthma: a conference report. J Allergy Clin Immunol 85:1098–1111
39. Mapp CE, Boschetto P, Dal Vecchio L et al. (1987) Protective effect of antiasthma drugs on late asthmatic reactions and increased responsiveness induced by toluene-diisocyanate in sensitized subjects. Am Rev Respir Dis 136:1403–1407
40. Tossin L, De Marzo N, Crescioli S, Mapp CE, Fabbri LM (1989) Ketotifen does not inhibit asthmatic reactions induced by toluene diisocyanate in sensitized subjects. Clin Exper Allergy 19:177–182
41. Chan-Yeung M (1988) Occupational asthma update. Chest 93:407–411
42. Warren CPW, Boulet L-P, Broder I et al. (1989) Occupational asthma: recommendations for diagnosis, management, and assessment of impairment. Can Med Assoc J 140:1029–1032

Exercise and Hyperventilation Provocation Challenges

S. Anderson[1], P. Tessier[2], C. M. Smith[1], and J. L. Malo[2]

[1] Department of Respiratory Medicine, Royal Prince Alfred Hospital,
  Camperdown, New South Wales, Australia
[2] Department of Chest Medicine, Hopital du Sacre-Coeur, Montreal, Canada

Introduction

Exercise and hyperventilation are two stimuli which are known to provoke acute airway narrowing in patients with clinically recognised asthma. The sensitivity of a subject to the effects of exercise or hyperventilation is often expressed by symptoms of cough, dyspnea or wheezing and frequently occur as the first sign of asthma, particularly in childhood.

Most patients with clinically recognized asthma manifest a state of non-allergic bronchial hyperresponsiveness (NABHR) and a laboratory challenge with a nonallergic stimulus such as exercise and hyperventilation has become popular for diagnosis and assessing the severity of bronchial hyper-responsiveness.

There are a number of advantages in using exercise or hyperventilation rather than pharmacological stimuli as tests of NABHR. Exercise is a common stimulus to airway narrowing in everyday life and the major factors which determine the severity of the airway response, that is, ventilation rate, water content, and temperature of the inspired air, can be measured easily in the laboratory. Thus documentation of severity of airway narrowing in response to hyperpnea, and the benefit afforded by pharmacological agents has direct clinical relevance to the treatment of the patient.

Although it was recognised as early as the seventeenth century that exercise could provoke an attack of asthma [88], it was only 40 years ago that hyperventilation was suggested as the initiating stimulus [56]. It was not until 1962 that considerable attention was given to exercise [60] and later to hyperventilation as provoking stimuli in patients with asthma [32, 116]. Although many of the findings suggest that these two challenges act via the same stimulus, there is sufficient debate to advise that a distinction should be made when describing these challenges and this is discussed in detail below.

Background to the Techniques for Challenge with Hyperpnea

When air is inspired there is a need to condition this to alveolar temperature, 37 °C, and water content, 44 mg/liter. In most climates inhabited by humans, the air is drier and cooler than alveolar air and the process of conditioning air requires the loss of heat and water from the airways. At resting levels of ventilation and under temperate or tropical conditions, the air is mostly conditioned before it reaches the pharynx [59]. During exercise or hyperventilation the rate of ventilation is increased and the nose by-passed to reduce resistance at high flow rates. Some of the burden to heat and humidify the air passes to the intrathoracic airways which must then provide sufficient heat and water to protect the alveoli from dehydration and cooling. The cooler and drier the air, the greater the number of generations of airways involved in the conditioning process [37]. As 80% of the heat lost during the conditioning of temperate air comes about through the evaporation of water, considerable attention has been focussed on the loss of water from the respiratory tract as the stimulus to airway narrowing provoked by hyperpnea [13, 44, 54]. Since the airway narrowing in response to hyperpnea can be prevented or inhibited by inhaling humid air during hyperpnea [7, 33, 98] the airway lumen has been thought to be the site of action for the stimulus to induce airway narrowing.

Although there is general agreement that the loss of water from the airways is the primary stimulus to airway narrowing, there is debate as to whether it is the cooling or the drying effects of water loss which is more important [5, 8]. Initially cooling of the airways was considered the most important event [33, 36, 37, 72, 98, 99] but later this theory was modified to incriminate rewarming and vascular engorgement after cooling as the critical event [50, 73]. A major argument against rewarming is that for many asthmatic subjects the attack of asthma comes on during hyperventilation or exercise at a time when the airway temperature is reduced and before rewarming has a chance to occur [8, 19, 93]. Furthermore recent studies in children have not supported rewarming as universal for provoking exercise-induced asthma (EIA) [96] and the hypothesis has been brought into question [8, 48]. Other groups of investigators have questioned the role of cooling alone [13, 44, 54] and suggested that drying and the consequent change in osmolarity of the periciliary fluid layer may be the primary factor involved [4, 54, 92]. Similar conclusions have been made with respect to the cough which follows exercise [20] even though it may not be accompanied by airway narrowing.

If mast cell release of histamine and other mediators is relevant to the airway narrowing provoked by hyperpnea [5, 65], then there is evidence to support an argument for both cooling and changes in osmolarity being important. Thus in vitro studies of histamine release from human lung mast cells show that the optimal conditions for release is a temperature of 32°C and an osmolarity of 640 msmol [43]. The temperature of the airways during exercise and hyperventilation with temperate air is about 32°C, while by breathing subfreezing air it is less [74]. The delay in the onset of the response after breathing subfreezing air may relate to the need for optimal temperature conditions for hyperosmolar release of histamine and in this respect rewarming per se rather than increased mucosal blood flow may be important. So potent is the hyperosmolar stimulus for provoking airway narrowing in patients with exercise- [16, 24, 94] and hyperventilation- [92, 93] induced attacks of asthma that challenge with inhaled aerosols of hyperosmolar saline are now used to identify subjects responsive to the effects of hyperpnea.

Methods: General Comments for Both Challenges

Conditions of Inspired Air

The two physical properties of the inhaled air which are relevant to provoking bronchoconstriction with exercise and hyperventilation are the water content and temperature of the inspired air. There is general agreement in the literature that dry air is more potent than air containing any moisture [13, 37, 44, 54, 84, 92, 110]. In many laboratories compressed air (exercise) or compressed air containing 4.9% carbon dioxide (hyperventilation) is used and it is assumed that this air is dry. Some investigators [21, 57] prefer to dry the air by circulating it through a chamber containing hydrophilic products.

There are different opinions as to whether the air should be cooled to subfreezing temperatures [37, 44]. Furthermore it is not known whether challenge with air of subfreezing temperature is providing the same stimulus as challenge with dry air at ambient to hot temperatures. The difference may be in the direction of changes in osmolarity. Thus dry warm or dry hot air may increase osmolarity whereas cold air may cause substantial cooling of the airways leading to condensation of water on the airway mucosa and thus decreasing airway osmolarity.

The use of cold air is, of course, relevant to geographical areas where cold air is a stimulus to bronchoconstriction. There are, however, many places where the inspired air never reaches subfreezing temperatures or is never completely dry. It would seem unwise in these circumstances to use a false stimulus to evaluate the effects of a natural one.

In laboratories which use cold air, the production of the cold air is carried out in a similar way. A heat exchanger allows for the contact of air with a cooling agent such as isopropyl alcohol [18], methanol [81], ethylene glycol [99], freon [68] and a mixture of ice and acetone [38].

Measurement of Respiratory Heat and Water Exchange

In 1979 Deal and coworkers [37] reintroduced and validated the equation first proposed by the French workers Houdas and Colin in 1966 [58].

$$RHE = VE \times HC(T_E - T_I) + HV(C_E H_2O - C_I H_2O)$$

where RHE is the respiratory heat exchange (usually a loss); VE, the minute ventilation; HC, the heat capacity of air; T_E and T_I, expired and inspired air temperature; C_E and C_I H_2O, water content of the expired and inspired air and HV, latent heat of vaporization.

The equipment required to make accurate measurements of inspired and expired temperature at frequencies of breathing associated with high levels of exercise and hyperventilation is expensive. Moreover when air of sub-freezing temperatures is inspired, accurate measurement is rendered more difficult by the potential of the expired water vapour to condense and to freeze the thermocouple or thermistor and thus dampen the response. Thermistors which may normally be considered to have rapid response may be limited when the frequency of breathing exceeds 30 breaths/min [13]. If measurements of both inspired and expired air temperatures are needed, it is recommended to use a divided valve to modify some of these problems but technically accurate measurements can be difficult.

It does appear that over a fairly wide range of inspired air temperatures which may be encountered in temperate, tropical and arid conditions (26°–42 °C) and 4–12 mg H_2O/liter that the expired air temperature and water content remain fairly stable during exercise [4, 13, 44, 101]. When the inspired air is hot and completely dry, however, there is a reduction in expired water vapour pressure [101]. We have also found during hyperventilation with dry air, that the mean expired water content of the air is stable around 29 mg/liter [92]. In our study [92] expired ventilation was measured and the expired water was collected and weighed in order to avoid the problems encountered with the accurate measurement of expired temperature. There is no necessity to measure or report values for heat and water loss for challenge with hyperpnea. Indeed there are several problems with global measurements of heat and water loss. The first is when comparing the same subjects under different inspired air conditions a twofold difference can occur in respiratory heat loss while the airway response remains the same [5, 37]. The second is that the proportion of the total heat and water which is lost below the pharynx is not known and is difficult to measure. Although there are reports of measurements of temperature in the airways [50], direct measurements of water have not been made and it is likely that water fluxes would change in response to a foreign object so that accurate measurement may be difficult. Finally there is considerable argument as to whether the expired temperature reflects a gradient in temperature from the alveoli to the mouth. The question as to whether there is abnormal cooling of the airways when T_E on exercise exceeds T_E at rest is as yet unresolved [12, 114].

Expressing the Results

Expressing the results in terms of minute ventilation, respiratory heat or water loss does not seem to affect the outcome of the test [13, 92, 105, 108]. The average physician or medical practitioner or respiratory scientist has no understanding of how the values of respiratory heat and water loss relate to daily life. They can, however, relate to the level of ventilation. Thus giving mea-

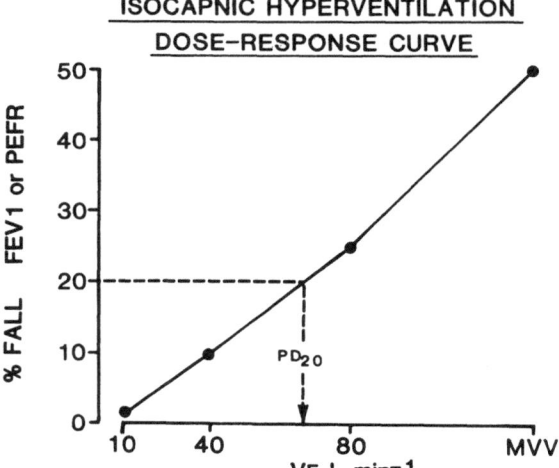

Fig. 1. The reduction in the forced expiratory volume in 1 s (FEV$_1$) after isocapnic hyperventilation with compressed air containing 4.9% carbon dioxide for 3 min, at 30% and 60% and at 100% of maximum voluntary ventilation in an asthmatic patient; PEFR, peak expiratory flow rate; VE, minute ventilation

surements in terms of ventilation while clearly stating the temperature and water content of the inspired air is more easily understood and is all that is required for routine investigation (Fig. 1).

Measuring the Airway Response

The selection of lung function measurement to assess the response may depend on the technical and physiological characteristics of the stimulus and on the specific need of the study. Forced expiratory volume in 1 s (FEV$_1$) and peak expiratory flow rate (PEFR) have been used more commonly than the measurement of specific conductance (sG_{aw}) or specific airways resistance (sR_{aw}). There are important reasons for this. For example, the measurement of FEV$_1$ and PEFR are more reproducible than measurements of resistance [10] and they are much easier and cheaper to assess because they require less sophisticated equipment. FEV$_1$, however, is superior to PEFR because it includes a large proportion of the flow volume curve whereas PEFR records only one point in this curve [9, 34]. PEFR measurements are useful to record changes during exercise when it is difficult to have a prolonged forced expiration.

In performing the FEV$_1$ and PEFR manouvers the subject is required to take a maximal inhalation to total lung capacity. In doing so bronchodilation may occur and so affect the measurement of airway caliber in response to inhalation of cold or dry air [66, 67]. However, this bronchodilation occurs only in subjects with mild bronchial hyperresponsiveness. Although it may result in a false negative tests in subjects with borderline abnormality, it has minimal effect in those with markedly increased bronchial hyperresponsiveness.

Some investigators use measurement of pulmonary and airway resistance and specific airway conductance, the measurement of which requires little effort from the patient. While these measures are generally accepted as being more sensitive for detecting changes, they are probably not superior in this regard to the measurement of flow in the mid and lower portions of the vital capacity [11, 29, 34]. Changes in resistance and conductance represent obstruction or narrowing of the large airways [111] and may be affected by variation in laryngeal caliber. Assessment of airway resistance is influenced by the lung volume at which it is measured, thus it is important to take into account this volume, and the use of sG_{aw} and sR_{aw} are based on this principle.

Three methods are commonly used for the assessment of airway resistance; body plethysmography, by interruption of the airflow, and, the most recent method, forced oscillometry. They all share the disadvantage of requiring complex, cumbersome and expensive apparatuses. Recently, there has been an interest in assessing airway caliber with flow oscillometry. Preliminary results [64] have shown a good correlation between the results assessed by the FEV_1 and those measured with oscillometry.

Performing the Test

As the index used to measure the response to hyperventilation and exercise is usually based on the prechallenge or baseline value, this measurement is important. The subject should be familiar with the manoeuvre used to measure airway caliber and the manouver should be repeated often enough to obtain a reproducible measurement. There are arguments for and against taking the lowest, highest or mean of the baseline values. In our laboratories we select the best measurement recorded as the baseline value.

Exercise and Hyperventilation – Are They the Same Challenge?

There have been a number of observations made which have contributed to the thinking that exercise and hyperventilation act to induce narrowing of the airways via the same mechanism. For example, the severity of asthma provoked by exercise and hyperventilation is the same providing that the ventilation and the temperature and water content of the inspired air are the same [36, 62, 63, 84, 116]. Indeed the magnitude of the reduction in airway temperature has been reported to be the same when both hyperventilation and exercise are performed at the same flow rates [74]. This suggests that heat and water fluxes are similar despite differences in cardiac output and possibly bronchial blood flow during these two challenges.

The time-course for the development of the maximal response is also the same [32, 69]. Many of the drugs which block exercise induced asthma similarly prevent hyperventilation asthma [6, 14, 28, 40, 61, 70, 83, 95] although there are recent reports which show responses to antihistamines may be different [107]. Not all patients are refractory to repeated challenge, by either exercise [90] or hyperventilation [85, 110]. In patients with asthma, sensitivity to methacholine is related to sensitivity to both exercise and hyperventilation [81, 94, 108] and is reported not to be changed significantly by challenge with hyperpnea [53, 87, 104] although this has not been observed by others [1, 100]. When changes in sensitivity have been reported they are small and often observed in those who did not have EIA as well as those who did [100].

The major differences between challenge by exercise and hyperventilation relate to the cardiovascular, metabolic, hematological and biochemical changes, most of which occur and have been measured in response to exercise and not hyperventilation [4, 6]. The release of catecholamines and changes in cyclic AMP have previously been thought to account for the dilatation observed during exercise and the delay in the responses after exercise [5]. Recent data, however, brings these conclusions into question because bronchodilatation occurred during the first few minutes of hyperventilation challenge which does not include catecholamine release [93].

It is the refractory period which follows these two challenges that has been shown to be markedly different. Godfrey and colleagues demonstrated that a refractory period could be induced after exercise which did not cause bronchoconstriction because heat and water loss was prevented by inhaling humid air [25]. They were unable to show the same after hyperventilation [21] and for this and other reasons have argued that the challenges are different [22, 26, 52].

In a recent study by Margolskee et al. [71] it was shown that, in contrast to exercise, the refractory period was not ablated after hyperventilation when subjects were pretreated with indomethacin. This finding suggests that either the mediators released in response to these two forms of hyperpnea are not the same or that their clearance from the airways by the bronchial blood flow is different.

Methodology for Exercise Tests

When exercise was first introduced as a stimulus for provoking an attack of asthma, there was considerable debate about the nature of the exercise, its intensity, and the duration for which it was performed [15]. Many publications appeared about the standardization of exercise taking into account these factors [34, 42, 91, 109]. When it was realized that the level of ventilation reached and sustained and the heat and water content of the air were the most important determinants, many of the earlier observations could be understood in this context. It is still thought by some experts in the field that the intensity of the exercise determines the response and that climatic conditions only modify it [79] and that type of exercise is important [23]. For routine laboratory testing, however, it would now seem that any form of exercise can be used to provoke an attack, providing it raises ventilation high enough and the inspired air is dry enough.

The most commonly úsed form of exercise has been running, either free range or on a motor driven treadmill. Cycling exercise on an electrically or mechanically braked bicycle is also used for challenge. Running or cycling for 6–8 min in an environment where the water content is less than 10 mg per liter with an exercise intensity sufficient to reach and sustain 70%–80% of predicted maximum oxygen uptake and 90% of predicted maximum heart rate, has been recommended [11]. This is probably the most common form of exercise for children and is likely to elicit a response in 70%–80% with clinically recognised asthma [34, 75]. Aiming for an intensity of exercise to achieve 40%–60% of maximum voluntary ventilation (MVV) and maintaining this for a minimum of 4 min in a relatively dry environment may improve the sensitivity of the test. For safety it is always advisable to measure heart rate and this also confirms the intensity of the exercise for each subject. The exercise test must be performed using a nose-clip to ensure mouth breathing. Thus while maintaining a relatively constant ambient temperature (variation of 3°–4°C) and a relatively constant water content (variation of 3–4 mg/l), which is less than 12 mg/liter and by measuring ventilation it is possible to get reproducible falls in FEV_1. This technique has some advantages in that it does not require sophisticated equipment to change the condition of the air. Under these conditions the drawback of not having cool or completely dry air can be overcome simply by increasing the duration of the exercise test to 8 min.

We have observed that it usually requires 4 min and maybe up to 6 min of cycling to achieve 60% or 70% of MVV, even when the intensity of work is high. Once this level of ventilation is achieved it should be maintained for 4 min. It is likely that running may be associated with a square wave, that is rapid response for ventilation, whereas for cycling the ventilation increases progressively even though the workload remains constant [13].

It is best to perform exercise uninterrupted by measurements of lung function. However a measurement can be made just before the patient stops exercising to assess if the attack of asthma has started. The occurrence of a reduction in lung function before the end of exercise depends on the duration for which exercise is performed. While it is most unlikely that by 4 min the lung function value is less than prechallenge, this is not the case if 8 min of exercise is performed at the same intensity [8]. Even if the value is lower at 8 min than prechallenge the lung function is likely to continue to fall for at least another 5–7 min in children and for up to 12 min in adults. It is recommended that measurements be made in duplicate at 1, 3, 5, 7, 10, and 15 min after exercise. The time of the test is 20–30 min.

The % fall index has been the one most commonly used to quantify the severity of EIA. The % rise index describes the bronchodilation during exercise. Both of these indices are illustrated in Fig. 2. The % fall index is obtained by subtracting the lowest FEV_1 or PEFR, recorded in the 15 min after

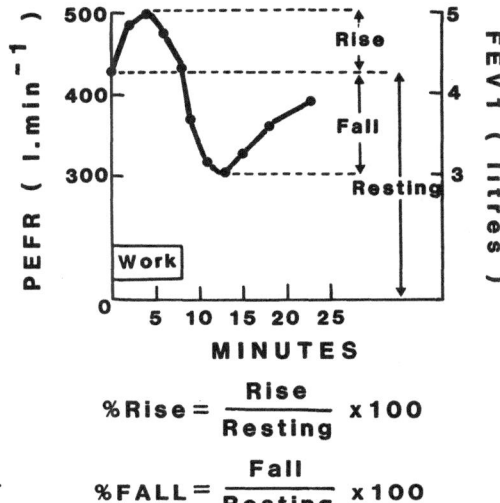

Fig. 2. Changes in peak expiratory flow rate (*PEFR*) and forced expiratory volume in 1 s (*FEV₁*) typically recorded during and after running exercise in an asthmatic patient who has some airways obstruction at rest. The highest and lowest and resting values used to assess the % rise and % fall are shown by the *broken lines*. (From [6])

$$\%\,Rise = \frac{Rise}{Resting} \times 100$$

$$\%\,FALL = \frac{Fall}{Resting} \times 100$$

exercise, from the value measured immediately before exercise and expressing it as a percentage of this value.

One of the major criticisms for the % fall index is in the comparison of the severity of EIA, either within the same patient, or between patients who may have the same predicted value or the same % fall but who start at a different level of lung function before exercise. For this reason, in addition to reporting the % fall index, it is recommended that the FEV_1 values measured before and after exercise should also be reported in terms of percentage of the predicted normal. When both the % fall in FEV_1 and the FEV_1 given in % predicted are reported, the clinical importance and physiological relevance of a fall in lung function can be more easily ascertained. Furthermore the separate effects of drugs on lung function and EIA are better understood (Fig. 3).

The % fall in FEV_1 and PEFR has been measured in response to exercise in many hundreds of healthy subjects [3, 30]. A value of 10% or more is generally accepted as abnormal because it represents the mean ±2 SD of the mean value for % fall, recorded in normal subjects. Although a 10% fall in FEV_1 may be diagnostic of EIA, the physiological significance of the response depends on the person concerned. For a competing athlete a 10% fall in FEV_1 can markedly reduce maximum ventilation and work performance. This point is highlighted when one considers that a 10% fall in FEV_1 is equivalent to a 20%–30% fall in the flow rate in the middle half of the vital capacity [11]. Since this is the part of the flow volume curve used to increase tidal volume, a reduction in these flow rates can have a marked effect on maximal exercise performance. Thus even a relatively small reduction in FEV_1 should be prevented, particularly if it is documented during as well as after exercise.

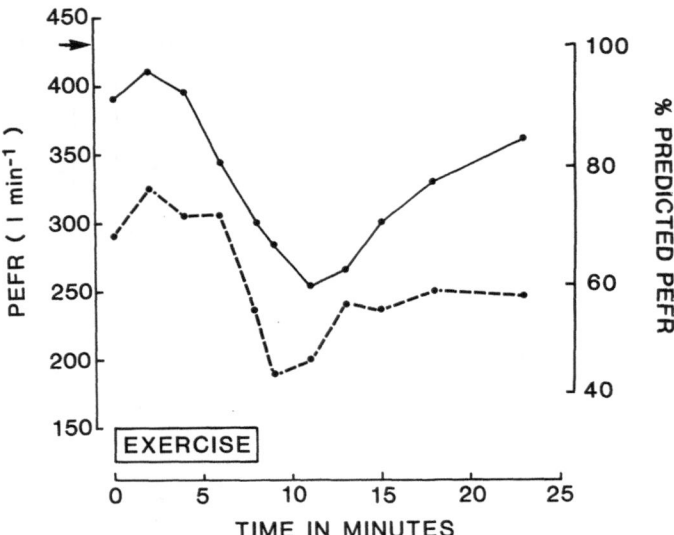

Fig. 3. Peak expiratory flow rate (*PEFR*) before, during and after running exercise in a 19 year old girl with a predicted PEFR of 430 liters/min. Exercise was performed 90 min after an oral placebo had been given (*broken line*) and again 2 h later 90 min after the administration of 4 mg of salbutamol. The % fall in PEFR was 34.5% after placebo and 34.6% after salbutamol. Before exercise after placebo, the PEFR was 67% of predicted normal, before exercise after the active drug it was 91% of predicted normal. (From [11])

The % fall in FEV_1, when exercise is performed repeatedly under the same conditions, has a coefficient of variation of 21% [14]. Thus for a drug to be considered efficacious against EIA, there should be an inhibition of 50% or more in the % fall in FEV_1 compared with the response after placebo. A similar degree of inhibition should be exhibited when a refractory period is being identified. It is also recommended that subjects used in clinical trials of medication should have at least a fall in FEV_1 of 20% or more. If exercise is to be repeated on the same day, a minimum of 2 h should elapse between tests.

To evaluate EIA in a patient, the time of last medication must be taken into account and a suitable period should elapse. The time may vary depending on whether a short or long acting bronchodilator is being used. At present we recommend 4–6 h after a short acting bronchodilator or sodium cromoglycate as the protective effect of these drugs against challenge by hyperpnea is remarkable short and nearly always less than 4 h [95, 11]. The duration of action for the newer bronchodilators, salmeterol and formoterol, is not presently known. We recommend 12 h after oral medication and 24 h after drugs given in sustained release preparations. We make every attempt to encourage a subject to keep a regular interval between medication and testing if they are requested to exercise on more than one occasion. When a refractory period is being identified it is important that nonsteroidal anti-in-flammatories are not taken for at least 3–4 days [71, 80].

The major disadvantage of challenge by exercise is that only one response is elicited; thus a dose-response curve cannot be obtained. This is one of the reasons that challenge by hyperventilation was developed.

Summary

To assess the presence and severity of EIA and to obtain a reproducible response it is recommended that:

1. The FEV_1 or PEFR before exercise is greater than 75% of predicted or similar before each challenge.

2. No aerosol medications have been taken for 6 h or oral medications for 12 h and the interval since the last medication should be constant.

3. The duration of exercise is 6–8 min;

4. The intensity of exercise is sufficient to raise the ventilation to 40%–60% of predicted maximum voluntary ventilation, based on FEV_1, and maintain this for a minimum of 4 min.

5. The water content of the inspired air is less than 10 mg/liter and preferably less than 4 mg/liter;

6. A nose-clip is used to ensure that ventilation during exercise is by mouth.

7. A period of at least 2 h has passed since last exercise challenge.

8. The results are expressed in terms of the % fall index; the values for lung function before and the lowest value after are expressed as a percentage of the predicted normal value and a time course of response curve is constructed.

9. Patients chosen for drug trials should have at least a 20% fall in FEV_1.

Methodology for Hyperventilation Tests

There are, in the literature, almost as many descriptions of techniques to perform hyperventilation challenges as centers with interest in the tests. This has come about because of the different aims investigators had for using the tests. For example, a rapid test is needed for use in a routine pulmonary function laboratory to identify a responder. By contrast a dose-response technique, which is much slower, may be used to evaluate the protection afforded by pharmacological agents. The precise details of all these techniques are available in previous publications cited in this text and only some will be described in detail here, together with some of the technical aspects of these challenges which we think are the most important.

Hyperventilation tests can be administered in different ways. First, a single dose can be used and this is usually hyperventilation at a set percentage of the predicted or MVV [95]. This has been used in epidemiological surveys for ease of administering the test and studying large numbers of subjects [102]. Using this technique only one value for airway response is obtained in response to the test. Second, hyperventilation using progressively higher ventilation rates can be used (Fig. 1). Third, the rate of ventilation can be kept constant but performed for intervals of 1 min with a measurement of response being made between each exposure [93, 115]. These last two techniques allow a dose-response curve to be examined. Due to the potential to administer higher doses or a longer duration of challenge using these last two techniques, the sensitivity of the test for detecting an abnormal response is likely to be improved using dose-response challenges. Furthermore, as the response develops slowly, it is possible to terminate the test as required, which makes it safer than the single exposure technique. By obtaining a dose-response curve it is also possible to characterize the response in terms of different indices, i.e. threshold of the response, slope of the dose-response curve, dose inducing a predetermined fall in FEV_1 or sG_{aw}, or increase in sR_{aw} (Fig. 1).

Control of Ventilation

In order to achieve fixed levels of ventilation which can allow the tracing of dose-response curves and the comparison of subjects, different methods can be used. Deal and coworkers [35] have described a system which can act as a target for the subjects to breathe at a preset level of ventilation. The expired air accumulates in a reservoir which is a balloon of known volume. This reservoir is emptied with a vacuum at a speed corresponding to the level of ventilation which is expected. The subject attempts to keep the reservoir filled, which stimulates him or her to breath at the same speed as the calibrated vacuum, i.e. at the desired level of ventilation. A modification of this system has been developed by Phillips and coworkers [84], who put a balloon reservoir between the subject and the source of compressed air (Fig. 4). The flow is determined and the subject has to prevent the filling of the balloon [92, 95]. Other laboratories [77, 110] use instead a mechanism which allows the subject to visualize his or her minute-ventilation on an apparatus. Some centers prefer to simulate frequency of breathing with a metronome [44] or with respiratory noises recorded on a tape [68]. Tidal volume is then adjusted by direct reading for the technician to get the desired minute ventilation.

Control of End-Tidal Carbon Dioxide

Hyperventilation or air can lead to hypocapnia. This hypocapnia has two deleterious effects on hyperventilation tests. Firstly, it may cause symptoms of dizziness which can lead to syncope. Secondly, hypocapnia has bronchoconstrictor effects [97] which can affect the results of the test on its own. Thus CO_2 has to be added to the inspired air to keep isocapnia or eucapnic. Iso-

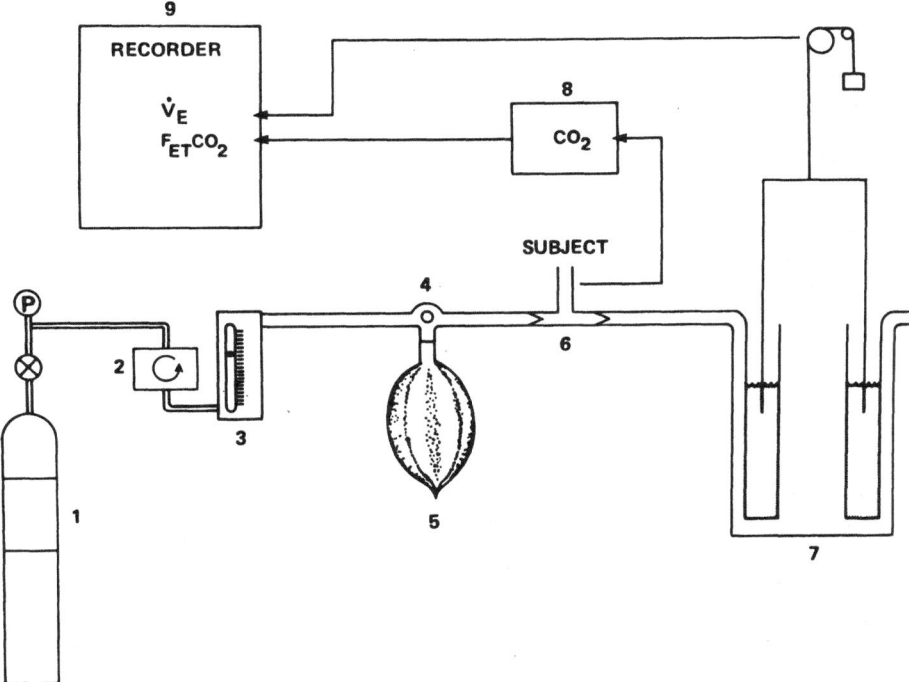

Fig. 4. The circuit used for isocapnic hyperventilation challenge with dry air as described by Smith and Anderson [92]. The technique was modified from that described by Phillips et al. [84]. *1*, compressed gas tanks (compressed air at rest and a mixture of 5% CO_2, 21% O_2 and 74% N_2 for $\dot{V}_E > 30$ liters/min); *2*, demand valve; *3*, rotameter; *4*, 3-way tap; *5*, target balloon; *6*, low resistance 2-way valve; *7*, 350 liter Tissot gasometer; *8*, CO_2 meter measuring end-tidal CO_2; *9*, chart recorder

capnia refers to the CO_2 level remaining constant throughout the challenge. Eucapnia refers to a normal state of CO_2 being maintained. The value for eucapnic end-tidal CO_2 could be argued. If it is to remain eucapnic for rest, values of 38–42 mm Hg would be acceptable. If, however, the values are eucapnic for exercise, values may be as low as 35 mm Hg and be eucapnic. The quantity of CO_2 can be adjusted by assessing end-tidal CO_2 of the expired air. Phillips and coworkers [84] have shown that a fixed amount of CO_2 (4.9%) added to the inspired air maintains isocapnia just as well on the whole scale of minute ventilation ordinarily necessary for the hyperventilation test. However, it is not known for each subject if this end-tidal CO_2 is eucapnic for the subject exercising 30–105 liters/min. The Phillips method substantially reduces the cost of the tests as no CO_2 assessment is required and simplifies the tests. It is now routinely used in the Royal Prince Alfred Hospital laboratory and recommended for use in adults. Its use is limited in children because a minimum ventilation rate of 35 liters/min is required to maintain isocapnia. Its use in children, however, has been reported [86].

Hyperventilation with Air at Room Temperature

A technique which has been used to obtain a dose-response curve, and one we recommend, is as follows. Initially the subject has a 3 min exposure to dry compressed air at resting ventilation. This serves as a baseline measurement [92]. The subsequent hyperventilation challenge is carried out breathing compressed air containing 4.9% CO_2 according to the method described by Philips et al. [84]. The expired ventilation is measured in a gasometer, gasmeter, or by a pneumotachograph, and expired and inspired air temperature can be recorded if necessary using a divided valve. The subjects are asked to breath between 30 and 40 liters/min (or 30% of MVV) for 3 min and the 60–80 liters/min (or 60% of MVV) for 3 min and finally at MVV for 3, or even 6 min. After each exposure FEV_1 is measured at 0.5, 1.5 and 3 min and then at 2 min intervals until it reaches a plateau. This technique is slow and it may take 20–30 min to complete the test [92].

We have found several modifications of this technique useful for reducing the time of the test. We have used 2–4 min isocapnic hyperventilation at 60% of MVV, based on FEV_1 measured before challenge ($FEV_1 \times 37.5$). Measurements of FEV_1 are made in triplicate before, and in duplicate 1, 3, 5, 7, 10, and 15 min after challenge. This relatively short test has allowed us to challenge people repeatedly throughout a day to evaluate the duration of protection of pharmacological agents. Since the test is only 4 min maximum duration, the subjects do not become easily fatigued with repeated challenge. Thus the level of ventilation attained and sustained during challenge on the first test of the day is the same as the last test [95]. This single level of ventilation test should only be used in subjects whose sensitivity to the test has been assessed using a dose-response technique.

Another technique we have used [93] is adopted from the work of Zach and Polgar [115]. For this challenge repeated 1 min hyperventilation at 60% of MVV is used and immediately on cessation a measurement of FEV_1 is made. The hyperventilation for 1 min is repeated until a 'plateau' is observed for FEV_1. This 'plateau' during challenge represents approximately 56% of the maximal response which is obtained within 3–5 min after the final minute of hyperventilation. This test usually takes less than 12 min. This technique is slower than the single challenge of 2–4 min but has an advantage in that multiple points are obtained on a dose-response curve. The 'plateau' obtained during challenge serves as a useful endpoint. However, it is not the same as the 'plateau' described by Woolcock et al. [112] for those pharmacological agents in which multiple exposure to high doses induces no more response. It is usually obtained after six to eight 1 min bouts of hyperventilation but may take up to 15 min and therefore may be more of interest for use in the research laboratory.

Hyperventilation with Air at Subfreezing Temperatures

For challenge with cold air the duration of inhalation is also relevant. Bronchoconstriction seems to be maximal and to reach a plateau after 3 min of inhalation, being less after 2 min and only marginally superior after inhaling for 4 min [19, 31]. Assessment of airway caliber is performed 30 s, 1 min and at 1 min intervals until the lowest value is obtained. Analysis of the time-course of recovery of bronchoconstriction caused by cold air using lung resistance has shown that the maximum bronchoconstriction is usually seen between 1 and 3 min but always before 5 min after ending the inhalation [69].

With the method we have proposed elsewhere [105] (Fig. 5) and which has been modified from works by O'Byrne and coworkers [81], cold air is produced with a freon heat exchanger (Air Jet Breathing Device, FTS Systems, Stoneridge, New York). We use a mixture of compressed air and CO_2 to preserve isocapnia. This system allows a fixed volume of cold air to be delivered. Two thermocouples are located on either side of the valve (in-

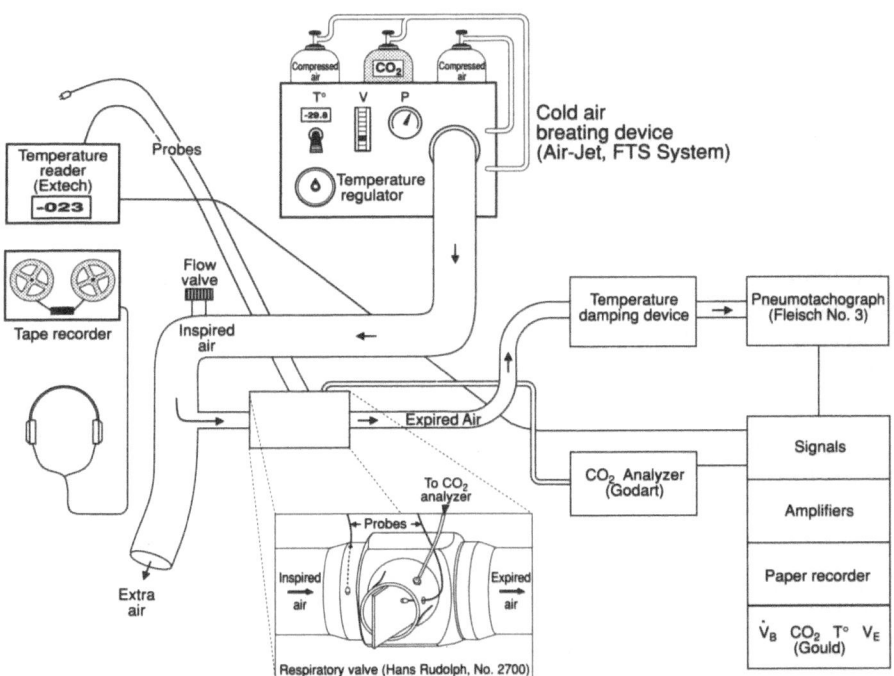

Fig. 5. The cold air breathing device is shown. Compressed air or compressed air mixed with CO_2 is used. The conditioned air is directed to the respiratory valve shown in close-up. This valve is separated by a plexiglass wall to prevent contamination of inspired and expired air. The expired air is directed to a damping device and then to a pneumotachograph to derive minute ventilation. Buccal flow, end tidal CO_2, inspired and expired temperatures, and minute ventilation are continuously recorded during the test

spiratory and expiratory sides) to assess temperatures of the inspired and expired air. A small sample of air is also taken on the expiratory side to assess end-tidal CO_2. After leaving the valve, the expired air is directed through a pneumotachograph. Electrical transformation of flow is carried out to derive volume. Tidal volume is thus continuously recorded. Minute ventilation is obtained by multiplying tidal volume by frequency. All the data (volume of expired air, content in CO_2 of expired air, inspiratory and expiratory temperatures) are recorded on paper during the tests. In order to obtain a dose–response curve by increasing the volume of air at each step, the subject is asked to breath less, or more deeply, by observing tidal volume on the paper recording. Breathing frequency is obtained by asking the subject to hear a tape recording of breathing noises and following the rhythm of these noises.

Although it would be more precise to draw the dose–response curve by increasing the levels of minute ventilation from 5 liters/min by steps of 5 liters/min (for example), this method is time consuming. Therefore the steps which are commonly used are 7.5 liters/min, 15 liters/min, 30 liters/min, 60 liters/min and MVV [81]. Whereas it is relatively easy to get the desired level for lower levels of ventilation (7.5 and 15 liters/min), differences between the obtained and the expected levels of ventilation are wider at 30 and 60 liters/min [41, 106].

Drawing the Dose–Response Curve

Several points can be interpolated from the dose–response curves. Setting a point at a 10% change in FEV_1 (PD_{10}) has been shown to be less reproducible than for 15% (PD_{15}) and 20% (PD_{20}) changes in FEV_1 (Table 1). This also corresponds to what has been found for pharmacological agents [78]. Moreover, the dose–response curve to hyperventilation has a linear portion beyond a fall in FEV_1 close to 15% in every instance for which it was asses-

Table 1. Reproducibility of hyperventilation tests as expressed by the 95% confidence intervals of the mean for subjects based on a single determination (from [105])

	Within-day	Between-day
Log_e RHE		
$\quad PD_{10}$	±0.59	±0.38
$\quad PD_{15}$	±0.40	±0.34
$\quad PD_{20}$	±0.39	±0.32
Log_e VE		
$\quad PD_{10}$	±0.64	±0.41
$\quad PD_{15}$	±0.43	±0.35
$\quad PD_{20}$	±0.43	±0.28

Data expressed on a log_e scale represent the 95% confidence interval for which a single value sampled at random would belong to the population. RHE, respiratory heat exchange; VE, minute ventilation.

sed [105]. The threshold of the response, i.e. the point at which the curve steadily departs from baseline, was greater than 10% in some instances. For these reasons it seems preferable to select PD_{15} or PD_{20} and not PD_{10} in assessing the response to hyperventilation with cold air.

A small cumulative bronchospastic reaction has been documented when the test is performed with progressively increasing levels of ventilation [68]. However, this effect is of small magnitude.

Either a logarithmic or a nonlogarithmic scale can be used. Indeed, the complete scale of levels of ventilation lie from approximately 5 liters/min to a value close to 100 liters/min. Expressing the results on a linear or a logarithmic scale for such a rather narrow range of values does not make much difference. This is different from pharmacological agents for which the length of the scale is much broader (from 0.03 to 16, or even 128 mg/ml).

Other Techniques

Other aspects of the hyperventilation test have been examined by Assoufi and coworkers [19]; varying the time intervals between each inhalation and the pattern of ventilation (different rates but similar levels of ventilation) do not affect the result of the test; subfreezing air ($-15\,^{\circ}C$) yielded more pronounced bronchoconstriction than dry room air ($21\,^{\circ}C$).

A technique for cold dry air in infants has also been developed [49]. Forced expiratory flow measurements were obtained by the modified thoracic compression technique [103].

Recently there has been an investigation to compare the effects of hypocapnic hyperventilation with isocapnic hyperventilation [39]. These workers concluded that free hypocapnic hyperventilation with ambient air is as reliable as the more sophisticated controlled isocapnic tests. This finding is important as it would allow a more wide spread application of these challenges.

Standardising the Test

Every diagnostic test in medicine should go though a process of rigorous standardisation before being used for clinical purposes. Reproducibility of the test should first be assessed in individual laboratories. The within-subject between-day reproducibility of the cold air inhalation test among subjects with similar initial airway caliber is comparable to what has been found for pharmacological agents. The 95% confidence intervals for the reproducibility of the test corresponds to approximately one third to the entire dose range [105] (Table 1).

The question of sensitivity and specificity of the test has also to be addressed as these allow comparisons of normal and abnormal subjects. Selecting PD_{10} may show that the test is as sensitive as PC_{20} histamine or methacholine in identifying subjects with symptoms compatible with asthma, al-

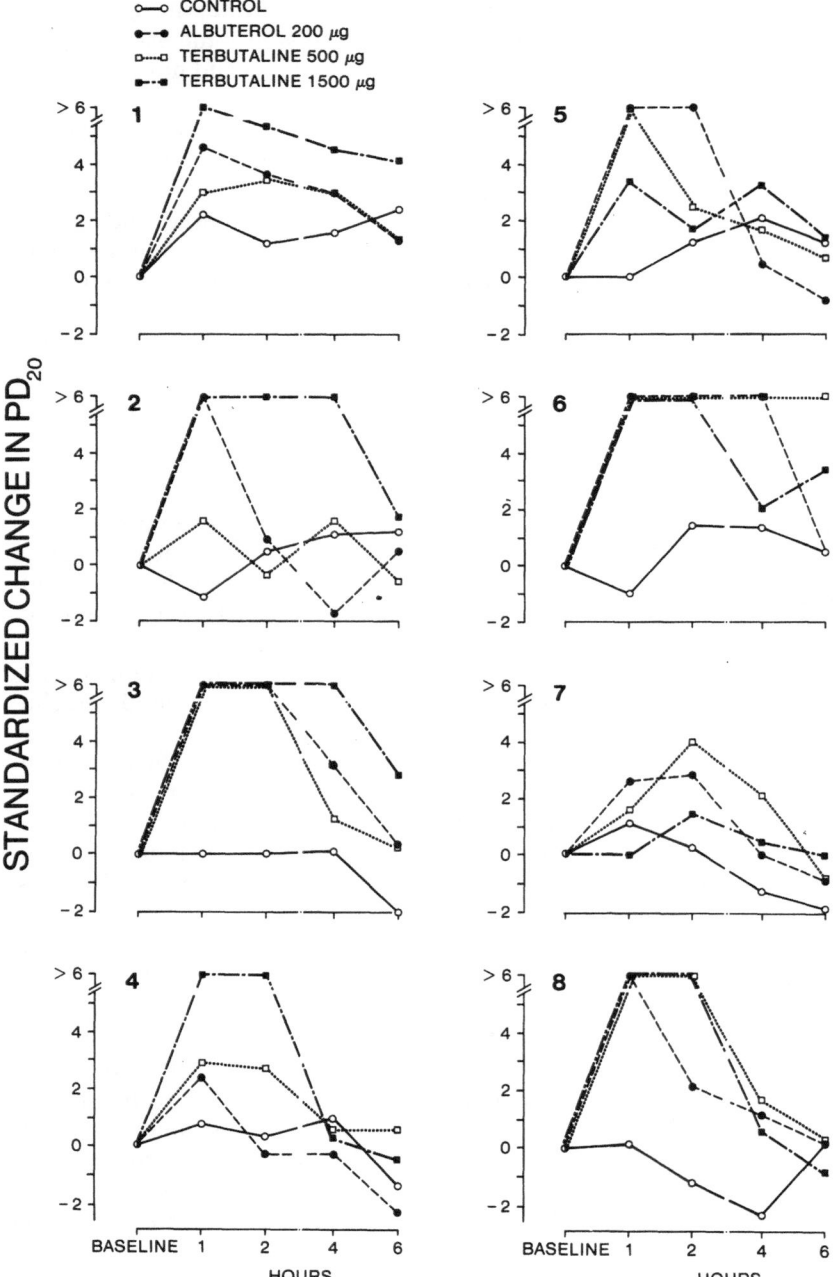

Fig. 6. Example of the usefulness of hyperventilation tests in assessing the time-course of the blocking effect of inhaled β-2 adrenergic agents on the response. Individual results for changes in standardized PD_{20} values on the baseline day and the three treatment days are shown. Complete and partial blockades are respectively defines as changes $\geq$ and from 2 to 6. (From [70])

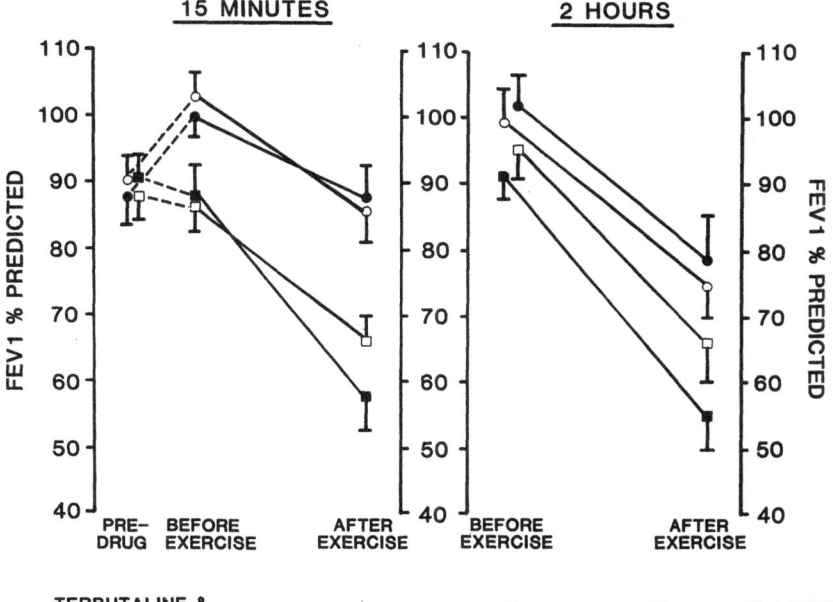

Fig. 7. Mean ± 1 SEM for forced expiratory volume (FEV_1) expressed as a percentage of predicted value immediately before and 15 min after the administration of 2 mg of sodium cromoglycate and 0.5 mg of terbutaline sulphate alone or in combination. Values given are those measured immediately before administration of the drug, immediately before exercise and the lowest values measured after exercise. The exercise took place 15 min and 2 h after administration of the drug. (From [113])

though subjects who react to one stimulus do not necessarily react to the other [41, 46, 89]. While a 10% fall in response to exercise may be considered abnormal, as pointed out earlier, a 10% change in FEV_1 may well be spurious [106] for hyperventilation.

Clinical Usefulness

Hyperventilation and exercise are natural stimuli, which makes them useful in assessment of the efficacy of a drug on NABHR. This point is interesting as anti-asthmatic medication needs assessment not only of its effect on baseline lung function but also of its effect on NABHR [2, 40, 70, 76, 82, 83]. The efficacy and duration of action of bronchodilators have been examined by assessing their effect on NABHR to inhalation of unconditioned air during hyperventilation (Fig. 6) and exercise (Fig. 7). From a technical point of view, the factors that limit the effect of inhaled particles, for example, the output of the nebulizer and the deposition of inhaled particles, do not play a role when using hyperventilation or exercise. However, the apparatus needed for exercise and hyperventilation tests is more complex than for pharmacological agents. A PD_{10} obtained with exercise and hyperventilation can be as sensitive as a PC_{20} using pharmacological agents to identify NABHR. However albeit more specific than a PD_{10}, a PD_{20} is less sensitive than a PC_{20}. These factors limit the clinical use of exercise and hyperventilation tests [41]. Finally these tests require the cooperation from the subject who is asked to breathe at progressively increasing levels of ventilation or to work at 70%–80% of predicted maximum work load for 6–8 min. The level of ventilation and work which is reached is most often inferior to the theoretical obtainable value [41, 105] particularly in untrained subjects.

Correlations Between the Response to Different Stimuli

There are many investigators who have compared the sensitivity to exercise and hyperventilation with other nonspecific challenges. The techniques used to analyse the data have not been uniform so that correlations have been made using actual data (Pierson) and ranking data (Spearmans). It is perhaps for this reason that there has been so much variation in the reported findings. The correlation between responses to exercise and histamine is satisfactory for some [17] but not for others Belcher et al. [24]. The response to hyperventilation as compared to the response to a pharmacological agent has been found to be variable, from excellent [81, 94] to moderate [106, 108] to poor [51]. There is a satisfactory correlation between the response to ultrasonically nebulized distilled water and hyperosmolar solutions and hyperventilation or exercise in asthmatic subjects [45, 47, 92, 94]. No significant correlation between the response to hyperosmolar saline and methacholine in asthmatic subjects [27] is found when the osmotic stimulus is progressively increased but there is a correlation when a constant stimulus is used [94]. It might well be that the NABHR of asthma can find its expression through different mechanisms which are not equivalent in any given subject.

Table 2. Tests for the assessment of bronchial hyperresponsiveness: advantages and disadvantages (modified from [55])

	Histamine/ methacholine	Exercise	Hyperventilation of unconditioned air
Stimulus	Artificial	Natural	Natural
Dose-response curve	Yes	No	Yes
Sensitivity	High	Moderate	Moderate
Reproducibility	High	Moderate	High
Clinical usefulness	High*	Moderate	Moderate
Cooperation of patient	Little	Moderate	Much
Technical aspects	Simple	Variable	Variable
Equiment cost	Low	Variable	Variable
Research tool	Variable	Moderate	High

* High negative predictive value, low positive predictive value

If one has to assess NABHR, several points should be considered. Table 2, modified from Hargreave and coworkers [55], lists the advantages and disadvantages of pharmacological agents, exercise and hyperventilation of unconditioned air. While pharmacological agents may be the preferred means for assessing NABHR for clinical purposes, exercise and hyperventilation of unconditioned air represent natural stimuli to which asthmatic subjects are often exposed in their daily life. Thus challenge by hyperpnea might be preferable in certain circumstances, particularly for testing the efficacy of a bronchodilator in an acute situation for a subject who presents without significant alteration in airway caliber.

Recommendations for Choice of Challenge

An exercise challenge should be used to:

1. Make a diagnosis of EIA in asthmatic patients who give a history of breathlessness during or after exertion
2. Confirm that the drug prescribed prevents EIA and permits normal exercise performance
3. Select the appropriate combination of drugs for patients whose EIA is not controlled by a single drug
4. Assess duration of action of drugs used to control EIA
5. Evaluate long-term therapy and whether it affects the severity or the amount of drugs needed to control EIA

Isocapnic hyperventilation should be used to:

1. Make a diagnosis of EIA in a superfit patient and in patients for whom exercise is contraindicated
2. Obtain a dose-response curve for comparing change in sensitivity with time or in response to treatment
3. Document cough and assess the effect of treatment
4. Compare sensitivity to water loss with sensitivity to inhaled agents

References

1. Ahmed T, Danta I (1988) Effect of cold air exposure and exercise on nonspecific bronchial reactivity. Chest 93:1132–1136
2. Ahrens RC, Bonham AC, Maxwell GA, Weinberger MM (1984) A method for comparing the peak intensity and duration of action of aerosolized bronchodilators using bronchoprovocation with methacholine. Am Rev Respir Dis 129:903–906
3. Anderson SD (1972) Physiological aspects of bronchoconstriction. Ph D Thesis, University of London
4. Anderson SD (1984) Is there a unifying hypothesis for exercise-induced asthma. J Allergy Clin Immunol 73:660–665

5. Anderson SD (1985) Issues in exercise-induced asthma. J Allergy Clin Immuol 76:763–772
6. Anderson SD (1988) Exercise-induced asthma. In: Middleton E, Reed C, Ellis E, Adkinson NF, Yunginger JW (eds) Allergy: Principles and Practice, vol 2, 3rd edn. Mosby, St Louis, pp 1156–1175
7. Anderson SD, Daviskas E, Schoeffel RE, Unger SF (1979) Prevention of severe exercise-induced asthma with hot humid air. Lancet 2:629
8. Anderson SD, Daviskas E, Smith CM (1989) Exercise-induced asthma: a difference in opinion regarding the stimulus. Allergy Proc 10:215–226.
9. Anderson SD, McEvoy JDS, Bianco S (1972) Changes in lung volumes and airway resistance after exercise in asthmatic subjects. Am Rev Respir Dis 106: 30–37
10. Anderson SD, Schoeffel RE (1983) The importance of standardizing exercise tests in the evaluation of asthmatic children. In: Oseid S, Edwards A (eds) The asthmatic child in play and sport. Pitman Medical London, pp 145–158
11. Anderson SD, Schoeffel RE (1985) Standardization of exercise testing in the asthmatic patient: a challenge in itself. In: Hargreave FE, Woolcock AJ (eds) Airway responsiveness: measurement and interpretation. Proceedings of a workshop, edited by Astra Pharmaceuticals Canada, Ontario, pp 51–59
12. Anderson SD, Schoeffel RE, Black JL, Daviskas E (1985) Airway cooling as the stimulus to exercise-induced asthma. A re-evaluation. Eur J Respir Dis 67: 20–30
13. Anderson SD, Schoeffel RE, Follet R, Perry CP, Daviskas E, Kendall M (1982) Sensitivity to heat and water loss at rest and during exercise in asthmatic patients. Eur J Respir Dis 63:459–471
14. Anderson SD, Seale JP, Ferris L, Schoeffel RE, Lindsay DA (1979) An evaluation of pharmacotherapy for exercise-induced asthma. J Allergy Clin Immunol 64:612–624
15. Anderson SD, Silverman M, Konig P, Godfrey S (1975) Exercise-induced asthma. A Review. Br J Dis Chest 69:1–39
16. Anderson SD, Smith CM (1989) The use of nonisotonic aerosols for evaluating bronchial hyperresponsiveness. In: Spector SL (ed) Provocating challenge procedures: background and methodolgy. Futura, Mt Kisco, pp 227–252
17. Anderton RC, Cuff MT, Frith PA, Cockcroft DW, Morse JLC, Jones NL, Hargreave FE (1979) Bronchial responsiveness to inhaled histamine and exercise. J Allergy Clin Immunol 63:315–320
18. Aquilina AT (1983) Comparison of airway reactivity induced by histamine, methacholine, and isocapnic hyperventilation in normal and asthmatic subjects. Thorax 38:766–770
19. Assoufi BK, Dally AJ, Newman-Taylor A, Denison DM (1986) Cold air test: a simplified standard method for airway reactivity. Bull Eur Physiopathol Respir 22:349–357
20. Banner AS, Green J, O'Connor M (1984) Relation of respiratory water loss to coughing after exercise. N Engl J Med 311:883–886
21. Bar-Yishay E, Ben-Dov I, Godfrey S (1983) Refractory period after hyperventilation-induced asthma. Am Rev Respir Dis 127:572–574
22. Bar-Yishay E, Godfrey S (1984) Mechanisms of exercise-induced asthma. Lung 162:195–204
23. Bar-Yishay E, Gur I, Inbar O (1982) Differences between running and swimming as stimuli for exercise-induced asthma. Eur J Appl Physiol 48:387–397
24. Belcher NG, Lee TH, Rees PJ (1979) Airway responses to hypertonic saline, exercise and histamine challenges in bronchial asthma. J Allergy Clin Immunol 63:315–320
25. Ben-Dov I, Bar-Yishay E, Godfrey S (1982) Exercise-induced asthma without respiratory heat loss. Thorax 37:630–631
26. Bon-Dov I, Gur I, Bar-Yishay E, Godfrey S (1983) Refractory period following

induced asthma: contributions of exercise and isocapnic hyperventilation. Thorax 38:849–853

27. Boulet LP, Legris C, Thibault L, Turcotte H (1987) Comparative bronchial responses to hyperosmolar saline and methacholine in asthma. Thorax 42: 953–958

28. Breslin FJ, McFadden ER, Ingram RH (1980) The effects of cromolyn sodium on the airway response to hyperpnea and cold air in asthma. Am Rev Respir Dis 122:11–16

29. Buckley JM, Souhrada JF (1975) A comparison of pulmonary function tests in detecting exercise-induced bronchoconstriction. Pediatrics 56:883–889

30. Burr NL, Eldridge BA, Borysiewicz LK (1974) Peak expiratory flow rates before and after exercise in schoolchildren. Arch Dis Child 49:923–926

31. Caire N, Cartier A, Ghezzo H, Malo JL (1989) Influence of the duration of inhalation of cold dry air on the resulting bronchoconstriction in asthmatic subjects. Eur Respir J 2:741–745

32. Chan-Yeung MM, Vyas MN, Grzybowski S (1971) Exercise-induced asthma. Am Rev Respir Dis 104:915–923

33. Chen WY, Horton DJ (1977) Heat and water loss from the airways and exercise-induced asthma. Respiration 34:305–313

34. Cropp GJ (1975) Grading, time course, and incidence of exercise-induced airway obstruction and hyperinflation in asthmatic children. Paediatrics 56: 868–879

35. Deal EC, McFadden ER, Ingram RH, Breslin F, Jaeger JJ (1980) Airway responsiveness to cold air and hyperpnea in normal subjects and in those with hay fever and asthma. Am Rev Respir Dis 121:621–628

36. Deal EC, McFadden ER, Ingram RH, Jaeger JJ (1979) Hyperpnea and heat flux: initial reaction sequence in exercise-induced asthma. J Appl Physiol Respir Environ Exercise Physiol 46:476–483

37. Deal EC, McFadden ER, Ingram RH, Strauss RH, Jaeger JJ (1979) Role of respiratory heat exchange in production of exercise-induced asthma. J Appl Physiol Respir Environ Exercise Physiol 46:467–475

38. Decramer M, Demedts M, van de Woestijne KP (1984) Isocapnic hyperventilation with cold air in healthy non-smokers, smokers and asthmatic subjects. Bull Eur Physiopathol Respir 20:237–243

39. Dejaegher P, Rochette F, Clarysse I, Demedis M (1987) Hypocapnic hyperventilation versus isocapnic hyperventilation with ambient air or with dry air in asthmatics. Eur J Respir Dis 70:102–109

40. Dente FL, Del Bono L, Del Bono W (1986) Cold-air isocapnic hyperventilation test in the study of the effects and duration of action of duovent. Comparison with fenoterol, salbutamol, disodium cromoglycate and placebo. Respiration 50 [Suppl 2]:196S–200S

41. Desjardins A, De Luca S, Cartier A, L'Archeveque J, Ghezzo H, Malo JL (1988) Nonspecific bronchial hyperresponsiveness to inhaled histamine and hyperventilation of cold dry air in subjects with respiratory symptoms of uncertain etiology. Am Rev Respir Dis 137:1020–1025

42. Eggleston PA (1975) Exercise-induced asthma in children with intrinsic and extrinsic asthma. Pediatrics 56:856–859

43. Eggleston PA, Kagey-Sobotka A, Lichtenstein LM (1987) A comparison of the osmotic activation of basophils and human lung mast cells. Am Rev Respir Dis 135:1043–1048

44. Eschenbacher WL, Sheppard D (1985) Respiratory heat loss is not the sole stimulus for bronchoconstriction induced by isocapnic hyperpnea with dry air. Am Rev Respir Dis 131:894–901

45. Fabbri LM, Mapp CE, Hendrick DJ (1984) Comparison of ultrasonically nebulized distilled water and hyperventilation with cold air in asthma. Ann Allergy 53:172–177

46. Filuk RB, Serrette C, Anthonisen NR (1989) Comparison of responses to methacholine and cold air in patients suspected of having asthma. Chest 95: 948–952
47. Foresi A, Mattoli S, Corbo GM, Polidori G, Ciappi G (1986) Comparison of bronchial responses to ultrasonically nebulized distilled water, exercise, and methacholine in asthma. Chest 90:822–826
48. Freed AN, Kelly LJ, Menkes HA (1987) Airflow-induced bronchospasm. Imbalance between airway cooling and airway drying. Am Rev Respir Dis 136: 595–599
49. Geller DE, Morgan WJ, Cota KA, Wright AL, Taussig LM (1988) Airway responsiveness to cold, dry air in normal infants. Pediatr Pulmonol 4:90–97
50. Gilbert IA, Fouke JM, McFadden ER (1987) Heat and waterflux in the intrathoracic airways and exercise-induced asthma. J Appl Physiol 63:1681–1691
51. Gillioz F, Orehek J (1983) Reponse bronchique au carbachol et a l'hyperventilation isocapnique dans l'asthme. Bull Eur Physiophathol Respir 19:563–566
52. Godfrey S (1989) Bronchial challenge by exercise or hyperventilation. In: Spector SL (eds) Provocative challenge procedures: background and methodology. Futura, Mt Kisco, pp 365–394
53. Hahn A, Anderson SD, Morton AR, Black JL, Fitch KD (1984) A re-interpretation of the effect of temperature and water content of the inspired air in exercise-induced asthma. Am Rev Respir Dis 130:575–579
54. Hahn AG, Nogrady SG, Tumulty DMcA, Lawrence SR, Morton AR (1984) Histamine reactivity during the refractory period after exercise induced asthma. Thorax 39:919–923
55. Hargreave FE, Dolovich J, Boulet LP (1983) Inhalation provocation tests. Semin Respir Med 4:224–236
56. Herxheimer H (1946) Hyperventilation asthma. Lancet 1:83–87
57. Hodgson WC, Cotton DJ, Werner GD, Cockcroft DW, Dosman JA (1984) Relationship between bronchial response to respiratory heat exchange and nonspecific airways reactivity in asthmatic patients. Chest 85:465–470
58. Houdas Y, Colin J (1966) Echanges thermiques et hydriques par les voies respiratoires de l'homme. Pathol Biol 14:229–238
59. Ingelstedt S (1956) Studies on conditioning of air in the respiratory tract. Acta Otolaryngol (Stockh) 131:1S–80S
60. Jones RS, Buston MH, Wharton MJ (1962) The effect of exercise on ventilatory function on the child with asthma. Br J Dis Chest 56:78–86
61. Juniper EF, Latimer KM, Morris MM, Roberts RS, Hargreave FE (1986) Airway responses to hyperventilation of cold dry air: duration of protection by cromolyn sodium. J Allergy Clin Immunol 78:387–391
62. Kilham H, Tooley M, Silverman M (1979) Running, walking, and hyperventilation causing asthma in children. Thorax 34:582–586
63. Kivity S, Souhrada JF (1980) Hyperpnea: the common stimulus for bronchospasm in asthma during exercise and voluntary isocapnic hyperpnea. Respiration 40:169–177
64. Lebecque OP, Spiers S, Lapierre JG, Lamarre A, Zinman R, Coates AL (1987) Histamine challenge test in children using forced oscillation to measure total respiratory resistance. Chest 92:313–318
65. Lee TH, Assoufi BK, Kay AB (1983) The link between exercise, respiratory heat exchange, and the mast cell in bronchial asthma. Lancet i:520–522
66. Lim TK, Pride NB, Ingram RH (1987) Effects of volume history during spontaneous and acutely induced air-flow obstruction in asthma. Am Rev Respir Dis 135:591–596
67. Malo JL, L'Archeveque J, Cartier A (1990) Comparative effects of volume history on bronchoconstriction induced by hyperventilation and methacholine in asthmatic subjects. Eur Respir J 3:639–643

68. Malo JL, Cartier A, L'Archeveque J, Ghezzo H, Martin RR (1986) Cold air inhalation has a cumulative bronchospastic effect when inhaled in consecutive doses for progressively increasing degrees of ventilation. Am Rev Respir Dis 134:990–993
69. Malo JL, Cartier A, L'Archeveque J, Ghezzo M, Martin RR (1988) Kinetics of the recovery from bronchial obstruction due to hyperventilation of cold air in asthmatic subjects. Eur Respir J 1:384–388
70. Malo JL, Ghezzo H, Trudeau C, Cartier A, Morris J (1989) Duration of action of inhaled terbutaline at two different doses and of albuterol in protecting against bronchoconstriction induced by hyperventilation of dry cold air in asthmatic subjects. Am Rev Respir Dis 140:817–821
71. Margolskee DJ, Bigby BG, Boushey HA (1988) Indomethacin blocks airway tolerance to repetitive exercise but not to eucapnic hyperpnea in asthmatic subjects. Am Rev Respir Dis 137:842–846
72. McFadden ER, Ingram RH (1979) Exercise-induced asthma. Observations on the initiating stimulus. N Engl J Med 301:763–769
73. McFadden ER, Lenner KAM, Strohl KP (1986) Postexertional airway rewarming and thermally induced asthma. New insights into pathophysiology and possible pathogenesis. J Clin Invest 78:18–25
74. McFadden ER, Pichurko BM (1985) Intraairway thermal profiles during exercise and hyperventilation in normal man. J Clin Invest 76:1007–1010
75. Mellis CM, Kattan M, Keens TG, Levison H (1978) Comparative study of histamine and exercise challenges in asthmatic children. Am Rev Respir Dis 117:911–915
76. Meriand N, Cartier A, L'Archeveque J, Ghezzo H, Malo JL (1988) Theophylline minimally inhibits bronchoconstriction induced by cold dry air inhalation in asthmatic subjects. Am Rev Respir Dis 137:1304–1308
77. Nagakura T, Lee TH, Assoufi BK, Newman-Taylor AJ, Denison DM, Kay AB (1983) Neutrophil chemotactic factor in exercise and hyperventilation-induced asthma. Am Rev Respir Dis 128:294–296
78. Neijens HJ, Hofkamp M, Degenhart HJ, Kerribijn KF (1982) Bronchial responsiveness as a function of inhaled histamine and the methods of measurement. Bull Eur Physiopathol Respir 18:427–438
79. Noviski N, Bar-Yishay E, Gur I, Godfrey S (1987) Exercise intensity determines and climatic conditions modify the severity of exercise-induced asthma. Am Rev Respir Dis 136:592–594
80. O'Byrne PM, Jones GL (1986) The effect of indomethacin on exercise-induced bronchoconstriction. Am Rev Respir Dis 134:69–72
81. O'Byrne PM, Ryan G, Morris M, McCormack D, Jones NL, Morse JLC, Hargreave FE (1982) Asthma induced by cold air and its relation to non specific bronchial responsiveness to methacholine. Am Rev Respir Dis 125:281–285
82. O'Byrne PM, Thomson NC, Morris M, Roberts RS, Daniel EE, Hargreave FE (1983) The protective effect of inhaled chlorpheniramine and atropine on bronchoconstriction stimulated by airway cooling. Am Rev Respir Dis 128:611–617
83. Patel KR, Berkin KE, Kerr JW (1982) Dose-response study of sodium cromoglycate in exercise-induced asthma. Thorax 37:663–666
84. Phillips YY, Jaeger JJ, Laube BL, Rosenthal RR (1985) Eucapnic voluntary hyperventilation of compressed gas mixture. A simple system for bronchial challenge by respiratory heat loss. Am Rev Respir Dis 131:31–35
85. Rakotosihanaka F, Melaman F, d'Athis P, Florentin D, Dessanges JF, Lockhart A (1986) Refractoriness after hyperventilation-induced asthma. Bull Eur Physiopathol Respir 22:581–587
86. Reisman J, Mappa L, De Benedictis F, McLaughlin J, Levison H (1987) Cold air challenge in children with asthma. Pediatr. Pulmonol 3:251–254
87. Rosenthal RR, Laube B, Jaeger JJ, Phillips YY, Norman PS (1984) Methacholine sensitivity is unchanged during the refractory period following an exercise or isocapnic challenge. J Allergy Clin Immunol 73 [Suppl]:281A

88. Sakula A (1984) Sir John Floyers's "A treatise of the asthma" (1698). Torax 39: 248–254
89. Scharf SM, Heimer D, Walters D (1985) Bronchial challenge with room temperature isocapnic hyperventilation. A comparison with histamine challenge. Chest 88:586–593
90. Schoeffel RE, Anderson SD, Gillam I, Lindsay DA (1980) Multiple exercise and histamine challenge in asthmatic patients. Thorax 35:164–170
91. Silverman M, Anderson SD (1972) Standardization of exercise tests in asthmatic children. Arch Dis Child 47:882–889
92. Smith CM, Anderson SD (1986) Hyperosmolarity as the stimulus to asthma induced by hyperventilation? J Allergy Clin Immunol 77:729–736
93. Smith CM, Anderson SD (1989) A comparison between the airway response to isocapnic hyperventilation and hypertonic saline in subjects with asthma. Eur Respir J 2:36–43
94. Smith CM, Anderson SD (1990) Inhalational challenge using hypertonic (4.5%) saline in asthmatic subjects: a comparison with responses to hyperpnea, methacholine, and water. Eur Respir J 3:144–151
95. Smith CM, Anderson SD, Seale JP (1988) The duration of action of the combination of fenoterol hydrobromide and ipratropium bromide in protecting against asthma provoked by hyperpnea. Chest 94:709–717
96. Smith CM, Anderson SD, Walsh S, McElrea M (1989) An investigation of the effects of heat and water exchange in the recovery period after exercise in children with asthma. Am Rev Respir Dis 140:598–605
97. Sterling GM (1968) The mechanism of bronchoconstriction due to hypocapnia in man. Clin Sci 34:277–285
98. Strauss RH, McFadden ER, Ingram RH, Deal EC, Jaeger JJ, Stearns D (1978) Influence of heat and humidity on the airway obstruction induced by exercise in asthma. J Clin Invest 61:433–440
99. Strauss RH, McFadden ER, Ingram RH, Jaeger JJ (1977) Enhancement of exercise-induced asthma by cold air. N Engl J Med 297:743–747
100. Suzuki S, Chonan T, Sasaki H, Takishima T (1985) Bronchial hyperresponsiveness to methacholine after exercise in asthmatics. Ann Allergy 54:136–141
101. Tabka Z, Ben Jebria A, Guenard H (1987) Effect of breathing dry warm air on respiratory water loss at rest and during exercise. Respir Physiol 67:115–125
102. Tager IB, Weiss ST, Munoz A, Welty C, Speizer FE (1986) Determinants of response to eucapnic hyperventilation with cold air in a population-based study. Am Rev Respir Dis 134:502–508
103. Tepper RS, Morgan WJ, Cota K, Taussig LM (1986) Physiologic growth and development of the lung during the first year of life. Am Rev Respir Dis 134: 513–519
104. Tessier P, Cartier A, Ghezzo H, Martin RR, Malo JL (1988) Bronchoconstriction due to exercise combined with cold air inhalation does not generally influence bronchial responsiveness to inhaled histamine in asthmatic subjects. Eur Respir J 1:133–138
105. Tessier P, Cartier A, L'Archeveque J, Ghezzo J, Martin RR, Malo J-L (1986) Within- and between-day reproducibility of isocapnic cold air challenges in subjects with asthma. J Allergy Clin Immunol 78:379–787
106. Tessier P, Ghezzo H, L'Archeveque J, Cartier A, Martin RR, Malo JL (1987) Shape of the dose-response curve to cold air inhalation in normal and asthmatic subjects. Am Rev Respir Dis 136:1418–1423
107. Walden SM, Britt EJ, Permutt S, Bleecker ER (1985) The effect of alpha-adrenergic and antihistaminic blockade on conditioned cold air and exercise-induced asthma. Chest 87:195S–197S
108. Weiss JW, Rossing TH, McFadden ER, Ingram RH (1983) Relationship between bronchial responsiveness to hyperventilation with cold and methacholine in asthma. J Allergy Clin Immunol 72:140–144

109. Wilson BA, Evans JN (1981) Standardization of work intensity for evaluation of exercise-induced bronchoconstriction. Eur J Appl Physiol 47:289–294
110. Wilson NM, Barnes PJ, Vickers H, Silverman M (1982) Hyperventilation-induced asthma: evidence for two mechanisms. Thorax 37:657–662
111. Woolcock AJ, Permutt S (1986) Bronchial hyperresponsiveness. In: Fishman AP, Macklem PT, Mead J, Geiger SR (eds) The respiratory system. Mechanics of breathing (Handbook of physiology, vol 3, section 3). Williams and Wilkins, Baltimore, pp 727–736
112. Woolcock AJ, Salome CM, Yan K (1984) The shape of the dose-response curve to histamine in asthmatic and normal subjects. Am Rev Respir Dis 130:71–75
113. Woolley M, Anderson SD, Quigley B (1990) The duration of the protective effect of terbutaline sulphate and sodium cromoglycate alone, and in combination on exercise-induced asthma. Chest 97:39–45
114. Zawadski DK, Lenner KA, McFadden ER (1988) Comparison of intraairway temperatures in normal and asthmatic subjects after hyperpnea with hot, cold, and ambient air. Am Rev Respir Dis 139:1553–1558
115. Zach MS, Polgar G (1987) Cold air challenge of airway hyperreactivity in children: dose-response interrelation with a reaction plateau. J Allergy Clin Immunol 80:9–17
116. Zeballos RJ, Shturman-Ellestein R, McNally JF, Hirsch JE, Souhrada JF (1978) The role of hyperventilation in exercise-induced bronchoconstriction. Am Rev Respir Dis 118:884–887

Mediators in Bronchial Provocation Tests

N. DEL BONO and L. DEL BONO

Centro per lo Studio dell' Asma e delle Allergopatie Respiratorie, Pisa, Italy

Introduction

Three major pathogenetic components characterize bronchial asthma: (1) atopy, i.e., increased levels of IgE and increased degranulation of mast cells and basophils triggered by IgE-mediated or non-IgE-mediated stimuli; (2) allergic inflammation, which damages to varying extents the bronchial wall components (epithelium, vessels, submucosal glands, respiratory nerve endings, and smooth muscle); (3) bronchial hyperreactivity (BH) to physical, chemical, and allergic stimuli, which trigger bronchial obstruction by bronchospasm, vasodilation, mucosal edema, and mucous hypersecretion.

The reaction of asthmatic subjects with bronchospasm or a true asthmatic crisis to allergic or nonallergic stimuli has been reported present in the anecdotical history of asthma [46], but a precise methodology and maximal accuracy in respiratory function studies were needed to discriminate between the different responses to stimuli, not only between patients or in the variable expressions of asthmatic syndrome, but also in the same subject during the course of his/her disease.

In the history of nonspecific bronchial provocation tests, "physiologic" mediators were used at first: acetylcholine [40, 143], as a direct contraction mediator on smooth muscle; and histamine, as the first known allergic mediator [37].

For a long period of time, these two mediators, histamine and acetylcholine (or the similar cholinergic substances carbachol and methacholine), were the only two triggers in bronchial provocation tests [77], and the preferences for the one or the other were principally determined by traditional use (histamine in America, methacholine in Europe).

As the know-how grew, many other mediators were shown to have important effects in the pathogenesis of asthma (phlogogenic effects on bronchial mucosa and constrictive action on smooth muscle): prostaglandins (PGs), Leukotrienes (LTs), platelet-activating factor (PAF), and bradykinin. Furthermore, every single one of these mediators has been proposed as a trigger stimulus in bronchial provocation tests, but the discrepancy between techniques employed makes the comparison between new tests and better standardized old tests very difficult. In addition, these mediators, which are not easily purified and are rapidly inactivated, are expensive; thus they cannot be proposed for routine bronchial provocation tests in clinics. They do play a role, however, in studying the pathogenesis of asthma and of BH or in evaluating efficacy and mode of action of new antiasthmatic drugs.

In this chapter we report in detail on the technical aspects of bronchial provocation tests with the following bronchoconstrictor mediators: histamine, $PGF_{2\alpha}$, LTC_4, LTD_4, LTE_4, PAF, bradykinin, and methacholine. The latter is not a physiologic mediator but is the most frequently used because it mimics the actions of acetylcholine on muscarinic receptors without collateral effects.

The only way to get mediators into the bronchi is by aerosol. Therefore the correct method to obtain good and reproducible results from bronchoprovocation tests with mediators, is to standardize preparation and administration of the aerosol, i.e., standardization of nebulizer delivery systems, inhalation techniques, and preparation and storage of all solutions. Moreover, the choice of the respiratory function parameters to be evaluated is of obvious importance to show the effect of the particular mediator. Finally the best method to process the data must be chosen in order to optimalize expression, analysis, and comparison of data.

We will summarize some aspects of these important considerations here; for additional information, complete descriptions are available elsewhere [109, 126, 133], and in this volume.

General Principles of Aerosols and Some Advice About Standardizing Methods

The two principal aerosol delivering techniques in bronchoprovocation tests are: (1) the continuously and (2) the intermittently generated aerosol. In the former the mediator-containing aerosol, in fixed or increasing concentrations, is generated continuously by a nebulizer and inhaled for a preset time by tidal volume [33] or for a preset number of breaths taken slowly from functional residual capacity (FRC) to near total lung capacity (TLC) [27].

The second technique uses dosimeters (Rosenthal-French, Mefar, Spira Elektro 2, etc.), which are breath- or manually actuated to push air into the nebulizer for a preset time (0.5–1 s) and for a preset number of breaths (generally five breaths) [24]. When the subject inhales from the mouthpiece, the change in mouth pressure opens the solenoid valve of the dosimeter, which allows air into the nebulizer (breath-actuation). Manual actuation can be performed by the operator with a starting pulse when the subject signals he is ready to inhale from FRC [95].

The dosimeter methods have the advantage that the doses of aerosol are delivered for a short and always equal time, independently of the minute volume of the subject, which interferes with tidal techniques; thus, the doses of inhaled aerosol can be accurately determined. A third type of nebulizer-delivery system (reservoir or storage method) has been proposed by Tiffeneau [143] and is still used in France [109]: the subject inhales a fixed volume from a container (generally the bell of the spirograph) which has been filled with aerosol by a nebulizer immediately before every step of the test.

In a fourth technique (spray method) the mediator (histamine) is delivered by a metered dose aerosol [94] like those commonly used in β_2-adrenergic agonist topical treatment.

The best nebulizer delivery systems have compressors, which produce a 7–8 liters/min air flow and push air into the nebulizer at variable pressure. In continuous nebulization, pressure is kept constant during nebulization (8–20 psi according to the compressor's power). In the dosimeter methods, pressure reaches the greatest values while the solenoid valve remains closed (20 psi in the Rosenthal and 1.65 kg/cm^2 in the Mefar dosimeter). After opening of the valve, the pressure reduces itself from the beginning to the end of each nebulization, but the reduction is negligible (-8% in 1 s) and does not interfere with the result.

The most important thing is that the air flow in the nebulizer should be constant, since it affects the output (i.e., the quantity of aerosol that is delivered per unit time or during the time of every inhalation). Also the particle or droplet size is affected by air flow variations.

To control the air flow it is sufficient to connect the delivery system to the bell of a spirograph and let in the air for 1 min. To measure the average output, the container of the nebulizer is filled with the same amount of solution needed in the test (usually 3–5 ml) and the nebulizer is weighed before and after 1 min of nebulization (when the test uses continuous nebulization) or after ten nebulizations, each prolonged for the preset time as indicated by the method (0.6 s or 0.8 s or 1 s) when a dosimeter is used.

From the difference between the two weighings the output per unit time or during each preset nebulization by the dosimeter can be calculated. It is necessary to use high precision electronic balances (± 0.1 mg) and to repeat the weighings many times to obtain a very precise mean value.

The terms "MMD" (mass median diameter) and "AMMD" (aerodynamic mass median diameter) are used to indicate the particle size. The "GSD" or geometric standard deviation (GSD) of the two former measures is a useful indication of particle size variability. Since particle size changes according to the type of the nebulizer, and the evaluation of particle diameter is very complex, these values should be given with every nebulizer, as is the case with the De Vilbiss, Wright, and Mefar nebulizers. In the nebulizers with ventilation openings (vents), e.g., the De Vilbiss 646, the open vent increases the particle size.

The increases in flow pressure increase considerably the size of the particles, which partly adhere to the glass of the nebulizer and partly stop in the mouth. (Droplets >10 µm in diameter are mainly deposited in the mouth or pharynx, those >5–10 µm are deposited in the trachea and in the bronchi until the 5th–6th bifurcation and the particles of 1–4 µm reach the smaller bronchi.)

Proper cleaning of the nebulizer, keeping it in a vertical position during the inhalation, repeated tapping on the nebulizer to periodically bring drops adhering to the walls, to the bottom and at least five initial practice nebulization are all expedients to make the technique uniform and the test reproducible.

The pattern of breathing is an important determinant of aerosol deposition: the greater the inhaled volume and slower the inspiration, the more peripheral is the deposition of the particles. Moreover, deposition of the aerosol is an exponential function of the breath-holding time. An increase in inspiratory flow rate increases the inertial impact on the pharynx and in the trachea. However, these variables in breathing pattern are less crucial when a dosimeter is used [133].

The delivered dose is the most important variable. Indeed the response is based on the provocative dose. The following circumstances can alter the results or make their interpretation impossible:

1. The baseline measurements of pulmonary function are not reproducible or there is a significant fall ($>10\%$ vs baseline) after diluent inhalation.

2. The baseline forced expiratory volume in 1 s (FEV_1) is lower than 80% of normal and specific airways conductance (sG_{aw}) is lower than $0.9\ s^{-1} \times kPa^{-1}$ compared to the predicted normal value when the tests are used for research purposes. For clinical requirements, bronchoprovocation tests can be cautiously conducted in subjects whose FEV_1 is lower, provided that the FEV_1 is within 80% of their previously recorded best value.

3. Many factors and drugs that alter the results of the tests are reported in Tables 1 and 2, as proposed by the SEPCR (European Society of Clinical Respiratory Physiology) working group [50]. Moreover, the circadian variations in outcomes [45, 119] and the necessity to repeat the tests (always at the same time and preferably in the morning) should be considered.

It is necessary to instruct the subject in the procedure: He or she should be trained to correctly execute a full inspiration and expiration when the measurements are made by forced expiratory flows. In measurements made

Table 1. Factors affecting bronchial responsiveness (from [50])

Factor	Recommended interval
Upper and lower respiratory infection	6 Weeks
Vaccination with live attenuated influenza virus	3–6 Weeks
Specific antigen exposure with late response	1 Week (longer if late response severe or lasts for more than 24 h)
Occupational sensitizers	Several months
Cigarette smoke	2 h
Atmospheric pollutants	At least 1 week

Table 2. Drugs affecting bronchial responsiveness (from [50])

Drug	Responsiveness	Duration of drug action (h)
β_2-Adrenergic agonist aerosols	↓	12
Anticholinergic aerosols	↓	12
Cromolyn[a,b]	?	8 ?
Oral Drugs		
β_2-Adrenergic agonist	↓	12
Theophyllines	↓	48
H_1-Receptor antagonists[c]	↓	48
Corticosteroids (inhaled or oral)	No effect	–

[a] Single dose immediately before challenge.
[b] After long-term administration cromolyn decreases responsiveness even if the drug has been stopped for many days.
[c] H_1-receptor antagonists decrease responsiveness only in the histamine bronchoprovocation test and in allergic challenge.

at low flow rates, a nose clip is compulsory, and the cheeks should be supported by the hands during plethysmographic procedures. If a tidal volume method is used, the subject should be instructed to breathe through the face mask (or mouthpiece) wearing the nose clip and to keep a regular frequence and rhythm (a metronome could be helpful breathing guid). In dosimetric methods, the duration and the depth of the inspiration do not modify the delivered dose, but, in order to standardize the distribution of the particles in the airways, it is useful to protract the inspiration from FRC to TLC, and the breath holding for 2–5 s. Whatever the method used, at least three baseline measurements of the pulmonary function parameters are necessary in order to consider the higher value as baseline.

The parameters may be measured after adequate inhalation of diluent (for 2 min in tidal volume methods, for five inhalations if a dosimeter is used). A fall $>10\%$ of FEV_1 vs baseline advises against performance of the test. The postdiluent value is very important, since with it may be compared the fall in the values of the parameters after each mediator dose. Thus, three postdiluent measurements should be recorded at 1–2 min intervals.

There are discordant opinions about which of the three values may be considered as the control, the highest or the lowest. Since vital capacity maneuvers may induce bronchoconstriction in some subjects, causing the consecutive values to decrease, it is preferable to take the highest value, which is also less affected by a possible lack of cooperation.

The goal of the bronchoprovocation test with mediators is to verify an increased bronchial response to these substances. In order to explain the results it is necessary to compare the quantity of the mediator (dose), with the intensity of the response (degree of bronchoconstriction).

Obviously, calculation of inhaled dose is founded on exact knowledge of the base substance's concentration in the test solution (if a salt is used, it is necessary to compare the molecular weight of the salt with that of the pure substance for the calculation) and of the quantities of solution delivered at every step, i.e., during the 2 min of continuous aerosolization in the tidal volume methods or during each breath if the test is performed with a preset number of breaths.

In the tidal volume methods the quantity of the stimulus is expressed by the concentration that has caused a fall in the preestabilished parameter vs the baseline value, the *provocative concentration* (PC, i.e., $PC_{20} FEV_1$). The *threshold dose* is the lowest dose which causes a percent fall greater than or equal to the fixed percent fall in baseline value, as listed in Table 3. The *pre-threshold* dose is the immediately preceding dose, which does not yet produce the fixed fall. These two values are necessary to obtain PC by the intercept on the dose-response curve or by an algebraic formula [34].

In methods involving the number of breaths, the doses can considered as *breath units* (BUs, i.e., one BU is one inhalation of 1 mg/ml of the base substance, as in the method of Chai and coworkers [24] or as *dose units* (DU, which is the concentration of mediator (mg/ml) × number of inhalations).

Any reported dose might indicate a single dose, inhaled during each step, or the cumulative dose, i.e., the sum of all single doses which have been inhaled till the particular step of the test.

The cumulative dose is a correct indication if the mediator is not rapidly inactivated in the airways and the doses are additive in effect. If we want to consider the single dose, each successive step may start only when the value of the parameter has returned to near baseline (80%–90%). When the return time at 90% of baseline (RT_{90}) is very long, it conditions the rapidity of the test.

Among the numerous pulmonary function parameters proposed to estimate airways caliber in vivo, those listed in Table 3 are the most useful to measure the degree of response during bronchoprovocation. Table 3 indi-

Table 3. Pulmonary functional parameters and minimal required changes after bronchoprovocation tests

Parameter	Change from baseline (%)
FVC	−10
PEF	−20
FEV_1	−20
FEF_{25-75}	−30
V_{30-P}	−30
V_{60-P}	−30
sG_{aw}	−35

FVC, forced vital capacity; PEF, peak expiratory flow; FEV_1, forced expiratory volume in 1 s; FEF_{25-75}, forced expired flow from 25% to 75% of the forced vital capacity; V_{30-P}, V_{60-P}, maximum partial expiratory flow at 30% or 60% of the forced vital capacity above residual volume; sG_{aw}, specific conductance

cates the minimal percent fall of each parameter vs baseline needed to demonstrate a positive response.

The sG_{aw} is a more sensitive index of airways caliber than FEV_1, with a coefficient of variation about 7% in normal subjects and >20% in asthmatic patients. The limitation in its use comes from the high cost of body plethysmograph, the necessity to very qualified operators, the not insignificant loss of time to calibrate the plethysmograph, and the indispensable need to repeat the measurements.

The sG_{aw} dose-response curve is prolonged till a 35%–45% fall in this parameter is observed.

Among the parameters that can be obtained from a forced expiration, i.e. forced vital capacity (FVC), FEV_1, peak expiratory flow (PEF), and forced expiratory flow (FEF_{25-75}), the FEV_1 is the most widely used. It is recommended because of the low cost of the apparatus, the easy recording of values (so that the dose-response curves can be rapidly drawn) and its reproducibility (coefficient of variation 0%–8%). Since it is less sensitive than sG_{aw}, the FEV_1 makes the bronchoprovocation tests more discriminating (i.e., between asthmatics with BH and allergic rhinitics without BH).

The dose-response curve, usually relating to the PC_{20}, can be prolonged to PC_{35}, in order to adequately confirm the negative response in normal subjects or in normoreactive patients.

Since the FEV_1 is effort-dependent in its first portion and can be influenced by the subject's cooperation, the 25%–75% portion of the FVC or FEF_{25-75} [84] has been reconsidered, but it has a high coefficient of variation in normal subjects as well. The dose-response curves obtained with this parameter are prolonged till to PC_{30}.

PEF is widely used, especially in children, because of the simplicity in measuring it. Falls $\geq 20\%$ of PEF are considered significant in a dose-response curve. PEF is effort-dependent, can be greatly influenced by the subject's cooperation, and has a high coefficient of variation.

Some of the flow volumes obtained by a FVC curve, if performed by pneumotachograph, are useful in examining the state of the smaller airways. These volumes are indicated "at isoflow," because they are measured starting from the same portion of FVC (30%, 60%) above the residual volume (RV). Measurement of the parameters V_{30-P}, V_{60-P}, etc., do not require, as does FEV_1, a deep inspiration before the maximal expiration to perform FVC; thus they do not produce changes in the small airways. Indeed, the parameters which require maximal expiration flow volume (MEFV) can produce bronchodilation in the small airways of normal subjects and variable effects on the small airways of asthmatics.

With the volumes at isoflow PGs, LTs, and PAF, which have a more potent effect on the smaller bronchi, may be studied. The utility of V_{30-P} and V_{60-P} is less in a bronchoprovocation test with histamine and methacholine. A 30% fall in these parameters during bronchoprovocation tests is considered to be a significant response.

Numerous approaches have been advocated to express and analyze the response: the most simple is to record the first dose that produces a fall of predetermined magnitude of the parameter (threshold dose), and if at this dose the fall should be greater than that previously fixed, the provocative dose can be calculated with the formula: $PD_N = (\text{threshold dose} \times N)/F$ where PD_N is the provocative dose at (N) fixed fall (%) and F is the fall (%) at threshold dose.

The most commonly used approach is the multiple dose-response curve, obtained by plotting the falls (%) in the particular parameter against the dose (or, better, against the log dose) of mediator. The dose of mediator producing a fixed percent fall in the parameter vs baseline value (PD) is derived from the intercept of the line that joins the last two points of the dose-response curve (at prethreshold and threshold, i.e., those bracketing the 20% fall in FEV_1) with the line traced from the fixed percent fall.

The response curve can be expressed as a single or cumulative dose. It has been demonstrated [34] that the PD can be calculated by an algebraic formula, which for accuracy and simplicity is preferred over graphically interpolating PD.

The following formula can be used to calculate the PD_{20} FEV_1: $PD_{20} = [(20 - F_1) \times (C_2 - C_1)/(F_2 - F_1)] + C_1$ where C_1 is the prethreshold concentration of mediator, C_2 is the threshold concentration, F_1 is the fall % at C_1, and F_2 is the fall % at C_2.

Another modality considers the value of the area under the parabolic dose-response curve [66], which provides useful parametric data on all examined subjects and discriminates among subjects who might otherwise all be classified as responders if the responses are expressed as PC_{20} FEV_1.

The area under parabolic curve must not be confused with the area under the expiratory flow-volume curve (AEFV), which expresses the functional changes of a whole expiration after a single dose of mediator [140].

Histamine Bronchoprovocation Tests

Histamine (5-β-imidazolylethylamine) is the most abundant amine in humans [18]. It is synthesized from L-histidine by decarboxylation and stored preformed in mast cells and basophils [123]. In humans it is present in the epidermis, the gastrointestinal tract, and the central nervous system as a non-mast cell-associated compound. Histamine is rapidly metabolized by N-methyltransferase to N-methylhistamine and by diamine oxidase into imidazole acetic acid.

The association of histamine with asthma has long been known [68, 136, 154] and, although many mediators are involved in the pathogenesis of asthma [150], its effects are preeminent. These include: (a) contraction of bronchial smooth muscle by direct stimulation of H_1-receptors. The indirect bronchoconstrictive effect of histamine mediated through the vagal reflex has been demonstrated in dogs [43, 134] but is unclear in humans [128]; (b) a double effect on pulmonary vessels: vasodilation by vascular H_1-receptors; vasoconstriction by vascular H_2-receptors [21]; (c) an increase in the permeability of bronchial epithelium (whether this effect is mediated by H_1 or H_2 receptors is unknown) [22, 25]; (d) stimulation of the IgE-dependent release of PGE_2 and $PGF_{2\alpha}$ from pulmonary cells [112]; and (e) stimulation of cytokines production with inhibitory effects on allergic inflammation [16, 125].

Preparation of Histamine Solutions

Histamine is purchased as the dry hydrosoluble powder histamine diphosphate (molecular weight 307) or histamine dihydrochloride (molecular weight 184.08). The compounds must be stored at 0°C in their original containers. Stock solutions are prepared with isotonic phosphate buffered saline (PBS) (pH 7.4) and the appropriate quantity of histamine salt to obtain the desired stock solutions. The amount of histamine (molecular weight 111) required to prepare a 10% stock solution (100 mls in PBS) is 16.60 g of histamine dihydrochloride or 27.66 g of histamine diphosphate (Table 4). In Table 5 are listed the necessary concentrations of the two salts to prepare the histamine solutions that are used in the principal bronchoprovocation methods. Table 6 lists some of the indications to prepare the scalar H-solutions.

The solutions must be made under strict sterile conditions, because bacterial contamination affects the stability of histamine, especially at lower concentrations. However, at concentrations from 2.76 to 22.10 mg/ml histamine diphosphate, the solutions are stable over a 4 month period when stored at 12°C. Concentrations lower than 2.76 mg/ml are not stable after 2 months [115].

Table 4. Buffered phosphate solution

Diluent solution:	solution A (1000 ml) + solution B (200 ml)
Solution A	$Na_2HPO_4 \cdot 2 H_2O$ (14.2 g) Distilled H_2O qs to 1000 ml
Solution B	$Na_2HPO_4 \cdot H_2O$ (2.76 g) Distilled H_2O qs to 200 ml
Stock solutions	containing histamine (10%)
	Histamine diphosphate 27.66 g Diluent solution qs to 100 ml
	Histamine dihydrochloride 16.60 g Diluent solution qs to 100 ml

The stock solutions remain stable at least 4 months in white glass and at +4°C. Sterilize through micropore filter (Aerodisc, Gelman no. 4192,02).

Table 5. Histamine concentrations of the histamine diphosphate and histamine dihydrochloride solutions used in the principal bronchoprovocation methods

Histamine content (mg/ml)	Method (reference)	Histamine diphosphate (mg/ml)	Histamine dihydrochloride (mg/ml)
0.03	24, 33	0.08	0.05
0.06	24, 33	0.17	0.10
0.12	24, 33	0.33	0.20
0.25	24, 33	0.69	0.42
0.50	24, 33	1.38	0.83
1.00	24, 33	2.76	1.66
2.00	33	5.53	3.32
2.50	24	6.92	4.15
3.13	156	8.66	5.20
4.00	33	11.06	6.64
5.00	24	13.83	8.30
6.25	156	17.29	10.38
8.00	33	22.13	13.28
10.00	24	27.66[a]	16.60[a]
16.00	33	44.26	26.56
20.00	24	55.32	33.20
25.00	156	69.15	41.50
50.00	156	138.30	83.00

[a] Stock solutions: histamine 10 g% PBS, histamine diphosphate 27.66 g% PBS, histaine dihydrochloride 16.60 g% PBS

Table 6. Preparation of histamine solutions

Solution number	Histamine content (mg/ml)	Method (reference)	Preparation Solution No. or stock	Volume (ml)	Diluent (ml)
1	0.03[a]	24, 33	2	5	5
2	0.06[a]	24, 33	3	5	5
3	0.12[a]	24, 33	4	5	5
4	0.25[a]	24, 33	5	5	5
5	0.50[a]	24, 33	6	5	5
6	1.00	33	7	50	50
	1.00	24	12	10	90
7	2.00	33	9	50	50
8	2.50	24	10	50	50
9	4.00	33	11	50	50
10	5.00	24	Stock (10%)	5	95
11	8.00	33	13	50	50
12	10.00	24	Stock (10%)	10	90
13	16.00	33	Stock (10%)	16	84
14	20.00	24	Stock (10%)	20	80
15	3.13	156	16	50	50
16	6.25	156	Stock (10%)	6, 25	93,75
17	25.00	156	Stock (10%)	25	75
18	50.00	156	Stock (10%)	50	50

[a] Prepare as needed.

Histamine Inhalations Test Techniques

Here, we will limit ourselves to a description of the principal, i.e., more commonly used, techniques and will neglect the numerous variants when they do not make substantial differences.

Tidal Breathing Method

Proposed by Cockcroft et al. [33], this method is used at the Chest and Allergy Clinic at St. Joseph's Hospitals (Hamilton, Ontario, Canada).

The solutions and nebulizer-delivery system consist of:

1. PBS, pH 7.4
2. Histamine acid phosphate in doubling concentrations to obtain solutions from 0.03 mg/ml to 8 mg/ml of histamine (or 16–32 mg/ml when necessary for epidemiological studies).
3. A Wright nebulizer with 5 ml of PBS or test solution in the nebulizer container. An oxygen flow of 7 liters/min, output 0.13 ml/min, and particle size AMMD 1.3 μm (GSD 2.11) are some characteristics of the nebulizer-delivery system in the original method.
4. Face mask and nose clip. Instead of a face mask a Hans Rudolph inspiratory-expiratory valve box with mouthpiece can be used: it does not influence the response when aerosol is inhaled by tidal breathing [73].

Each solution is inhaled by tidal breathing for 2 min, with the speed of inhalation approximately 0.5 liters/s, while aerosol is delivered continuously during inspiration and expiration; total available dose 260 μl. The responses are measured by FEV_1 at 30 and 90 s after each inhaled dose, and the test is continued until there is a decrease in $FEV_1 \geq 20\%$ of the post-saline value or until the maximum dose has been given. Spirometry is repeated 3 and 5 min after stopping the test. FEV_1 may be preferable to sG_{aw} because of better separation of asthmatics from other groups [31].

The results are expressed as PC_{20} (provocative concentrations of histamine required to produce a 20% fall in FEV_1, as calculated from the log dose-response curve, by linear interpolation between the last points). The interpolation may be performed by mean of the algebraic formula given above. The formula is preferable to manual (graphical) determination for reasons of both accurancy and simplicity.

Intermittently Generate Doses (Dosimeter Method)

This method was developed by Chai and coworkers [24] and has been recommended by the National Institute of Allergic and Infectious Diseases and by the National Institute of Health.

The solutions and nebulizer-delivery system consist of:

1. Buffered diluent, which according to the original method contains 0.5% sodium chloride, 0,275% sodium bicarbonate, and 0.4% phenol (pH 7.0).

2. Histamine phosphate dilution to obtain doubling concentrations from 0.03 mg/ml to 10 mg/ml histamine (more precisely 0.03, 0.06, 0.12, 0.25, 1.00, 2.50, 5.00 and 10.00 mg/ml).

3. A number 42 De Vilbiss nebulizer (original method) with production of particles of MMAD 3.8 μm (GSD 2.8), with 5 ml of PBS or testing solution in the nebulizer container. Nebulizer number 646 is now used in many laboratories. It produces particles 2.6 μm in MMAD (GSD 2.7). The MMAD is very variable in different 646 De Vilbiss nebulizers; indeed, particles of MMAD 1.32 μm (2.55 GSD) have been reported [133].

4. A Rosenthal-French dosimeter, which allows air at 20 psi into the nebulizer for a preset time (0.6 s) and for a preset number of breaths (5 breaths); output 9.04 ± 0.43 μl with air flow 7 liters/min: approximately 45 μl/5 breaths. The dosimeter may be started manually or by changes in mouth pressure at the beginning of inspiration.

5. Mouthpiece and nose clip.

The subject inhales solutions by mouthpiece (starting from FRC to near TLC, with 2–5 s breath-hold) for five consecutive breaths (rate of inhalation 0.5–1.2 liters/s).

The pulmonary parameters are measured before, 3, and 5 min after the five inhalations of diluent (this postdiluent value is used as control), and then immediately, 3, and 5 min after each dose of histamine. The test proceeds until there is a decrease in $FEV_1 \geq 20\%$ from postdiluent value or until the maximum concentration is inhaled.

The results are expressed in arbitrarily defined "histamine inhalation breath units" (H-BUs), in which 1 H-BU equals one inhalation of the solu-

Table 7. Cumulative doses of histamine in bronchial inhalation challenge at five breaths per dilution

Concentration (mg/ml)	Inhalation (units/5 breaths)	Cumulative dose (inhalation units)
0.03	0.15	0.15
0.06	0.30	0.45
0.12	0.60	1.05
0.25	1.25	2.30
0.50	2.50	4.80
1.00	5.00	9.80
2.50	12.50	22.30
5.00	25.00	47.30
10.00	50.00	97.30

One inhalation unit = one breath of solution with 1 mg of drug/ml.

tion containing 1 mg/ml of histamine in diluent. The calculations for cumulative inhaled H-BUs are presented in Table 7. The dose-response curve may be deduced from the log concentrations vs percent fall in FEV_1.

Rapid Dosimeter Method

A rapid method using the Mefar M B3 dosimeter has been proposed by Michel and coworkers from Hopital Universitaire St. Pierre in Brussels [94]. Only three histamine concentrations (8, 16, and 32 mg/ml) are inhaled. The dosimeter is preset at 0.6 s (duration of each air flow in the nebulizer) and at five inhalations for every step. In the three steps 120, 240, and 480 μg are inhaled (cumulative doses 120, 360, and 840 μg).

Rapid, Portable, Manual Method

Proposed by Yan and coworkers [156], this method is used at the Department of Medicine at the University of Sydney. It is a simple, rapid method, particularly useful for studies on a large number of subjects

The solutions and nebulizer-delivery system consists of:

1. Saline solution (0.9% NaCl) as diluent.
2. Histamine diphosphate solutions: 3.13, 6.25, 25, and 50 mg/ml.
3. Five De Vilbiss number 40 nebulizers, each used to administer saline and the four histamine solutions. The air in the nebulizer is manually pushed at the beginning of inspiration, when the operator gives the bulb of the nebulizer one firm squeeze. Output 3 μl (1.8–4.2) with 1 ml of solution in the nebulizer container.

FEV_1 is measured before and after three breaths of saline solution from the first nebulizer. The postsaline value of FEV_1 is the control value. The subject inhales slowly from FRC to TLC during 1–2 s and a breath-hold of 3 s. The successive steps (number of inhalations and histamine concentrations with cumulative dose delivered) are listed in Table 8. When a dose re-

Table 8. Dose schedule for rapid histamine inhalation

Dose number	1	2	3	4	5	6	7	8
Histamine concentration (mg/ml)	3.13	3.13	6.25	6.25	25	25	25	50
Inhalations (*n*)	1	1	1	2	1	2	4	4
Cumulative dose delivered								
μg	9	19	37	75	150	300	600	1.200
μmol	0.029	0.061	0.122	0.244	0.488	0.977	1.954	3.910

quires more than one inhalation, the breaths are consecutive. The test is stopped when the FEV_1 decreases $\geq 20\%$ from postdiluent or when the maximum dose is reached. The test usually takes 7–8 min.

Britton and coworkers compared this method with Cockcroft's method, and no significant difference was found [23]. Miller and coworkers, however, have reported results that indicate important sources of experimental error with hand-driven nebulizers [41].

Spray Method

This method is based on the delivery of histamine by a metered dose aerosol [94]. Every puff delivers 120 μg of histamine diphosphate acid (pH 5.2) in particles of 5 μm MMD.

Pulmonary function parameters are measured before and 2 min after delivery of each dose. The first dose is 120 μg (one puff), the following doses are 240 μg (two puffs), and 480 μg (four puffs); intervals between the doses are 3 min. The test is discontinued when FEV_1 decreases $\geq 20\%$ (sG_{aw} $\geq 35\%$) or the maximum dose has been inhaled (maximal cumulative dose 840 μg).

The distribution of bronchial responsiveness to histamine, as to various other stimuli, depends on the tested subject and how bronchial responsiveness is defined. Since BH is not a characteristic that perfectly discriminates bronchial asthma from other manifestations of the asthmatic syndrome and asymptomatic asthmatics from allergic rhinitics or from some normal subjects, there is not an absolute threshold dose of histamine or other agents by which all asthmatic subjects will respond and all normal or nonasthmatic patients will fail to respond [144].

Cockcroft and coworkers [32] pointed out the unimodal distribution of the responsiveness to inhaled histamine the asthmatic subjects representing a subgroup within the hyperresponsive distribution tail and not a group with a separate peak, as would be the case if the distribution was bimodal. However, there is increased responsiveness to histamine associated with a decreased level of pulmonary function and severity of asthma. Importantly, although in asthmatic subjects (or in allergic rhinitics) the response to histamine could be absent outside the allergy season, bronchoprovocation with histamine can still demonstrate the presence of BH by inducing an exaggerated response, also when spirographic parameters are normal.

Histamine has not shown a cumulative effect when administered repeatedly at 5 min intervals [72], and this could provide more precise data on the threshold dose. However, a cumulative effect of histamine phosphate, when inhaled at 5 min intervals, might be present, but only for the pre-threshold doses and not for the complete scale of the dose-response curve [145].

Tachyphylaxis to inhaled histamine has been demonstrated in asthmatic subjects when repeated challenges are performed, and this loss of responsiveness has been ascribed to release of inhibitory PGs [79]. However, several well-conducted studies have failed to point out tachyphylaxis being a frequent phenomenon, and significant tachyphylaxis could not be demonstrated when three histamine challenges were performed at 1 h intervals [83, 132].

Methacholine Bronchoprovocation Tests

Acetylcholine, carbachol, and methacholine (MC) cause contraction of airway smooth muscle by activation of muscarinic cholinergic receptors M_3 [9] and breakdown of membrane phosphoinositides with release of intracellular calcium [12, 28, 55].

The major response to the lowest dose of cholinergic agent by asthmatic subjects could be due to the extensive permeability of tracheobronchial epithelium, damaged by the allergic inflammation. Thus the cholinergic mediators easily reach the smooth muscle below (hypersensibility). Moreover, the basal muscular hypertonia, always present in these patients, could facilitate the exaggerated bronchoconstrictor response to cholinergic agonists (hyperreactivity). No significant increase in M_3 receptors has been demonstrated in bronchial smooth muscle of asthmatics; on the contrary, a reduction in muscarinic receptors has been reported in lung homogenates of patients with chronic obstructive lung disease [118]. A decreased activity of muscarinic M_2 receptors, localized in airway cholinergic efferent nerves at the prejunctional level where they block acetylcholine release via feedback inhibition [97, 98] (autoreceptors), probably accounts for the increased response to cholinergic agents by asthmatics.

M_1 and M_2 muscarinic receptors are present in ganglia of efferent cholinergic nerves,the former, located on postganglionic neurons, facilitates passage of impulses from pre- to postganglial fibers [20], the latter, located on preganglionic neurons, blocks acetylcholine release and impulse transmission (negative feedback) [81].

Muscarinic receptors are also found on airway epithelium and in submucosal glands [10]. In animals, cholinergic agonists stimulate ion transport across bronchial epithelium, and this effect has also been shown in vitro in human airways [70, 102]; in submucosal glands cholinergic agonists are potent stimulants of mucous and serous cells (M_1 and M_2 receptors) [14].

Preparation of Methacholine Testing Solutions

We have already stated why MC is the cholinergic agonist more often used in bronchoprovocation tests. We will only discuss methods that employ MC.

MC-chloride (acetyl-β-methylcholine chloride) (molecular weight 195.59) is available as a white crystalline solid or powder.

MC has strong hygroscopic properties; indeed, the apparent weight of dried powder may increase by 10% or more when exposed to ambient humidity [3]. Strict attention must be paid to careful dessication before weigh-

Table 9. Preparation of methacholine solutions

Solution number	Methacholine content (mg/ml)	Method (reference)	Preparation Solution No. or stock	Volume (ml)	Diluent (ml)
1	0.025	82	9	10	90
2	0.031	72	3	50	50
3	0.062	72	6	50	50
4	0.075	24	·7	50	50
5	0.100	64	16	5	95
6	0.125	72	9	50	50
7	0.156	24	10	50	50
8	0.200	64	16	10	90
9	0.250	82, 103	17	10	90
		72	11	50	50
10	0.312	24	13	50	50
11	0.500	72	16	25	75
		76	14	50	50
12	0.600	64	20	10	90
13	0.625	24	15	50	50
14	1.00	76	16	50	50
		27	19	20	80
15	1.25	24	17	50	50
		8	22	12.5	87.5
16	2.00	72, 76	18	50	50
		64	24	10	90
17	2.50	24, 82, 103	25	10	90
18	4.00	72, 76	21	50	50
19	5.00	24, 27	B	5	95
20	6.00	64	28	10	90
21	8.00	72, 76	23	50	50
22	10.00	24, 82	B	10	90
		8	27	25	75
23[a]	16.00	72=142	26	50	50
		72, 76	B	16	84
24	20.00	64	B	20	80
25	25.00	24, 27, 82, 103	B	25	75
26[a]	32.00	72=142	29	50	50
27	40.00	8	B	40	60
28	60.00	64	B	60	40
29[a]	64.00	72=142	30	50	50
30[a]	128.00	72=142	31	50	50
31[a]	256.00	72=142	A	51.2	48.8

A, stock solution A = methacholine 50 g in 100 ml PBS.
B, stock solution B = methacholine 10 g in 100 ml PBS.
[a] Solution used only in epidemiologic studies; in clinical studies the higher concentration is 8 or 16 mg/ml. Thus, solution B will be the best stock solution.

ing out the required amount to prepare the stock solution. MC must be stored in its original unopened container at 4°C. All weighings must be made rapidly and, once the container of MC is opened, all unused material should be discarded. However, if the remaining MC powder should be used a second time, it should be spread thinly on filtered paper and dessicated in a dessicator for at least 24 h before weighing and then dissolved in a previously prepared volume of diluent.

If adequately prepared and stored at 4°C, solutions from 1.25 to 20 mg/ml are stable for at least 4 months (if frozen, the stock solutions of MC retain their stability for years) [36]. This is extremely convenient, since when patients are to be tested at different times a reproducible dose can be assured by using the same stock solution.

Table 9 lists the concentrations of testing solutions used in the principal testing methods and some indications for their preparation.

Techniques of Methacholine Inhalation Tests

The proposed techniques for MC bronchoprovocation tests are usually based upon two principal modalities of agent nebulization: continuous aerosol which is inhaled at tidal volume (in a variant, with a present number of inhalations from FRC) or intermittent aerosol with a dosimeter, in which the time of nebulization and the number of breaths are preset. Many of the methods are the same, or very similar to, those already described for histamine inhalation. Therefore, we will deal with them only briefly.

Tidal Volume Methods

Hamilton school's method [59, 72] is the same as Cockcroft's method for histamine provocation testing [33] and the same doubling concentrations in testing MC solutions (from 0.03 to 8 mg/ml) are used; but, because inhaled MC is tolerated better than histamine, higher concentrations can be inhaled (256 mg/ml, as cited in Rasmadall and coworkers study on the protective effect of formoterol) [120].

The method of Kennedy et al. [76] is used at the General Hospital of Vancouver and is a variant of the preceding method, from which it differs in delivery system (Bennet-Twin nebulizer) oxygen flow (5 liters/min), output (0.25 ml/min), particle size (MMD 3.1 μm), and intervals of spirographic measurements ($^{1}/_{2}$ and 3 min after each dose). Also, the doubling concentrations are different: 0.5, 1.0, 2.0, 4.0, 8.0, and 16.0 mg/ml. As in Cockcroft's method [33], each dose is inhaled during 2 min at tidal volume.

The method of Chatham et al. [27] is an abbreviated MC inhalation challenge that is used in Baltimore (at the City and The Good Samaritan hospitals). The subject slowly inhales the aerosol during 6 s from FRC through a face mask attached to a De Vilbiss 646 nebulizer. The nebulizer delivery

Table 10. Abbreviated methacholine challenge protocol

Dose	Concentration (mg/ml)	Inhalations (n°)	Dose (μmol)	Cumulative dose (μmol)
Diluent	0	5	0	0
1	1	1	0.330	0.330
2	5	1	1.65	1.98
3	5	4	6.59	8.58
4	25	1	8.23	16.8
5	25	4	33.0	49.8

Delivered doses calculated using a De Vilbiss 646 nebulizer (output 0.0645 ± 0.0077 ml) and inhalations 6 s in duration from FRC.

system is manually activated by the operator when the patient signals he is ready to inhale from FRC (breath-hold 2 s). The successive doses consist of: (a) 5 mg/ml solution (1 inhalation); (b) 5 mg/ml solution (4 inhalations); (c) 25 mg/ml solution (1 inhalation); (d) 25 mg/ml solution (4 inhalations). In Table 10, from O'Connor and coworkers [106], the nebulized doses (the first is not inhaled in the original method) and the corresponding molar concentrations are listed.

Dosimetric Methods

Technical characteristics of test using different dosimeters, i.e., Rosenthal-French, Spira Elektro 2, or Mefar MB 3, will be discussed here.

The method of Chai and coworkers [24] is the same used for histamine inhalation testing. Table 11 lists the testing concentrations, inhaled BUs at every step, and the corresponding cumulative BUs. Table 12 (from O'Connor) [106], starting concentration 0.156 mg/ml) lists the corresponding concentrations in μmoles.

Table 11. Cumulative doses of methacholine in bronchial inhalation challenge at five breaths per dilution

Concentrations (mg/ml)	Units/5 breaths	Cumulative units/5 breaths
0.075	0.375	0.375
0.15	0.750	1.125
0.31	1.55	2.68
0.62	3.10	5.78
1.25	6.25	12.0
2.50	12.50	24.5
5.00	25.00	49.5
10.00	50.00	99.5
25.00	125.00	225.0

One breath unit = 1 inhalation of 1 mg/ml.

Table 12. Standard methacholine challenge protocol

Dose	Concentration (mg/ml)	Inhalations (n)	Dose (µmoles)	Cumulative (µmoles)
Diluent	0	5	0	0
1	0.156	5	0.0973	0.0973
2	0.312	5	0.195	0.292
3	0.625	5	0.390	0.682
4	1.25	5	0.782	1.46
5	2.50	5	1.56	3.02
6	5.00	5	3.12	6.13
7	10.0	5	6.23	12.4
8	25.0	5	15.6	28.0

The method of Laube et al. [82] is used in the Division of Allergy and Clinical Immunology in Baltimore and is an abbreviation of Chai's method [24]; Only five concentrations are used (0.025, 0.25, 2.5, and 10 mg/ml).

The method of Hopp et al. [64] is used at the University of Creighton, in the Allergic Diseases Center. The technique is another variant of Chai's method [24] with respect to the concentration of the testing solution (0.1, 0.2, 0.6, 2.0, 6.0, 20.0, and 60.0 mg/ml) and in the output (22 µl). The authors advise prolonging the MC challenge until FEV_1 decreases $\geq 35\%$, compared to the postdiluent value, or until the maximum dose is inhaled; however, their results are expressed as the $PD_{20} FEV_1$, which is determined by linear interpolation of the points on the dose-response curve above and below a

Table 13. Single and cumulative methacholine doses in method of Hopp and coworkers [64, 65]

Concentration (mmol/ml)	Concentration (mg/ml)	Breaths[a]		Cumulative
		n	BUs	BUs
0.51	0.1	5	0.5	0.5
1.02	0.2	5	1.0	1.5
3.06	0.6	5	3.0	4.5
10.22	2.0	5	10.0	14.5
30.66	6.0	5	30.0	44.5
102.20	20.0	5	100.0	144.5
306.60	60.0	5	300.0	445.5
306.60	60.0	6	360.0	805.5

With the De Vilbiss 646, used by Hopp and coworkers [64, 65], each breath delivered 0.031 ± 0.010 ml (mean output of eight nebulizers) when the Rosenthal-French dosimeter was activated by a 0.6 s burst of compressed air at 6 liters/min and methacholine volume in the nebulizer container maintained at 2.0 ml. For different characteristics in nebulizer-delivery system, the breath unit (BU) inhaled at every dose may be recalculated.
[a] One breath unit (BU) = one inhalation of 1 mg/ml.

20% drop. In two more recent articles [65, 66] the same Baltimore group demonstrated that expressing results as area beneath a dose-response curve provides more discriminant data among subjects than results that might otherwise be expressed solely as PD_{20}. The area beneath a dose-response curve and the higher MC concentrations are very useful in epidemiological studies. As listed in Table 13, the maximal cumulative dose increases to 805.5 BUs.

The method of Nieminen et al. [103] is used in the Department of Pulmonary Diseases at the University of Tempere (Finland) and employs the Spira Elektro 2 dosimeter, preset for a time flow of 0.5 s and with an output 7.1 ± 0.5 μl. The particle size is 1.6 μm AMMD (1.4 GSD). Only two testing concentrations are used: 2.5 and 25 mg/ml. The spirographic parameters are measured 3 min after saline, and then 3 min after each dose. The number of inhalations and the cumulative dose at every step are listed in Table 14.

Table 14. Methacholine doses delivered by the method using the Spira Elektro 2 dosimeter

Dose	Concentrations (mg/ml)	Inhalations (n)	Cumulative dose (μg)
Diluent	0	5	0
1	2.5	1	18
2	2.5	1	36
3	2.5	2	72
4	2.5	2	110
5	2.5	4	180
6	25.0	1	360
7	25.0	1	530
8	25.0	2	890
9	25.0	4	1600
10	25.0	4	2300

Table 15. Characteristics of the Mefar dosimeter and corresponding methacholine inhalation test

Volume in the nebulizer container	3 ml
Compressed air	1.65 kg/cm^2
Particles size	0.5–5 μm
Air flow	7–7.5 liters/min
Nebulization time	0.8 ± 0.2 s
Output	5 ± 0.2 μl
Starting inspiratory volume	FRC
Breath-hold	5 s
Intervals between each inhalation	10 s
Intervals between each dose	5 min
Intervals between each dose and measurement of respiratory parameters	1.5 and 3 min
Methacholine concentration of testing solutions	1.25, 10.0 and 40.0 mg/ml
Number of inhalations per dose	1–8
Mouthpiece and nose clip	Yes

Table 16. Methacholine doses delivered by the Mefar dosimeter method (from [8])

Dose	Concentration (mg/ml)	Inhalations (n)	Cumulative dose (μg)
Diluent	0	5	0
1	1.25	1	6.25
2	1.25	1	12.5
3	1.25	2	25.0
4	1.25	4	50.0
5	10.00	1	100.0
6	10.00	2	200.0
7	10.00	4	400.0
8	40.00	2	800.0
9	40.00	4	1600.0
10	40.00	8	3200.0

In Italy the most commonly used dosimeter is the Mefar. Balzano et al. [8] were among the very first to employ this dosimeter and from their method we list the characteristics of the Mefar dosimeter and some information about the corresponding MC inhalation test [7, 8] (Table 15). In Table 16 the number of inhalations and the concentration used for each dose are given.

Bronchoprovocation Tests with Arachidonic Acid Metabolites

Out of the great number of mediators generated under normal physiologic conditions or during inflammation, those derived from oxygenation of arachidonic acid are very important. Their increase is tightly associated with an influx of inflammatory cells, predominantly neutrophils and eosinophils.

This correlation has also been observed in asthmatic subjects [44, 47] and in experimental models of asthma [48, 49, 63, 89]; moreover, the importance of PGs, thromboxanes, and LTs in the pathogenesis of asthma has been amply proved. In particular, it has been shown that the slow reacting substance of anaphylaxis (SRS-A) – already known as the mediator responsible for the late and protracted bronchoconstriction after allergic challenge – is a mixture of LTs [85, 86, 100, 110]. However, it has long been well known that $PGF_{2\alpha}$ could be an important factor in asthma, given its bronchoconstrictive effect in isolated human bronchi in vitro [141], or in normal subjects [61] and particularly in asthmatics [91] in vivo.

Many of the relevant studies have been carried out by using arachidonic acid metabolites in bronchoprovocation tests.

Before we describe the protocols used in these studies, it should be noted that results can vary according to the respiratory function parameter that has been chosen to measure the response. Indeed, PGs and LTs show a selective effect at various levels in airways. For example, the selective effect of $PGF_{2\alpha}$ explains its bronchoconstrictive effects both in central and peripheral airways by direct action on tracheobronchial smooth muscle [90]; it can also cause reflex bronchospasm by sensibilization [105] and stimulation [35] of ending afferent vagal fibers in tracheal and bronchial epithelium. These effects can be measured by using both sG_{aw} or FEV_1, and there are little differences between the doses necessary to significantly reduce sG_{aw} and those required to obtain significant reductions of FEV_1.

The LTs are potent bronchoconstrictive mediators which act predominantly on peripheral airways, so that the most useful parameters to study their effects are the partial flows V_{P-30} and V_{P-60}. These indexes can be obtained from partial expiratory flow volumes initiated at about 30% or 60% of vital capacity above RV and are sensitive to alterations in the state of peripheral airways, but are not misrepresented, as is the FEV_1, from the bronchodilation that, especially in normal subjects, follows a deep inspiration [101].

Since the provocative dose to obtain significant reduction of such parameters is very variable, there is substantial overlap in LT responsiveness among normals and asthmatics when V_{30-P} and V_{60-P} are used as bronchoconstrictor indexes, whereas there is little overlap between asthmatic and normal subjects when FEV_1 is used in LT inhalation tests [48].

Bronchoprovocation Tests with Prostaglandins

Inhalation Tests with PGF$_{2\alpha}$

The first PG used in bronchoprovocation tests was $PGF_{2\alpha}$. We will report four techniques, differing in the delivery of mediator and in the doses and bronchoconstrictor indexes used.

The ultrasonic nebulizer method of Mathe' et al. [91] was one of first methods employed for studying the effects of $PGF_{2\alpha}$ in humans and has been used in the Department of Physiology at the Karolinska Institute (Stockholm) and in the Department of Psychiatry and Pharmacology at Boston University. A stock solution of $PGF_{2\alpha}$, as the tromethamine salt (5 mg/ml free acid), is diluted with normal saline to prepare testing solutions that range in doubling concentration from 0.2×10^1 to 1×10^6 ng in 0.5 ml. The ultrasonic nebulizer (LKB Medical, Stockholm, in the original method) produces an aerosol fog with a 2 μm median particle size. The subject inhales at his tidal volume for 1 min before diluent and after each testing solution at 30–45 min intervals, until approximately a 50% reduction of sG_{aw} is obtained. The sG_{aw} is recorded 1, 5, and 15 min after each dose and then every 15 min until the lowest value of sG_{aw} is obtained. With this method, significant falls of sG_{aw} (50%) have been recorded after 250–1000 μg $PGF_{2\alpha}$ in healthy subjects and after 4–512 ng $PGF_{2\alpha}$ in asthmatics. The doses are not cumulative.

The tidal volume method of Thomson et al. [142] is similar to that already proposed by Hamilton's school for histamine and MC inhalation tests. Normal saline with benzyl alcohol (1.5%) is inhaled first (for control) followed

Table 17. Noncumulative inhalation units in the steps of $PGF_{2\alpha}$ inhalation test (from [54])

Steps	Inhalation (n)	Concentration $PGF_{2\alpha}$ (mg/ml)	Inhalation units
Diluent	1	0	0
1	1	0.01	1
2	5	0.01	5
3	1	0.1	10
4	5	0.1	50
5	10	0.1	100
6	20	0.1	200

by the testing concentrations (from 0.00007 to 5 mg/ml) at 5 min intervals between each dose. The FEV_1 is recorded at 30 and 90 s after each dose and the test stopped when FEV_1 falls by 20% or more. The greatest reduction of FEV_1 is usually obtained at 3 min after each dose. The PC_{20} is extremely variable (from 0.0001 to more than 5 mg/ml), but in the same subjects the responses to $PGF_{2\alpha}$ are highly reproducible. With this method there a significant cumulative dose effect.

The preset number of inhalations method of Georgopoulos et al. [54] is used in the Pulmonary Clinic at the University of Thessaloniki and is based on dose determination by the number of inhalations and by the concentrations of the test solutions. Only two dilutions (0.01 and 0.1 mg/ml, in normal saline) are prepared from $PGF_{2\alpha}$ (obtained as a solid) and delivered by the Maxi Mist type compressor (Mead-Johnson Co, Evansville, IN, in original method), with 9 liter/min flow and a De Vilbiss 646 nebulizer. FEV_1 is recorded before and after diluent inhalation and then 3 min after each dose of $PGF_{2\alpha}$. The subject, while wearing a nose clip, breathes through a mouthpiece from FRC to TLC for 5 s. The start of the inhalations is synchronized with the onset of inspiration. The response is expressed in inhalation units (1 IU = one inhalation of 0.01 mg/ml $PGF_{2\alpha}$) required to cause a 20% fall of FEV_1 and calculated by a coordinate system. The steps of the test with concentration of testing solutions, numbers of breaths for every dose, and noncumulative IUs are listed in Table 17.

Bronchoprovocation Test with PGD_2

PGD_2, the principal cyclooxygenase product of mast cells in humans [87], is produced by a number of different tissues and has a variety of actions in animals: it is a potent bronchoconstrictor [151, 152], potentiates the effects of histamine in the inflammatory reaction [51], inhibits platelet aggregation [138], and increases platelet cAMP content [96]. Moreover PGD_2 causes peripheral vasodilation [26] and pulmonary vasoconstriction [57, 151], and increases bronchial hyperreactivity. Elevated levels of PGD_2 are present in bronchoalveolar lavage fluid of mild asthmatics [88].

PGD_2 is metabolized to compounds reflecting its reduction, dehydrogenation, or oxygenation. A metabolite of PGD_2, a diastereoisomer of $PGF_{2\alpha}$, is formed by action of PGF synthase in the lung [26].

The effects of inhaled PGD_2 have been studied in humans by two groups: the first compared effects of PGD_2 and $PGF_{2\alpha}$ on specific airway conductance in normal and asthmatic subjects [58]; the second used PGD_2 in nasal provocation in hay fever patients [93].

PGD_2 for bronchoprovocation tests is dissolved in methanol at a concentration of 40 mg/ml and stored at $-20°C$ under nitrogen. Immediately before use, the desired concentrations are made with a 150 mM PBS buffer (pH 7.4) in doubling concentrations from 3.9 to 500 µg/ml.

In the original method the subject, wearing a nose clip, inhales the aerosol through a mouthpiece during tidal breathing for 1 min: first PBS diluent, then increasing concentrations of PGD_2 at 5 min intervals. sG_{aw} is measured after diluent (control) and 1, 2.5, and 4 min after each dose. In normal subjects PGD_2 caused only a 20% ($\pm 6\%$) fall in sG_{aw}, even with the highest doses (250 and 500 µg/ml). In asthmatic subjects the mediator caused a dose-related fall in sG_{aw} starting at a concentration of 4 µg/ml. In this study PGD_2 was 3.5 times more potent than $PGF_{2\alpha}$ [58].

Bronchoprovocation Tests with Leukotrienes

In a bronchoprovocation test LTs were first employed by Holroyde and coworkers [62] in two normal subjects. Since that time a great variety of methods has been proposed, with either negligible or substantial differences.

Bronchoprovocation Tests with LTC$_4$

Two principal techniques are employed: continuous nebulization at tidal volume and dosimetric inhalations.

The tidal volume method has been used by Barnes and coworkers [11] at the Chest Unit of King's College Hospital in London. The stock solution, containing 1.4 mmol/liter, is diluted in normal saline to give up to a tenfold increased concentration. The starting dose of LTC_4 is 14 nmol/liter. In the original method, a Wright nebulizer containing 2 ml of testing solution was used; the flow rate was 7 liters/min producing a 0.165 ml/min output. After each dose, inhaled for 2 min by tidal volume, the sG_{aw} and V_{30-P} (the most sensitive parameters) are measured at 6, 11, and 16 min. When a 35% or greater fall in sG_{aw} occurs, no further dose is given and further sG_{aw} and V_{30-P} measurements are made after 30, 45, and 60 min. With this method the geometric mean of PC_{35} was 73 µmol/liter in normal subjects, in whom LTC_4 caused bronchoconstriction that was more potent and longer lasting than that induced by histamine.

Regarding the dosimetric method, we report only on the technique with the Mefar dosimeter, used at the Department of Respiratory Medicine, at the Western Infirmary, Glasgow, by Albazzaz and coworkers [2]. The stock solution of LTC_4, containing 100 μg of LTC_4, is diluted with PBS to prepare the testing solutions (from 0.5 to 16 nmol/liter). The subject inhales ten breaths at each concentration from FRC to TLC and airway responses are measured at 2, 5, 10, and 15 min and then for as long as 60 min if the fall in FEV_1 is ≥20%. In the original method, FEV_1 was the parameter recorded but the V_{30-P} could be substituted.

Bronchoprovocation Tests with LTD₄

For this mediator we also report on two techniques: one at tidal volume with continuous nebulization [11, 124] and the other with a dosimeter [139]. A third modality is based on mediator stocks of known quantities placed in a plastic chamber, by which the subject inhales the aerosol. We will not describe this method and we refer the reader to the original paper [17].

The tidal volume method is the same as the one used by Barnes and coworkers for LTC_4 [11]. The stock solution, containing 2 mmol/liter, is used to prepare the up to tenfold increased test concentrations. The starting concentration is 20 nmol/liter. In normal subjects the geometric mean PC_{35} sG_{aw} was 80 μmol/liter. A similar technique, but with different doses, is used by Roberts and coworkers [124] at the Department of Respiratory Medicine, Western Infirmary, Glasgow. A Wright nebulizer (50 psi, flow rate of 8 liter/min to produce an output of 0.15 ml/min) and increasing concentrations of LTD_4 from 0.4 to 50 μg/ml (0.4, 0.8, 1.6, 3.2, 6.4, 12.8, 25, 50 μg/ml) are used. Each test solution is inhaled for 2 min. Inhalations are repeated every 15 min until PC_{10} FEV_1 has been recorded or the maximum concentration has been inhaled. Results are expressed as PC_{10} FEV_1., PC_{35} sG_{aw}, or PC_{30} V_{30-P}.

The dosimeter technique is similar to Chai's method for histamine and MC [24]. It has been used by Smith and coworkers at the University of Chicago [139]. A De Vilbiss 646 nebulizer is attached to a Rosenthal-French dosimeter. An output 0.023 ml of solution is delivered during 0.6 s. The stock solution (1 mg/ml of LTD_4 dipotassium salt) is prepared from lyophilized material and then diluted with PBS (pH 7.4). The dilutions (0.5, 1, 5, 10, 50, 100, and 500 μg/ml) are sterilized, injected into vials filled with argon gas, and kept at −70°C until immediately before being placed in the nebulizer. The subject takes five consecutive breaths of diluent, each beginning at FRC and ending just below TLC, and pulmonary function tests are performed (the authors prefer sG_{aw}, V_{30-P}, and FEV_1) and repeated at 2–5 min after five breaths of each dilution, the intervals between the doses being 10–12 min (in the test that considers cumulative doses) or 45–90 min (if the pulmonary function parameters are measured until they return to 90% of baseline, RT_{90}).

Normal subjects showed $PC \geq 100$ μg, rhinitic subjects $PC \leq 50$ μg, and asthmatics PC 1 μg (with dose-response curves to identify the concentration of LTD_4 that produces a 35% decrease in sG_{aw} and a 30% decrease in V_{30-P}). With this method, using LTD_4, there is less overlap between normals, rhinitic subjects, and asthmatics than with MC.

Bronchoprovocation Tests with LTE$_4$

Drazen's group [41] was the first to study the bronchoconstrictor effects of LTE_4 in normal and asthmatic subjects. However, in contrast to LTC_4 and LTD_4, there are few studies with LTE_4, probably because this mediator has not been commercialized and was prepared by total chemical synthesis by those authors using LTE_4 in bronchoprovocation tests. Arm's group in London studied the effects of LTE_4 in humans [4, 5, 108] and the method was similar. The starting concentration was 0.1 mM (0.01 in asthmatics) using Drazen's technique and 0.18 μg/ml in Arm's, successive concentrations being increased threefold. Inhalation challenges were performed with a nebulizer (De Vilbiss 42 in Drazen's technique, Hudson in Arm's) linked to a breath-activated dosimeter (Rosenthal-French). Delivery of air to the nebulizer was regulated to a pressure of 20 psi and the pulse of compressed air provided by the dosimeter with the onset of inspiration was 0.6 s in duration. At the beginning the subject inhaled ten consecutive breaths of the diluent and performed sG_{aw} and/or V_{30-P} (control). After each dose of LTE_4 (ten consecutive breaths) the responses were measured every 5 min for 20 min, and, if the desired decrease of sG_{aw} ($\geq 35\%$) and V_{30-P} ($\geq 30\%$) was not achieved within 20 min, the subject inhaled the successive concentration until PC was achieved. The PC_{30} of V_{30-P} was 0.30 (± 1.460) nM LTE_4 in normal subjects and 0.058 (± 1.63) nM in asthmatics. LTE_4 had more potent bronchoconstrictor effects than histamine (39-fold in normal subjects, 14-fold in asthmatics). As measured by the dose which produced a fall in sG_{aw}, PD_{35} ranged from 0.06–24.4 (± 4.1) nmol in asthmatic subjects and from 39.0–370 (± 105) nmol in normals. In subjects with aspirin-induced asthma, the airway responsiveness to LTE_4 was increased vs nonaspirin-sensitive asthmatics [41].

Bronchoprovocation Tests with Platelet-Activating Factor

The sulfide-peptide LT PAF has potent inflammatory properties [147] and may play a role in several diseases, including asthma [15, 111].

When inhaled, PAF can produce bronchoconstriction in both normal and asthmatic subjects [38, 70, 130, 131] and airway hyperreactivity in normal subjects [38, 70, 75], but it does not sensitize the airways of asthmatics [131]. The ability of PAF to induce airway hyperresponsiveness to MC is unclear

[70]; however, recently [75], it has been confirmed that this mediator increases airway reactivity, which was maximal at 1 day and persisted for 14 days.

The effects of PAF are mediated through a specific receptor in cellular membranes, including membranes from human lung tissue [67], and many antagonists with competitive inhibition of PAF binding provide further evidence for a putative PAF receptor site [92].

PAF is rapidly inactivated in the lung [60]; therefore it probably acts by indirect pathways: (a) in animals, PAF is able to initiate a cascade leading to LT [148] and thromboxane [116] generation; (b) the effects of PAF on eosinophil function result in epithelial damage (caused by eosinophil cytotoxic mediator [52]) and consequent hyperreactivity by exposure of local nerve networks [80] or by loss of epithelium-derived substances with inhibiting effects on smooth muscle tone [146]; (c) the wide spectrum of effects also includes vascular events [99], neutrophil [39] and eosinophil [149] chemotaxis, degranulation and mediator secretion [107, 148], and reduction of tracheobronchial mucus velocity [6].

The effects of inhaled PAF in humans have been studied with dosimeter techniques and the differences in methodology are very small. The dosimeters were the Rosenthal-French, Mefar, or Spira Elektro 2. The airways function was studied with V_{30-P} or sG_{aw}, because they are more sensitive than FEV_1.

In the protocol of Chung et al. at Brompton Hospital in London [30], the Mefar dosimeter delivered 6 μl per breath of a PAF solution (1.5 mg/ml in saline with 0.03% of human serum albumin to minimize adherence to the nebulizer). Equal doses of mediator (18 μg) are inhaled every 15 min in each of five or six steps (the subject inhales per 3 s from FRC to TLC with a breath hold of 7 s). Measurements of V_{30-P} are made at 1, 3, 5, 10, and 15 min after each dose of PAF and the responses expressed as the percent fall from baseline (postdiluent) value; the total dose administered can be up to 90–108 μg.

In the protocol of Rubin et al. in the Pulmonary Section at Chicago's Northwestern University [131] of the Rosenthal-French dosimeter was used, according to the method of Chai [24], with a De Vilbiss 646 nebulizer that delivered approximately 0.023 ml of solution per inhalation. The subject takes five inhalations of five- or tenfold increasing concentrations of PAF (0.1–1000 μg/ml) at 10 min intervals; 2 min after each inhalation, pulmonary function tests are performed (sG_{aw}).

In the protocol of Nieminen and coworkers [104], at the Departments of Pulmonary Diseases and Biomedical Sciences, University of Tempere, Finland, the dosimeter used was the Spira Elektro 2, with a volume output of 7.1 μl/breath (mean ±0.5 SD) in 0.5 s nebulization periods.

The PAF dilution (3.6 mg/ml with 0.9% saline and 0.25% human serum albumin) is delivered with the dosimeter in four successive doses: 25, 50, 150, and 275 μg (respectively 1, 2, 6, and 11 inhalations) with 3 min intervals between each dose. The cumulative dose is 500 μg. FEV_1 and FVC were utilized in obtaining the pulmonary function data. This protocol is very simple, but it would be better to use V_{30-P} or sG_{aw}.

Bronchoprovocation Tests with Bradykinin

Bradykinin (BK) is a nine amino acid peptide that is generated from kininogens by action of neutral proteases, including kallikrein (kinogenase) which is stored in plasma and in various tissues as inactive prekallikrein [121]. Once generated BK acts locally and then is rapidly inactivated by a kinase and by angiotensin converting enzyme (ACE). Two distinct BK receptors, B_1 and B_2, have been described; the former is activated by Arg-BK, the latter is potently stimulated by BK [122]. BK is able to elicit vasodilation [155], with increased vascular permeability, edema, and mucus hypersecretion [42, 56, 135]. It has been also demonstrated that BK stimulates histamine release from mast cells in vitro [69, 71] and may modulate production of arachidonic acid metabolites (thromboxane [129], $PGF_{2\alpha}$, PGI [13], etc.). BK stimulates sensory unmyelinated nerve endings (C fibers) [74].

The exact role of BK in the pathogenesis of allergic asthma and rhinitis is not well understood: After bronchial or nasal allergic challenge, BK, immunoreactive kinins, and kinogenase activity has been demonstrated in bronchoalveolar lavage fluid or in nasal washings obtained from asthmatic and rhinitic subjects [29, 117]. When inhaled, BK causes bronchoconstriction in asthmatics but not in normals [137]; however, a direct contractile effect on airways smooth muscle (where the presence of BK receptors has not been confirmed) is unlikely, because in vivo BK has a tenfold more potent bronchoconstrictive effect than histamine and MC and in vitro it is 1000-fold less potent than carbachol in inducing contraction of bronchial smooth muscle [19, 137].

Finally, in sheep it has been shown that peptide analogue antagonists of BK block BK-induced bronchoconstriction and the antigen-induced increase in the inflammatory response and associated hyperresponsiveness [1].

These findings suggest that BK may be involved in secondary cell influx and in inflammatory mediator release (thromboxane, $PGF_{2\alpha}$, PGI_2). Neither flurbiprofen nor terfenadine block the bronchoconstrictive effect of BK in humans in vivo [114]. Thus, the most probable action of BK on bronchial smooth muscle is through a cholinergic vagal reflex mechanism caused by damage to airway epithelium with its subsequently diminished protective role (lack of barrier effect, decreased release of epithelial relaxant factors).

In normal and asthmatic subjects, BK causes cough and retrosternal discomfort [53].

Bradykinin Inhalation Test

We will report on the dosimetric method of Polosa and Holgate at Southampton University, England [113]. It uses five preset breaths for each concentration, as in Chai's technique for histamine and MC [24]. BK-triacetic acid in 10% ethanol is diluted in 0.9% sodium chloride to produce a stock solution of 8 mg/ml. Doubling concentrations of testing solution, from 0.015

to 8 mg/ml (0.012–6.5 mmol/ml), contain bovine or human serum albumin to avoid adherence to glass surfaces. To avoid losing BK through oxidation, the solutions should be stored at 4°C and used within 30 min of reconstitution. The nebulizer delivery system in the original method was Inspiron mini nebulizer (CR Bard International, Sunderland UK), but another group has used a Mefar dosimeter [153]. With an aerosol starting volume of 3 ml in the nebulizer container (compressed air at 8 liters/min, output 0.48 ml/min, MMD 4.7 μm), the subject inhales from FRC to TLC in 3 s (five breaths for each dose) through a mouthpiece while wearing a nose clip. The parameters FEV_1 and V_{30-P} are recorded before and postdiluent and then in 5 min intervals between doses. The test is stopped when FEV_1 has fallen by 20% or V_{30-P} by 30% of the postsaline value.

References

1. Abraham WM, Burch RM, Farmer SG, Sielczak MW, Ahmed A, Cortes A (1991) A bradykinin antagonist modifies allergen-induced mediator release and late bronchial responses in sheep. Am Rev Respir Dis 143:787–796
2. Albazzaz MK, Patel KR, Shakir S, Dargie HJ, Reid JM (1989) Effect of inhaled leukotriene C_4 on cardiopulmonary function. Am Rev Respir Dis 139:188–193
3. Alberts WM, Ferguson PR, Ramsdell JW (1983) Preparation and handling of methacholine chloridre testing solutions: effect of the hygroscopic properties of methacholine. Am Rev Respir Dis 127:350–351
4. Arm JP, O'Hickey SP, Spur BW, Lee TH (1989) Airway responsiveness to histamine and leucotriene E_4 in subjects with asthma. Am Rev Respir. Dis 140:148–153
5. Arm JP, Spur BW, Lee TH (1988) The effects of inhaled leukotriene E_4 on the airway responsiveness to histamine in subjects with asthma and normal subjects. J Allergy Clin Immunol 82:654–660
6. Aursudkij B, Rogers DF, Evans TW, Alton EWFW, Chung KF, Barnes PJ (1987) Reduced tracheal mucus velocity in guinea-pig in vivo by platelet-activating factor. Am Rev Respir Dis 135:A160
7. Balzano G, Delli Cari I, Gallo C, Cocco G, Melillo G (1989) Intrasubject between-day variability of PD_{20} methacholine assessed by the dosimeter inhalation test. Chest 95:1239–1243
8. Balzano G, Schiano M, Cocco G et al. (1984) Me. Far dosimeter in bronchial provocation testing with pharmacological agents. Respir News Bull 26:3–5
9. Barnes PJ (1989) Muscarinic receptor subtypes: implications for lung disease. Thorax 44:161–167
10. Barnes JP, Nadel JA, Roberts JM, Basbaum CB (1982) Muscarinic receptors in lung and trachea: autoradiographic [^{3}H] quinuclidinyl benzilate. Eur J Pharmacol 86:103–106
11. Barnes NC, Piper PJ, Costello JF (1984) Comparative effects of inhaled leukotriene C_4, leukotriene D_4 and histamine in normal human subjects. Thorax 39:500–504
12. Baron CB, Cunnigham M, Strauss JF, Coburn RF (1984) Pharmacomechanical coupling in smooth muscle may involve phosphatidylinositol metabolism. Proc Natl Acad Sci USA 81:6899–6903
13. Barrow SE, Dollery CT, Heavey DJ, Hickling NE, Ritter JM, Vial J (1986) Effect of vasoactive peptides on prostacyclin synthesis in man. Br J Pharmacol 87:243–247

14. Basbaum CB, Ueki I, Berzina L, Nadel JA (1981) Tracheal submucosal gland serous cells stimulated *in vitro* with adrenergic and cholinergic agonists. Cell Tissues Res 220:481–498
15. Basran GS, Page CP, Paul W, Morley J (1984) Platelet activating factor: a possible mediator of the dual response to allergen. Clin Allergy 14:75–79
16. Beer DJ, Rocklin RE (1984) Histamine-induced suppressor-cell activity [Postgraduate course]. J Allergy Clin Immunol 73:439–452
17. Bel EH, van der Veen H, Dijkman JH, Sterk PJ (1989) The effect of inhaled budesonide on the maximal degree of airway narrowing to leukotriene D_4 and methacholine in normal subjects *in vivo*. Am Rev Respir Dis 139:427–431
18. Best CH, Dale HH, Dudley HV, Thorpe WV (1927) The nature of dilator constituents of certain tissue extracts. J Physiol 62:397–417
19. Bhoola KD, Collier HOJ, Shachter ML, Shorley PG (1962) Actions of some peptides on bronchial muscle. Br J Pharmacol 19:190–197
20. Bloom JW, Yamamura HI, Baumgartener C, Halonen M (1987) A muscarinic receptor with high affinity for pirenzepine mediates vagally induced bronchoconstriction. Eur J Pharmacol 133:21–27
21. Boe J, Boe MA, Simonsson BG (1980) A dual action of histamine on isolated pulmonary arteries. Respiration 40:117–122
22. Braude S , Royston D, Coe C, Barnes PJ (1984) Histamine increases lung permeability by an H_2 receptor mechanism. Lancet ii:372–374
23. Britton J, Mortagy A, Tattersfield A (1986) Histamine challenge testing: comparison of three methods. Thorax 41:128–132
24. Chai H, Farr RS, Froehlich LA, Matheson DA, McLean JA, Rosenthal RR, Sheefer AL, Townley RG (1975) Standardization of bronchial inhalation procedures. J Allergy Clin Immunol 56:323–327
25. Chan TB, Eiser N, Shelton D, Rees PJ (1987) Histamine receptors and pulmonary epithelial permeability. Br J Dis Chest 81:260–267
26. Chapnick BM, Feigen LP, Hyman AL, Kadowitz PJ (1978) Differential effects of prostaglandins in the mesenteric vascular bed. Am J Physiol 235:H 326
27. Chatham M, Bleecker ER, Norman P, Smith PL, Mason P (1982) A screening test for airways reactivity. An abbreviated methacholine inhalation challenge. Chest 18:15–18
28. Chilvers ER, Barnes PJ, Nahorski SR (1998) Muscarinic receptor stimulated turnover of polyphosphoinositides and inositol polyphosphates in bovine tracheal smooth muscle. Br J Pharmacol 95:778P
29. Christiansen SC, Proud D, Cochrane CG (1987) Detection of tissue kallikrein in the bronchoalveolar lavage fluid of asthmatic subjects J Clin Invest 79:188–197
30. Chung KF, Minette P, Mc Cusker M, Barnes PJ (1988) Ketotifen inhibits the cutaneous but not the airway responses to platelet-activating factor in man. J Allergy Clin Immunol 81:1192–1198
31. Cockcroft DW, Berscheid BA (1983) Measurement of responsiveness to inhaled histamine: comparison of FEV_1 and sG_{aw}. Ann Allergy 51:374–377
32. Cockcroft DW, Berscheid BA, Murdock KY (1984) Unimodal distribution of bronchial responsiveness to inhaled histamine in a random human population. Chest 83:751–754
33. Cockcroft DW, Killian DN, Mellon JJA, Hargreave FE (1977) Bronchial reactivity to inhaled histamine: a method and clinical survey. Clin Allergy 7:235–243
34. Cockcroft DW, Murdock KY, Mink JT (1983) Determination of histamine PC_{20}. Comparison of linear and logarithmic interpolation. Chest 84:505–506
35. Coleridge HM, Coleridge JCG, Ginzel KH et al. (1976) Stimulation of "irritant" receptors and afferent C-fibers in the lung by prostaglandins. Nature 264:451–453
36. Cropp GJA, Bernstein IL, Boushey HA et al. (1980) Guidelines for bronchial inhalation challenges with pharmacologic and antigenic agents. ATS New Spring 6:11–19

37. Curry JJ (1946) The action of histamine on the respiratory tract in normal and asthmatic subjects. J Clin Invest 25:785–791
38. Cuss FM, Dixon CMS, Barnes PJ (1986) Effects of inhaled platelet activating factor in man. Lancet ii:189–192
39. Czarnetski BM, Benveniste J (1981) Effect of synthetic PAF-acether on human neutrophil function. Agents Actions 2:549–552
40. Dautrebande L, Philippot E (1941) Crisi d'asthme expérimental par aérosols de carbaminoylcholine chez l'homme, traitée par dispersat de phénylaminopropane. Etude de l'action sur la respiration de ces substances par la détermination du volume respiratoire utile. Presse Méd 49:942–946
41. Davidson AB, Lee TH, Scanlon PD, Solvay J, McFadden ER Jr, Ingram RH Jr, Corey EJ, Austen KF, Drazen JM (1987) Bronchoconstrictor effects of leukotriene E_4 in normal and asthmatic subjects. Am Rev Respir Dis 135:333–337
42. Davis B, Roberts AM, Coleridge HM, Coleridge JCG (1982) Reflex tracheal gland secretion evoked by stimulation of bronchial C-fibers in dogs. J Appl Physiol 53:985–991
43. De Koch MA, Nadel JA, Zuri S, Colebatch HJH, Olsen CR (1966) New method for perfusing bronchial arteries: histamine bronchoconstriction and apnoea. J Appl Physiol 21:185–194
44. De Monchy JGR, Kauffman HF, Venge P, Koeter GH, Jansen HM, Sluiter HJ, De Vries K (1985) Bronchoalveolar eosinophilia during allergen-induced late asthmatic reactions. Am Rev Respir Dis 131:373–376
45. De Vries K, Goei JT, Booij-Noord H, Orie NGM (1962) Changes during 24 hours of the lung function and histamine hyperreactivity of the bronchial tree in asthmatic and bronchitic patients. Int Arch Allergy 20:93–101
46. Del Bono N (1982) L'asma e la sua storia. Sandoz, Milano
47. Diaz P, Gonzalez MC, Galleguillos FR, Ancic P, Cronwell O, Shepherd D, Durham SR, Gleich GI, Kay AB (1989) Leukocytes and mediators in bronchoalveolar lavage during allergen-induced late-phase asthmatic reactions. Am Rev Respir Dis 139:1383–1389
48. Drazen JM (1986) Inhalation challenge with sulfidopeptide leukotrienes in human subjects. Chest 89:414–419
49. Dworski R, Sheller JR, Wickershan NE, Oates JA, Brigham KL, Roberts LJ, Fitzgerald GA (1989) Allergen-stimulated release of mediators into sheep bronchoalveolar lavage fluid: effect of cyclooxygenase inhibition. Am Rev Respir Dis 139:46–51
50. Eiser NM, Kerrebijn KF, Quanjer PH (1983) Guidelines for standardization of bronchial challenges with (non specific) bronchoconstricting agents. Bull Eur Physiopathol Respir 19:495–514
51. Flower RJ, Harvey EA, Kingston WP (1976) Inflammatory effects of prostaglandin D_2 in rat and human skin. Br. J Pharmacol 56:229–233
52. Frigas E, Gleich GJ (1986) The eosinophil and the pathology of asthma. J Allergy Clin Immunol 218:286–288
53. Fuller RW, Dixon CMS, Cuss FMC, Barnes PJ (1987) Bradykinin-induced bronchoconstriction in humans. Mode of action. Am Rev Respir Dis 135:176–180
54. Georgopoulos D, Giulekas D, Ilonidis G, Sicletidis L (1989) Effect of salbutamol, ipratropium bromide and cromolyn sodium on prostaglandin $F_{2\alpha}$-induced bronchospasm. Chest 96:809–814
55. Grandordy BM, Cuss FM, Sampson AS, Palmer JB, Barnes PJ (1986) Phosphatidylinositol response to cholinergic agonists in airway smooth muscle: relationship to contraction and muscarinic receptor occupancy. J Pharmacol Exp Ther 238:273–279
56. Griesbacher T, Lembeck F (1987) Effect of bradykinin antagonists on bradykinin-induced plasma extravasation, venoconstriction, prostaglandin E_2 release, nociceptor stimulation and contraction of the iris sphincter muscle in the rabbit. Br J Pharmacol 92:333–340

57. Gruetter C, McNamara D, Hyman A, Kadowitz P (1978) Contractile effects of a PGH$_2$ analog and PGD$_2$ on intrapulmonary vessels. Am J Physiol 234: H 139–145
58. Hardy CC, Robinson C, Tattersfield AE, Holgate ST (1984) The bronchoconstrictor effect of inhaled prostaglandin D$_2$ in normal and asthmatic men. N Engl J Med 311:209–213
59. Hargreave FE, Ryan G, Thomson NC, O'Byrne PM, Latimer K, Juniper EF, Dolovich J (1981) Bronchial responsiveness to histamine or methacholine in asthma: measurement and clinical significance. J Allergy Clin Immunol 68:347–355
60. Haroldsen PE, Voelkel NF, Henson JE, Henson PM, Murphy RC (1987) Metabolism of platelet-activating factor in isolated perfused rat lung. J Clin Invest 79:1860–1867
61. Hedqvist P, Holmgren A, Mathe' AA (1971) Effect of prostaglandin F$_{2\alpha}$ on the airway resistence in man. Acta Physiol Scand 82:29A
62. Holroyde MC, Altounyan REC, Cole M, Dixon M, Elliot EV (1981) Bronchoconstriction produced in man by leukotrienes C and D. Lancet ii:17–18
63. Holtzman MJ, Fabbri LM, O'Byrne PM, Gold BD, Aizawa H, Walters EH, Alpert SE, Nadel JA (1983) Importance of airway inflammation for hyperresponsiveness induced by ozone in dogs. Am Rev Respir Dis 127:686–690
64. Hopp RJ, Bewtra AK, Nair NM, Townley RG (1984) Specificity and sensitivity of methacholine inhalation challenge in normal and asthmatic children. J Allergy Clin Immunol 74:154–158
65. Hopp RJ, Bewtra AK, Nair NM, Watt GD, Townley RG (1986) Methacholine inhalation challenge in a selected pediatric population. Am Rev Respir Dis 134: 994–998
66. Hopp RJ, Weiss SJ, Nair NM, Bewtra AK, Townley RG (1987) Interpretation of the results of methacholine inhalation challenge test. J Allergy Clin Immunol 80:821–830
67. Hwang SB, Lam MH, Shen TY (1985) Specific binding sites for platelet activating factor in human lung tissues. Biochem Biophys Res Commun 128:972–979
68. Ishizaka T (1981) Analysis of triggering events in mast cells for immunoglobulin E-mediated histamine release. J Allergy Clin Immunol 67:90–96
69. Ishizaka T, Iwata M, Ishizaka K (1985) Release of histamine and arachidonate from mouse mast cells induced by glycosylation-enhancing factor and bradykinin. J Immunol 134:1880–1887
70. Jenkins JR, Lai CKW, Holgate ST (1989) Effect of increasing doses of platelet activating factor (PAF) on normal human airways (abstract). J Allergy Clin Immunol 83:282
71. Johnson AR, Erdos EG (1973) Release of histamine from mast cells by vasoactive peptides. Proc. Soc Exp Biol Med 142:1252
72. Juniper EF, Frith PA, Dunnet C, Cockcroft DW, Hargreave FE (1978) Reproducibility and comparison of responses to inhaled histamine and methacholine. Thorax 33:705–710
73. Juniper EF, Syty-Golda M, Hargreave FE (1984) Histamine inhalation tests: inhalation of aerosol via a face mask versus a valve box with mouthpiece. Thorax 39:556–557
74. Kaufman MP, Coleridge HM, Coleridge JCG, Bauer DG (1980) Bradykinin stimulates afferent vagal C-fibres in intrapulmonary airways of dogs. J Appl Physiol 48:511–517
75. Kaye MG, Smith LJ (1990) Effect of inhaled leucotriene D$_4$ and platelet-activating factor on airway reactivity in normal subjects. Am Rev Respir Dis 141: 993–997
76. Kennedy SM, Burrows B, Vedal S, Enarson DA, Chan-Yeung M (1990) Methacholine responsiveness among working populations. Relationship to smoking and airway caliber. Am Rev Respir Dis 142:1377–1383

77. Klein RC, Salvaggio JE (1966) Nonspecificity of the bronchoconstricting effect of histamine and acetyl methylcholine in patients with obstructive airway disease. J Allergy 37:158–168
78. Knowles M, Murray G, Shallal J, Askin F, Ranga V, Gatzy J, Boucher R (1984) Bioelectric properties and ion flow across excised human bronchi. J Appl Physiol 56:868–877
79. Krzanowski JJ, Anderson WH, Polson JB, Szentivanji A (1980) Prostaglandin mediated histamine tachyphylaxis in subhuman primate tracheal smooth muscle. Arch Int Pharmacodyn 247:155–162
80. Laitinen LA, Heino M, Laitinen A, Kava T, Haatela T (1985) Damage of the airway epithelium and bronchial reactivity in patients with asthma. Am Rev Respir Dis 131:599–606
81. Lammers J-W, Minette P, McCusker M, Barnes JP (1989) The role of pirenzepine-sensitive (M_1) muscarinic receptor in vagally mediate bronchoconstriction in humans. Am Rev Respir Dis 139:446–449
82. Laube BL, Adams GK III, Norman PS, Rosenthal RR (1985) The effect of inspiratory flow rate regulation on nebulizer output and on human airway response to methacholine aerosol. J Allergy Clin Immunol 76:708–713
83. Lemire RE, Cartier A, Malo JL, Pineau L, Ghezzo H, Martin RR (1984) Effect of sodium cromoglycate on histamine inhalation tests. J Allergy Clin Immunol 73:234–239
84. Leuallen EC, Fowler WS (1955) Maximal midexpiratory flow. Am Rev Tuberc 72:783–800
85. Lewis RA, Austen KF (1984) The biologically active leukotrienes. Biosynthesis, metabolism, receptors, functions and pharmacology. J Clin Invest 73:889–898
86. Lewis RA, Drazen JM, Austen KF, Clark DA, Corey EJ (1980) Identification of the c(6)-S-coniugate of leukotriene A with cysteine as a naturally occurring slow-reacting substance of anaphylaxis (SRS-A). Importance of the 11-cis geometry for biological activity. Biochem Biophys Res Commun 96:271–277
87. Lewis RA, Soter NA, Diamond PT, Austen KF, Oates JA, Roberts LJ II (1982) Prostaglandin D_2 release after activation of rat and human mast cells with anti IgE. J Immunol 129:1627–1631
88. Liu MC, Blecker ER, Lichtenstein LM, Kagey-Sobotka A, McLemore TL, Permutt S, Proud D, Hubband WC (1990) Evidence for elevated levels of histamine, prostaglandin D_2, and other bronchoconstricting prostaglandins in the airways of subjects with mild asthma. Am Rev Respir Dis 142:126–132
89. Marsh WR, Irwin CG, Murphy KR, Behrens BL, Larsen GL (1985) Increases in airway reactivity to histamin and inflammatory cells in bronchoalveolar lavage after the late asthmatic response in an animal model. Am Rev Respir Dis 131:875–879
90. Mathe' AA, Hedqvist P, Strandberg K, Leslie CA (1971) Aspects of prostaglandin function in the lung. N Engl J Med 296:850
91. Mathe' AA, Hedqvist P, Holmgren A, Svanborg N (1973) Bronchial hyperreactivity to prostaglandin $F_{2\alpha}$ and histamine in patients with asthma. Brit J Med 1:193–196
92. Meade CJ, Heuer H (1991) PAF antagonism as a approach to the treatment of airway hyperreactivity. Am Rev Respir Dis 143:S 79–S 82
93. Miadonna A, Tedeschi A, Leggieri E, Fabbri C, Lorini M, Qualizza R, Pastorello E, Froldi M, Zanussi C (1986) Effetto della provocazione nasale con istamina, leucotriene C_4 e prostaglandina D_2 nei pazienti affetti da rinite allergica da pollini di graminacee. Folia Allergol Immunol Clin 33:279–284
94. Michel O, Sergysels R, Duchateau J (1989) Comparison de deux modes d'administration de l'histamine sur la résponse bronchomotrice chez l'asthmatique. Rev Mal Respir 6:251–254
95. Miller MR, Tarin C, Madan I (1991) The effect of a subject's inhalation on the output of hand driven nebulizers (abstract). Am Rev Respir Dis 142:S 427

96. Mills DCB, Macfarlane DE (1974) Stimulation of human platelet adenylate ciclase by prostaglandin D_2. Thromb Res 5:401–412
97. Minette PA, Barnes PJ (1988) Prejunctional inhibitory muscarinic receptors on cholinergic nerves in human and guinea-pig airways. J Appl Physiol 64: 2532–2537
98. Minette PA, Lammers J-W, Barnes PJ (1988) Is there a defect in inhibitory muscarinic receptors in asthma? Am Rev Respir Dis 137 [Suppl]:239
99. Mojarad M, Hamasaki Y, Said I (1983) Platelet-activating factor increases pulmonary microvascular permeability and induces pulmonary oedema. Bull Eur Physiopathol Respir 19:253–257
100. Murphy RC, Hammarstrom S, Samuelsson B (1979) Leukotriene C: A slow-reacting substance from murine mastocytoma cells. Proc Natl Acad Sci USA 76:4275–4279
101. Nadel JA, Tierney DF (1961) Effect of a previous deep inspiration on airway resistence in man. J Appl Physiol 16:717–719
102. Nadel JF, Widdicombe JG, Peatfield AC (1985) Regulation of airway secretion, ion transport and water movement. In: Fishman AP, Fisher AB (eds) Handbook of physiology, vol 1, sect 3: the respiratory system. American Physiological Society, Bethesda, pp 419–445
103. Nieminen MM, Lahdensuo A, Kellomaeki L, Karvonen J, Muittari A (1988) Methacholine bronchial challenge using a dosimeter with controlled tidal breathing. Thorax 43:896–900
104. Nieminen MM, Moilanen EK, Nyholm J-EJ, Koskinen MO, Karvonen JI, Metsä-Ketelä TJ, Vapaatalo H (1991) Platelet-activating factor impairs mucociliary transport and increases plasma leukotriene B_4 in man. Eur Respir J 4:551–560
105. O'Byrne PM, Aizawa H, Bethel RA et al. (1984) Prostaglandin $F_{2\alpha}$ increases responsiveness of pulmonary airways in dogs. Prostaglandins 28:537–543
106. O'Connor G, Sparrow D, Taylor D, Segal M, Weiss S (1987) Analysis of dose-response curves to methacholine. An approach suitable for population studies. Am Rev Respir Dis 136:1412–1417
107. O'Flaherty JT (1985) Neutrophil degranuation: evidence pertaining to its mediation by the combined effects of leukotriene B_4, platelet-activating factor, and 5-HETE. J Cell Physiol 122:229–239
108. O'Hickey SP, Arm JP, Rees PJ, Spur BW, Lee TH (1988) The relative responsiveness to inhaled leukotriene E_4, methacholine and histamine in normal and asthmatic subjects. Eur Respir J 1:913–917
109. Orehek J, Gayrard P (1976) Les tests de provocation bronchique non specifiques dans l'asthme. Bull Eur Physiopathol Respir 12:565–598
110. Orning L, Hammarstrom S, Samuelsson B (1980) Leukotriene D: a slow reacting substance from rat basophilic leukemia cell. Proc Natl Acad Sci USA 77: 2014–2017
111. Page CP, Paul W, Dewar A, Wood L, Basran GS, Morley J (1982) PAF-acether: a putative mediator of asthma and inflammation. Agents Actions [Suppl] 13:177–183
112. Platshon LF, Kaliner M (1978) The effect of the immunologic release of histamine upon human lung cyclic nucleotide levels and prostaglandin generation. J Clin Invest 62:1113–1121
113. Polosa R, Holgate ST (1990) Comparative airway response to inhaled bradykinin, kallidin and [des-Arg⁹]bradykinin in normal and asthmatic subjects. Am Rev Respir Dis 142:1367–1371
114. Polosa R, Phillips GD, Lai CKW, Holgate ST (1990) Contribution of histamine and prostanoids to bronchoconstriction provoked by inhaled bradykinin in atopic asthma. Allergy 45:174–182
115. Pratter MR, Marwaha RK, Irwin RS, Johnson BF, Curley FG (1985) Stability of stored histamine diphosphate solutions. Clinically useful information. Am Rev Respir Dis 132:1130–1131

116. Pretolani M, Lefort J, Malanchere E, Vergaftig BB (1987) Interference by the novel PAF-acether antagonist WEB 2086 with the bronchopulmonary responses to PAF-acether and to active and passive anaphylactic shock in guinea pigs. Eur J Pharmacol 140:311–321

117. Proud D, Togias A, Nacleiro RM, Crush SA, Norman PS, Lichtenstein LM (1983) Kinins are generated in vivo following nasal airway challenge of allergic individuals with allergen. J Clin Invest 72:1678–1685

118. Raaijmakers JAM, Terpstra GK, Van Rozen AJ, Witter A, Kreukniet J (1984) Muscarinic cholinergic receptors in peripheral lung tissue of normal subjects and of patients with chronic obstructive lung disease. Clin Sci 66:585–590

119. Rachiele A, Malo JL, Cartier A, Pineau L, Ghezzo H, Martin RR (1983) Circadian variations of airway response to histamine in asthmatic subjects. Bull Eur Physiopathol Respir 19:465–469

120. Ramsdale EH, Otis J, Kline PA, Gontovnik LS, Hargreave FE, O'Byrne PM (1991) Prolonged protection against methacholine-induced bronchoconstriction by the inhaled β_2-agonist formoterol. Am Rev Respir Dis 143:998–1001

121. Regoli D, Barabe J (1980) Pharmacology of bradykinin and related peptides. Pharmacol Rev 32:1–46

122. Regoli D, Barabe J, Park WK (1977) Receptors for bradykinin in rabbit aorta. Can J Physiol Pharmacol 55:855–867

123. Riley JF, West GB (1953) The presence of histamine in tissue mast cells. J Physiol 120:528–537

124. Roberts JA, Rodger IW, Thomson NC (1987) In vivo and in vitro human airway responsiveness to leukotriene D_4 in patients without asthma. J Allergy Clin Immunol 80:688–694

125. Rocklin, RE (1977) Histamine induced suppressor factor (HSF): effect on migration inhibitory factor (MIF) production and proliferation. J Immunol 118:1734–1740

126. Romano C (1990) Importanza della standardizzazione degli aerosoli nei test di broncoprovocazione. In: Del Bono L, Del Bono N (eds) I test di broncoprovocazione. Essetre, Roma, pp 106–121

127. Roseman TJ, Yalkowsky SH (1973) Physicochemical properties of prostaglandin $F_{2\alpha}$ (tromethamine salt): solubility behavior, surface properties, and ionization constants. J Pharm Sci 62:1680–1685

128. Rosenthal RR, Norman PS, Summer WR, Permutt S (1977) Role of the parasympathetic nervous system in antigen-induced bronchospasm. J Appl Physiol 42:600–606

129. Rossoni G, Omini C, Vigano T, Mandelli V, Folco GC, Berti F (1980) Bronchoconstriction by histamine and bradykinin in guinea-pigs: relationship to thromboxane A_2 generation and the effect of aspirin. Prostaglandins 20:547–557

130. Rubin AE, Smith LJ, Patterson R (1987) Platelet activating factor (PAF)-induced bronchoconstriction in man: mechanism of action (abstract). Am Rev Respir Dis 135:A 158

131. Rubin AE, Smith LJ, Patterson R (1987) The bronchoconstrictor properties of platelet-activating factor in man. Am Rev Respir Dis 136:1145–1151

132. Ruffin RE, Alpers JH, Crocket AJ, Hamilton R (1981) Repeated histamine inhalation tests in asthmatic patients. J Allergy Clin Immunol 67:285–289

133. Ryan G, Dolovich MB, Eng P, Obminski G, Cockcroft DW, Juniper EF, Hargreave FE, Newhouse MT (1981) Standardization of inhalation provocation tests: influence of nebulizer output, particle size, and method of inhalation. J Allergy Clin Immunol 67:156–161

134. Samson SR, Vidruk DH (1979) The nature of the receptor mediating stimulant effects of histamine on rapidly adapting vagal afferents in the lung. J Physiol (Lond) 287:509–518

135. Saria A, Lundberg JM, Skofitsch G, Lembeck F (1983) Vascular protein leakage in various tissues induced by substance P, capsaicin, bradykinin, serotonin,

histamine and by antigen challenge. Naunyn Schmiedebergs Arch Pharmacol 324:212–218

136. Schild HO, Hawkins DF, Momgar JL, Herxheimer H (1951) Reactions of isolated human asthmatic lung and bronchial tissue to a specific antigen: histamine release and muscolar contraction. Lancet ii:376–382

137. Simonsson BG, Skoogh BE, Bergh NP, Anderson R, Svedmyr N (1973) *In vivo* and *in vitro* effect of bradykinin on bronchial motor tone in normal subjects and in patients with airway obstruction. Respiration 30:378–380

138. Smith JB, Silver MJ, Ingerman CM, Kocsis JJ (1974) Prostaglandin D_2 inhibits the aggregation of human platelets. Thromb. Res 5:291–299

139. Smith LJ, Greenberger PA, Patterson R, Krell RD, Bernstein PR (1985) The effect of inhaled leukotriene D_4 in humans. Am Rev Respir Dis 131:368–372

140. Sovijärvi ARA (1983) Area under the flow-volume curve: a new sensitive index to asses bronchodilation. IRCS Med Sci 11:1104

141. Sweatman WJF, Collier HOG (1968) Effects of prostaglandins on human bronchial muscle. Nature 217:69

142. Thomson NC, Roberts R, Thech M, Bandouvakis J, Newball H, Hargreave FE (1981) Comparison of bronchial response to prostaglandin $F_{2\alpha}$ and methacholine. J Allergy Clin Immunol 68:392–398

143. Tiffeneau R, Beauvallet M (1945) Épreuve de bronchoconstriction et de bronchodilation par aérosols. Emploi pour le dépistage, la mesure et le controle des insuffisance respiratoires chroniques. Bull Acad Méd Paris 129:165–168

144. Townley RG, Hopp RJ (1988) Measurement and interpretation of nonspecific bronchial reactivity. Chest 94:452–454

145. Tremblay C, Lemire I, Ghezzo H, Pineau L, Martin RR, Cartier A, Malo JL (1984) Histamine phosphate has a cumulative effect when inhaled at five minute intervals. Thorax 39:946–951

146. Vanhoutte PM (1989) Epithelium-derived relaxing factor(s) and bronchial reactivity. J Allergy Clin Immunol 83:855–861

147. Vargaftig BB, Chignard M, Benveniste J, Lefort J, Wal F (1981) Background and present status of research on platelet-activating factor (PAF-acether). Ann NY Acad Sci 370:119–137

148. Voelkel NF, Worthen S, Reeves JT, Henson PM, Murphy RC (1982) Non immunological production of leukotrienes induced by platelet-activating factor. Science 218:286–289

149. Wardlaw AJ, Moqbel R, Cromwell O, Kay AB (1986) Platelet-activating factor. A potent chemotactic and chemokinetic factor for human eosinophils. J Clin Invest 78:1701–1706

150. Wasserman ST (1983) Mediators of immediate hypersensitivity. J Allergy Clin Immunol 72:101–105

151. Wasserman MA, Du Charme DW, Griffin RL, De Graaf GL, Robinson FG (1977) Bronchopulmonary and cardiovascular effects of prostaglandin D_2 in the dog. Prostaglandins 13:255–269

152. Wasserman M, Griffin RL, Marsalisi FB (1980) Potent bronchoconstrictor effects of aerosolized prostaglandin D_2 in dogs. Prostaglandins 20:703–715

153. Watanabe K, Iguchi Y, Iguchi S et al. (1986) Stereospecific conversion of prostaglandin D_2 to (5Z,13E)-(15S)-9α,11β,15-trihydroxyprosta-5,13-dien-1-oic-acid-(9α, 11β-prostaglandin f_2) and of prostaglandin H_2 to prostaglandin $F_{2\alpha}$ by bovine lung prostaglandin F synthase. Proc Natl Acad Sci USA 83:1583–1587

154. Weiss S, Robb GP, Ellis LB (1932) The systemic effects of histamine in man with special reference to the response of the cardiovascular system. Arch Intern Med 49:360–396

155. Wilhelm DL (1971) Kinins in human disease. Annu Rev Med 22:63–84

156. Yan K, Salome CM, Woolcock AJ (1983) Rapid method for measurement of bronchial responsiveness. Thorax 38:760–765

Part VI

Diagnostic Use of Bronchodilators

Long- and Short-Term Reversibility Tests

N. E. MOAVERO

Institute of Respiratory Diseases, School of Medicine, University of Milan, Milano, Italy

Bronchial obstruction is the consequence of several factors: (a) broncho-spasm with or without bronchial smooth muscle hypertrophy; (b) inflammatory cells infiltration; (c) vascular congestion and mucosal edema; (d) hypersecretion of mucus with changes in its viscoelastic properties; (e) degenerative processes such as fibrosis and/or alveolar disruption. All these features are usually present, each one contributing differently according to the specific disease.

The definition of bronchial obstruction varies among investigators [1–4]. Nonetheless, bronchial obstruction in chronic bronchitis is mainly caused by mucus, infiltration, and edema with, to some extent, bronchospasm and loss of the structural components (ciliated cells) of the bronchial wall and of the alveoli, while in asthma the paramount cause of obstruction is broncho-spasm. In emphysema, obstruction is mainly due to external compression of airways because of the decrease in lung elastic recoil. In each case, the result is airflow limitation with airways narrowing during expiration, leading to an obstructive ventilatory defect.

Criteria for the lower case differential diagnosis of chronic bronchitis, asthma, and emphysema are based on ventilatory function differences, the most important criterion being reversibility. Reversibility is the ability of bronchoconstriction to return to normal spontaneously (during remission of asthma) or acutely in response to administration of bronchodilator aerosols, indicating smooth muscle spasm to be the main component in the pathogenesis of obstruction. In fact, although it may be found in other obstructive diseases, reversibility is characteristic of bronchial asthma, which since the Ciba symposium in 1959 has been defined as "a widespread narrowing of the airways which alters in severity either spontaneously or in response to treatment" [5]. This concept of reversibility is still a hallmark of asthma, in spite of several different subsequent definitions, based on newer and more complete knowledge of the pathogenetic mechanisms and the overall pathology of the disease.

A more extensive use of the term reversibility indicates the reversal of obstruction not only spontaneously or after a single administration of bronchodilator but also after a certain period of treatment with drugs that act on the components of obstruction other than bronchospasm. Thus "early" reversibility (after a single administration of bronchodilator), indicating a major role for bronchospasm in the obstruction, as mainly occurs in bronchial asthma, could be distinguished from "late" reversibility (after any other treatment), indicating a major role for factors other than bronchospasm, as mainly occurs in chronic obstructive pulmonary disease (COPD). The absence of reversibility (early and late) would be suggestive of degenerative irreversible obstruction, as occurs mainly in emphysema. A finding of partial reversibility is suggestive of the simultaneous presence of bronchospasm and other "inflammatory" determinants of bronchoconstriction, which may or may not be overcome by treatment. Only in the former will late reversibility be found, confirming irreversible bronchial obstruction in the latter. Therefore, reversibility becomes an essential point in the differential diagnosis of bronchial obstruction.

In the literature, "reversibility" is more frequently used to indicate the reversal of bronchoconstriction as a consequence of the administration of a spasmolytic agent, therefore implicating bronchospasm in the pathogenesis of obstruction. According to this point of view, detection of reversibility has become a major test in the differential diagnosis of asthma.

Bronchoconstriction can be studied using several parameters of pulmonary function: (a) airway resistance (R_{aw}) can be directly measured plethysmographically and expressed as specific airway conductance (sG_{aw}) or specific airway resistance (sR_{aw}); (b) airway patency can be derived from indirect evaluation of resistance, i.e., measuring forced expiratory volume at 1 s (FEV_1), forced vital capacity (FVC), FEV_1/VC, FEV_1/FVC, peak expiratory flowrate (PEFR), or maximum expiratory flow (MEF) at different values of expired (or residual) pulmonary gas volume.

The plethysmographic parameters have some advantages compared to the spirometric ones as, for example, normal breathing or just panting, so avoiding problems due to forced expiration which, in some subjects, can trigger bronchospasm with a progressive decrease in FEV_1 and FVC [6]. Moreover, plethysmographic measurements include information from thoracic gas volume (usually FRC) measurement, especially sG_{aw}. Although some investigators have shown R_{aw} and sG_{aw} to be more sensitive than spirometry in detecting changes in airway patency [7–9], the additional time required for the procedure and the cost of plethysmography have excluded these parameters from routine evaluation of bronchial obstruction.

By contrast, FEV_1 is a very good indicator of bronchoconstriction, is well-tolerated by the patient, and relatively easily performed. Furthermore, FEV_1 can be easily obtained from many different types of devices, such as bell spirometers, pneumotachographs, and even low cost instruments including computerized spirometers (e.g., turbine spirometers). FEV_1 has a high degree of within- and between-individual reproducibility, its variability being below 5%.

From the same forced expiratory maneuver PEFR and MEF at different values of expired FVC (or at different values of pulmonary residual volume) can be derived. However, the high degree of intra- and interindividual variability of these parameters [10], especially MEF at different lung volumes makes them unsuitable for assessing reversibility. Moreover, measurement of maximal flows at different values of expired FVC can be misleading if, as a consequence of the bronchodilator, FVC increases. In fact, in spite of bronchodilation, MEF values could come out lower than the initial values because of a shift of the point at which the measurement is done [11, 12].

For routine purposes, the most widely used parameter to define bronchial obstruction is FEV_1. The choice of the criterion to establish the lower limit of FEV_1 is a matter of debate. The practice of classifying values less than 80% of predicted as abnormal may be misleading [13, 14] for FEV_1 and especially for instantaneous flows [10]. According to the American Thoracic Society (ATS) recommendations, spirometric values less than the fifth percentile must be interpreted as being below the lower limit of normal [15, 16]. As a consequence, bronchial obstruction may be defined by an FEV_1 less than that limit.

Once obstruction has been detected, checking for reversibility is mandatory in order to reveal a potential bronchospastic component and to quantify it. After a basal measurement, the patient is given a single dose of bronchodilator, usually a β_2-agonist by inhalation.

One of the most popular drugs currently used in Europe to check for reversibility is salbutamol, with other β_2-adrenergic agents being far less popular. Salbutamol is inhaled at a dose of 200 μg., i.e., two actuations of 100 μg, one puff every 1–2 min. Obviously, the way the patient inhales is crucial: at the very beginning of inspiration, after a full expiration, the patient actuates a metered-dose inhaler, always continuing inspiration up to the maximum (to total lung capacity), at which he holds his breath for a few seconds. After a normal expiration and a few breathing cycles, a second inhalation takes place. The metered-dose inhaler is preferably held in front of the open mouth, about 5 cm from the lips (on this point there is no general agreement). In any case, it is preferable that the metered-dose inhaler is actuated by a skilled laboratory operator, in order to best coordinate drug administration with the patient's respiratory movements.

Bronchodilation starts very quickly, within few minutes after inhalation, 80%–90% of the maximal response being achieved in about 10 min. Bronchodilation reaches its maximum level, with a plateau 15–20 min later. At this time, functional measurement is repeated and reversibility calculated.

According to the more extensive meaning of reversibility, if only a partial early reversibility or none has been found, the next step is to check for late reversibility. The patient is administered an other suitable drug in an attempt to treat all the components of bronchoconstriction. This treatment is maintained for a proper period after which functional measurements are repeated. If the treatment results in normalization or a further partial improvement in pulmonary function, the conclusion can be drawn that factors other than bronchospasm were responsible for bronchoconstriction. The component of bronchoconstriction that persists despite therapy has to be considered as a consequence of structural changes of the lung (emphysema, fibrosis).

As for bronchial obstruction, reversibility can be studied using several parameters. Although plethysmographic measurement of R_{aw} and sG_{aw} have the advantage of avoiding triggering bronchospasm in susceptible individuals, there is no agreement on their ability to provide additional (to FEV_1 measurement) information about reversibility [17, 18]. Therefore FEV_1 measurement has become the most widely used means to routinely check for reversibility, other parameters being used according to circumstances.

There is a controversy in the literature with regard to the reversibility value that may be considered significant. Generally speaking, reversibility is diagnosed if the change of any measured parameter after bronchodilator inhalation is higher than the normal variability of that parameter [19–21]. Using FEV_1 measurements (as well as any other suitable parameter) reversibility can be expressed as: (a) the absolute difference: postBD − preBD; (b) a percent of the initial value: postBD − preBD/preBD × 100; or (c) a percent of the predicted value: postBD − preBD/predicted value × 100 (postBD being the functional measurement after and preBD the functional measurement before bronchodilator therapy). Expressing reversibility as a percent of the predicted value has been reported to have some advantages over the other two methods [1, 22]. More frequently, reversibility is related to the basal value of bronchoconstriction. In general, the greater the degree of obstruction, the greater the degree of reversibility expected (if, obviously, the main component of obstruction is bronchospasm) [23, 24].

The bronchodilator response appears inversely correlated with FEV_1 when reversibility is expressed as a percent of the initial value; this inverse correlation does not occur when it is calculated as a percent of predicted or as absolute value. If calculated as a percent of the initial value of FEV_1, reversibility can be overestimated in more obstructed patients, the same small absolute change in FEV_1 being larger when expressed as a percent of the initial than of the expected value. In fact, it seems that, in some patients, there may be a real negative correlation between response and baseline spirometry, while in general this correlation is mostly due to regression towards the mean [1].

A lesser degree of functional obstructive impairment is followed by a lesser degree of reversibility after bronchodilation. The effect of the degree of obstruction in the response to a bronchodilator must be pointed out; 15 % reversibility in a very obstructed and a near normal patient is not comparable [1]. As a consequence, attention must be paid in comparing different bronchodilator studies when the same drug has been used on groups of obstructive patients with different degrees of obstruction, especially if reversibility has been calculated as a percent of the initial value. Differences due to methodological problems may appear as being due to treatment, thereby leading to misinterpretations [1].

In general, a significant response should be more than twice the coefficient of variation of that baseline measurement, namely, 10 %–20 % for R_{aw} [25–28], 9 % for sG_{aw} [29, 30], 0 %–8 % for FEV_1 [31], and 3 %–32 % for MEF_{50} and MEF_{75} [31]. Using the percent difference from the basal value, a change of more than 12%–15% in FEV_1 is needed for reversibility to be diagnosed, an increment up to 8% considered to be within measurement variability [1, 32]. According to ATS recommendations, FEV_1 must increase more than 12% of baseline, together with an absolute increase of 200 ml [16], while the American College of Chest Physicians (ACCP) [33] recommends a 15%–25% increase of FEV_1 over baseline in at least two of three tests (because of possible false negative results).

In COPD patients, because of the intrinsic variability of measurements, significant improvement after bronchodilator therapy has been defined as an increase from baseline of more than 15% for FEV_1 and FVC and 20% for forced expiratory flow (FEF_{25-75}) [17]. The same change of 15% was considered significant for TLC, FRC and residual volume (RV), and a change of over 20% for R_{aw} and sG_{aw}.

Finally, attention must be paid to the within-individual variability of reversibility, which makes confirmation of the diagnosis of asthma somewhat hazardous after just one measurement. Nonetheless, checking for reversibility when an obstructive ventilatory impairment has been detected helps in the differential diagnosis of obstructive diseases, as schematically shown in Fig. 1.

If, after just a single inhaled dose of bronchodilator, FEV_1 reverses to normal, it means that bronchoconstriction is basically due to bronchospasm, a finding consistent (but not conclusive) with the diagnosis of bronchial asthma.

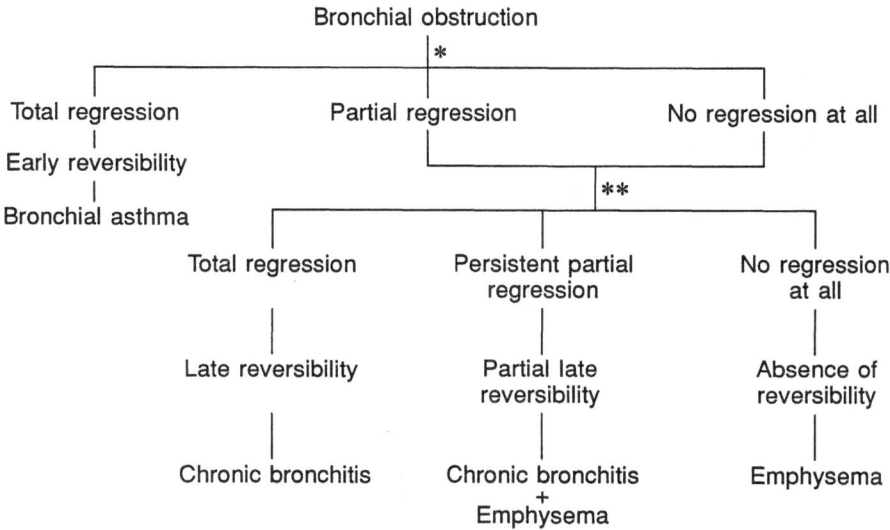

Fig. 1. How reversibility can aid in the differential diagnosis of obstructive diseases. If there is not total regression of obstruction after a single dose of β_2-agonist (*), measurement is repeated after suitable treatment (**)

If FEV_1 reverses only partially or does not reverse at all, this would reveal the presence of inflammatory factors of obstruction needing treatment other than bronchodilators. This could lead to provisional diagnosis of chronic bronchitis or emphysema, being aware, however, that some asthmatic patients with fully reversible airway obstruction may initially fail to respond to inhaled bronchodilators [34, 35] but respond after treatment with corticosteroids [36, 37]. Only the control measurement after treatment will clarify the functional diagnosis.

If FEV_1 does not reverse at all neither after bronchodilator nor after other treatments, this will indicate that bronchial obstruction is not based on bronchospasm. In this case the diagnosis could be chronic bronchitis or emphysema, according to other clinical aspects.

References

1. Eliasson O, Degraff AC (1985) The use of criteria for reversibility and obstruction to define patient groups for bronchodilator trials. Am Rev Respir Dis 132: 858–864
2. Eaton ML, Green BA, Church TR, McGowan T, Niewohner DE (1980) Efficacy of theophylline in "irreversible" airflow obstruction. Ann Intern Med 92:758–761
3. Mendella LA, Manfreda J, Warren CPW, Anthonisen NR (1982) Steroid response in stable chronic obstructive pulmonary disease. Ann Intern Med 96: 17–21
4. Detels R, Tashkin DP, Simmons MS et al. (1982) The UCLA population studies of chronic obstructive respiratory disease. 5: Agreement and disagreement of tests in identifying abnormal lung function. Chest 82:630–638
5. Anonymous (1959) A report of the conclusions of a Ciba Guest Symposium: terminology, definitions and classifications of chronic pulmonary emphysema and related conditions. Thorax 14:286–299
6. Gimeno F, Berg WC, Sluiter HJ, Tammeling GJ (1972) Spirometry-induced bronchial obstruction. Am Rev Respir Dis 105:68–74
7. Anthonisen NR, Wright EC, IPPB trial group (1986) Bronchodilator response in chronic obstructive pulmonary disease. Am Rev Respir Dis 133:814–819
8. Lloyd TC, Wright GW (1963) Evaluation of methods used in detecting changes in airway resistance in man. Am Rev Respir Dis 87:529–537
9. Watanabe S, Renzetti AD, Begin R (1974) Airway responsiveness to a bronchodilator aerosol. Am Rev Respir Dis 109:530–537
10. Knudson RJ, Lebowitz MD, Holberg CJ, Burrows B (1983) Changes in the normal maximal expiratory flow-volume curve with growth and aging. Am Rev Respir Dis 127:725–734
11. Olive JT, Hyatt RE (1972) Maximal expiratory flow and total respiratory resistance during induced broncho-constriction in asthmatic subjects. Am Rev Respir Dis 106:366–376
12. Stanescu DC, Brasseur L (1973) Maximal expiratory flow rates and airway resistance following histamine aerosols in asthmatics. Scand J Respir Dis 54:333–340
13. Oldham PD (1979) Percent of predicted as the limit of normal in pulmonary function testing: a statistically valid approach. Thorax 34:569
14. Miller MR, Pincock AC (1988) Predicted values: how should we use them? Thorax 43:265–267
15. Crapo RO, Morris AH, Gardner RM (1981) Reference spirometric values using techniques and equipment that meet ATS recommendations. Am Rev Respir Dis 123:659–664

16. American Thoracic Society (1991) Lung function testing: selection of reference values and interpretative strategies. Am Rev Respir Dis 144:1202–1218
17. Berger R, Smith D (1988) Acute postbronchodilator changes in pulmonary function parameters in patients with chronic airway obstruction. Chest 93:541–546
18. Light RW, Conrad SA, George RB (1977) The one best test for evaluating the effects of bronchodilator therapy. Chest 72:512–516
19. Hruby J, Butler J (1975) Variability of routine pulmonary function tests. Thorax 30:548–553
20. Garcia JG, Hunninghake GW, Nugent KM (1984) Thoracic gas volume measurement: increased variability in patients with obstructive ventilatory defects. Chest 85:272–275
21. Pelzer AM, Thompson ML (1966) Effect of age, sex, stature and smoking habits on human airway conductance. J Appl Physiol 21:469–476
22. Brand PLP, Quanjer PH, Postma DS et al. (1990) A comparison of different ways to express bronchodilator response, part 2. Am Rev Respir Dis 141:A20
23. Tinkelman DG, Avner SE, Cooper DM (1977) Assessing bronchodilator responsiveness. J Allergy Clin Immunol 59 (2):109–114
24. Lorber DB, Kaltenborn W, Burrows B (1978) Response to isoproterenol in a general population sample. Am Rev Respir Dis 118:855–861
25. Lord PW, Brooks AGF (1977) A comparison of manual and automated methods of measuring airways resistance and thoracic gas volume. Thorax 32:60–66
26. Lord PW, Brooks AGF, Edwards JM (1977) Variation between observers in the estimation of airways resistance and thoracic gas volume. Thorax 32:67–70
27. Lord PW, Edwards JM (1978) Variation in airways resistance when defined over different ranges of airflows. Thorax 33:401–405
28. Zedda S, Sartorelli E (1971) Variability of plethysmographic measurements of airway resistance during the day in normal subjects and in patients with bronchial asthma and chronic bronchitis. Respiration 28:158–166
29. Eiser NM, Mills J, McRae KD, Snashall PD, Guz A (1980) Histamine receptors in normal human bronchi. Clin Sci 58:537–544
30. Pelzer AM, Thompson ML (1969) Body plethysmographic measurements of airway conductance in obstructive pulmonary disease. Am Rev Respir Dis 99:194–204
31. Becklake MR, Permutt S (1979) Evaluation of tests of lung function for "screening" of early detection of chronic obstructive lung disease. In: Macklem PT, Permutt S (eds) Lung Biology in Health and Disease, vol 12: The lung in the transition between health and disease. Dekker, New York, pp 345–387
32. Tweeddale PM, Alexander F, McHardy GJR (1987) Short term variability in FEV_1 and bronchodilator responsiveness in patients with obstructive ventilatory defect. Thorax 42:487–490
33. American College of Chest Physicians (1974) Report of the Committee on Emphysema. Criteria for the assessment of reversibility in airway obstruction. Chest 65:552–553
34. Rebuck AS, Read J (1971) Assessment and management of severe asthma. Am J Med 51:788–798
35. Shenfield GM, Hodson ME, Clarke SW, Paterson JW (1975) Interaction of corticosteroids and catecholamines in the treatment of asthma. Thorax 30:430–435
36. Kalsner S (1969) Mechanism of hydrocortisone potentiation of responses to epinephrine and norepinephrine in rabbit aorta. Circ Res 24:383–395
37. Davies AO, Lefkowitz RJ (1980) Corticosteroid-induced differential regulation of beta-adrenergic receptors in circulating human polymorphonuclear leukocytes and mononuclear leukocytes. J Clin Endocrinol Metab 51:599–605

Part VII

Anatomical Structures Involved in Asthma: Methodology

In Vivo Experimental Methods for Assessing Muscle Tone Involvement in Bronchial Constriction

P. C. BRAGA

Center for Respiratory Pharmacology, School of Medicine, University of Milan, Milano, Italy

Introduction

Tests of pulmonary mechanical function provide information about the state of the lungs, both airways and parenchyma, and about smooth muscle involvement in asthma. Information about the latter can be obtained from measurements in laboratory animals. Several *in vivo* techniques have been described for the investigation of pulmonary function; these can also be used to study the effects of drugs in reversible airways disease.

Changes in smooth muscle tone, especially in small caliber airways, interfere greatly with airway mechanics and flow and induce changes in airway resistance.

Animals of small size are frequently used, with the guinea pig one of the most common. The tests were based on similar ones used to diagnose and manage patients with lung diseases. The major difference is that human pulmonary function is usually measured in awake cooperating individuals, while the animals do not cooperate and are frequently anesthetized. In addition, the measurement of respiratory events in small animals requires both sensitive equipment, because the signals are frequently small, and rapidly responding equipment.

Invasive Methods of Analysis of Smooth Muscle Tone

Methods Involving Anesthesia and Cannulation

Methods involving anesthesia (ether, chloroform, urethane) and minor surgery (tracheal cannulation) are often required and these influence certain respiratory parameters in the recording [1–4].

Konzett and Rossler's method [5] can be used to investigate the action of bronchodilating drugs in guinea pigs with induced bronchoconstriction. Resistance to lung inflation is measured by the overflow technique [5], in which air not entering the animal on inspiration overflows to a pneumotachograph. This method requires deep anesthesia and artificial ventilation of the animals.

Amdur and Mead [6] proposed methods to measure the tidal volume by an air pressure transducer, the intrapleural pressure by a liquid filled intrapleural catheter connected to a transducer to measure transpulmonary pressure, and the rate of flow in the guinea pig lung. This data, obtained with a body plethysmograph, can be used to calculate the pulmonary flow-resistance and compliance. This isovolume technique was applied by Amdur and Mead [6] and originally introduced by Neergard and Wirz [7].

For simple measurement of tidal volume and respiratory rate some physical restraint and anesthesia of the animal are often required [8–11]. Under light ether anesthesia, a catheter is inserted at the level of the sixth intercostal space, near the posterior midline. The catheter is then flushed through regularly with saline containing a small amount of heparin and connected to a pressure transducer to measure intrapleural pressure.

Tidal volume is measured by recording the pressure changes produced by animal breathing in a body plethysmograph connected to a 5 liter reservoir bottle in which a copper sponge is placed to provide a large heat sink, in an attempt to approach isothermal conditions during pressure changes associated with normal breathing.

Rates of air flow in and out of the respiratory system are obtained from electrical differentiation of the volume signals plotted against time.

Figure 1 shows respiratory recordings from a guinea pig [6]. At the time of zero airflow, at the beginning of inspiration and at the end of expiration, no air moves into or out of the respiratory system, so the flow-resistive component drops out and any pressure change must be related to elastic forces alone [6].

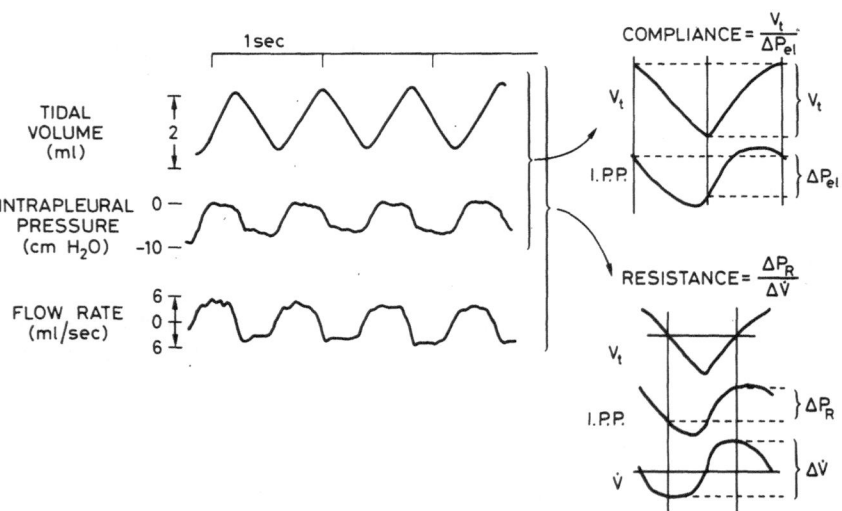

Fig. 1. Graphical method of measuring compliance and pulmonary flow resistance from respiratory tracings (guinea pig)

Lung compliance is the amount of lung expansion (volume changes) per unit of pleural pressure change when the pressure and volume changes are measured at zero airflow.

In conscious humans, this measure can be made during breath holding and is called "static lung compliance." In spontaneously breathing animals, the compliance must be measured as indicated above during cyclic breathing and this measure ($V_t/\Delta P_{el}$ = compliance) is called "dynamic lung compliance (C_{dyn})." It is not a "pure" measurement of lung compliance because the instant of flow reversal may be too short for pressure to reach equilibrium throughout the lungs [12].

During breathing an additional pleural pressure change is required to drive air in or out of the airways. The ratio between this additional pressure drop, across lungs and airways, and the airflow rate is called "pulmonary resistance" [12].

To eliminate the influence of lung expansion on the caliber of airways, the resistance (R_{aw}), which is $\Delta P_R/\Delta \dot{V}$, was measured at points of equal volume. The intrapleural pressure changes between two such points must be related chiefly to resistance to flow in the lungs and airways (see Fig. 1) [6].

Table 1 lists the respiratory parameters, with resistance and compliance obtained for 200 guinea pigs [6].

Breath-by-breath evaluation of the mechanical changes is tedious and time-consuming and a computer computation program has been devised [13].

Comparison of normal and tracheotomized animals suggests that in the guinea pig the upper airway accounts for about 45% of the total resistance to airflow. The tidal volume was decreased and the frequency increased in tracheotimized animals, while the minute volume remained unchanged [6].

The method of Amdur and Mead [6] has also been used successfully over the last 30 years to investigate lung responses to respiratory irritants [14–20]. The advantages of the technique are that it requires minimal equipment and

Table 1. Comparison between resistance and compliance in different situations in guinea pig and humans (from [6])

Parameters	Guinea pig		Human	
	Normal	Tracheotomy	Adult	Infant
Body weight	209 ± 30	192 ± 25	70 (kg)	3.04 (kg)
Respirations/minute	81 ± 13	104 ± 26**		
Tidal volume (ml)	1.07 ± 0.1	1.3 ± 0.3**		
Minute volume (ml)	137 ± 23	125 ± 26		
Resistance	0.69 ± 0.18	0.38 ± 0.16**		
(cm H_2O/ml/s)	(0.35–1.19)			
Compliance	0.22 ± 0.05	0.24 ± 0.04	0.18	0.005
(ml/cm H_2O)	(0.10–0.34)		(l/cm H_2O)	(l/cm H_2O)

** $p \le 0.01$

that it is rapidly and easily performed. The disadvantage of this approach is that differences in inspiratory or expiratory resistance cannot be determined with ease. The limiting factors for these techniques are that they require the use of some sort of anesthesia and surgical preparation.

A second technique, "electrical subtraction" [21], for measuring pulmonary resistance displays the signals of transpulmonary pressure and flow on the x and y axes of an oscilloscope.

A signal proportional to volume change is then electrically subtracted from the total pressure signal until a closed "loop" is obtained.

The advantage of this technique is that inspiratory and expiratory resistance can be separated, and resistance at a specific flow rate and lung volume can be determined. The disadvantage is that rapidly changing pulmonary resistance values may be hard to follow and record without special equipment [22].

Methods Without Anesthesia

Investigating lung mechanics was improved after it was found that the intraesophageal pressure, measured by an esophageal catheter, reflects the intrathoracic pressure rather closely and therefore can be used interchangeably in investigations of lung mechanics [23–26].
Skornik et al. [27] reported a method for measurement of pulmonary mechanics using plethysmography and esophageal pressure to determine total volume, compliance, resistance, frequency, and minute volume in the guinea pig. The procedure is not surgical, does not require anesthesia, and can be used for repeated measurements in the same animal. The plethysmographic method of Amdur and Mead [6] was adopted with one major modification, substitution of the intrathoracic catheter with a nose cone which seals around the head.

Through a port in the nose cone a liquid-filled intraesophageal catheter is inserted through a short length of brass tubing, which prevents the animal's biting through the catheter. Its location in the stomach is ascertained when the pressure swings are positive with respect to the ambient pressure [27].

Pulmonary compliance and resistance are determined by the classical zero-crossing method, based on breath-to-breath data [6]. Measurements of respiratory mechanics were also made in the ferret, with the animal supine and sealed in a pressure plethysmograph with an esophageal cannula [28]. In the zero-crossing method, (dynamic) compliance is defined as the volume change produced by a unit of pressure change averaged over two extreme points which coincide with zero airflow. Thus compliance is computed by dividing the volumetric change (full inspiration and full expiration) during each breath by the corresponding differential pressure. Pulmonary resistance is similarly calculated as the ratio of flow or peak flow, as determined at selected test points, to the corresponding pressures. Data are analyzed by computer, and pressure-flow and pressure-volume loops are obtained. In this way a population of animals can be screened prior to the study to determine those animals which may differ substantially from the group [27].

Other plethysmographic methods use different approaches, for instance, head-out body plethysmography with pleural catheterization [17] or head-out body plethysmography with esophageal catheterization [27]. In addition, there are whole-body plethysmography with tracheal cannulation [29, 30] and body plethysmography using two chambers [31–33].

Noninvasive Methods of Analysis of Smooth Muscle Tone

Plethysmographs are generally subdivided into pressure, volume, and barometric plethysmographs.

A pressure plethysmograph is a closed system that encloses the animal's body either at the neck or at an extension of the trachea (by transoral or intratracheal cannula). As the animal breathes to the outside, the expansion and contraction of its thorax cyclically compresses and decompresses the gas inside the sealed box. The resulting pressure changes can be measured by a transducer and, when calibrated as volume, can be used to determine ventilation during tidal breathing or to estimate volume changes during an imposed maneuver [34]. Pressure plethysmographs are convenient to use because pressure and volume are directly proportional so long as the system is functionally isothermal or functionally adiabatic. Since the volume of a plethysmograph for small animals is generally small, variations of heat (during respiration) are too fast, making adiabatic function impossibile, so the alternative is to try to make the system behave isothermally [35]. The most commonly used method is to fill the reservoir attached to the animal chamber portion of the plethysmograph with a material which has a high heat capacity and a large surface area. Copper sponges have been used for this purpose, since they will quickly absorb and release the heat and the system will be nearly isothermal [26, 35].

A volume or flow plethysmograph is essentially similar to a pressure plethysmograph except that it has an opening (calibrated) to the outside which can be connected directly to a spirometer to measure volume changes. A resistance element (stainless steel mesh of known resistance) is placed across the hole in the box and the flow should be proportional to the pressure drop across this element. Volume is obtained by electronically integrating this flow signal [36, 37].

A barometric plethysmograph, the third type of plethysmograph, requires only a sealed box, a pressure transducer, an unrestrained animal, and temperature and humidity sensors [38]. If an animal is in a closed chamber, the gas entering its lungs is warmed and humidified and therefore expands. This results in a pressure change in the system which is proportional to the tidal ventilation [35, 39]. Animal movements, gross breathing, changes in room temperature and humidity, and difficulty of calibration are some of the factors that limit extensive use of this plethysmograph.

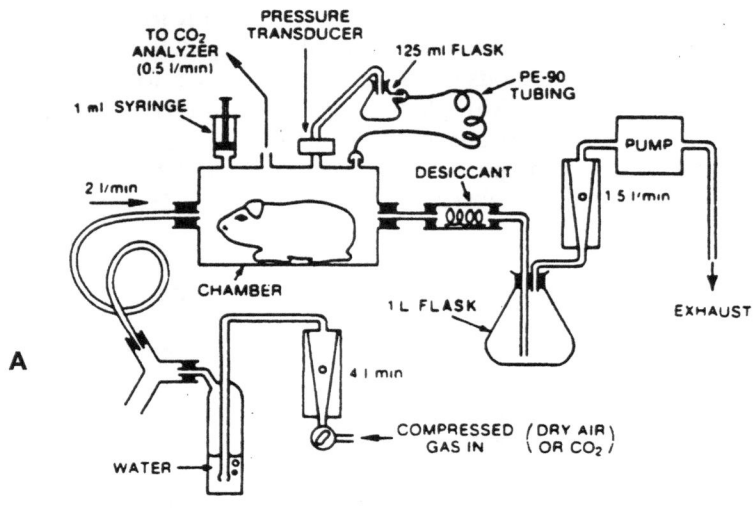

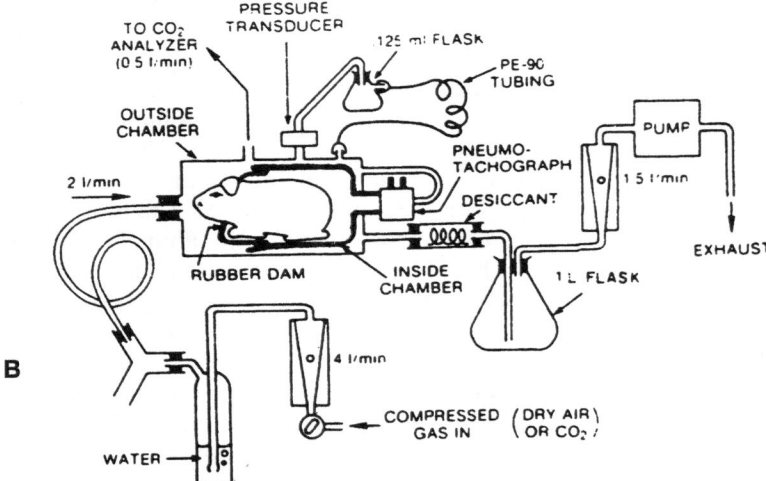

Fig. 2. A Whole body plethysmograph with a flow-through arrangement which permits measurement of ΔP_c, proportional to V_T, of an unanesthetized guinea pig breathing room air or a mixture containing various concentrations of CO_2 in 20% O_2 with the balance being N_2. When testing the CO_2 response during challenge with an aerosol, an absolute filter should be placed before the flow meter; such a device will not interfere with performance of the system.
B Arrangement of a body plethysmograph (*inside chamber*) inside a whole body plethysmograph (*outside chamber*) to verify that ΔP_c increases during CO_2 challenge are proportional to V_T, which was determined from integration with time of airflow, measured by a pneumotachograph, created by thoracic displacement in the inside chamber. (From [42])

Functional assessment of a smaller animal requires measurement of rapid events of minute amplitude. This means sensitivity and responsiveness, so the system must have linear behavior (the box must act either isothermally or adiabatically) and phase concordance, especially between the transducers, whose outputs should be phase matched [34].

When an animal is in a body plethysmograph (a hermetically closed chamber), we can observe a change in pressure in correspondence with each breath. The pressure amplitude for each cycle is proportional to tidal volume and is produced by the fact that the air, at 20°–24 °C, in the plethysmograph is humidified and heated to body temperature (37.5 °C) in the lung, thus creating an increase in pressure in the whole body plethysmograph. The reverse occurs during expiration [28, 40–43].

The pressure changes in the plethysmograph (Fig. 2A) are measured by a differential pressure transducer [43].

One port of the transducer is attached directly to one port of the whole body plethysmograph, while the other port of the transducer is connected to another port of the whole body plethysmograph through 125 cm of PE-90 tubing in series with a 125 ml flask [43]. The long time constant (8–10 s) created by the narrow tubing and flask connected to port 2 of the differential pressure transducer makes it possible ot not to use the reference chamber system [44] and keeps the baseline very stable during long periods of recording [45].

A body plethysmograph inside a whole body plethysmograph system has been used (Fig. 2B) [43] to verify that the pressure changes in the plethysmograph are accurate reflections of tidal volume both in normal conditions and during exposure, for instance, to 10% CO_2 [43].

A body plethysmograph method for measuring respiratory changes in conscious mice and rats has also been described [46–49].

Double plethysmography is another recent method proposed for measurement of pulmonary mechanics without prior surgery. The adopted procedures enable measurement of a new parameter called "specific airway resistance" or specific airway conductance (sG_{aw}). One is the reciprocal of the other.

Specific airway resistance is not a pure resistance but is the product of resistance times volume. The volume is the thoracic gas volume (TGV), which is to say, the tidal volume plus the functional residual capacity.

Airway resistance is defined as the pressure difference between the alveoli and mouth divided by airflow and it is dependent upon the volume of air in the lungs, the thoracic gas volume (TGV). sG_{aw} is the reciprocal of airway resistance per unit of TGV [50].

Agraval [51] measured sG_{aw} in a constant volume plethysmograph without the need to occlude airflow to obtain alveolar pressure [52] or to measure TGV [53]. In this method the snout of an unanesthetized unrestrained guinea pig is pushed into a cone connected with a pneumotachograph which measures the airflow. The entire animal plus pneumotachograph is enclosed within a sealed box (barometric plethysmograph) (Fig. 3).

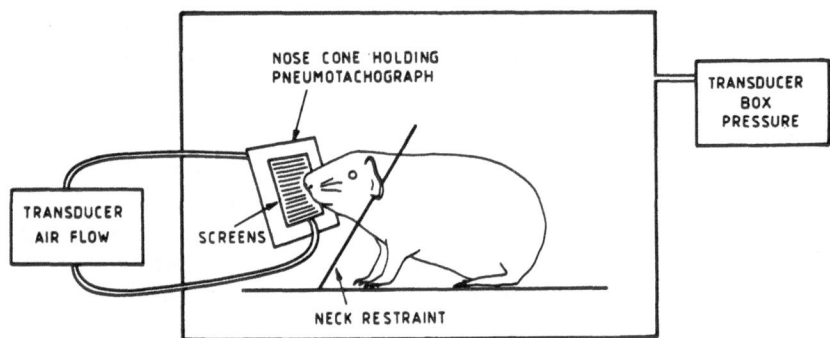

Fig. 3. Box configuration to measure specific airway resistance according to method of Agraval [56]. Box pressure and nasal flow are measured. (From [61])

Variations in box pressure are measured by a pressure transducer as differences between chest volume changes and air volume respired at atmospheric pressure and fed to the x axis of an x–y recorder. The airflow signal was fed to its y axis. A loop was formed [51].

The slope of the flow-volume loop as expiration goes into inspiration is proportional to specific airway conductance and that is the reciprocal of specific airway resistance. The decline in sG_{aw}, after a static exposure to histamine in the nose chamber, was interpreted as an indication of bronchoconstriction [51].

Temperature and humidity changes of respired air during the respiratory cycle affected the measurement of airway resistance. In a constant volume sealed plethysmograph these factors directly affect the box pressure value (Boyle's law). To overcome the errors due to these factors, some possibilities have been proposed, e.g., an electronic compensation proportional to the respired air volume [54], warming and humidification of inspired air to achieve constant body temperature, pressure, and saturation (BTPS) conditions [55], and panting through a heated pneumotachograph [53].

During normal breathing there are only very small changes in lung volume at the points of reversal of respiration. Thus, resistance measurements made at this point will be virtually free of temperature and humidity artifacts [56]. sG_{aw} measurements are made at the point of reversal of respiratory flow (end expiration), which avoids the need for complicated methods of controlling the temperature-humidity artifact (Fig. 4).

For long-term measurements a bias flow system can be adopted. These criteria are also followed by Clay and Thompson [57] and by Griffiths-Johnson et al. [58], who use a face mask, an animal restrainer, and a plethysmograph,

Dorsch et al. [33] used double chamber plethysmography, one a body chamber and the other a respiratory chamber fixed around the head of the guinea pig. The volume changes in the respiratory chamber were plotted against those of the body chamber by an x–y plotter. If gases were to be

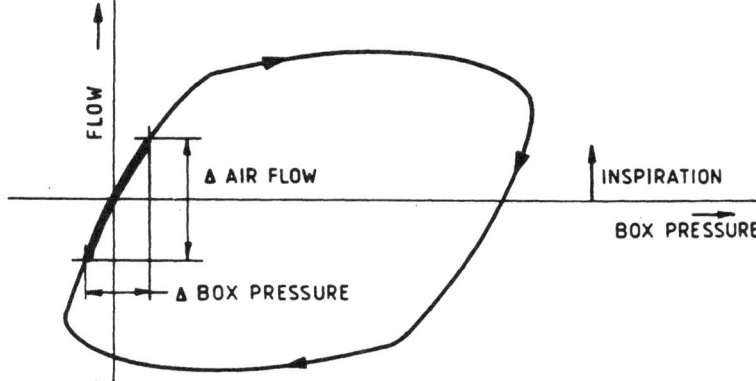

Fig. 4. Example of the loop obtained by plotting airflow vs box pressure. The slope of the loop at the transition of expiration to inspiration is proportional to specific airway conductance. (From [61])

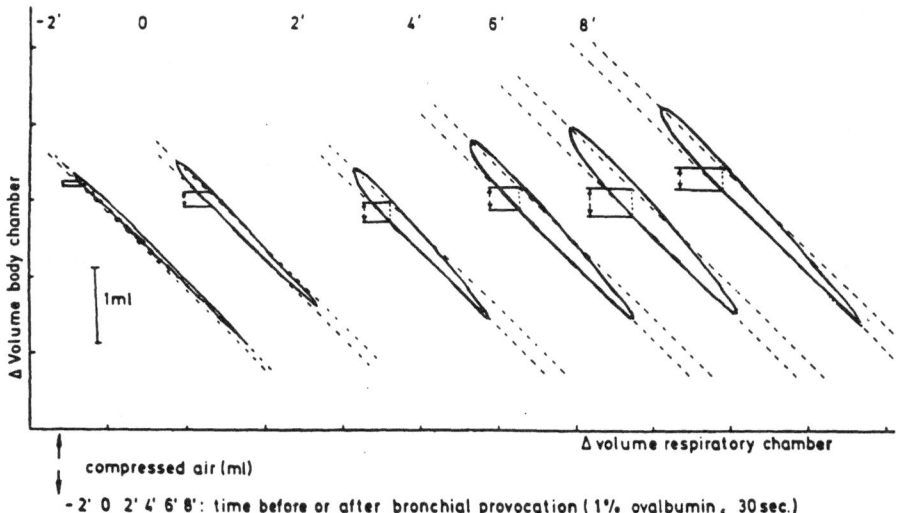

Fig. 5. Measurement of compressed air during an inhalation allergen challenge in a sensitized guinea pig; compressed air is defined as the deviation of the respiratory loop from the *dotted expiratory* −*45° line*; we used the maximal amount of compressed air in a respiration loop as a measure of bronchial obstruction. (From [32])

transported without any resistance from one to the other chamber, the x–y recorder would draw a straight −45° line.

However, in overcoming the physiological airway resistance, intrapulmonary air must be compressed during expiration and expanded during inspiration. This phenomenon is reflected by small deviations from the −45 °C line, with the result that a losed loop is drawn (Fig. 5) [33]. The area enclosed by

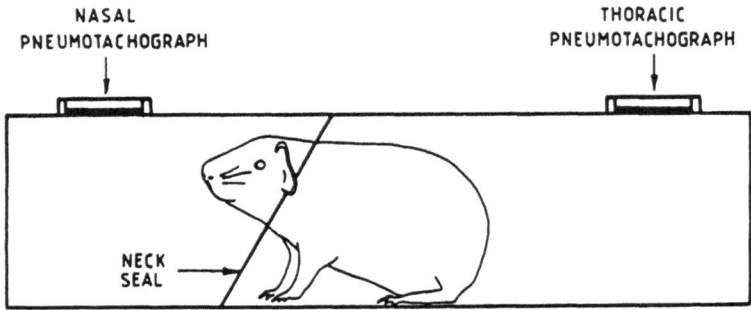

Fig. 6. Plot of a double chamber plethysmograph. (From [60])

the loop reflects the degree of airway obstruction [33]. In pharmacological tests, the parameter compressed air was more than ten times as sensitive as specific airway conductance for indicating bronchial obstruction [33].

Matijak-Schaper et al. [59] simplified and improved on the Agraval design by adding a high resistance port in the barometric plethysmograph to reduce baseline drift and by using the head chamber as a dynamic exposure system [34]. Another system is that of Pennock [60], who used a double body box. The animal is held by a neck seal in a thoracic chamber and thoracic movements are measured through a pneumotachograph. The head is placed in another chamber and nasal flow is measured with another pneumotachograph (Fig. 6). When the animal's chest expands, a breath is drawn but there is a time-lag between when the animal's diaphragm initiates the breath and the instant that the air flows into the animal. That time lag is proportional to the resistance of the airways and the pulmonary system and to the total volume of air (TGV) within [61].

Another approach is that of Silbaugh et al. [62], who used a standard head-out pressure plethysmograph placed inside a barometric plethysmograph. They calculated the ratio of V_t from the pressure plethysmograph to prime V'_t, from the barometric plethysmograph and correlated V_t/V'_t and dynamic compliance (using the Amdur-Mead technique).

The above mentioned methods provide information on airway smooth muscle tone and have the advantage of being noninvasive. The animal can be tested repeatedly. At the same time, they require an environment of relatively stable temperature and humidity. Phase-matching problems can arise in double plethysmograph techniques and they provide only relative measures of pulmonary function.

References

1. Berendt RF (1968) The effect of physical and chemical restraint on selected respiratory parameters of macace mulatta. Lab Anim Care 18:391–394
2. Richardson PS, Widdicombe JG (1969) The role of the vagus nerve in the ventilatory responses to hypercapnia and hypoxia in anesthetized and unanesthetized rabbits. Respir Physiol 7:122–135
3. Dixon W, Brodie TG (1903) Contribution to the physiology of the lungs. I. The bronchial muscles, their innervation, and the action of drugs upon them. J Physiol 24:97–173
4. Dale HH, Laidlaw PP (1910) The physiological action of β-imidazolylethylamine. J Physiol 41:318–344
5. Konzett H, Rossler R (1940) Versuchsanordnung zu Untersuchungen an der Bronchialmuskulatur. Naunyn-Schmiedebergs Arch Pharmakol 195:71–74
6. Amdur MO, Mead J (1958) Mechanics of respiration in unanesthetized guinea-pigs. Am J Physiol 192:364–368
7. Neerrgard K, Wirz K (1927) Die Messung der Strömungswiderstände in den Atemwegen des Menschen, insbesondere beim Asthma und Emphysem. Z Clin Med 105:51–82
8. Guyton AC (1947) Measurement of the respiratory volumes of laboratory animals. J Appl Physiol 150:70–77
9. Ekberg DR, Hance HE (1960) Respiration measurements in mice. J Appl Physiol 15:321–324
10. Mead J (1960) Control of respiratory frequency. J Appl Physiol 15:325–336
11. Crosfill ML, Widdicombe JG (1961) Physical characteristics of the chest and lungs and the work of breathing in different mammalian species. J Physiol 158:1–14
12. Douglas JS, Dennis MW, Ridgway P, Bouhuys A (1972) Airway dilatation and constriction in spontaneously breathing guinea pigs. J Pharmacol Exp Ther 180:98–109
13. Dennis MW, Douglas JS, Casby JU, Stolwijk JA, Bouhuys J (1969) On-line analog computer for dynamic lung compliance and pulmonary resistance. J Appl Physiol 26:248–252
14. Comroe JH, Nisell OI, Nims RG (1954) A simple method for concurrent measurement of compliance and resistance to breathing in anesthetized animals and man. J Appl Physiol 7:225–228
15. Amdur MO (1959) The physiologic responses of guinea pigs to atmospheric pollutants. Int J Air Pollut 1:170–183
16. Amdur MO (1966) Respiratory absorption data and SO_2-response curves. Arch Environ Health 12:729–732
17. Amdur MO, Dubriel M, Creasia DA (1978) Respiratory response of guinea pigs to low levels of sulphuric acid. Environ. Res. 15:418–423
18. Costa DL, Amdur MO (1979) Effect of oil mists on irritancy of sulphyr dioxide. I. Mineral oil and light lubricating oil. Am Ind Hyg Assoc J 40:680–785
19. Costa DL, Amdur MO (1979) Respiratory response of guinea pigs to oil mists. Am Ind Hyg Assoc J 40:673–679
20. Nayler RA, Mitchell HW (1987) Airways hyperreactivity and bronchoconstriction induced by vanadate in the guinea-pig. Br J Pharmacol 92:173–180
21. Mead J, Whittenberger JL (1953) Physical properties of human lungs measured during spontaneous respiration. J Appl Physiol 5:779–796
22. Drazen JM, Loring SH, Regan R (1976) Validation of an automated determination of pulmonary resistance by electrical subtraction. J Appl Physiol 40:110–114
23. Fry DL, Stead WW, Ebert RW, Lulbin RI, Wells HS (1952) The measurement of intraesophageal pressure and its relationship to intrathoracic pressure. J Lab Clin Med 40:664–673

24. Cherniak RM, Farhi LE, Armstrong BW, Proctor DF (1956) A comparison of esophageal and intrapleural pressure in man. J Appl Physiol 8:203–211
25. Palace KF (1969) Measurement of ventilatory mechanics in the rat. J Appl Physiol 27:149–156
26. Koo KW, Leith DE, Shester CB, Snider GL (1976) Respiratory mechanics in normal hamsters. J Appl Physiol 40:936–942
27. Skornik WA, Heimann R, Jaeger RJ (1981) Pulmonary mechanics in guinea pigs: repeated measurements using a nonsurgical computerized method. Toxicol Appl Pharmacol 59:314–323
28. Vinegar A, Sinnett E, Kosch PC (1982) Respiratory mechanics of small carnivore: the ferret. J Appl Physiol 52:832–837
29. Gjuris V, Heicke R, Westermann E (1964) Über die Stimulierung der Atmung durch Bradykinin und Kallidin. Naunyn-Schmiedebergs Arch Exp Pathol Pharmakol 247:429–444
30. Koller EA (1962) Die Wirkung von Micoren auf Atmung und Blutdruck. Helv Physiol Acta 20:47–102
31. Johanson WG Jr, Pierce AK (1971) A noninvasive technique for measurement of airway conductance in small animals. J Appl Physiol 30:146–150
32. Gordont B, Pistorius D (1974) Tierexperimentelle Lungenfunktions-analysen während Inhalation von Zinkoxidstaub. Zentralbl. Bakteriol (Naturwiss, Abt 1) A277:166–120
33. Dorsch W, Waldherr U, Rosmanith J (1981) Continuous recording of intrapulmonary "compressed air" as a sensitive noninvasive method of measuring bronchial obstruction in guinea-pigs. Pflügers Arch 391:236–241
34. Costa DL, Tepper JS (1988) Approaches to lung function assessment in small mammals. In: Gardner DE, Crapo JD, Massaro EJ (eds) Toxicology of the lung. Raven, New York, pp 147–174
35. O'Neil JJ, Raub JA (1984) Pulmonary function testing in small laboratory mammals. Environ Health Perspect 56:11–22
36. Sinnett EE, Jackson AC, Leith DE, Butler JP (1981) Fast integrated flow plethysmograph for small mammals. J Appl Physiol 50:1104–1110
37. Jackson AC, Vinegar A (1979) A technique for measuring frequency response of pressure, volume and flow-transducers. J Appl Physiol 47:462–467
38. Chapin JL (1954) Ventilatory response of the unrestrained and unanesthetized hamster to CO_2. Am J Physiol 17:146–148
39. Drorbaugh JE, Fenn WO (1955) A barometric method for mesuring ventilation in newborn infants. Pediatrics 16:81–86
40. Chapin H (1954) The ventilatory response of the unrestrained hamster to carbondioxide. Am J Physiol 179:146–148
41. Drobaugh JE, Fenn WO (1955) A barometric method for measuring ventilation in newborn infants. Pediatrics 16:81–87
42. Bargeton D, Gauge P (1959) Observation barometrique de la ventilation pulmonaire chez l'homme sous contact instrumental. J Physiol 51:395–396
43. Wong KL, Alaire Y (1982) A method for repeated evaluation of pulmonary performance in unanesthetized, unrestrained guinea pigs and its application to detect effects of sulfuric acid mist inhalation. Toxicol Appl Pharmacol 63:72–90
44. Jacky JP (1978) A plethysmograph for long-term mesurements of ventilation in unrestrained animal. J Appl Physiol 45:644–647
45. Karol MH, Stadler J, Underhill D, Alayre Y (1981) Monitoring delayed-onset pulmonary hypersensitivity in guinea pigs. Toxicol Appl Pharmacol 61:277–285
46. Kokka N, Elliott HW, Way WL (1965) Some effects of morphine on respiration and metabolism of rats. J Pharmacol Exp Ther 148:386–392
47. Nelson RB, Elliott MW (1967) A comparison of some central effects of morphine, morphinone and the brain on rats and mice. J Pharmacol Exp Ther 155:516–520
48. Oktay S, Onur R, Ilhan M, Turker RK (1981) Potentiation of the morphine-in-

duced respiratory rate depression by captopril: Eur J Pharmacol 70:257–262
49. Kigasawa K, Saitoh K, Tanizaki A, Ohkubo K, Iirino O (1984) A new method for measuring respiration in the conscious mouse. J Pharmacol Methods 12:183–189
50. Tattersfield AE, Keeping IM (1981) Assessing change in airway calibre-measurement of airway resistance. In: Howell JL, Tattersfield AE (eds) Respiratory system – methods in clinical pharmacology, vol 2. MacMillan, New York, pp 25–38
51. Agrawal KP (1981) Specific airway conductance in guinea pigs: normal values and histamine induced fall. Respir Physiol 43:23–30
52. Von Neergaard J, Wirz K (1927) Die Messung der Strömungswiderstände in den Atemwegen der Menschen, insbesondere bei Asthmas und Emphysema. Z Klin Med 105:51–82
53. Du Bois AB, Botelho SY, Comroe JH (1956) A new method for measuring airway resistance in man using a body plethysmograph. J Clin Invest 35:327–325
54. Bargeton G, Barres G, Lefebvre des Noettes, Gauge P (1957) Resistance des voies aeriennes de l'homme au cours du cycle respiratoire. C R Soc Biol 151: 427–432
55. Jaeger MJ, Ottis AB (1964) Measurement of airway resistance with a volume displacement body plethysmograph. J Appl Physiol 19:813–820
56. Agrawal KP, Kumar A (1980) Fall in specific airway conductance at residual volume in small airway obstruction. Respir Physiol 40:65–78
57. Clay TP, Thompson MA (1983) Plethysmographic determination of histamine independent lung dysfunction following antigen provocation of conscious guineapigs. Br J Pharmacol 79:418P
58. Griffiths-Johnson DA, Nicholls PJ, McDermott M (1988) Measurement of specific airway conductance in guinea pigs. A noninvasive method. J Pharmacol Methods 19:233–242
59. Matijak-Schaper M, Wong KL, Alaire Y (1983) A method to rapidly evaluate the acute pulmonary effects of aerosols in unanesthetized guinea pigs. Toxicol Appl Pharmacol 69:451–460
60. Pennock BE (1987) A double flow body plethysmograph for measuring specific airflow conductance. In: Zink R (ed) Mess- und Auswerteanlage zur Bestimmung von Parametern der Atemmechanik. Atmung und Beamtung Biomesstechnik. Sachs, Freiburg, pp 75–104
61. Lomask MR (1987) Respiratory mechanics analyzer for noninvasive measurements on conscious animals. In: Zink R (ed) Atmung und Beatmung Biomesstechnik. Sachs, Freiburg, pp 216–226
62. Silbaugh SA, Mauderly JL, MacKenc A (1981) Effects of sulfuric acid and nitrogen dioxide on airway responsiveness of the guinea pig. J Toxicol Environ Health 8:31–45

In Vitro Experimental Methods for Assessing Tracheobronchial Smooth Muscle Contraction

P. C. BRAGA

Center for Respiratory Pharmacology, School of Medicine, University of Milan, Milano, Italy

Introduction

Both the physiological and pathological changes in the mechanical behavior of tracheobronchial smooth muscles (shortening or development of tension) have been widely studied. There have been many studies to characterize and to reproduce the muscular aspects of the "asthma phenomenon" and pharmacological correction of it.

Tracheal and bronchial smooth muscle (like other muscle) are complex biological systems and the changes which lead to a contraction are the last step of a specific event involving an increase in membrane conductance, membrane depolarization and hyperpolarization, and changes in firing, all of which change the complex viscoelastic properties of the system.

In vitro and *in vivo* methods have been developed to investigate the functioning of smooth muscles. In this chapter the *in vitro* methods are reviewed.

Since the introduction of *in vitro* studies with isolated organs by Magnus in 1904 [1] many different *in vitro* preparations of bronchial tissue from different animals have been proposed. *In vitro* experimental studies of the mechanical behavior of tracheal or bronchial smooth muscle require: (1) an appropriate tissue specimen, (2) a container able to maintain vital physiological properties, and (3) a lever-transducer-recorder system to measure muscle force and variations in length. Even the best combination of the several components of this apparatus requires the acceptance of some technical and experimental compromises, with conflicting theoretical physical and physiological requirements.

Tissue Sampling

The tracheobronchial musculature of all common laboratory animals and of humans has been investigated.

For animals general anesthesia (ethylurethane, pentobarbital, etc.) is used to anesthetize the animal before the trachea is dissected and cut from the larynx to the carina or other pulmonary tissue removed. Otherwise, for small animals cervical dislocation or stunning and exsanguination are frequently used. For larger animals (pig, sheep, etc.) trachea and lungs can be obtained from the local slaughterhouse. Human samples of lung tissue can be obtained, always by permission, from patients with carcinoma during surgery or during other lung surgery. Post-mortem material can be used, after appropriate control of its reactivity, but is not easy to obtain it fresh enough except occasionally from fatal accident cases. Another source could be human fetuses from therapeutic abortions, from which preparations can be made from the trachea and primary bronchi [2].

The validity of the recorded data depends on the state of functioning and the conditions of maintenance of the tissue specimen, so particular care must be taken during dissection of the tissue specimen not to pull or stretch it during mounting of the preparation in the bath and connecting it to the lever system. If the lever is not properly balanced, the tissue may suddenly be grossly overloaded and damaged. Biological tissues are very sensitive to metals, especially iron, copper, and mercury. Attention must be paid to the types of material in contact with the tissue during preparation and maintenance (forceps, scissors, pins, etc.).

Organ Bath

The organ bath is a particular type of glass (Pyrex) container in which the tissue under investigation is placed and maintained in stable conditions, theoretically as close as possible to physiological conditions.

Figure 1 shows some examples of organ baths. The shape is generally cylindrical. The volume of the bath can vary according to the volume of the tissue and the requirements of the study. A small glass hook at the bottom of the bath ensures attachment of the tissue; it can also be attached to a stainless steel tube of appropriate shape inserted in the bath. The organ bath generally has a port in its lower part into which the feeding medium is introduced, while the volume in excess is discharged from the upper part of the

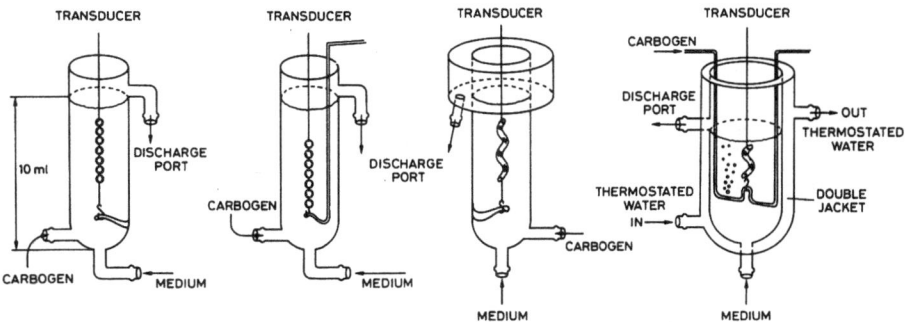

Fig. 1. Different types of organ baths used to investigate tracheobronchial smooth muscle contraction

bath through another port. Washing by upward gentle displacement and overflow is recommended to prevent damage that can occur to some tissues during downward draining. Another port is generally present to introduce a carbon dioxide-oxygen mixture to keep the pH balanced. The shape and the volume of the organ bath can be varied according to the kind of investigation.

The organ bath is generally placed in a larger container filled with water and thermostatically controlled (generally to 37°C) to maintain a stable temperature of the medium inside the bath. The vital functions of mammalian and avian tissue may last longer in vitro at lower temperatures than 37°C, but their sensitivity to drugs is often markedly altered by changes in temperature, even as small as 1°C. It is therefore essential to use a thermostat to maintain the temperature within 0.5°C.

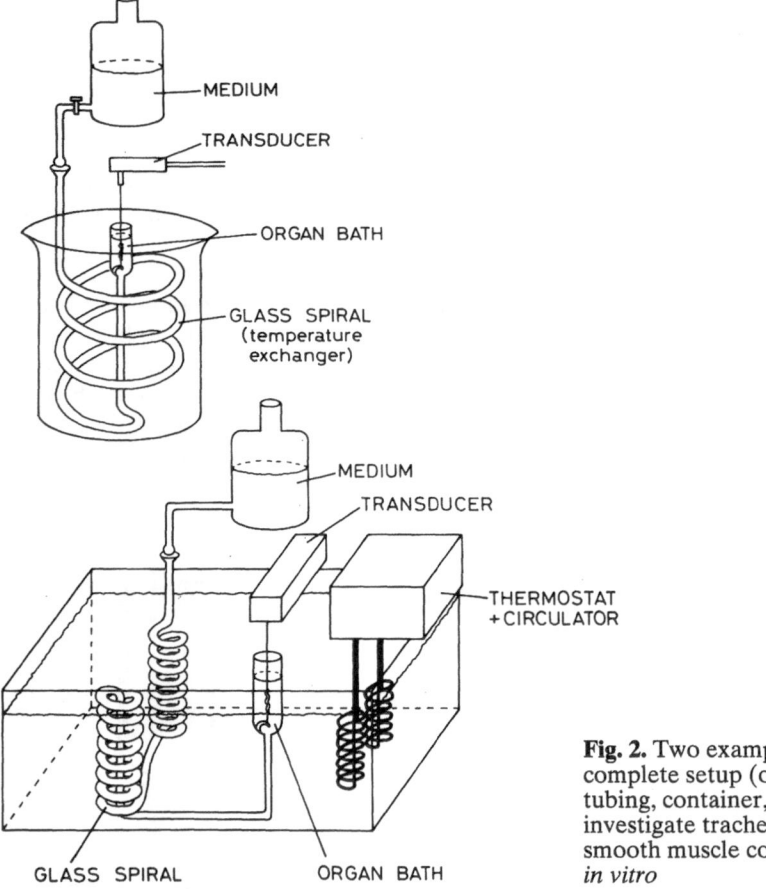

Fig. 2. Two examples of the complete setup (organ bath, tubing, container, etc.) to investigate tracheobronchial smooth muscle contraction *in vitro*

In the container shown in Fig. 2, there is also a long spiral tube of glass, to reduce the overall length, in which the medium from the container (Mariotte bottle) flows to warm the cold medium and maintain its temperature to avoid thermal shock to the tissue when the organ bath is flushed out.

The volume of fluid in this tube must be two or, better, three times the corresponding volume of the organ bath, to avoid temperature shock while washing the organ bath. Washing consists of displacing the fluid in the bath with fresh prewarmed and preaerated (with O_2-CO_2) Kreb's solution.

Tubing connecting the glass coil, the bath, and every other item in contact with physiological solutions must be free of toxic materials, such as the filler or antioxidant contained in rubber or plastic tubing.

The whole setup, organ bath, tubing, and container, must be cleaned and washed with distilled water after use to inhibit the growth of microorganisms. The glass parts should be periodically cleaned with detergents or in chromic acid. Chromic acid can be prepared from a saturated solution of sodium dichromate, adding sufficient concentrated sulphuric acid to redissolve the CrO_3 which is formed.

The solution must be made up in a Pyrex glass container and is dangerous because it is very caustic. Glassware should not be left in chromic acid for more than about 12 h and must be rinsed thoroughly (first with water and then with distilled water) to remove traces of chromium[3].

Tissue Preparation Techniques

Chains of Tracheal or Bronchial Rings

Castillo and de Beer [4], in 1947, introduced the use of an isolated bronchial muscle preparation, consisting of a chain of guinea pig tracheal rings, to investigate the effect of bronchoconstricting and bronchodilating drugs.

Basically the method consists of isolating the trachea, as described above, and then cutting the tissue in the spaces between the cartilaginous rings (Fig. 3A) to obtain single isolated tracheal rings that are then tied together with cotton loops with the muscular parts of the rings in alignment and mounted in a bath (Fig. 3B).

Due to the small size of the muscles, only small amounts of tone relaxation can be obtained. Other experimental difficulties are the relatively slow response to drugs and recovery (generally long) and the wide variation in the sensitivities of individual animals.

Akcasu [5] opened the tracheal rings by cutting through the cartilage, and this maneuver increased the sensitivity to drugs by a factor of three (Fig. 3C). Subsequently, he cut away most of the cartilage and tied the remaining cartilaginous ends together [6]. Interindividual variability between chains was reduced by Foster's expedient [7] of forming a chain in which the odd numbered rings from one animal (guinea pig) were tied to the even numbered rings from a second animal (a third animal can also be used) (Fig. 3D).

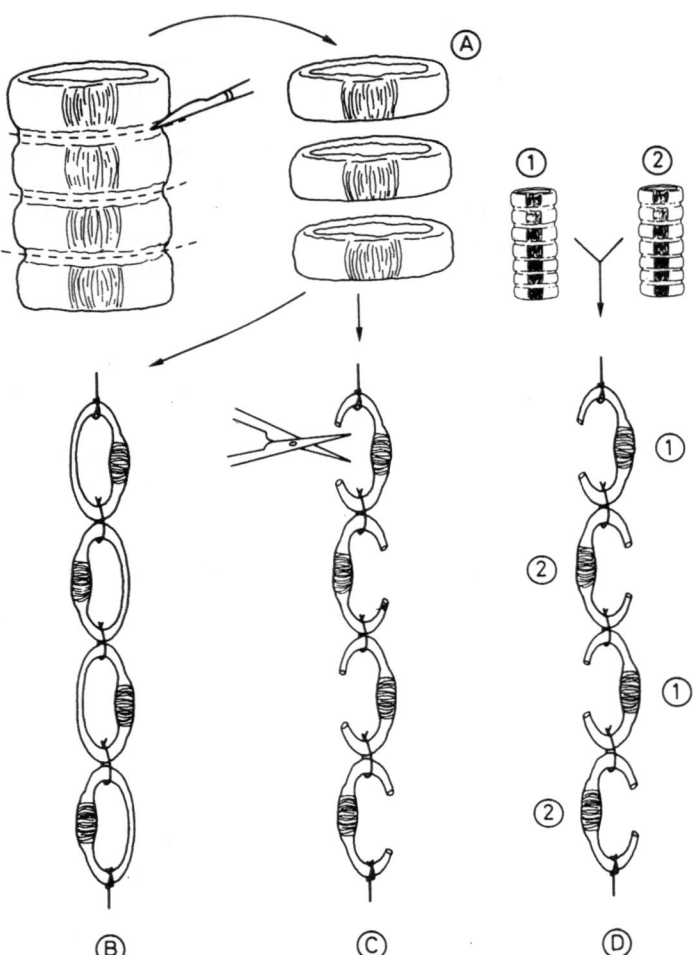

Fig. 3. A–D. Procedure to obtain a chain of tracheal or bronchial rings. *A* Cutting of the tracheal rings; *B* chain of rings tied together; *C* opening the cartilaginous part of the ring to increase the sensitivity; *D* how to reduce the interindividual variability, odd rings from one animal (*1*) even rings from a second animal (*2*)

Each ring is opened by cutting through the cartilage. The remaining rings can be pooled to form a second preparation, which in this construction is identical with the first.

The technique of combining tracheal or bronchial rings from different experimental animals or from humans (from secondary bronchi lumen, diameter 6–8 mm, to fifth order bronchi lumen, diameter about 1 mm) [2] has been widely used to investigate drug action during sessions of several hours [8].

Tracheal or Bronchial Spirals

The preparation and manipulation of the tracheal chain is laborious and the magnitude of the recorded responses is small [9]; the spirally cut tracheal strip can overcome these problems.

To obtain this preparation the excised trachea or bronchus, with a small glass or stainless steel rod inserted in the trachea as a support, is cut from end to end spirally with two or three separated segments of cartilage in each turn of the spiral [9] (Fig. 4). Depending on the length, the entire spiral can be used or it can be cut in half to obtain two preparations from one donor. The tracheal or bronchial spirals are generally left in the bath for 1 h to equilibrate, with the tension depending on the kind of specimen. During the equilibration period, the bathing medium must be changed three to four times.

The imposed tension is necessary because the tissue is not homogeneous and the cut, semicircular, cartilaginous ring exerts an elastic recoil. Therefore, to clearly demonstrate contraction of the muscular part, the spiral must be straightened out by applying tension, for instance 5 g for a tracheal spiral from guinea pig [9] or 1 g for a bronchial spiral from chicken [10]. Attention must also be paid to applying appropriate resting tension, because an erroneous resting tension to stretch the muscle could lead to inconsistent results when testing drugs, because of poor contraction.

The angle of the cutting spiral must always be the same, to avoid increasing the variability of the responses evoked. Cutting of the spiral should theoretically be done always by the same experienced person [11].

In humans, lung tissue is usually obtained from autopsies up to 14 h postmortem and from thoracotomies performed because of bronchial carcinoma. In the first tissue the influence of hypoxia is not easy to evaluate, so the latter type of tissue is used more frequently.

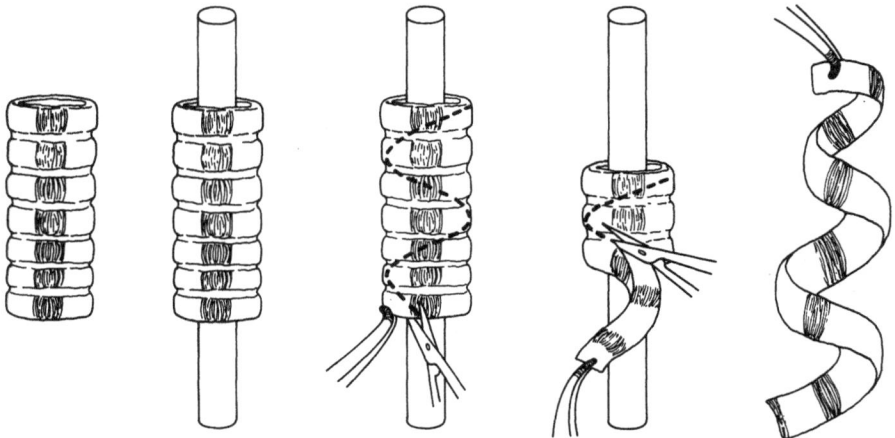

Fig. 4. Step by step procedure to produce a tracheal or bronchial spiral to investigate smooth muscle contraction

In human lung tissues obtained from surgery, some normal lung tissue, is present and often contains airways (bronchioles) of 1–2 mm in diameters. In 1951 Rosa and McDowell [12], and recently De Jongste et al. [11], have used human bronchioles in this technique.

The basic technique for preparation of the spiral was the same as described above. Due to the small size of bronchioles, care was taken to not squeeze, stretch, or apply any force to the tissue, as this is deleterious to its contractile function. Thin surgical silk threads were tied to both ends of the spiral and it was then mounted in the bath in the conventional fashion.

A particular detail of this preparation is that the spirals were stored overnight in cooled (4°C) Krebs buffer containing penicillin (3×10^{-5} g/liter) and tobramycin (5×10^{-3} g/liter). CO_2-O_2 was bubbled through the buffer and a perfusion pump continuously changed the total bath volume every hour to wash out both substances possibly liberated during the preparation procedure and those administered to the patient during narcosis and preparation for surgery (e.g., atropine, thiopental, fentanyl, O_2/NO_2, halothane, pancuronium) [11].

The following day, 20 h postoperatively, the bronchioles were mounted in 10 ml organ baths containing Krebs buffer at 37°C, aerated with CO_2-O_2 (pH 7.35, pCO_2 35 mm Hg, pO_2 540 mm Hg). A resting tension of 500 mg was applied through the isometric force transducer. The viability of the bronchioles after storage and the reproducibility of responses were studied over a 55 h period [11].

Tracheal or Bronchial Strips

The information given for the spiral preparation is also applicable to strips of trachea or bronchus, the only difference being that the trachea (guinea pig)

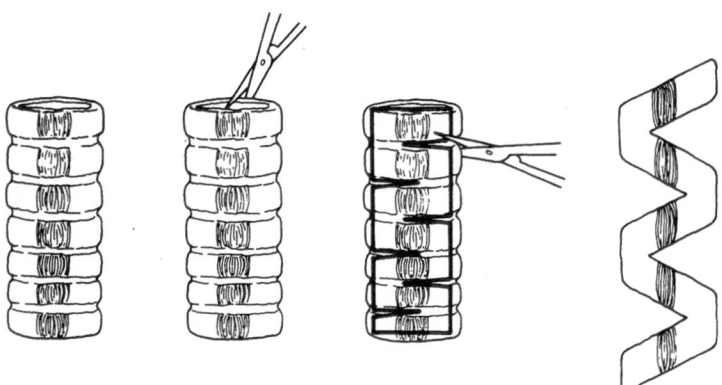

Fig. 5. Step by step procedure to produce a tracheal or bronchial strip to investigate smooth muscle contraction

must be opened (leaving the muscular part intact) and then a zig-zag cut must be done as shown in Fig. 5. In this way it is possible to obtain not a spiral but a zig-zag strip that can be used in the same way as a spiral; this is simpler than preparing a spiral.

Tracheal, Bronchial, or Bronchiolar Segments

Another possible method to investigate tracheal or bronchial muscle contraction is to use a segment of respiratory channels or a simple ring (for samples with airways of large caliber diameter). This is a simple and less manipulated in vitro preparation than the chains of rings or the spirals.

The preparation basically involves positioning a segment of the trachea or the bronchus of predetermined length, or for large diameter samples even a single ring, in a horizontal position instead of vertically, as for the other preparations described above [13–16].

To keep the specimen submerged in the bath in a horizontal position, two small wires (platinum, tungsten, aluminum) are inserted in the lumen of the specimen. One is connected to the bottom of the bath and one is connected to the force transducers (Fig. 6). The organ bath, in this case, is a different shape than the usual one, in that it is oriented in the horizontal axis, although it is possible to also use vertical baths with a rod bearing the specimen (Fig. 6).

For better use of this kind of preparation the force-transducer should be positioned and displaced with accurate movements in the vertical direction by means of a micrometer to measure the stretch and tension imposed [16]. After being mounted in the bath, the segment or single ring must be gently stretched (three to five times), and then a resting tension must be applied to better demonstrate the action of the drugs.

Sterling et al. [15] showed that it is possible to use short segments of lobar and primary segmental bronchi of dog even after storage for 24–48 h at 4°C in a Krebs-Ringer solution containing dextrose (5 mM). The results were qualitatively similar to those obtained with fresh segments. Using this kind of preparation, Stephens et al. [14] investigated length-tension relationships and measured several indices of isometric contraction, such as active tension, peak tension, maximum rate of tension development (dp/dt_{max}), and time to peak tension.

This technique can also be used with very small bronchi, such as intralobular bronchi of the guinea pig, with segments about 1 mm long and 0.2 mm in internal diameter. Specimens with such small dimensions cannot be investigated in ring or strip preparations.

Advenier et al. [17] inserted two tungsten wires 25 μm in diameter into the lumen of the bronchus and then connected one to a micrometer and the other to the force transducer, essentially the same preparation as for larger airway segments. The organ bath was 4 ml in volume and a mean static tension of 180 mg was applied.

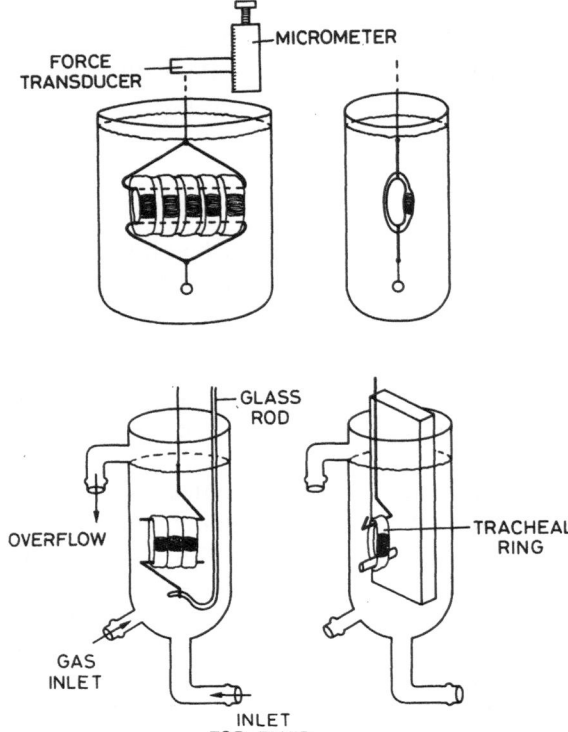

Fig. 6. Different ways to set up tracheobronchiolar segments or rings in a horizontal position in an organ bath

Hooker et al. [18] described another variation of this technique using two 30-gauge needles bent into shape to mount bronchial rings of very small diameter (about 1 mm) for isometric recording.

Jongejan et al. [19] compared the isotonic responses (load 250 mg) to methacholine of human bronchiolar segments and spiral strips. Segments had greater intrinsic contractile activity than spiral strips. Moreover, segment contraction theoretically more closely reflected the physiological luminal narrowing than did chains of rings or spiral strips, in which cutting can interfere with the configuration and the mechanics of the smooth muscle bundles [19].

Muscle Strips from Trachea or Bronchi

This preparation is different from the one above because the cartilaginous component is removed and only muscle is investigated. The preparation is simple: the cartilage is carefully cut without damage to the muscular portion of the trachea or bronchi, and this tissue is mounted in a bath. This manoeuver is in general easily done with large caliber airway segments [20, 21], but even small pieces of tissue from guinea pig trachea mounted in a microbath of 5 ml have been investigated [22, 23].

Canine trachealis muscle (m. trachealis transversus) is frequently used in this preparation because it can be easily separated from the mucosa, has parallel fibers, a small resting tension, no spontaneous activity, can be tetanized, [24] and is the "purest" muscle preparation of the bronchial tree (75% muscle) [25]. Trachealis muscle has been used for studies of smooth muscle mechanics [26], drug action [27] and electrophysiological studies, alone [28–30] and together with tension recording [31, 32].

Strips from Lung Parenchyma

The isolated lung strip has been proposed as a possible model for investigating the direct effects of drugs on the smooth muscle located in the peripheral part of the lung.

The first step is to carefully excise the lungs, which are then placed in Krebs solution. Sections of lung tissue, about 3 mm in width, are dissected quickly from a lower lobe with the longitudinal axis of the strip cut parallel to the bronchus. This is then divided into two or more thin strips with approximate dimensions of $20 \times 3 \times 3$ mm (Fig. 7) [33]. With threads attached to each end, strips are mounted in organ baths. A load of between 2.0 and 2.5 g force is applied to gently stretch the tissue and changes in tension are measured isometrically [33]. The size of the organ generally permits many strips to

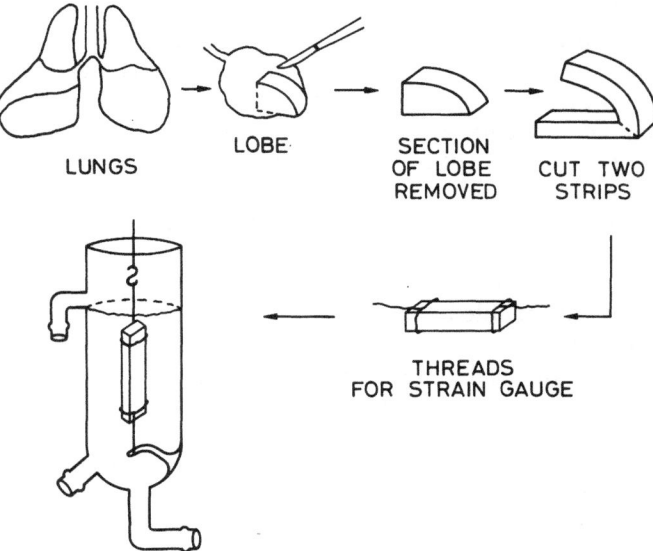

LUNGS   LOBE   SECTION OF LOBE REMOVED   CUT TWO STRIPS

THREADS FOR STRAIN GAUGE

Fig. 7. Procedure to produce a strip from lung parenchyma

Table 1. Comparison of the activity of different drugs between lung strips and trachea of the cat (modified from [33])

Substances	Lung strip (pD$_2$)	Trachea (pD$_2$)
Isoprenaline	7.34 ± 0.02	6.74 ± 0.25
Adrenaline	6.07 ± 0.03	5.46 ± 0.02
Noradrenaline	4.22 ± 0.04	5.53 ± 0.03
Terbutaline	6.05 ± 0.08	4.59 ± 0.15
Salbutamol	6.34 ± 0.06	4.11 ± 0.23
Ascaris extract [a, b] (mg/ml)		
0.01	43, 0, 10	63, 0, 2
0.1	50, 14, 15	57, 2, 6
1.0	68, 42, 14	61, 17, 7
10.0	106, 74, 17	62, 31, 11

pD$_2$ is defined as the negative log EC$_{50}$ (mean $\pm$ SEM).
[a] Response expressed as the percentage of the peak isometric tension elicited by a maximal concentration of acetylcholine (1 mM).
[b] Response from each of three cats.

be obtained, providing an adequate number of control and test strips. Table 1 shows a comparison of drug activities in lung strips and in the trachea of the cat [33].

Since 1976, when Lulich et al. [33] investigated the lung parenchymal strip from the cat, lung strips from many other animals, guinea pig [34, 35], rat [36, 37], cat [38], dog [39], pig [40], ox [41] and humans [42] have been used.

The lung strip preparation was claimed to reflect the direct effects of drugs on peripheral small airways, but, unfortunately, in lung parenchymal strips there is not only bronchiolar smooth muscle [33] but also other contractile elements, such as blood vessel smooth muscle [33, 36, 43] and alveolar interstitial myofibroblasts [44]. Thus the net pharmacological response of a lung strip is related to the integrated responses of one or more of these components. Moreover, there are interactions between different (potentially) reactive components. One component might contract, while the other might relax and the net response could be zero [45]. The proportions of different contractile components could differ in lung strips from the same animal and in those from smaller or larger animals [46].

Stereological analysis of parenchymal lung strips from humans [47] revealed that 46.4% of the lung strip was tissue, while the remainder was alveolar air space. Of the tissue part, vascular wall smooth muscle accounted for about 8.4%, bronchiolar wall smooth muscle made up about 3.5%, and alveolar parenchyma accounted for about 78.4%.

Table 2 shows different pharmacological profiles of lung strip preparations from different mammalian species [45]. Lung strips had pharmacological characteristics in common with both central airways and vascular smooth

Table 2. Profile of pharmacological reactivity of lung strip preparations from humans and animal species: relative effects on resting tension (from [45])

	Humans	Rat	Guinea pig	Rabbit	Cat	Dog	Pig	Sheep	Cow	Monkey
Spontaneous tone	Yes	Yes[a]/No[b]	Yes	No	Yes	No	Yes	No	No	
Carb/ACh	++	++	++	++	++	+++	++	++	+	+++
Hist H$_1$	++	0	+++	++	+++	+++	+++	+++	++	+++
Hist H$_2$		0	--	0	-	-	0			0
α-Agonists	++	++	++	+++	+		++		+++	
β-Agonists	---	---	---	---	---	---	---	---	---	
5-HT	{ ++ / --	+	+	+	++	+	0	0	+	
Bk		0	++	+		+				
PGF$_2$	+++	0	+'++	+	+++	++				
PGE$_1$		0	---	---	-	--				
PGE$_2$		0	--			--				

Carb, carbachol; Ach, acetylcholine; Hist, histamine, 5-HT, serotonin (5-hydroxytryptamine); Bk, bradykinin; PG, prostaglandin; +, contraction; -, relaxation; 0, no response.
[a] Superfused.
[b] Incubated.

muscle. The anatomical complexity of the mammalian lung strip preparation reduces and limits its value as a preparation with which to study peripheral airways pharmacology [45].

Isolated Whole Trachea

Instead of cut rings, spiral strips, or segments, the tracheal tube can be used in toto to measure drug effects. The trachea is isolated and dissected from extraneous tissue, the two ends are generally tied tightly around cannulas and the system is then filled with Krebs fluid, care being taken to exclude air bubbles from the system. The system is positioned in an organ bath so that the physiological salt solutions are in contact with the inner and outer surfaces of the trachea without direct contact between these fluids, and the actions of drugs are evaluated by measuring the change in the pressure of the liquid inside the system caused by contraction or relaxation of the smooth musculature of the isolated intact trachea (Fig. 8).

This is the basic preparation and the intraluminal pressure variations can be sensed by a capillary tube manometer [47] or by a pressure transducer [48]. Drugs can be administered into the organ bath or into the intraluminal system and the trachea in toto can also be stimulated by transmural electrical stimulation with alternating square wave pulses [48, 49].

Contraction is due to excitation of postganglionic parasympathetic nerves, since the response is blocked by atropine and hemicholinium-3, but

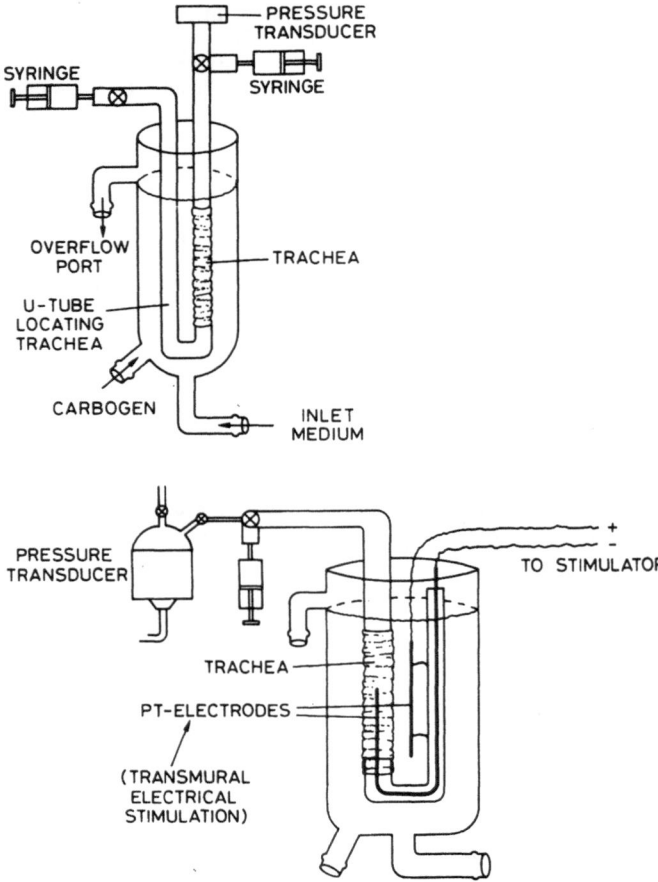

Fig. 8. Two different set-ups to insert a whole isolated trachea in organ baths. Intraluminal pressure variations can be sensed by transducers. Transmural electrical stimulation can also be performed

not by hexamethonium [48]. The preparation showed the expected sensitivity to a variety of drugs known to inhibit contractile responses of tracheobronchial smooth muscle [48].

Superfusion and Cascade Techniques

An alternative to the classic organ bath for in vitro pharmacological experimentation is the superfusion technique. Here, the sample of tissue, instead of being immersed in a physiological saline solution to keep it vital, has the fluid continuously running over it, drop by drop, which forms a liquid layer over the surface of the tissue suspended in air or, better, placed in a bath or in a temperature-controlled chamber, which protects it from surrounding interference. The technique was introduced by Finkleman in 1930 [50] and subsequently developed by Gaddum [51] for assay of biologically active substances.

Figure 9 is a schematic drawing of the superfusion chamber, in which it is possible to test an isolated tracheal strip (guinea pig) and other kinds of smooth muscles [52]. The superfusion fluid can be pumped, for instance, at a rate of 2 ml/min through a jacketed glass heat-exchanger. Drugs can be added to the stream of fluid running over the tissue or, alternatively the flow can be stopped for a standard interval of time and the solution containing the drug applied undiluted to the surface of the tissue (bronchial smooth muscle). The latter method of administration provides greater sensitivity [51].

Indomethacin can be added in the Krebs superfusion solution to inhibit endogeneous prostanoid synthesis and a resting tension of 1 g can be applied to the preparation [52].

Bipolar platinum electrodes may be introduced through the roof of the chamber, and positioned parallel in close proximity to the superfused tissue. Electrical field stimulation with 10 s trains of square wave pulses of 0.1 ms duration and just maximal voltage every 2 min resulted in spike contractile responses that are pulse frequency-dependent (1–20 Hz) [52].

Spasmolytic agents reduced the amplitude of electrically induced spike responses, which were completely inhibited by atropine but not by hexamethonium, suggesting that the contractions resulted from stimulation of postganglionic cholinergic nerves within the tissue [52].

There is evidence that adrenergic inhibitory nerves were also stimulated, as the amplitudes of contractile spike responses were increased on administration of propranolol and inhibited by the indirectly acting sympathomimetic amine, tyramine [52]. Spasmolytic agents can also be tested against $PGF_{2\alpha}$-induced tone ($PGF_{2\alpha}$ in the Krebs). The differences between superfusion and the immersed technique may be due to the rapid removal of potentially

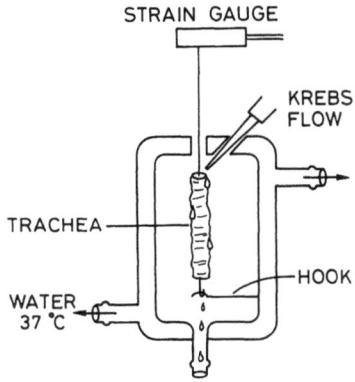

Fig. 9. A superfusion chamber to test isolated trachea or other kinds of smooth muscle preparations

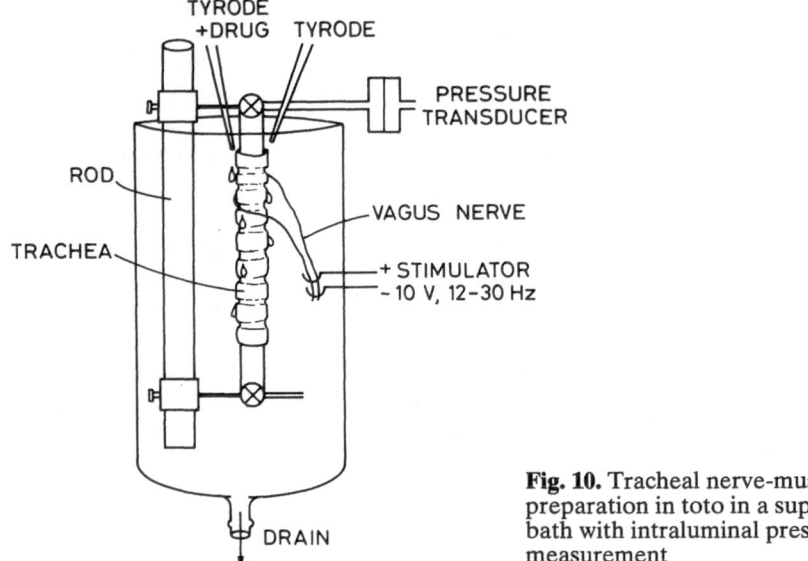

Fig. 10. Tracheal nerve-muscle preparation in toto in a superfusion bath with intraluminal pressure measurement

toxic metabolites, which thus do not accumulate within the tissue. No repeated washing procedures are necessary, as they are in immersion experiments. Finally, rates of onset and offset of drug action are easily measured [52].

A superfusion method with a tracheal nerve-muscle preparation in toto has also been developed by Bouhuys [53] and can be used to assess the interaction between mediators and the efferent vagus nerve (Fig. 10).

The superfusion method can be modified for simultaneous use of more than one tissue, to have different tissues in series [54]. This technique is called "cascade superfusion" which is a multiple tissues assay system [5].

Along with the different tissues investigated (e.g., rat fundus strip, rat duodenum, rat colon, rat bladder strip, guinea pig ileum, guinea pig proximal colon, rabbit stomach strip), rabbit celiac, mesenteric artery and aortic strip) guinea pig tracheal chains and other tracheal preparations can be used, but this technique is mainly used for identification and assay of prostaglandins and prostaglandin-like substances [56–59].

Transmural and Vagal Electrical Stimulation

The preparations described above can also be investigated with alternating electrical stimulation, which induces contraction and relaxation of the tracheal or bronchial smooth muscles. The electrical stimulation can be used to increase the intrinsic tone of these preparations, which in general have the disadvantage of low intrinsic muscular tone [48], or to investigate the response to intrinsic nerve stimulation [49] or vagal stimulation [60]. The most frequently used preparation is the isolated whole trachea, because measurement of changes in the intraluminal pressure gives reliable information about the narrowing induced by mediators and drugs.

To electrically stimulate an isolated organ or tissue preparation, there are two main techniques: direct electrical stimulation by applying electrodes to the organ or the tissue and indirect stimulation by transmural field stimulation or by stimulating the nerve fibers previously isolated that innervate the tissue being studied.

The organ bath has the same shape (Fig. 8) as those described in the section on isolated, whole, intact trachea, with some modifications to allow the positioning of stimulating electrodes. Intraluminal pressure can be recorded during electrical stimulation of the whole trachea.

For field stimulation, platinum or silver chloride wires can be used as electrodes and are positioned in the organ bath near the organ but not in contact with it. Field stimulation requires high-intensity voltage or current stimulation.

Electrical parameters for stimulation must be adapted for each set-up: for instance, rectangular pulses of 0.3–1 ms duration and supramaximal voltage (40–60 V) applied in a train of pulses are used. Transmural electrical stimulation of the trachea causes an initial contraction and a rapid increase in the intraluminal pressure, followed by relaxation in the absence of stimulus.

Spasmolytic, anticholinergic and sympathomimetic agents were able to reduce the intraluminal pressure. The electrically induced contractions were blocked by atropine, hemicholinium-3, and tetrodoxin, but not by hexamethonium, suggesting that they resulted from excitation of postganglionic cholinergic nerves within the tissue [48, 52]. The inhibitory effect of isoprenaline was prevented by propranolol [48]. Cumulative dose-effect curves can be studied.

Single pulses of excessive duration must be avoided because they can induce production of gas at the electrode surfaces. The production of gas on the intraluminal electrode can cause an increase in the intraluminal pressure, thus causing an error in reading basal values [48].

The other possibility is to stimulate vagus nerves in a tracheal nerve-muscle preparation in which vagus nerves have been carefully dissected free from surrounding tissue 10–15 mm from the laryngeal end and removed attached to the trachea [60]. The preparation is mounted on a holder and transferred to an organ bath (Fig. 10). A bipolar electrode or a suction electrode can be used. Bilateral stimulation of the vagus nerves increased the intratracheal pressure more than stimulation of either nerve alone and the resultant response was about 70 % of the algebraic sum [60]. With this preparation one can differentiate between pre- and postjunctional sites of action of pharmacological agents.

Tracheal Preparation with Epithelium Removed

It has been observed that the damage or loss of airway epithelium results in airway hyperreactivity, and this is probably due to an exposure of afferent receptors to the environment, leading to increased sensitivity of these receptors and increased reflex bronchoconstriction [61–63].

It has been postulated that, in many species including humans, the airway epithelial cells produce one or more inhibitory substances that can modulate smooth muscle responsiveness [63].

It was first demonstrated in dogs [64] that loss of the epithelial layer augments contractile responses of isolated airways to various agents. Experiments were performed on third or fourth generation bronchi taken from mongrel dogs. Bronchial segments (4–6 mm O.D., 8–10 mm long) were dissected, and paired ring segments (4–5 mm long) were prepared from each segment. The tips of a pair of watchmaker's forceps were inserted into the lumen and the epithelial layer was removed by gently rolling the preparation back and forth over saline-soaked filter paper [64]. Similar results were obtained by inserting a cotton swab into the lumen of the bronchial rings. The removal of the epithelium was confirmed histologically. The segments were suspended horizontally between two stainless steel wires, as previously described.

In this study transmural nerve stimulation was also performed. Concentration-effect curves for exogenous agonists were constructed and ED_{50} were calculated. The sensitivity to drugs was greater than that of a preparation still having epithelium.

The gentle mechanical rubbing technique to remove the epithelial layer had previously been used to remove the endothelium in isolated blood vessels [65, 66]. Another method was to remove the trachea (e.g., guinea pig), cut it open longitudinally through the ventral cartilage and carefully dissect a cartilage strip of about 1 mm in width (mainly from the portion close to the bronchus) avoiding mechanical damage to the laminal surface as much as possible [67]. Epithelial cells were removed by 20 gentle rubbings of the laminal surface with a cotton swab [68]. The presence or absence of epithelium was confirmed by microscope examination of the preparations after hematoxylin-eosin staining. Each strip was mounted vertically in an organ bath and the mechanical response were measured isometrically. This kind of preparation was made from several animal species including guinea pigs [68–71, 75], dogs [67, 76], rabbits [72], cows [73], and humans [74]. The various species exhibited different effects of epithelium removal on airway responsiveness to bronchodilator drugs [63].

Isolated Perfused Lungs

The isolated perfused lung can be considered as a cross between in vitro and in vivo techniques, because the methodology for maintenance is closer to

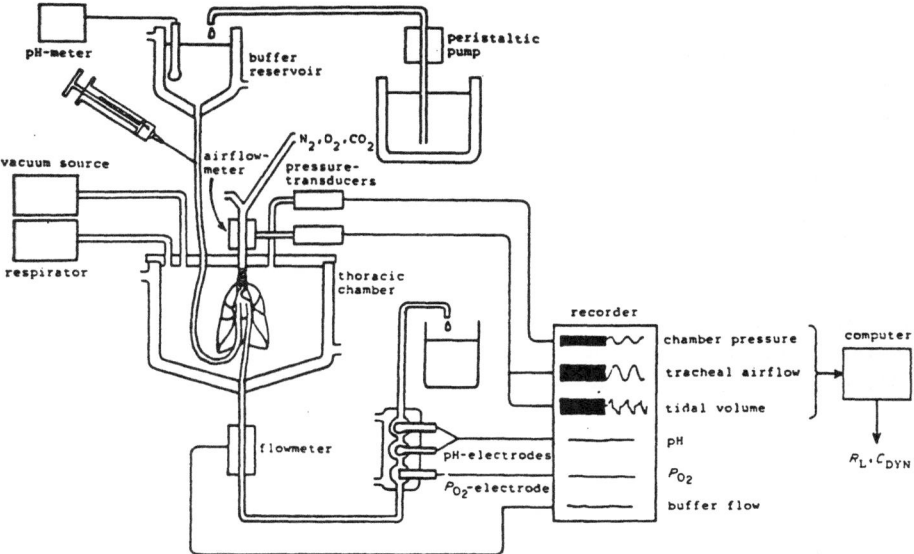

Fig. 11. The isolated perfused lung set-up (From [80])

that for in vitro preparations and the function of the organ is closer to that of in vivo preparations. This type of preparation is rather complicated and can be maintained without deterioration of function for only a short period of time, on the average 4–5 h [77]. Therefore, it is not frequently used for investigation of mechanical behavior of respiratory smooth muscle ex vivo; rather it is more often used in toxicological or metabolic studies and for investigation of uptake and distribution of exogenous and endogenous substances. For these reasons this preparation is only mentioned, not discussed extensively. Further information can be found in recent papers [78, 79]. Very recently, there was a report on the use of this preparation for measurement of lung resistance and dynamic compliance [80]. A schematic drawing of the isolated perfused lung set-up is shown in Fig. 11.

The Measuring System

Experimental studies of the mechanical behavior of smooth muscle generally require measurement and control of muscle force and length with an apparatus containing electrical transducers, levers, and various mechanical supports [81].

The classic methods of transduction or translation of these muscle responses involve a mechanical lever system on which the muscle is mounted in the organ bath with one end connected to a lever arm attached to a transducer (the lever arm acts as a cantilever beam). This system can operate in conjunction with a strain gauge, photocell, or some other device that enables recordings to be made [82]. The lever must have a small mass and a negligable moment of inertia. There are equations for calculation of mass, inertia, stress distribution, strain, deflection curve, compliance, and resonant frequency of uniform and nonuniform cantilever beams made of structural materials of different density or elastic moduli [81].

Early systems used some form of lever system in conjunction with kymographic recording, while modern systems, although based on the same physical principles as the early devices, have combined these with some kind of electrical "sensor" to produce an electrical signal suitable for display purposes on either a pen recorder or an oscilloscope [83]. The classic leverage systems are: isometric, isotonic, and auxotonic (Fig. 12).

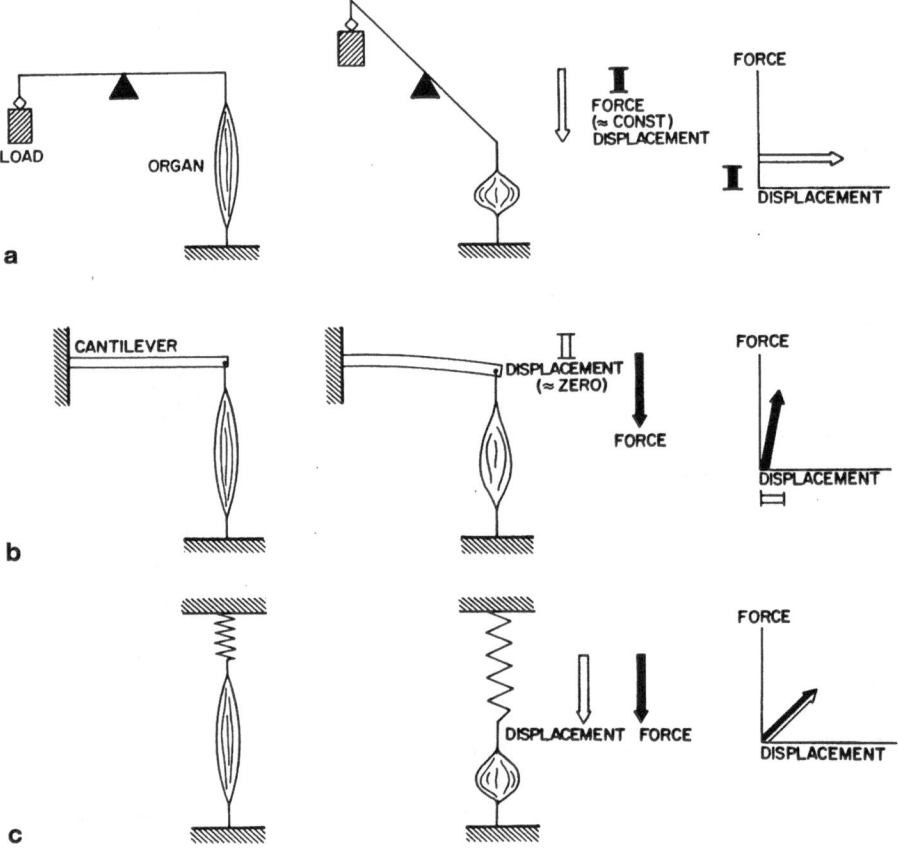

Fig. 12. a-c. Isotonic, isometric, or auxotonic conditions and leverages. The force displacement graphs are also shown. **a** Isotonic contraction lever; **b** isometric contraction: flat spring (rigid); **c** auxotonic contraction: coil spring (flexible). (From [83a])

When investigation of the strength or the tension developed by the muscle during contraction is required, an isometric lever, which measures only the tension changes while the appearance of the tissue remains unchanged, must be used. Resting tensions of different strength can be applied to the preparation. Relaxation of tension after contraction is relatively rapid, since the restoration force increases with contraction. A dose-response curve can also be generated.

When investigation of the change in the length of the muscle during contraction is required (e.g., ileum preparation), an isotonic lever, which measures the shortening of the muscle during its contraction against a load, must be used. With smooth muscle, isotonic recording probably is a more physiological type of investigation from a theoretical point of view than an isometric one [84]. In most situations smooth muscle shortens considerably during its response and it may also be an advantage that, even though the spontaneous tone in the muscle changes during an experiment, the load does not alter as the muscle length changes [84].

Nonetheless, isotonic recording also has certain practical and theoretical disadvantages. Under physiological conditions smooth muscles can shorten considerably and the active tension developed is, as with other muscles, a function of the length. Isotonic recording, using a constant load at the expense of varying length, implies recording the active state at varying points on its length-tension curve. Moreover, the choice of the load is arbitrary and it is not easy to combine sensitivity to low doses of a drug with the ability to record maximal or near maximal responses [84]. Alternatively, the maximal response can be made possible, but to do this a considerable isotonic load is required and this reduces the sensitivity and imposes a considerable tension even under resting conditions. With lightly loaded levers relaxation from larger contractions may be slow, since the external restoration force does not increase with increased shortening. With isotonic recording it is not possible to simultaneously independently vary the loading of the tissue and its length: the length, whether physiological or not, is set by the load chosen [84].

An auxotonic lever is a compromise. The preparation is allowed to shorten significantly, but the restoration force increases with the degree of shortening [84]. Santesson, in 1891 [85], indicated that the tension developed by a muscle during shortening increases continuously while the muscle stretches a cantilever beam (auxotonic). This lever maintains some of the advantages of isometric recording, namely that: (a) any initial length or load may be chosen, regardless of the sensitivity of the system; (b) relaxation is facilitated after a stimulus is withdrawn; and (c) a full range of responses can readily be recorded. An isotonic lever can be converted to an auxotonic one by attaching a small weight below the pivot point to function as a pendulum [86]. An isometric lever can be converted to an auxotonic one by attaching a spring between the transducer and the preparation. With springs weaker than those strong enough to make the lever approximately isometric, it is possible to obtain an auxotonic lever [87], in which the load on the muscle increases as it shorten. The spring can have any strength within the limits set by isotonic recording, on the one hand, and isometric recording on the other [84].

Force displacement transducers which are connected to the different types of lever use many different sensing probes or circuits to convert the measurements to electric signals, e.g., mirrors, light or laser beams [82, 85, 86, 88–94], inductive effects by differential transformers [95–98], differential capacitative effects [99–101], potentiometric effects [102], ultrasonic [83], dc excited strain-gauge, and resistance-bridges [98, 103–105].

The mechanical system of recording requires no compliance of the attaching system (thread, knots, etc.) and has a very low frictional torque, resistance to corrosion, a very low moment of inertia. It is protected against the entrance of solutions and is easy to mount and set up. Accuracy, linearity, and freedom from drift are essential requirements of the electrical specifications to maintain stable baselines.

Now that we have indicated the advantages, the disadvantages, and the limiting factors, how do we choose which of the different recording systems to use in pharmacological studies? Generally, for in vitro pharmacological

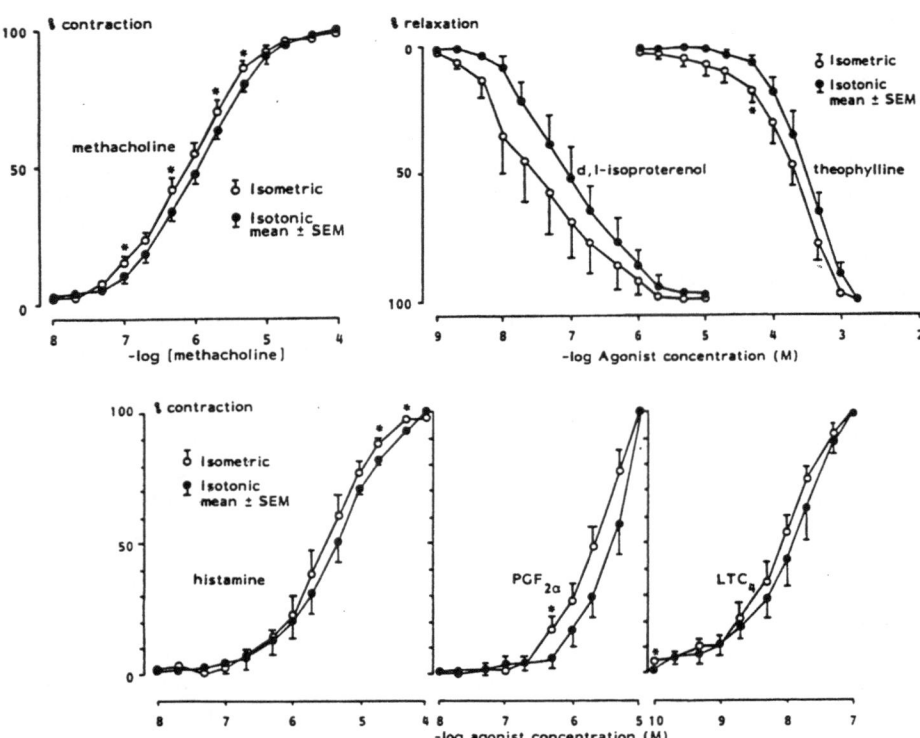

Fig. 13. Concentration-response curves (mean ± SEM) of bronchiolar strips obtained with challenge of different agents. (Modified from [110])

studies of airway smooth muscle, isometric fore transducers are commonly used, although isotonic systems have also been used. The comparisons between these two systems mainly concerned tension-length relationships and contraction kinetics [106–109] and have shown that isometric responses develop more rapidly and usually require greater stimuli than isotonic responses.

All tissues should be attached to tissue hooks with noncompliant materials, e.g., stainless steel wire of 37 SWG, to overcome the problem of stretching that is found with silk, braided silk, or cotton when they are wet with physiological saline [89].

Recently De Jongste et al. [110] have investigated the difference between the isometric and isotonic responses of human bronchiolar strips to a number of pharmacological agonists. Figure 13 shows the data from some of the recordings. The sensitivity to methacholine measured isometrically was slightly but significantly greater than the isotonically determined sensitivity. A similar trend was observed for other drugs, although no differences were significant, probably due to the limited number of observations [110]. Maximal force and shortening are related linearly. We can conclude that the observed differences are of little practical importance for conventional pharmacological investigations [110].

Maintenance Solutions

The aim of in vitro studies with different kinds of organs or parts of living organisms is to obtain information about their functional mechanisms in vivo and their pharmacological responses, specifically about direct actions of drugs without interference and under controlled conditions. Therefore in vitro conditions must be as close as possible to in vivo conditions.

A large number of bath solutions with well defined electrolyte composition (as close as possible to plasma) and with the ionic concentration and osmotic pressure necessary for cells to survive without damage are in use [111, 112]. Physiological, salt solutions must be carefully prepared in glass containers with pure chemicals (analytical grade) and distilled or deionized water. Solutions can be prepared with weighing out the salts and dissolving them in water every time a solution is required or can be prepared by dilution from concentrated stock solutions. In any case the errors involved in preparations should not exceed 1%. Special care must be taken with highly hygroscopic chemicals, such as $MgCl$ or $CaCl_2$, which must be maintained in antihygroscopic conditions. Physiological salt solutions can be kept for about 24 h, (it is better to store them in the refrigerator), but they are good media for the growth of microorganisms and must be kept cold [3]. The compositions of a number of solutions are shown in Table 3.

For in vitro studies, temperature, pH, pO_2, and pCO_2 must be under control in addition to ionic concentration and osmotic pressure:

Table 3. Composition of various physiological solutions

		Salts (w/o) water of crystallization										Aerating gas[a] (pH)
		NaCl	KCl	CaCl₂	MgCl₂	MgSO₄	NaHCO₃	NaH₂PO₄	KH₂PO₄	Glucose	Na-Pyruvate	
Tyrode (standard)	g/ml	8.0	0.2	0.2	0.1	–	1.00	0.05	–	1.0	–	100 Vol% O₂ (7.9)
	mmol/l	136.9	2.68	1.80	1.05	–	11.90	0.42	–	5.55	–	3 Vol% CO₂ (7.4) 5 Vol% CO₂ (6.8)
Tyrode (Ca⁺⁺-deficient)	g/ml	8.0	0.2	0.1	0.1	–	1.00	0.05	–	1.0	–	Carbogen[b] (7.2)
	mmol/l	136.9	2.68	0.9	1.05	–	11.90	0.42	–	5.55	–	
Tyrode (Mg⁺⁺-enriched)	g/ml	8.0	0.2	0.1	0.2	–	1.00	0.05	–	1.0	–	Carbogen[b] (7.2)
	mmol/l	136.9	2.68	0.9	2.10	–	11.90	0.42	–	5.55	–	
Gaddum's tyrode (K⁺-enriched, Mg⁺⁺-free)	g/l	9.0	0.42	0.06	–	–	0.50	–	–	0.5	–	Carbogen[b] (7.0)
	mmol/l	154.0	5.63	0.54	–	–	5.95	–	–	2.78	–	
Langendorff's tyrode (K⁺ and Ca⁺⁺-deficient)	g/l	8.0	0.075	0.1	–	–	0.05	–	–	1.0	–	
	mmol/l	136.9	1.01	0.9	–	–	0.6	–	–	5.55	–	
Locke	g/l	9.2	0.42	0.23	–	–	0.15	–	–	1.09	–	100 Vol% O₂ (8.5)
	mmol/l	157.4	5.63	2.09	–	–	1.78	–	–	5.55	–	1 Vol% CO₂ (6.8) 5 Vol% CO₂ (6.4)
Locke (modified)	g/l	9.2	0.42	0.23	Phosphate buffer[c]		–	–	–	–	–	100 Vol% O₂ (7.4)
	mmol/l	157.4	5.63	2.09			–	–	–	5.55	–	
Krebs-Henseleit	g/l	6.9	0.35	0.28	–	0.14	2.09	–	0.16	1.09	0.22	5 Vol% CO₂ (7.4)
	mmol/l	118.0	4.70	2.52	–	1.64	24.88	–	1.18	5.55	2.0	

Solution	Unit											Gassing [a]
Ringer	g/l	9.0	0.2	0.2	–	–	0.10	–	–	–	–	100 Vol% O_2 (8.4)
	mmol/l	153.9	2.68	1.80	–	–	1.19	–	–	–	–	1 Vol% CO_2 (6.7)
												5 Vol% CO_2 (6.1)
Ringer (modified)	g/l	9.0	0.2	0.2	Phosphate buffer [c]			–	–	–	–	100 Vol% O_2 (7.4)
	mmol/l	153.9	2.68	1.80				–	–	–	–	
De Jalon	g/l	9.0	0.42	0.06	–	–	0.5	–	–	0.5	–	Carbogen [b]
	mmol/l	154.0	5.63	0.54	–	–	5.95	–	–	2.78	–	
Sund	g/l	9.0	0.42	0.06	0.09	–	0.5	–	–	0.5	–	Carbogen [b]
	mmol/l	154.0	5.63	0.54	0.95	–	5.95	–	–	2.78	–	
Ringer (reptilian)	g/l	6.0	0.075	0.10	–	–	0.10	–	–	–	–	100 Vol% O_2 (8.4)
	mmol/l	102.6	1.01	0.91	–	–	1.19	–	–	–	–	
Ringer (reptilian, modified)	g/l	6.0	0.075	0.10	Phosphate buffer [c]			–	–	–	–	100 Vol% O_2 (7.4)
	mmol/l	102.6	1.01	0.91				–	–	–	–	

[a] Where Vol% CO_2 is given, the remainder of the aerating gas is O_2.

[b] Carbogen = 95% O_2 + 5% CO_2.

[c] Stock solutions for phospate buffer: solution I: 1.432 g $Na_2HPO_4 \cdot 12H_2O$/100 ml H_2O; solution II: 1.560 g $NaH_2PO_4 \cdot 2H_2O$/100 ml H_2O; 10 ml m/s of solution I and 1 ml of solution II per litre Ringer or Locke solution.

1. As previously discussed, there are several systems (see section "Organ Bath") that maintain the baths at $37 \pm 0.1°C$, which is the temperature usually adopted.

2. For pO_2, since there is no hemoglobin in in vitro experiments, the only resource is the physically absorbed oxygen in the surrounding fluids. This means that oxygen must be continuously bubbled through the bath fluid to keep the oxygen tension in the tissue bath at a constant an relatively high level (600–700 mm Hg) and to maintain the balance between the amount of O_2 consumed by the tissue in the bath and the amount of O_2 which passes from the air according to the atmospheric pressure. Oxygen tensions below 160 mm Hg reduce the noradrenaline-evoked contractions of rabbit arteries [115]. Reduction of oxygen tension from 700 to 150 mm Hg reduces the contraction of vascular smooth muscles caused by electrical field stimulation [111]. The active tension in isometric recordings of electrically stimulated bronchial canine segments varied with the pO_2 of the medium, decreasing sharply at values less than 135 mm Hg. Hypercapnic acidosis (pCO_2 78 mm Hg, pH 7.17, pO_2 630 mm Hg) also decreased the active evoked tension, but normocapnic acidosis and hypocapnic alkalosis were without effect [116].

3. The carbonate/bicarbonate buffer system present in physiological solutions, used to maintain stable pH, gradually loses CO_2. This results in an increase in pH, with a possible precipitation from a hypersaturated calcium solution. To reequilibrate the solutions, CO_2 should be added. The preferred method is to aerate the solutions by bubbling them through under pressure in a gas mixture containing 95% O_2 and 5% CO_2 (carbogen) [113]. Table 4 shows the efficacy of different flows of this gas [114].

4. Calcium salts play a critical role in maintaining the viability of isolated vertebrate muscle in vitro [117], but these salts can precipitate during the preparation or use of physiological salines. Precipitate can appear when the

Table 4. Efficiency of carbonation of a carbonate bicarbonate buffer at different gas flows (from [114])

Dispersion method	F_{low}		CO_2 supplied mol/mol Na[c]	Time (min) to reduce pH to 7.5
	mmol × liter^{-1} × h^{-1} [a]	ml × liter^{-1} × min^{-1} [b]		
Fritted gas	10	84	0.88	132
dispersion tube [d]	50	420	1.18	35
	150	1260	1.43	14
Pasteur pipette [e]	50	420	3.55	106

[a] mmol CO_2 × (liter solution with 25 mM neutralizable Na)$^{-1}$ × h^{-1}.
[b] ml 5% CO_2 in O_2 × (liter solution)$^{-1}$ × min^{-1}.
[c] mol CO_2 needed per mol neutralizable Na to reduce pH to 7.5 from initial value of 10.75.
[d] Porex Materials Corporation, distributed by Bel-Art Products, Pequannock, NJ, USA.
[e] Fisher Scientific Company, Pittsburgh, Pa, USA

only anions present are chloride and bicarbonate [118, 119], suggesting that the precipitate is probably calcium carbonate, or in the presence of phosphate [114]. In a recent study of this aspect Mac Conail [114] indicated that, at its physiological concentration of 1.6 mM, calcium precipitation also appeared in solutions of pH greater than 9. When phosphate was present the precipitate appeared immediately but redissolved once the pH was reduced below 7.8.

Since a bicarbonate stock solution gradually loses CO_2 and becomes alkaline, a protocol for mixing physiologic salines from alkaline bicarbonate stock was developed [114].

All constituents except that containing calcium are added to a volume of 80% of the final amount of water. Taking into account the volume of the still to be added calcium-containing stock, more water is then added. If [Ca] in the final solution is to be between 5.6 and 16 mM, then phosphate is omitted. Mix, then gas for 15 min with 500 ml/min of 5% CO_2 in 95% O_2 per liter of final solution volume, bringing the pH below 7.5. Add the calcium containing stock, make up to volume with water, and gas again for 5 min [114].

5. It has been observed [120] that exposure to cold during the preparation of isolated tissues can radically alter the ionic content of smooth muscle, so that if the experiment is then conducted at 37°C, for instance, there can be substantial changes in response to various stimuli during the initial period of study, depending on how long the cooling had lasted [84]. Therefore it is better that the whole procedure of preparation of trachea or bronchi is performed in a bath solution kept at 37°C to avoid thermal shock.

References

1. Magnus R (1904) Versuche am überlebenden Dünndarm von Säugetieren. Pflugers Arch Physiol 102:123
2. Hawkins DF, Schild HO (1951) The action of drugs on isolated human bronchial chains. Br J Pharmacol 6:682–690
3. Department of Pharmacology, University of Edinburgh (1968) Pharmacological experiments on isolated preparations. Livingstone, Edinburgh
4. Castillo JC, de Beer EJ (1947) A tracheal chain. 1. A preparation for the study of antispasmodics with particular reference to bronchodilator drugs. J Pharmacol 90:104–109
5. Akcasu A (1952) The actions of drugs on the isolated trachea. J Pharm Pharmacol 4:671–676
6. Akcasu A (1959) The physiologic and pharmacologic characteristics of the tracheal muscle. Arch Int Pharmacodyn Ther 122:201–207
7. Foster WR (1960) The paired tracheal chain preparation. J Pharm Pharmacol 12:189–191
8. McDougal MD, West GB (1953) The action of drugs on isolated mammalian bronchial muscle. Br J Pharmacol 8:26–29
9. Constantine JW (1965) The spirally cut tracheal strip preparation. J Pharm Pharmacol 17:384–385
10. Chand N, Eyre P (1978) Pharmacological study of chicken airway smooth muscle. J Pharm Pharmacol 30:432–435

11. De Jongste JC, van Strik R, Bonta IL, Kerrebijn KF (1985) Measurement of human small airway smooth muscle function in vitro with the bronchiolar strip preparation. J Pharm Methods 14:111–118
12. Rosa LM, McDowall JS (1951) The action of local hormones on the isolated human bronchus. Acta Allergol 4:293–304
13. Danko G, Tozzi S, Roth FE (1968) Determination of the adrenergic mechanism of the isolated guinea pig trachea utilizing a new technique. Fed Proc Fed Am Soc Exp Biol 27:351
14. Stephens NL, Meyers JL, Cherniack RM (1968) Oxygen, carbon dioxide, H^+ ion and bronchial length tension relationships. J Appl Physiol 25:376–383
15. Sterling GM, Holst PE, Nadel JA (1972) Effect of CO_2 and pH on bronchoconstriction caused by serotonin vs acetylcholine. J Appl Physiol 32:39–43
16. Souhrada JF, Dickey DW (1976) Mechanical activities of trachea as measured in vitro and in vivo. Respir Physiol 26:27–40
17. Advenier C, Freslon JL (1985 The guinea-pig isolated bronchus for the *in vitro* study of small calibre airway reactivity. Br J Pharmacol 86:367–373
18. Hooker CS, Calkins PJ, Fleisch JH (1977) On the measurement of vascular and respiratory smooth muscle responses in vitro. Blood Vessels 14:1–11
19. Jongejan RC, de Jongste JC, van Strik R, Raatgeep HR, Bonta IL, Kerrebijn KF (1988) Measurement of human small airway smooth muscle function in vitro. Comparison of bronchiolar strip and segments. J Pharmacol Methods 20:135–142
20. Trendelemburg P (1912) Physiologische und Pharmakologische Untersuchungen an der isolierten Bronchialmuskulatur. Arch Exp Pathol Pharmakol 69:79–107
21. Macht DI, Ting GC (1921) A study of antispasmodic drugs on the bronchus. J Pharmacol Exp Ther 18:373–398
22. Gaddum JH, Stephenson RP (1958) A microbath. Br J Pharmacol 13:394–497
23. Offermeier J, Ariens EJ (1966) Serotonin. 1. Receptors involved in its action. Arch Int Pharmacodyn Ther 164:192–215
24. Sperlakis N (1962) Contraction of depolarized smooth muscle by electric fields Am J Physiol 202:731–742
25. Stephens NL, Kroeger E, Mehta JA (1969) Force-velocity characteristics of respiratory airway smooth muscle. J Appl Physiol 26:685–692
26. Stephens NL (1975) Physical properties of contractile systems. Methods Pharmacol 3:265–296
27. Coburn RF, Tomita T (1973) Evidence for nonadrenergic inhibitory nerves in the guinea pig trachealis muscle. Am J Physiol 224:1072–1080
28. Kirkpatrick CT (1975) Excitation and contraction in bovine tracheal smooth muscle. J Physiol 244:263–281
29. Coburn RF, Yamaguchi T (1977) Membrane potential-dependent and -independent tension in the canine tracheal muscle. J Pharmacol Exp Ther 201:276–284
30. Cameron AR, Kirkpatrick CT (1977) A study of excitatory neuromuscular transmission in the bovine trachea. J Physiol 270:733–745
31. Yamaguchi T, Hitzig B, Coburn RF (1976) Endogeneous prostaglandins and mechanical tension in canine trachealis muscle. Am J Physiol 230:1737–1743
32. Bose R, Bose D (1977) Excitation-contraction coupling in multiunit tracheal smooth muscle during metabolic depletion: induction of rhythmicity. Am J Physiol 2:C8–C13
33. Lulich KM, Mitchell HW, Sparrow MP (1976) The cat lung strip as an in vitro preparation of peripheral airways: a comparison of β-adrenoceptor agonists, autacoids and anaphylactic challenge on the lung strip and trachea. Br J Pharmacol 58:71–79
34. Chand N, de Roth L (1979) Responses of guinea-pig lung parenchimal strips to prostaglandins and some selected autacoids. J Pharm Pharmacol 31:712–714
35. Siegl PKS, Rossi GV, Orzechowski RF (1979) Isolated lung strips of guinea pigs.

Responses to beta-adrenergic agonists and antagonists. Eur J Pharmacol 54:1–7

36. Burn JW, Doe JE (1978) A comparison of drug-induced responses on rat tracheal bronchial and lung strip in vitro preparations. Br J Pharmacol 64:71–74

37. Lulich KM, Paterson JW (1980) An in vitro study of various drugs on central and peripheral airways of the rat: a comparison with human airways. Br J Pharmacol 68:633–636

38. Chand N (1981) Reactivity of isolated trachea, bronchus and lung strip of cats to carbachol, 5-hydroxytryptamine and histamine; evidence for the existence of methysergide-sensitive receptors. Br J Pharmacol 73:853–857

39. Chand N, de Roth L, Eyre P (1979) Pharmacology of Schultz-Dale reaction in canine lung strip in vitro: possible model for allergic asthma. Br J Pharmacol 66:511–516

40. Goldie RG, Paterson JW, Wale JL (1982) Pharmacological responses of human and porcine lung parenchima, bronchus and pulmonary artery. Br J Pharmacol 76:515–521

41. Mirbahar KB, Eyre P (1980) Bovine lung parenchyma strip has both airway and vascular characteristics (Pharmacological comparison with bronchus, pulmonary artery and vein). Res Commun Chem Pathol Pharmacol 29:15–25

42. Ghelani AM, Holroyde MC, Sheard P (1980) Response of human isolated bronchial and lung parenchimal strips to SRS-A and other mediators of asthmatic bronchospasm. Br J Pharmacol 71:107–112

43. Drazen JM, Schneider MW (1978) Comparative responses of tracheal spirals and parenchimal strips to histamine and carbachol in vitro. J Clin Invest 61:1441–1448

44. Kapanci Y, Assimacopoulos A, Irle C, Zwahlen A, Gabbiani G (1974) Contractile interstitial cells in pulmonary alveolar septa: a possible regulator of ventilation/perfusion ratio? J Cell Biol 60:375–392

45. Goldie RG, Bertram JF, Papadimitriou JM, Paterson JW (1984) The lung parenchyma strip. Trends Pharmacol Sci 5:7–10

46. Eyre P, Mirbahar KN (1981) Is the lung parenchyma strip a true airway preparation? Agents Actions 11:173–177

47. Bertram JF, Goldie RG, Papadimitriou JM, Paterson JW (1983) Correlation between pharmacological responses and structure of human lung parenchyma strips. Br J Pharmacol 80:107–114

48. Farmer JB, Coleman RA (1970) A new preparation of the isolated intact trachea of the guinea-pig. J Pharm Pharmacol 22:46–50

49. Carlyle RF (1964) The response of the guinea pig isolated intact trachea to transmural stimulation and the release of an acetylcholine-like substance under conditions of rest and stimulation. Br J Pharmacol 22:126–136

50. Finkleman B (1930) On the nature of inhibition in the intestine. J Physiol 70:145–147

51. Gaddum JH (1953) The technique of superfusion. Br J Pharmacol Chemother 8:321

52. Coleman RA, Nials AT (1989) Novel and versatile superfusion system. J Pharmacol Methods 21:71–86

53. Bouhuys A (1974) Bronchial asthma. In: Bouhuys A (ed) Breathing, physiology, environment and lung disease. Grune and Stratton, New York, pp 441–489

54. Armitage AK, Vane JR (1964) A sensitive method for the assay of catecholamines. Br J Pharmacol Chemother 22:204–210

55. Henman MC, Naylor IL, Leach GDH (1978) A critical evaluation of the use of a cascade superfusion technique for the detection and estimation of biological activity. J Pharmacol Methods 1:13–26

56. Willis AL (1969) Parallel assay of prostaglandine-like activity in rat inflammatory exudate by means of cascade superfusion. J Pharm Pharmacol 1:126–128

57. Naylor IL (1977) A simple and inexpensive piece of apparatus for cascade superfusion procedures. Br J Pharmacol 59:529P

58. Hong E (1974) Differential pattern of activity of some prostaglandins in diverse superfused tissues. Prostaglandins 8:213–220
59. Gilmore N, Vane JR, Wyllie JH (1968) Prostaglandins released by the spleen. Nature 218:1125–1140
60. Widmark, E, Waldeck B (1986 Physiological and pharmacological characterization of an in vitro vagus nerve-trachea preparation from guinea-pig. J Auton Pharmacol 6:187–194
61. Empey DW, Laitinen LA, Jacobs L, Gold WM, Nadel JA (1976) Mechanisms of bronchial hyperreactivity in normal subjects following upper respiratory tract infection. Am Rev Respir Dis 113:131–139
62. Farmer SG (1986) Neutrophils and ozone-induced airway hyper-reactivity: cause or effect? Trends Pharmacol Sci 7:169–170
63. Farmer SG (1987) Airway smooth muscle responsiveness modulation by the epithelium. Trends Pharmacol Sci 81:8–10
64. Flavahan NA, Aarhus T, Rimele TJ, van Houtte PM (1985) Respiratory epithelium inhibits bronchial smooth muscle tone. J Appl Physiol 58:834–838
65. de Mey JG, van Houtte PM (1981) Role of the intima in cholinergic and purinergic relaxation of isolated canine femoral arteries. J Physiol 316:347–355
66. Furchgott RF, Zawdazki JV (1980) The obligatory role of endothelial cells in the relaxation of arterial smooth muscle by acetylcholine. Nature 288:373–376
67. Hisayama T, Takayanagi I, Nakazato F, Hirano F (1988) Epithelium selectively controls hypersensitization of the response of smooth muscle to leukotriene D_4 by endogenous prostanoid(s) in guinea-pig trachea. Naunyn-Schmiedebergs Arch Pharmacol 337:296–300
68. Goldie RG, Papadimitrious JM, Paterson JW, Rigby PJ, Self HM, Spina D (1986) Influence of the epithelium on the responsiveness of guinea-pig isolated trachea to contractile and relaxant agonists. Br J Pharmacol 87:5–14
69. Hay DWP, Farmer SG, Raeburn D, Robinson VA, Fleming WW, Fedan JS (1986) Airway epithelium modulates the reactivity of guinea-pig respiratory smooth muscle. Eur J Pharmacol 129:11–18
70. Holroyde MC (1986) The influence of epithelium on the responsiveness of guinea-pig isolated trachea. Br J Pharmacol 87:501–507
71. Hay DWP, Raeburn D, Farmer SG, Fleming WW, Fedant JS (1986) Epithelium modulates the reactivity of ovalbumin-sensitized guinea-pig airway smooth muscle. Life Sci 38:2461–2468
72. Raeburn D, Hay DWP, Robinson VA, Farmer SG, Fleming WW, Fedan JS (1986) The effect of verapamil is reduced in isolated airway smooth muscle preparations lacking the epithelium. Life Sci 38:809–816
73. Barnes PJ, Cuss FM, Palmer JB (1985) The effect of airway epithelium on smooth muscle contractility in bovine trachea. Br J Pharmacol 86:685–692
74. Raeburn D, Hay DWP, Farmer SG, Fedan JS (1986) Epithelium removal increases the reactivity of human isolated tracheal muscle to methacholine and reduces the effect of verapamil. Eur J Pharmacol 123:451–453
75. Fine JM, Gordon T, Sheppard D (1989) Epithelium removal alters responsiveness of guinea-pig trachea to substance P. J Appl Physiol 66:232–237
76. Aarrhus LL, Rimele TJ, van Houtte PM (1984) Removal of epithelium causes bronchial supersensitivity to acetylcholine and 5-hydroxytryptamine. Fed Proc 43:995–999
77. Niemeier RW, Bingham E (1972) An isolated perfused lung preparation for metabolic studies. Life Sci 11:807–820
78. Mehendale HM, Angevine LS, Ohmiya Y (1981) The isolated perfused lung: a critical evaluation. Toxicology 21:1–36
79. Niemeier RW (1984) The isolated perfused lung. Environ Health Perspect 56:35–41
80. Kroll F, Karlsson JA, Nilsson E, Persson CGA, Ryrfeldt A (1986) Lung mechanics of the guinea-pig isolated perfused lung. Acta Physiol Scand 128:1–8

81. McLaughlin RJ (1977) Systematic design of cantilever beams for muscle research. J Appl Physiol 42:786–794
82. Norris G, Carmeci P (1965) Isotonic muscle transducer. J Appl Physiol 20: 355–356
83. Illingworth DR, Naylor IL (1982) An improved, ultrasonic auxotonic transducer for use with isolated tissues. J Pharmacol Methods 8:59–71
83a.Blattner R, Classen HG, Dehnert H, Döring HJ (1978) Experiments on isolated smooth muscle preparations. HSE Biological Measuring Techniques. Sachs, Freiburg, p4
84. Paton WDM (1975) The recording of mechanical responses of smooth muscle. Methods Pharmacol 3:261–264
85. Santesson CG (1891) Studien über die allgemeine Mechanik des Muskels. Skand Arch Physiol 3:381–436
86. Paton WDM (1957) A pendulum auxotonic lever. J Physiol 137:35P–36P
87. Von Frey N (1908) Allegemeine muskelmechanik. In: Tigersted R (ed) Handbuch der physiologischen Methodik, vol 2. Hirzel, Leipzig, pp 87–119
88. Gaddum JH (1965) An improved microbath. Br J Pharmacol 23:613–619
89. Jewell BR, Wilkie DR (1958) An analysis of the mechanical components in frog's striated muscle. J Physiol 143:515–540
90. Lewis AF (1969) An improved isotonic transducer. J Physiol 203:15–17P
91. Mc Intosh M, Duggan DE, Watt DD, Goodson LH (1965) A photopotentiometric transducer for detecting in vitro muscle contractions. J Appl Physiol 20: 349–350
92. Ross SM, Brust M (1966) A photopotentiometric isotonic myogram. J Appl Physiol 21:293–294
93. Deby G, Espreux G, Topa C (1972) Appareil d'enregistrement electrique des contractions musculaires de faible amplitude. Experientia 28:114–115
94. Bucking J, Herbst M, Piontek P (1973) Ein optischer Messwertwandler zur Registrierung der Muskelkontraktion. Experientia 29:1311–1312
95. Erdos EG, Jackman V, Barnes WC (1962) Instrument for recording isotonic contractions of smooth muscles. J Appl Physiol 17:367–368
96. Hansom DN, Hughes IE, Letley E (1970) An isotonic transducer for general use. J Pharm Pharmacol 22:309–310
97. Jewell BR, Kretzschmar M, Woledge RC (1967) Length and tension transducer. J Physiol 191:10P–12P
98. Mellor PM (1984) A precision isotonic measuring system for isolated tissues. J Pharmacol Methods 12:259–264
99. Boucek RJ, Murphy WP, Paff GA (1959) Electrical and mechanical properties of chick embryo heart chambers. Circ Res 7:787–793
100. Cambridge GW, Haines J (1959) A new versatile transducer system inductance/capacitance change. J Physiol 149:2P–3P
101. Schilling MO (1960) Capacitance transducer for muscle research. Rev Sci Instr 31:1215–1217
102. Duxbury AJ (1971) A simple linear transducer for physiological and pharmacological applications. Med Biol Eng 9:719–720
103. Lewis AF (1969) An isometric strain-gauge transducer unit. J Physiol 203: 17P–19P
104. Feigl EO, Simon GA, Fry DL (1967) Auxotonic and isometric cardiac force transducers. J Appl Physiol 23:597–600
105. Hedlund L, Valentich F, Ralph CL, Cepko J, Lynch HJ (1971) Serotonin assay: a tissue chamber and recording lever for the fundus strip method. J Appl Physiol 30:787–791
106. Rosenblueth A, Alanis J, Robio R (1958) A comparative study of the isometric and isotonic contractions of striated muscle. Arch Int Physiol Biochem 66: 330–353
107. Taylor RR (1970) Active length-tension relations compared in isometric, after-

load and isotonic contractions of cat papillary muscle – their dependence on inotropic state. Circ Res 26:279–288

108. Michelson MJ, Shelkovnikov SA (1976) Isotonic and isometric responses of different tonic muscles to agonists and antagonists. Br J Pharmacol 56:457–467
109. Stephens NL, Van Niekerk W (1976) Isometric and isotonic contractions in airway smooth muscle. Can J Physiol Pharmacol 55:833–838
110. De Jongste JC, Mons H, van Strik R, Bonta IL, Kerrebijn KF (1987) Comparison of isometric and isotonic responses of human small airway smooth muscle in vitro. J Pharmacol Methods 17:165–171
111. Christensen JH, Østgaard SE, Andreasen F (1982) The influence of pO$_2$, pH and albumin on the in vitro contraction of vascular smooth muscle. J Pharmacol Methods 8:99–108
112. Lockwood APM (1961) Ringer solutions and some notes on the physiological basis of their ionic compositions. Comp Biochem Physiol 2:241–289
113. Perry WLM (1968) Pharmacological experiments on isolated preparations. Livingstone, Edinburgh
114. Mac Conail M (1985) Calcium precipitation from mammalian physiological salines (Ringer solutions) and the preparation of high [Ca] media. J Pharmacol Methods 14:147–155
115. Chang AA, Detar R (1980) Oxygen and vascular smooth muscle contraction revisited. Am J Physiol 238:H716–H728
116. Stephens NL, Meyer JL, Cherniack RM (1968) Oxygen, carbon dioxide, H$^+$ ion, and bronchial length-tension relationships. J Appl Physiol 25:376–383
117. Ringer S (1883) A further contribution regarding the influence of the different constituents of the blood on the contraction of the heart. J Physiol 4:249–254
118. Locke FS, Rosenheim O (1907) Contributions to the physiology of the isolated heart. The consumption of dextrose by mammalian cardiac muscle. J Physiol 36:205–220
119. Chenoweth MB, Koelle ES (1946) An isolated heart perfusion system adapted to the determination of nongasesous metabolites. J Lab Clin Med 31:600–608
120. Goodford PJ, Freeman-Narrod M (1962) Sodium and potassium content of the smooth muscle of the guinea-pig taenia coli at different temperatures and tensions. J Physiol 163:399–410

Evaluation of *In Vitro* Data on Agents Acting on Respiratory Smooth Muscle Tone

P. C. BRAGA

Center for Respiratory Pharmacology, School of Medicine, University of Milan, Milano, Italy

Introduction

When a chemical agent comes in contact (in different ways) with a biological structure there may be an interaction, with the final effect being a change from normal physiological function.

A drug can be characterized by investigating the changes induced by its administration in vivo or in vitro. In vivo studies are obviously closer to the true conditions of administration of a drug, but it is not usually possible to get information about its interaction with specific biological structures. With in vitro studies we can investigate this interaction under controlled conditions, without biological interference from other structures or organs (i.e., biotransformation, redistribution), assay drug-receptor interactions, and obtain dose-response curves with agonists and/or antagonists. Many different in vitro tissue preparations have been proposed for studying different kinds of drugs, but the method of analysis of the reciprocal interactions is the same and is based on the finding that the intensity of the pharmacological effect is a function of the number of receptors (in percent) occupied by the drug.

Dose–Effect Relationships

Figure 1A is a plot of the relationship between increasing concentrations of a drug and its effect [1]. The same phenomenon can also be plotted with the logarithm of the concentration on the abscissa. This gives a classical sigmoid curve (Fig. 1B).

The relationship between the drug (agonist) and the receptor, which is the basis of the pharmacological effect, depends on the number of receptors occupied, which is to say, on the concentration of agonist and the intrinsic activity of the agonist (potency). Dose–response curves can be obtained by measuring the effects of individual doses. The first dose chosen is added to the bath in a small volume and the effect is measured. When a stable level is reached the preparation is then washed to completely remove the drug and allowed to return to baseline. Increasing doses are then tested and the results

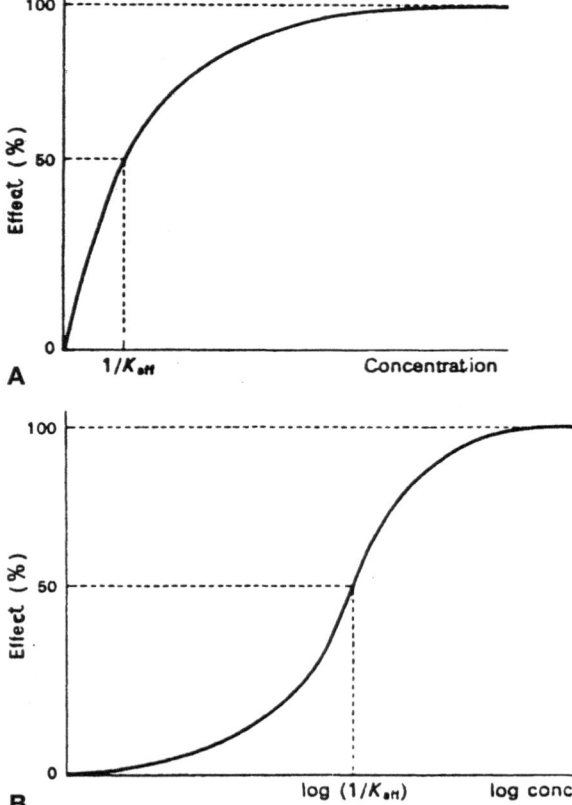

Fig. 1. A Relationship between concentration of a drug and its effect and **B** between the log of the concentration and its effect; a sigmoid curve is generated

plotted as in Fig. 2A. This approach is time-consuming but necessary for drugs that are easily degradable or that induce responses which are not stable over time.

For more stable drugs and more stable responses a cumulative dose–response curve (CRC) can be obtained. This means that when equilibrium has been reached, after the first dose, increasing doses can be added without washing [2]. A curve obtained in this way is shown in Fig. 2B.

The presentation of the doses on the abscissa depends on the variability of the preparation, on the accuracy of the recording, and on the slope of the dose–response curves. The time to reach equilibrium must also be considered. A logarithmic sequence of increasing doses, with steps of a factor of 10, is frequently used.

The effect obtained with every cumulative dose is measured in millimeters and calculated as a percentage of the maximum response (maximum height). The percentages are plotted on a linear scale on the ordinate against the doses plotted on a logarithmic scale on the abscissa.

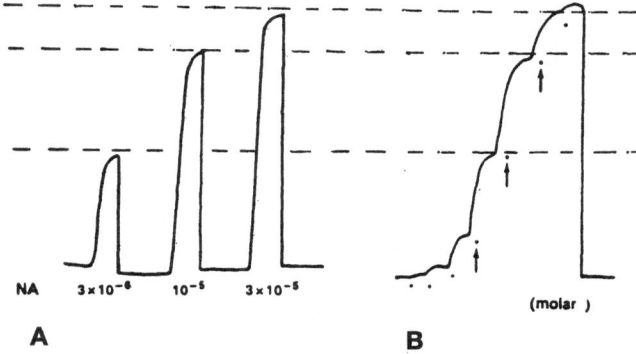

Fig. 2A, B. Increasing doses of an agonist induce a progressive increase in effects. **A** Washing between doses; **B** cumulative dose–response curve with the same doses

NA 3×10^{-6} 10^{-5} 3×10^{-5} (molar)

A   B

Evaluation of Agonist Action

Stimulant drugs are called agonists and have two characteristics, affinity for the receptor and intrinsic activity (potency). If the relationship between stimulus and effect is linear, the intrinsic activity and affinity can be determined directly from the dose–response curves [2].

The affinity is calculated from the position of the curve on the abscissa, as shown in Fig. 3 [1], and from the negative logarithm of the dose that produces 50% of the maximum effect. This magnitude is called the pD_2 [3].

$$pD_2 = -\log A_{50}$$

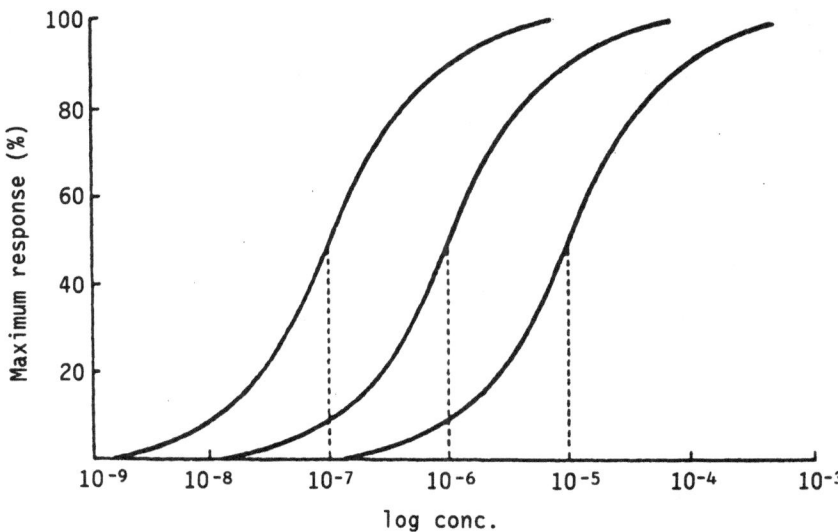

Fig. 3. Theoretical curves (dose–effect) of drugs with the same activity but with different receptor affinity. (From [1])

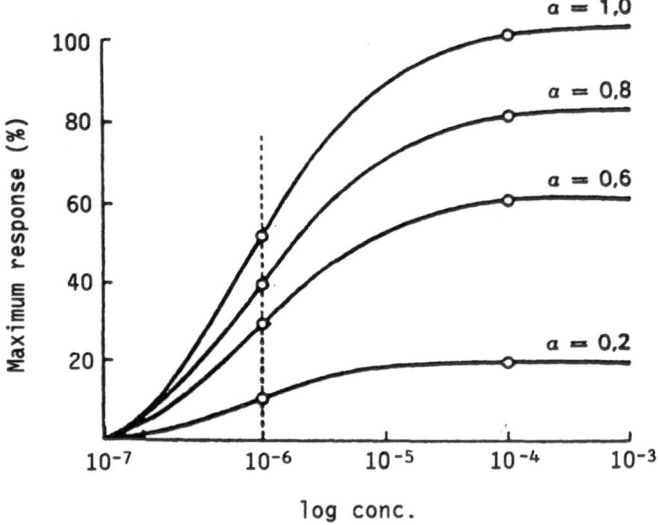

Fig. 4. Theoretical curves (dose–effect) of drugs with the same receptor affinity but with different activity. (From [1])

in which A_{50} is the molar concentration which produces 50% of the maximum response to the agonist. The dose of agonist producing the 50% effect ($E_{Am}/E_A = 2$; where E_{Am} = maximal effect of the drug A and E_m = maximal effect of the reference compound) for the agonist is determined by measuring the distance in millimeters between the position of the 50% effect point and a point ($10^{-q} M$) chosen on the abscissa to the left of the point measured ($pD_2 = q - \log A$).

The intrinsic activity (α) is calculated from the maximal effect that can be obtained with the drug, as shown in Fig. 4 [1], and is expressed as the ratio between the maximum effect E_{Am} of the drug A and the E_m of the reference compound [2]:

$$\alpha = E_{Am}/E_m$$

If different agonists have different affinities and intrinsic activities the dose–effect curves are not parallel, as shown in Fig. 5.

The dose–response curves of some drugs may show a maximum (peak) (autoinhibition). In that case, the drug also has affinity towards noncompetitive receptors at higher doses [2].

Evaluation of Antagonist Action

A chemical agent that reduces the effect of an agonist is called an antagonist. Antagonists have affinity for the specific receptors but no intrinsic activity

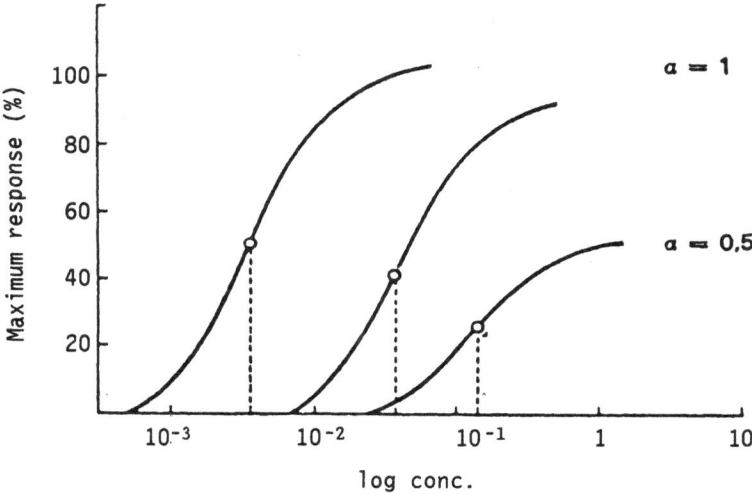

Fig. 5. Theoretical curves (dose–effect) of drugs with different receptor affinity and with different activity. (From [1])

and thus do not generate a stimulus. There are different forms of antagonism. A competitive antagonist is one that competes with the antagonist for the same receptors. Competitive antagonists can be studied by virtue of their influence on the effect of stimulant drugs. They are therefore always studied in combination with an agonist.

Whatever the relationship between stimulus and effect, the dose-response curve for the agonist in the presence of a constant concentration of the competitive drug has a shape essentially identical to the curve obtained without the antagonist, but the curves are shifted to the right on the log dose-axis.

The extent of a shift in the dose-response curve of a stimulant drug can be used to calculate the affinity of the antagonist.

Shild [4, 5] introduced a value called pA_x for comparing the potencies of antagonists. pA_x is the negative logarithm of the molar concentration of the antagonist (A):

$$pA_x = -(\log 1/B)$$

in which x is the ratio for equiactive doses of agonist with and without the antagonist, and B is the molar concentration of the agonist. When a double dose of the antagonist is required to reproduce the same initial effect of the agonist, the negative logarithm of this concentration is called pA_2.

The relationship between pA_x and pA_2 is a follows:

$$pA_2 = pA_x + \log(x-1)$$

Noncompetitive Antagonists

Noncompetitive antagonists have no affinity for the specific receptors of the agonist, but interact with different receptors and in this way influence either stimulus formation or stimulus effectuation. The main action of the noncompetitive antagonist is to depress the dose–response curve for the agonist. The negative logarithm of the molar concentration which produces such a depression is called the pD'_x value [6]. The negative logarithm of the molar concentration which causes a 50% depression ($x=2$) is called the pD'_2 value. $[pD'_2 = pD'_x + \log(x-1)]$.

Quantitative Assays

In vitro tissue preparations can also be used for quantitative assay of drugs or biological substances of unknown concentration. This use of the in vitro preparation received great theoretical and practical attention mainly between 1920 and 1970. Recently, sophisticated chemical and physical analytical methods have reduced their importance for this purpose. Nevertheless, the three-point assay and, even better, the four-point assay can be useful for the assay of agonists and or antagonists. The methods are well standardized and technical details are reported in pharmacological texts [1, 7].

Variability of In Vitro Tests

There is also biological variability of in vitro preparations. This means that different preparations can give different biological responses to stimuli of the same intensity. A dose that is applied successfully to one preparation of-

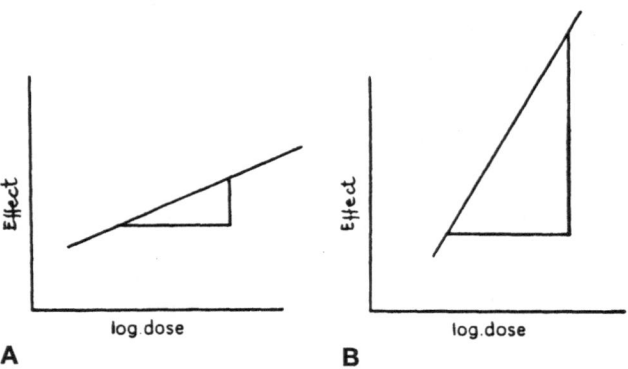

Fig. 6A, B. Relationship between the slope of the log dose–response line and the ability to discriminate between doses. **A** poor discrimination; **B** good discrimination. (From [7])

ten gives different results in another. Great care must be taken during: (a) excision of the trachea or bronchi, (b) manipulation for preparation, (c) maintenance in vitro, and (d) drug application. All of these steps must be well standardized and a control for good reproducibility of each step must be performed. Moreover, the sensitivity of the preparation can vary during the course of the experiment.

The slope of the log dose–response line provides information about the ability to discriminate between doses. When large differences in log dose produce only small differences in response, the preparation has a poor ability to discriminate (Fig. 6A). The opposite is shown in Fig. 6B: quite small differences in log dose produced large differences in response with great discrimination.

References

1. Bonaccorsi A (1972) Sperimentazione farmacologica su organi isolati. Boringhieri, Torino
2. Van Rossum JM (1963) Cumulative dose-response curves II. Technique for the making for dose-response curves in isolated organs and the evaluation of drug parameters. Arch Int Pharmacodyn 143:299–330
3. Ariens EJ, van Rossum JM (1957) pD_x, pA_x and pD'_x values in the analysis of pharmacodynamics. Arch Int Pharmacodyn 110:275–300
4. Schild HO (1947) pA_x, a new scale for the measurement of drug antagonism. Br J Pharmacol 2:189–207
5. Schild HO (1949) pA_x and competitive drug antagonism. Br J Pharmacol 4: 277–280
6. Stephenson RP (1956) A modification of receptor theory. Br J Pharmacol 11: 379–394
7. Department of Pharmacology of the University of Edinburgh (1968) Pharmacological experiments on isolated preparations. Livingstone, Edinburgh

Methods for Assessing Airway Blood Flow in Asthma

A. WANNER

Pulmonary Division, Schoof of Medicine, University of Miami, Miami FL, USA

Introduction

Since the tracheobronchial vasculature is the principal source of blood flow in the conducting airways, it can influence bronchial caliber [17], the bronchial response to thermal stress [4], the clearance of chemical mediators and other materials from the airway wall [18], the metabolism of circulating, biologically active substances before they reach the airway tissues [24], the distribution of systemically administered drugs to the airway, and the absorption of inhaled drugs from the airway. These functions may be relevant to the pathogenesis and treatment of bronchial asthma.

To appreciate the significance of the airway circulation, several of its physiologic and anatomic features should be pointed out. First, while airway blood flow in humans only constitutes 0.5–1% of cardiac output, the airways are highly perfused structures in comparison to other organs. In the trachea of sheep, for example, an animal species which does not use panting to control body temperature, blood flow values between 50 and 100 ml min^{-1} 100 g^{-1} wet tissue weight have been reported [40, 47]. Corresponding values for the brain and myocardium are 50 and 80 ml min^{-1} 100 g^{-1}, respectively. Second, airway circulation is under autonomic control, as suggested by the association of adrenergic, peptidergic, and, to a lesser extent, cholinergic nerves with bronchial vessels [10, 41] and by the ability to alter the perfusion and permeability of the airway circulation by efferent and afferent autonomic nerve stimulation and exogenous neurotransmitters [9, 26, 37]. Third, the microcirculation in the airway wall is strategically located between the surface epithelium, submucosal glands, and airway smooth muscle. Of the subepithelial tissue, the microvascular volume occupies 10% in the trachea and 20% in bronchioles, and as much as 85% of total tracheal blood flow has been reported to be directed to the subepithelial space in sheep [21, 35]. Thus, the airway circulation is well positioned to participate in the principal manifestations of bronchial asthma, i.e., mucosal dysfunction, airway smooth muscle contraction, and edema.

Alterations in blood flow and permeability are the two principal vascular responses in all vascular beds including the airway vascular bed. This brief review addresses blood flow responses. The experimental techniques required to measure airway blood flow are invasive and have therefore only been tried in animals. The experimental data pertaining to the participation of airway blood flow in airway disease have therefore been obtained primarily in animal models. Until less invasive methodologies which are suitable for use in human subjects have been developed, the significance of the airway circulation in the manifestations of bronchial asthma has to be deduced from the animal observations.

Methods

The blood supply to the trachea and larger bronchi is derived from systemic artieries which give rise to a plexus on the outside of the airway wall and another underneath the epithelium. The two plexus are connected by perforating branches [21]. Likewise, the veins form an inner and outer plexus, which are interconnected. In peripheral bronchioles, a distinction between the arterial and venous plexus is lost. The microvascular beds in the larger airways are interposed between arteries and veins while in peripheral bronchioles, the airway microvascular may anastomose with the pulmonary capillaries. Whereas the inflow of blood into the airway is supplied by the aorta and its branches, the venous drainage from the airway follows different paths along the length of the tracheobronchial tree. Venous blood from the trachea and larger bronchi drains via the azygous veins into the superior vena cava. The venous blood from the rest of the bronchial tree drains into pulmonary veins either directly or through pulmonary capillaries. The fraction of tracheobronchial blood flow which returns to the pulmonary veins is called anastomotic blood flow. Anastomotic blood flow occurs both through bronchial capillaries and arteriovenous connections bypassing the bronchial capillaries. There are interspecies differences in the anatomy of the airway circulation, but the basic pattern of nonanastomotic and anastomotic blood flow is present in most species studied.

The design of an outer and inner subepithelial vascular bed in the airway permits individual blood flow control through parallel resistors in the deep and subepithelial vascular beds. Therefore, the inflow of blood into the airway wall and subepithelial blood flow cannot be equated and have to be measured independently.

Total Blood Flow in the Tracheobronchial Tree

The term "total tracheobronchial blood flow" may be misleading since most methods used for its determination do not measure the entire blood supply to the conducting airways. For example, a flow probe placed around a bronchial artery would only reflect total blood flow if the artery is the sole source of blood supply to the tracheobronchial tree. This is never the case, although in certain species a major bronchial artery may invest more than 50%–70%

of the tracheobronchial tree. The blood flow measurement should therefore be considered as representative of rather than entirely representing total blood flow. Total tracheobronchial blood flow is generally used to denote the supply (inflow) of blood to the entire cross-section of the tracheal and bronchial wall, thereby differentiating it from microvascular blood flow at different depths of the airway wall.

Anastomotic Blood Flow

Bronchopulmonary anastomotic blood flow, i.e., the fraction of total bronchial arterial inflow that drains into the pulmonary circulation rather than the azygos vein, has been estimated to comprise two thirds of total bronchial arterial inflow [11]. Anastomotic bronchopulmonary flow can be determined by measuring right and left ventricular output separately. The difference between the two constitutes anastomotic blood flow. It amounts to approximately 1% of cardiac output in dogs and in humans [19, 20]. A higher value (3%) has been reported during cardiopulmonary bypass in humans where, after cross-clamping of the aorta, the only source of blood return to the left atrium is the bronchopulmonary anastomotic channels [7]. Blood flow through bronchopulmonary anastomoses has also been determined in lobes of open chested dogs by cannulating the labor branch of the pulmonary artery and the pulmonary vein and calculating the difference between the two [13].

Bronchial (Tracheal) Artery Cannulation

Bruner and Schmidt [12] cannulated the right bronchial artery of dogs and obtained an estimate of total bronchial blood flow of about 1% of cardiac output. Arterial cannulation has also been carried out in sheep, a species in which the bronchial artery provides most of the airway blood flow, and in the trachea of dogs (cranial tracheal artery) [14, 27]. In those studies, hemodynamic responses of the airway circulation were assessed by relating perfusion pressure to blood flow through the cannula under conditions of controlled pressure or flow. The possibility of administering vasoactive substances directly into the tracheal and bronchial arteries is a major advantage of this method.

Total bronchial blood flow can also be measured by creating an aortic pouch from which all bronchial arteries arise [25].

Flow Probes

In species with a large single bronchial artery which supplies the majority of airway blood flow (seal, pig, horse, sheep), a flow probe can be surgically placed around the bronchial artery to assess the hemodynamic responsiveness of the airway circulation without artificially altering it by the technique itself [1]. Magno and Fishman [33] placed an electromagnetic flow probe around the bronchoesophageal artery of sheep, ligated the esophageal branch, and found that 85% of airway blood flow was supplied by this artery; mean bronchial blood flow was 0.4% of cardiac output. Somewhat higher values (0.3%–3.3%) have been found by Long et al. [31] in the same species. Although the bronchial artery in sheep may contribute less than 85% to total airway blood flow, as suggested by other investigators [46], the flow probe method has retained its usefulness in physiologic studies involving the airway circulation [2, 32].

Video Densitometry

Parsons et al. [40] described a method to estimate bronchial arterial flow in intact sheep. An aortic catheter was placed with its tip near the origin of the bronchial artery and a radiopaque material (renographic) was injected through it. Radio density was then measured externally by fluoroscopy (with image intensifier) and videotaped for subsequent analysis using a window over the bronchial artery. The magnitude of bronchial blood flow (0.6% of cardiac output) was comparable to that obtained by other methods. Video densitometry can theoretically be used in humans; however, it remains to be shown if the technique is feasible in species, e.g. humans, with multiple arterial roots supplying the airway circulation.

Radiolabeled Microspheres

The determination of radioactivity in the lung removed from animals injected with 15 μm radiolabeled microspheres into the aorta can be used to calculate total airway blood flow. Due to the presence of peripheral arteriovenous shunts in the body, a fraction of the injected microspheres escapes trapping in the systemic microvascular bed, is recirculated through the pulmonary circulation, becomes trapped in the pulmonary microvascular bed, and contributes to the radioactivity of the lung. The microsphere technique, as originally described by Rudolph and Heyman [43], therefore has to be modified by ligating the pulmonary artery at a time after microsphere injection when systemic microvascular trapping has already occurred but pulmonary vascular trapping has not yet occurred. Employing this technique, airway blood flow to one lung has been reported to constitute 0.4% of cardiac output [8]. A correction for peripheral shunting of microspheres can also be made by obtaining timed reference samples from aorta and pulmonary artery after injection [34].

Pulmonary Gas Exchange

In the absence of pulmonary blood flow, gas exchange in a lung must be proportional to airway blood flow (vicarious pulmonary perfusion). Using this principle, airway blood flow to one lung after pulmonary artery ligation has been measured by CO and O_2 uptake, and CO_2 elimination in dogs [23, 30]. A wide range of airway blood flow to one lung was observed, depending upon the gas used (0.3%–3% of cardiac output).

Microvascular Blood Flow in the Tracheobronchial Tree

Microvascular blood flow in the conducting airways has been estimated or measured by laser doppler velocimetry (large airways), the uptake of a soluble inert gas (large airways), and radiolabeled microspheres (large and smaller airways). The former two have the advantage of assessing subepithelial blood flow in intact animals and humans, whereas the latter has the advantages of accuracy and localization of microvascular blood flow in the airway wall but the disadvantage of requiring tissue removal for analysis.

Radiolabeled Microspheres

Several investigators have used this method to measure microvascular blood flow in the airway of different species. Chih-Hsiung et al. [16] found that in sheep, airway microvascular blood flow to the entire airway wall, as measured with 15 μm microspheres, increased along the tracheobronchial tree from 16 ml min^{-1} 100 g^{-1} wet tissue in the trachea to 22 ml min^{-1} 100 g^{-1} wet tissue in the lung parenchyma (Table 1). The authors found blood flow in the subepithelial compartment of the trachea to be considerably higher. Likewise, tracheal mucosal blood flow in rabbits has been reported around 30 ml min^{-1} 100 g^{-1} wet tissue [38]. Tracheal subepithelial blood flow may be higher in dogs and possibly other species that utilize panting for body temperature control [3].

Soluble Gas Uptake

The steady-state uptake of a soluble gas from an isolated airway segment is governed by microvascular blood flow underneath the epithelium. A tracheal segment can be created *in vivo* by placing in it an endotracheal tube with two cuffs [47]. A soluble inert gas such as dimethyl-ether can then be introduced into the chamber and the uptake of dimethyl-ether from the chamber determined by a sensitive pneumotachograph connected to a catheter venting the chamber. Theoretically, this method can detected subepithelial microvascular blood flow to a tissue depth of 200 μm; in the trachea, this

Table 1. Microvascular blood flow in the airway wall

Anatomical location	Species	Blood flow ($ml\ min^{-1}\ 100\ g^{-1}$ wet tissue)	Method (reference)
Trachea			
Entire wall	Sheep	16	RM [16]
Mucosa	Sheep	95	RM [40]
	Sheep	52	SG [47]
	Rabbit	30	RM [38]
	Dog	54	RM [6]
Main Bronchus			
Entire wall	Sheep	17	RM [16]
Labor Bronchus			
Entire wall	Sheep	18	RM [16]
	Dog	28	RM [6]
Lung parenchyma	Sheep	22	RM [16]
	Dog	4	RM [4]

RM, radiolabeled microsphere technique; SG, soluble gas uptake technique

depth is within the mucosa. In lightly anesthetized sheep, the method has yielded an average blood flow of 52 ml min^{-1} 100 g^{-1} wet tissue [47]. This value was about 80% of tracheal mucosal perfusion as assessed by the radio-labeled microsphere technique.

Laser Doppler Velocimetry

Mucosal blood flow can also be measured with laser Doppler velocimetry [44]. Within the respiratory system, this method was first used in the nose [39]. Druce et al. [22] obtained in the human nose the value of 42 ml min^{-1} 100 g^{-1} wet tissue. Recently, a similar technique has been reported for the measurement of mucosal blood flow in the human trachea [5]. Absolute blood flow values were not obtained, but the method seems to be capable of detecting changes in tracheal mucosal blood flow. Since velocity is measured, the assumption has to be made that vascular diameters at the site of measurement undergo minor changes as flow increases or decreases.

Tracheobronchial Blood Flow in Asthma

Hyperemia of the bronchial mucosa is a characteristic endoscopic finding in patients with asthma. However, direct measurements of airway blood flow have thus far not been reported in human subjects. Inflammation appears to be an important feature of bronchial asthma, and an increase in airway blood flow can therefore be expected. Animal studies have suggested several possible mechanisms by which inflammation increases airway blood flow.

Airway anaphylaxis in animals has been the best studied model of the vascular responses in human bronchial asthma. In allergic sheep, inhalation challenge with specific antigen has been shown to lead to an increase in total bronchial blood flow which corresponds to the immediate increase in airflow resistance [32]. This change in airway blood flow appears to be independent of the mechanical effects of bronchoconstriction as demonstrated by the use of specific blocking agents. Mucosal blood flow also participates in this response [18]. The observation that intravenous sodium cromoglycate blunts the antigen induced increase of bronchial blood flow suggests the involvement of chemical mediators.

Inflammatory Mediators

The effects of several inflammatory mediators including amines, kinins, and lipid metabolites on airway blood flow have been evaluated in animals. Infused histamine has been found to lower tracheal vascular resistance in dogs and inhaled histamine to increase bronchial blood flow and tracheal mucosal blood flow in sheep [15, 28, 31]. Bradykinin is a potent vasodilator and increases permeability in systemic vascular beds including those in the airways [45]. The lipoxygenase and cyclooxygenase products of arachidonic acid, and platelet activating factor have also been shown to influence the airways vasculature. In the trachea, the sulfidopeptide leukotrienes have been shown to have variable effects on vascular resistance in different animal species [29, 42]. Prostaglanding B_1 and $F_{2\alpha}$, prostacyclin, and platelet activating factor are also vasodilators [28]. Finally, vasodilator prostanoids contribute significantly to the increase in bronchial blood flow which accompanies allergic bronchoconstriction in sheep [32]. Thus, several mediators released from inflammatory cells in the airway wall have the potential of increasing airway blood flow.

Neuropeptides

Laitinen et al. [28] showed that, in dogs, atropine pretreatment only partially blocked the decrease in tracheal vascular resistance during vagal nerve stimulation and that this was not blocked by hexamethonium. This suggested antidromic vagal vasodilation, presumably mediated by neuropeptides. The same authors showed that vasoactive intestinal peptide, substance P, and several other neuropeptides lower tracheal vascular resistance, with neurokinin-A being the most potent [26]. Of all the peptides tested, only neuropeptide tyrosine was found to be a vasoconstrictor. Noncholinergic vagally induced vasodilation in the bronchial tree has also been reported by another group of investigators [36]. The possibility therefore exists that local axon reflexes, via the release of vasoactive neuropeptides, control airway mucosal blood flow.

One might conclude from these animal studies that the role of airway perfusion in bronchial asthma merits further characterization. Hopefully, this research will not be limited to the physiological aspects of the airway circulation but also address its metabolic functions. Such information could advance our understanding of the mechanisms leading to airway disease and introduce new treatment modalities. However, a reliable noninvasive method for the assessment of airway blood flow in human subjects would first have to be developed.

References

1. Baier H, Long WM, Wanner A (1985) Bronchial circulation in asthma. Respiration 48:199–205
2. Baier H, Yerger L, Moas R, Wanner A (1985) Vascular and airway effects of endogenous cyclooxygenase products during lung inflation. J Appl Physiol 59: 884–889
3. Baile EM, Dahlby RW, Wiggs BR, Pare PD (1985) Role of tracheal and bronchial circulation in respiratory heat exchange. J Appl Physiol 58:217–222
4. Baile EM, Dahlby RW, Wiggs BR, Parsons GH, Pare PD (1987) Effect of cold and warm dry air hyperventilation on canine airway blood flow. J Appl Physiol 62:526–532
5. Baile EM, Godden DJ, Pare PD (1989) Effect of cold dry and warm humid air hyperventilation on tracheal wall blood flow in humans. Am Rev Respir Dis 139:A63 (abstract)
6. Baile EM, Guillemi S, Pare PD (1987) Tracheobronchial and upper airway blood flow in dogs during thermally induced panting. J Appl Physiol 63:2240–2246
7. Baile EM, Ling H, Heyworth JR, Hogg JC, Pare PD (1985) Bronchopulmonary anastomotic and noncoronary collateral blood flow in humans during cardiopulmonary bypass. Chest 87:749–754
8. Baile EM, Nelems JMB, Schulzer M, Pare PD (1982) Measurement of regional bronchial arterial blood flow and bronchial resistance in dogs. J Appl Physiol 53:1044–1049
9. Barker JA, Chediak AD, Baier HJ, Wanner A (1988) Tracheal mucosal blood flow responses to autonomic agonists. J Appl Physiol 65:829–834
10. Barnes P (1987) Neuropeptides in human airways: function and clinical implications. Am Rev Respir Dis 136:S77–S83
11. Berry JL, deBurgh Daly I (1931) The relationship between the pulmonary and bronchial vascular systems. Proc R Soc Lond [Biol] 109:319–336
12. Bruner HD, Schmidt CF (1947) Blood flow in the bronchial artery of the anesthetized dog. Am J Physiol 148:643–666
13. Charan NB, Albert RK, Lakshminarayan S, Kirk W, Butler J (1986) Factors affecting bronchial blood flow through bronchopulmonary anastomoses in dogs. Am Rev Respir Dis 134:85–88
14. Charan NB, Turk GM, Ripley R (1985) Measurement of bronchial arterial blood flow and bronchovascular resistance in sheep. J Appl Physiol 59:305–308
15. Chediak AD, Wanner A (1988) Effects of histamine on mucosal perfusion, water content and airway smooth muscle in the trachea: role of H_1 and H_2 receptors. Am Rev Respir Dis 137 (4):200 (abstract)
16. Chih-Hsiung Wu D, Lindsey C, Traber DL, Cross CE, Herndon DN, Kramer GC (1988) Measurement of bronchial blood flow with radioactive microspheres in awake sheep. J Appl Physiol 65:1131–1139
17. Csete ME, Abraham, WM, Wanner A (1990) Vasomotion influences airflow in peripheral airways. Am Rev Respir Dis (in press)

18. Csete ME, Chediak AD, Wanner A (1989) Mucosal blood flow influences the duration of allergic airway smooth muscle contraction in the trachea. Am Rev Respir Dis 139 (4): A228 (abstract)
19. Cudkowicz L, Calabresi M, Nims RG, Gray FD (1959) The simultaneous estimation of right and left ventricular outputs applied to a study of the bronchial circulation in patients with chronic lung disease. Am Heart J 58:743–749
20. Cudkowicz L, Calabresi M, Nims RG, Gray FD (1959) The simultaneous estimation of right and left ventricular outputs applied to a study of a bronchial circulation in dogs. Am Heart J 58:732–742
21. Deffebach ME, Charan NB, Lakshminarayan S, Butler J (1987) The bronchial circulation: small, but a vital attribute of the lung. Am Rev Respir Dis 135:463–481
22. Druce HM, Bonner RF, Patow C, Choo P, Summers RJ, Kaliner MA (1984) Response of nasal blood flow to neurohormones as measured by laser-Doppler velocimetry. J Appl Physiol 57:1276–1283
23. Fisher AB, Kollmeier H, Brody JS et al. (1970) Restoration of systemic blood flow to the lung after division of bronchial arteries. J Appl Physiol 29:839–846
24. Granthan CJ, Jackowski JT, Wanner A, Ryan US (1989) Merabolic and pharmacokinetic activity of the isolated sheep bronchial circulation. J Appl Physiol 67: 1041–1047
25. Horisberger B, Rodbard S (1960) Direct measurement of bronchial artery flow. Circ Res 8:1149–1156
26. Laitinen LA, Laitinen A, Salonen RO, Widdicombe JG (1987) Vascular actions of airway neuropeptides. Am Rev Respir Dis 136 [Suppl]: S59–S64
27. Laitinen LA, Laitinen A, Widdicombe J (1987) Effects of inflammatory and other mediators on airway vascular beds. Am Rev Respir Dis 135: S67–S70
28. Laitinen LA, Laitinen MA, Widdicombe JG (1987) Dose–related effects of pharmacological mediators on tracheal vascular resistance in dogs. Br J Pharmacol 92:703–709
29. Lee TH, Austen KF, Leitch AG et al. (1985) The effects of fish-oil-enriched diet on pulmonary mechanics during anaphylaxis. Am Rev Respir Dis 132:1204–1209
30. Lilker ES, Nagy EJ (1975) Gas exchange in the pulmonary circulation of dogs. Am Rev Respir Dis 11:615–620
31. Long WM, Sprung CL, El Fawal H et al. (1985) Effects of histamine on bronchial artery blood flow and bronchomotor tone. J Appl Physiol 59:254–261
32. Long WM, Yerger LD, Martinez H et al. (1988) Modification of bronchial blood flow during allergic airway responses. J Appl Physiol 65:272–282
33. Magno MG, Fishman AP (1982) Origin, distribution and blood flow of bronchial circulation in anesthetized sheep. J Appl Physiol 53:272–279
34. Malik AB, Tracy SE (1980) Bronchovascular adjustments after pulmonary embolism. J Appl Physiol 49:476–481
35. Mariassy AT, Gazeroglu H, Wanner A (1989) Morphometry of the subepithelial circulation in sheep airways: effect of vascular congestion. Am Rev Respir Dis 139 (4): A452 (abstract)
36. Martling C-R, Anggard A, Lundberg JM (1985) Noncholinergic vasodilatation in the tracheobronchial tree of the cat induced by vagal nerve stimulation. Acta Physiol Scand 125:343–346
37. McDonald DM (1987) Neurogenic inflammation in the respiratory tract: actions of sensory nerve mediators on blood vessels and epithelium of the airway mucosa. Am Rev Respir Dis 136: S65–S72
38. Nordin U, Lindholm C-E, Wolgast M (1977) Blood flow in the rabbit tracheal mucosa under normal conditions and under the influence of tracheal intubation. Acta Anaesthesiol Scand 21:81–94
39. Olsson P, Bende M, Ohlin P (1985) The laser doppler flowmeter for measuring microcirculation in human nasal mucosa. Acta Otolaryngol, (Stockh) 99:133–139
40. Parsons GH, Kramer GC, Link DP et al. (1985) Studies of reactivity and distribution of bronchial blood flow in sheep. Chest 87 [Suppl]: 180S–184S

41. Partanen M, Laitinen A, Hervonen A, Toivanen M, Laitinen LA (1982) Catecholamine- and acetylcholinesterase-containing nerves in human lower respiratory tract. Histochemistry 76:175–188
42. Peck MJ, Piper PJ, Williams TJ (1981) The effect of leukotrienes C_4 and D_4 on the microvasculature of guinea-pig askin. Prostaglandins 21 (2):315–321
43. Rudolph AM, Heymann MA (1967) The circulation of the fetus in utero: methods for studying distribution of blood flow, cardiac output and organ blood flow. Circ Res 21:163–184
44. Stern MD, Lappe DL, Bowen PD et al. (1977) Continuous measurement of tissue blood flow by laser-Doppler spectroscopy. Am J Physiol 232:H441–H448
45. Svensjo E, Persson CGA, Rutili G (1977) Inhibition of bradykinin induced macromolecular leakage from post-capillary venules by a B2-adrenoreceptor stimulant, terbutaline. Acta Physiol Scand 101:504–506
46. Turk GM, Charan NB, Czartolomny J (1985) Systemic arterial blood supply to the lung in sheep. Fed Proc 44:1757 (abstract)
47. Wanner A, Barker JA, Long WM, Mariassy AT, Chediak AD (1988) Measurement of airway mucosal perfusion and water volume with an inert soluble gas method. J Appl Physiol 65:264–271

Bronchoalveolar Lavage in Asthma

S. I. Rennard, A. A. Floreani, J. Linder, A. B. Thompson,
S. McGranaghan, and J. R. Spurzem

Department of Internal Medicine, Pulmonary and Critical Care,
University of Nebraska, Omaha, USA

Introduction

A number of methods are available for the assessment of airways inflammation in asthma: (1) Large samples of airways can be studied in material sampled at autopsy or at surgery. (2) Bronchoscopy provides a means to both inspect and sample the lower respiratory tract. (3) Expectorated sputum contains inflammatory cells and mediators which can be characteristic of asthma.

Each technique has its limitations. Histologic study of autopsy or surgical specimens has been very important in defining many of the features of both acute and chronic asthma [1, 2]. It is difficult, however, to obtain samples repeatedly in the same individual and to obtain samples at defined times after challenge or after therapeutic intervention. Sputum, of course, is (often) easier to obtain. It is not produced, however, except under conditions of exacerbation. Even then it may be expectorated variably and may be contaminated with oral or upper respiratory tract material. Recently, bronchoscopy to inspect and sample the lower respiratory tract has been applied more often than the other methods for the study of airway inflammation in asthma [3–7].

Bronchoscopy is an invasive technique but is generally well tolerated and can be performed repeatedly. It permits inspection of the airways down to about the sixth division [8]. In addition, airways can be sampled by a variety of techniques, which include biopsy of airway mucosa using transbronchoscopic forceps, collection of bronchial wall cells by brushing, and sampling of intraluminal contents by lavage. These methods complement each other in the study of inflammatory disorders of the airways. Lavage techniques have assumed a particularly important role because of the relative ease of the technique, the large number of airways sampled, the ability to recover viable cells, and the possibility to detect and quantify chemical mediators. The technique of bronchoalveolar lavage (BAL), particularly as it might be applied to asthma, forms the basis of this review.

Bronchoscopy

The flexible fiber optic bronchoscope, introduced by Ikeda in 1968, is the instrument generally used for research studies of asthmatics [3, 4, 8]. The rigid bronchoscope has also been used in asthmatics, but because it usually requires general anesthesia its use has been limited. Any of the currently available flexible fiber optic bronchoscopes can be used.

Bronchoscopy: Patient Safety, Preparation, and Monitoring
Bronchoscopy can precipitate episodes of bronchospasm in asthmatics, and fear of inducing such complications probably delayed the application of bronchoscopy to the study of asthma [9–12]. The safety of bronchoscopy and bronchoscopy with BAL, has been directly studied in asthmatics and in patients with other pulmonary diseases [13–15]. Rankin and colleagues examined expiratory flow rates, before and after bronchoscopy with lavage, in asthmatics and in nonsmoking control subjects. They found that the reductions in FVC, FEV_1 and $V_{max, 50\%}$ did not significantly differ between asthmatics and controls following lavage, though there was considerable variation in $V_{max, 50\%}$ for the entire group. Transiently after the procedure, inspiratory and expiratory wheezes were audible in asthmatics over lung areas lavaged [15]. Since, a number of investigators were interested in applying BAL to the study of asthma, the NIH convened a consensus conference which resulted in specific recommendations to insure that adequate margins of safety were assured and that study subjects had asthma that would be evaluable [16]:

1. Ages 18–45, healthy males and females, nonsmokers
2. History of mild seasonal or chronic asthma
3. Positive skin prick test to a putative allergen
4. Function evidence of reversible obstructive airway disease with or without specific or nonspecific airways challenge
5. FEV_1 before lavage of greater than or equal to 60% of predicted
6. No challenge in stable pulmonary function (spirometry) for 3 weeks

Other studies have since been conducted and serious complications were shown to be rare [17–24]. Bousquet and colleagues have studied a very large number of asthmatics, including many with relatively severe disease [19]. Despite the fact that these subjects have lung function worse than that recommended by the NIH guidelines, these investigators claim to have observed no serious complications. Thus, it appears that asthmatics can be safely studied.

Bronchoscopy can be performed with patients under general anesthesia and in awake subjects [25–27]. Topical anesthesia is generally preferred for research studies. To reduce the risk of aspiration during the procedure, the subject should have had no oral intake for 8 h to insure that the stomach is empty [27]. Some investigators will make exceptions to allow subjects to take their usual medicines as long as minimal volumes of fluid are consumed. If usual oral medicines are omitted, an alternate route for administration of medications is desirable.

Prior to commencing bronchoscopy, it is routine to establish venous access by the placement of an intravenous catheter. This allows the parental administration of narcotics and hypnotics while providing necessary venous access should emergency measures be necessary [16, 28]. Supplemental oxygen is generally given to all subjects undergoing bronchoscopy beginning at 2 liters/min through nasal prongs. Oxygen flow rates can be increased if needed [28–31].

Monitoring of all subjects undergoing bronchoscopy has greatly improved the margin of safety of the procedure. The most important monitoring modality is pulse oximetry which should be followed both during and in the first few hours after the procedure [28–32]. Monitoring of EKG and blood pressure may be helpful in selected cases [16, 28–32].

If BAL and inspection alone are to be performed, the procedure can be performed transnasally or transorally and does not generally require endotracheal intubation [27, 33, 34]. Intubation is indicated, however, if transbronchial biopsies or other procedures which may cause significant bleeding are to be performed [13, 35]. Intubation can also be helpful in certain patients who experience much cough or who have thick secretions which must be removed [27, 35]. In all these cases, the bronchoscopy is performed through the in-place endotracheal tube using a membrane adaptor. The endotracheal tube assures ready access to the lower respiratory tract and facilitates removal and reinsertion of the bronchoscope [13]. Use of small endotracheal tubes (less than 8.0 mm) may lead to significantly increased airway resistance and impaired ventilation since the bronchoscope will occlude a significant portion of the available airway [27]. With larger endotracheal tubes, this is generally not a problem.

Subjects are often premedicated with atropine and a narcotic or a hypnotic. The atropine has traditionally been given to prevent bradycardia and to reduce oral and airway secretions [36]. While most bronchoscopists are familiar with the use of atropine, the necessity for its use has not been determined experimentally. In theory, it could alter BAL results by changing the composition of lung epithelial lining fluid. It could also have a beneficial effect in asthmatics by blocking reflex bronchoconstriction. Some studies have been successfully performed without atropine, but its use must currently be considered standard [16, 37].

Narcotics and hypnotics are generally given to facilitate subject comfort. Narcotics may help suppress cough. A number of regimens have been suggested:some prefer codeine, others prefer morphine or demerol [36, 37]. Phenothiazines have been given to help suppress nausea and to potentiate the effect of narcotics. Naloxone (Narcan) can reverse narcotic effects if overdose is suspected. Benzodiazapine hypnotics often help with patient relaxation and frequently lead to amnesia for the procedure [36, 37].

Preparation of the patient for bronchoscopy and the bronchoscopic procedure itself is performed in the following manner at the University of

Nebraska Medical Center (Appendix A). Anesthesia of the pharynx and airways is achieved with the topical application of lidocaine. This can be administered via nebulizer and a β-agonist can be combined with the lidocaine to help reduce cough and bronchospasm. It is important to recognize that both the lidocaine and the β-agonist can potentially change the BAL results [3, 30, 31]. For this reason, some investigators have abandoned the use of these agents, but their use should still be considered standard. After administration of 3 ml of 4% lidocaine and 0.5 mg albuterol by jet nebulizer, additional 4% lidocaine is administered by direct spray into the pharynx until the gag reflex is completely blocked. Following this, the bronchoscope is inserted.

Under direct vision, the bronchoscope is passed between the vocal cords and into the trachea. Additional lidocaine is given directly through the bronchoscope to suppress cough. It is necessary to have cough adequately suppressed, but use of too much lidocaine can alter cellular results. Lidocaine is absorbed systemically when administered into the lung and overdose is a possibility [11, 29, 38]. In patients with hepatic insufficiency and reduced lidocaine clearance, this can be a particular problem [29, 38].

After adequate control of cough is achieved, a complete inspection of all airway segments should be systematically undertaken. It is possible to visually inspect the airways mucosa for signs of inflammation. A visual index of inflammation based on erythema, edema, secretions, and friability has been developed which allows for quantitative comparisons ([39], Table 1). This index has been used both to compare individual subjects at sequential time points and to compare various study groups. Secretions present in the large airways are generally removed by suction at the time of the general inspection. These can be collected into a specimen trap for later analysis. Care should be taken, however, to change to a fresh specimen trap when the lavage specimens are to be taken. If there is obvious contamination of the suction tubing with secretions, the tubing can be rinsed or changes. Keeping the length of tubing in the system to a minimum will be helpful in improving the quality of the samples collected [3].

Table 1. Bronchitis index: a visual score of airway inflammation (from [39])

Score	Erythema	Edema	Secretions	Friability
0	None	None	None	None
1	Light red	Blunting of airway bifurcations	Strands of clear mucus	Punctate submucosal hemorrhages with scope trauma
2	Red	Loss of airway wall indentations	Globs of mucus	Linear submucosal hemorrhages with scope trauma
3	Beefy red	Airway occluded	Airway occluded	Frank bleeding with scope trauma

After completing the inspection, the bronchoscope is advanced into a wedged position in preparation for the lavage. This should be done under direct vision, and it is important to continually visualize the lumen. In this manner, it is possible to prevent the airway mucosa from occluding the biopsy port of the bronchoscope and thereby decreasing fluid return during the procedure. Usually the caliber of the bronchoscope will match the caliber of the airway in a segmental or subsegmental airway, depending on the size of the subject. The technique most commonly used is to advance the bronchoscope gently with intermittent application of suction. When the scope is "wedged" the airway will be seen to collapse with the application of suction. It is important not to apply too much suction in the wedged position, however, as this could alter the composition of airway lining fluid [4, 30].

Generally it is easier to perform the lavage in an anterior segment as gravity will aid in the return of the fluid to the bronchoscope [4, 30, 40]. The right middle lobe and the lingula have become "standard" lavage sites both because they are more anteriorly located with the patient in a supine position and because they are easy to access bronchoscopically [4, 30]. Anterior segments of the lower lobes have also been widely used, although it is generally felt that returns are slightly less from the lower lobes [40]. Upper lobes can also be lavaged. Interestingly, returns from these sites appear to be slightly increased compared to the middle lobe and lingula. In a given study, therefore, it is probably important to perform the lavage in a consistent location.

A variety of fluids have been used for lavage, but the most common is unbuffered, sterile, isotonic saline. Buffered solutions have also been used, and these are felt to be of benefit for certain research applications. Warming the lavage solution to 37 °C is important as it reduces cough in all subjects and is felt to reduce bronchospasm in asthmatics [40, 41]. As noted above, a fresh specimen trap should be placed to collect lavage samples to minimize contamination from the large airways and the upper respiratory tract and the mouth.

A variety of aliquot sizes have been recommended generally ranging from 20 to 60 ml. The fluid can be allowed to "dwell" in the lung for various times prior to aspiration. While this is felt to increase slightly the yield of cells recovered, it also increases diffusion of material from the pulmonary interstitium and the blood into the lavage fluid [42, 43]. Most investigators, therefore, generally infuse and then immediately aspirate the fluid. Gentle suction should be used and can be applied by hand with a syringe, with a gravity siphon, or using vacuum suction [44, 45]. Care should be taken not to use too great a suction. This will cause collapse of the airway mucosa immediately distal to the tip of the wedged bronchoscope. If the airway mucosa collapses, fluid return will be reduced. In addition, too vigorous suction can traumatize the airway and lead to alteration of the epithelial lining fluid contents [4, 30].

Sequential aliquots are generally infused and aspirated at a single site. There is no standard volume of fluid used by all investigators, but a minimum of 100 ml is generally instilled to adequately sample a single wedged site [46, 47]. The studies have demonstrated mild fractional differences in cellular and biochemical components of aspirated lavage fluid when smaller (100 ml) volumes were instilled as compared to larger (240 ml) volumes for a single segmental lavage [48, 49]. The total volume of fluid to be used generally should not exceed 300–400 ml. Multiple segments can be lavaged during the same bronchoscopy if the total volume of fluid used is not excessive. The lavage fluid obtained after the initial bolus of saline is generally less than after subsequent aliquots of instilled saline. Overall, one should expect a 50% to 70% return of the saline volume infused during the lavage procedure. However, it is not unusual for lavage returns to be significantly attenuated in patients with obstructive lung diseases, such as emphysema, chronic bronchitis, or asthma [4, 50–53].

After completion of the lavage, the patient should continue to receive supplemental oxygen and continue to be monitored, since falls in arterial oxygen saturation can occur during bronchoscopy, and transient hypoxemia can continue following the procedure [54–56]. Bronchospasm, if present, should be treated appropriately. Oxygen can be slowly tapered beginning 1 h after the procedure if the patient is alert and oximetry is satisfactory. The patient should remain NPO until the gag reflex returns and is documented by direct examination. It seems prudent to maintain the venous access site until the patient is alert, is taking oral liquids, and has voided.

Postbronchoscopy fever develops in 20%–30% of subjects. The incidence increases with the volume of retained fluid [11, 14, 40, 57, 58]. The syndrome characteristically begins 4–6 h after the bronchoscopy with rigor, the onset of malaise, and fever to 39 °C. Both the rigor and the fever will often respond to meperidine or, more slowly, to acetaminophen [3, 4]. The syndrome is self-limited and symptomatic therapy is all that is required. Chest X-ray is not helpful. Nearly all subjects who undergo a lavage will have an infiltrate immediately after the procedure. This resolves gradually over the next 24 h, but up to 70% of patients may still have an infiltrate 4 h after the procedure [41, 57].

Postbronchoscopy fever should be resolved by 24 h following the procedure. Persistent fever raises the possibility of infection which, while rare, has been suggested to occur in about one subject in 1000 undergoing lavage. Postbronchoscopy pleuritis may also develop and also suggests the possibility of an infectious process. If these symptoms are present more than 24 h after the lavage, a chest X-ray is warranted and antibiotic therapy should be considered. Both aerobic and anaerobic infections can occur [11, 12, 14, 26, 58].

In patients with airways disease, superimposed worsening of airflow should be excluded. Monitoring of peak flows, therefore, should be performed in all patients [16]. When an inhalation challenge is performed prior to BAL, the patient should be monitored for at least 12 h after the procedure, for the possibility of a late-phase reaction [16].

Minor complications of bronchoscopy which can occur include sore throat, hoarseness, local problems at the intravenous insertion site, and problems associated with drugs used. Most are self-limited and should be resolved by 24 h after the procedure [11, 12].

Healthy subjects who have had no complications from the procedure may be discharged home when topical anesthesia has worn off, oral fluids are well tolerated, and supplemental oxygen is not required as documented by pulse oximetry. In patients who have received narcotics, it is advisable to be sure that voiding is no problem. There must be a competent adult at home with the subject during the first night following the procedure who can both render assistance and call for help should the need arise. Similarly, subjects who have received hypnotics or narcotics should be cautioned not to drive or consume alcohol for 24 h.

Specialized Lavage Techniques

It is thought that a wedged bronchoscope will subtend about one million alveoli and their conducting airways [28]. Since the fluid infused and subsequently aspirated samples the entire lumenal contents, both airways and alveolar material will be recovered. The alveolar surface area, of course, is very much larger than that of the airway. As a result, the standard BAL techniques probably reflect mostly alveolar contents [4, 43, 57]. Despite the fact that the airways contribution to the standard BAL is relatively small, characteristic findings have been reported in airways diseases [4, 48, 59, 60].

In an attempt to enrich for airways material, a number of investigators have sought to modify the BAL procedure. The most convincing of these is to isolate an airway segment using a double balloon catheter [61, 62]. The isolated segment of airway can then be lavaged without contamination by alveolar material. This technique has been applied both in animal and, more recently, in human studies including investigations of asthmatics (Table 2). An alternative method to enrich for airways material exploits the fact that

Table 2. Bronchial lavage cell population in normal nonsmokers and nonsmoking asthmatics

Normal nonsmokers		Nonsmoking asthmatics	
Cell population (means + SEM)	Linder and Rennard [3]	Echenbacher and Gravelyn [61]	Chan-Yeung et al. [148]
Total cells ($\times 10^6$)	4.1±0.6	0.2 to 1.0[a]	11.9± 6.5
Macrophages (%)	63±3	37.5±10.2	52.1±26.3
Neutrophils (%)	10±1	7.0± 8.9	1.9± 1.4
Eosinophils (%)	<1	0.7± 0.8	2.0± 2.5
Lymphocytes (%)	3±1	6.2± 3.8	3.2± 2.6
Epithelial cells (%)	19±2	48.2±16.2	32.9±24.2

[a] Average of three separate isolated segmental lavages.

the first fluid instilled through the bronchoscope reaches the proximal airways before reaching the more distal alveoli [63, 64]. If sufficiently small volumes of lavage fluid are instilled, the return from the first aliquot is enriched for bronchial contents while return from subsequent aliquots is enriched for alveolar material. Use of a 20 ml aliquot for this purpose results in significant enrichment for airways material ([65–69], Fig. 1). In contrast, use of a larger volume (50 ml) results in no significant enrichment for airways material. Lavage has also been performed using small volume lavages in an unwedged position. This technique also appears to result in a sample enriched for bronchial contents [70–74].

Each of the methods has advantages and disadvantages. The double balloon catheter provides convincing isolation of an airway segment. Unfortunately, the occluded airway is not available for ventilation during the procedure and this can both result in patient discomfort and prevent its use in patients with limited pulmonary reserve. This technique also requires special equipment, expertise, and that relatively small volumes of fluid be used during lavage. As a result, small numbers of cells are recovered with this technique [61, 62]. Small-volume sequential lavage has the advantages of simplicity and of providing both bronchial and alveolar samples for comparison. Its major disadvantage is that the separation is only partial. Unwedged lavage

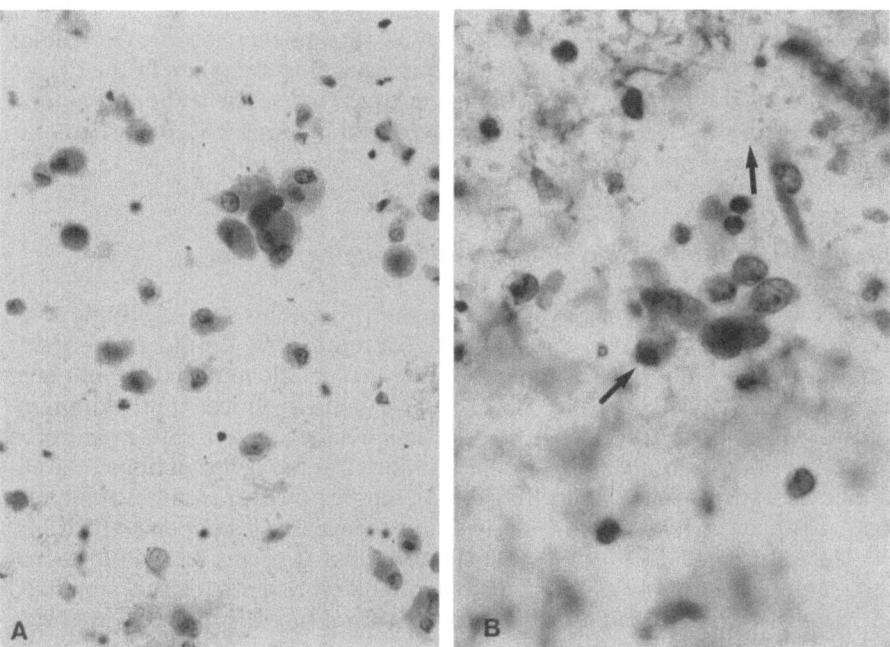

Fig. 1. A Normal lung. **B** Asthma: the background is inflammatory with reactive cell clusters (*arrow*), eosinophils, and Charcott-Leydon crystals (*arrowhead*). Papanicolaou, ×200

appears to give results similar to small volume wedged lavage. Unfortunately, fluid may be coughed proximally and then aspirated into adjacent segments. This confounds the use of serial sampling of various segments.

A number of investigators have also developed techniques for the direct challenge of airways with agents such as allergen administered through the bronchoscope [22, 24, 75–79]. These methods permit both the direct visualization of the response to challenge, at least in the large airways, and sampling of the lung for mediator release at very early times after challenge. When using these techniques, it is essential to first document that study subjects are sensitive to the antigen to be used [24]. In addition, use of graded challenges to prevent precipitation of severe bronchospasm is felt to be essential [24, 78]. The application of these methods promises to shed important light on the early events in asthma.

Bronchoscopy and BAL can also lead to artifacts. As noted above, drugs used in the preparation of the patient can alter airways secretions. Atropine and β-agonists are particularly active in this regard [80]. Lidocaine has been demonstrated to alter the function of cells recovered by BAL, and it is likely that other drugs will also affect BAL cell functions [81, 82]. Bronchoscopy and, in particular, BAL can also be a stimulus for airways inflammation [83]. Studies in a variety of animal species and humans have demonstrated acute airways and alveolar inflammation which develops in the few hours after a BAL and can take up to several days to resolve [83–85]. Longer term effects on other inflammatory parameters such as lymphocyte subsets or cellular function are, of course, also possible. Thus, care must be taken in the design and interpretation of studies involving multiple BALs. The standard method for the performance of BAL at the University of Nebraska Medical Center is summarized in Appendix A.

Bronchoalveolar Lavage Sample Processing

A number of methods are available for the processing of BAL fluids (Appendix B) [48, 86–89]. While some of the contents of BAL fluid are very stable, others are quite labile. Depending on the specific materials of interest, samples can be transported to the laboratory either on ice or at room temperature [30, 90]. Transporting the cells on ice has been reported to preserve certain mediators, but can result in alteration of some cell functions. Viability decreases with time. Cell differential counts, however, remain relatively similar for several hours and even overnight, permitting samples to be transported to a central facility [90, 91]. Nevertheless, it seems advisable to process samples as rapidly as possible. When labile mediators can be stabilized by the addition of specific preservatives, special modifications of the BAL handling procedures are warranted.

Microbiological studies can be performed on BAL samples. Some investigators use the first fluid returned for cultures, as this material is enriched for airways material and is most likely to be contaminated by oral contents.

However, many prefer to use subsequent aliquots of fluid recovered for microbiology.

Small aliquots of BAL fluid can be directly plated with a single dilution for the preparation of semiquantitative cultures [92, 93]. Alternatively, quantitative bacterial cultures can be prepared by making three serial dilutions (each 100-fold) of the original BAL specimen, followed by plating the sample after each dilution [94–96]. Evidence for true lower respiratory tract infection, rather than oropharyngeal contamination, has been described when the concentration of recovered organisms was $\geq 10^4$ CFU/ml from semiquantitative or quantitative cultures of BAL fluid [93, 96, 97]. Others have reported diagnostic semiquantitative or quantitative BAL cultures when the concentration of bacteria recovered was $> 10^5$ CFU/ml [92, 94].

Cytocentrifuge preparations of BAL cell populations can also be stained with a variety of rapid stains for the early detection of pathogens (Table 3). For example, the May-Grunwald-Giemsa stain or the more rapid version Diff-Quick stain (American Scientific Products, McGraw Park, IL) both effectively stain for intracellular organisms [3, 95, 97, 98]. These stains are commonly used in conjunction with the Gram reaction, since the latter stain better defines morphologic characteristics of bacteria [3, 95, 98]. BAL fluid can be utilized for the rapid detection of fungi, pneumocystis, legionella, mycobacteria, and viral antigen [99–111].

Finally, lavage fluid can be saved for cultures of the above types of organisms [102–111].

A cell count should be performed on the fluid before any processing since cells may be lost during handling. This count is best performed on a hemocytometer. Coulter counts have been reported to be unreliable, perhaps because of spontaneous cell clumping. Following counting, a differential count is performed. A number of stains are available which can be applied to BAL specimens (Table 3). The most commonly used technique is to prepare a cytocentrifuge specimen which then can be stained with a rapid modified Wright-Giemsa stain such as Leukostat or Diff-Quik [3, 95, 98, 111]. While these stains are rapid and convenient, they do not stain mast cells effectively. A special stain such as toluidine blue is required for the enumeration of mast cells [3].

The cytocentrifuge preparation slightly underestimates lymphocytes [86]. This appears to be due to a loss of lymphocytes during the centrifugation. An alternative method is to filter the BAL cells onto a Millipore filter which can then be stained with a Papanicolaou (PAP) stain or with hematoxylin and eosin. The PAP technique has the advantage of demonstrating nuclear detail, which facilitates cytological analysis of malignant and virally infected cells. In addition, the processing for the PAP method lyses red cells which occasionally are a problem with other methods [3]. The Millipore filter technique appears to accurately present lymphocytes, but neutrophils are lost, perhaps because some cells lyse and penetrate the filter [89].

Cytocentrifuge specimens can also be processed for special staining techniques including silver stains and iron stains, and can be used for some immunohistological and in situ hybridization studies (Table 3). The preservation and availability of antigen varies considerably from epitope to epitope, and each technique should be evaluated separately (3, 99–101, 106, 108–110, 113, 120, 121].

Samples of BAL fluid can also be centrifuged. This separates the remaining cells as a pellet from the supernatant BAL fluid. If the sample has been processed rapidly and excessive amounts of lidocaine have been avoided, viability of the recovered cells will exceed 80%. These cells can then be maintained in culture and utilized for a variety of functional studies (Appendix C) [30, 90].

Table 3. Frequently used stains for BAL specimens

Stain	Specimen stained or disorder sought	Comments	References
Wright-Giemsa or May-Grun-wald-Giemsa, Diff-Quik	Bronchial epithelial cells, macrophages, lymphocytes, neutro-phils, eosinophils, pneumocystis carinii (trophozoites)	Diff-quik is a more rapid modification, stains eosinophils less well	[3, 111, 112]
Papanicolaou	Same as above	Better for cytologic study of cells	[3]
Gram	Bacteria	Good for morpholo-gic characteristics of bacteria	[3, 95, 98, 111, 112]
Grocott or Gomori methen-amine silver stain, Toluidine blue	Fungal hyphae yeasts, pneumocystis carinii (cysts)	More rapid version of Grocott stain available (microwave method)	[3, 97, 99, 100, 101, 113]
Auramine-rhodamine, Acid-fast (Ziehl-Neelsen)	Mycobacterium ssp	Auramine-rhodamine is a good initial screen; if positive, needs con-firmation with acid-fast stain	[3, 97, 114, 115, 116]
Direct fluores-cence	Legionella ssp, cytomegalovirus, Herpes simplex	Direct fluorescence preferred method for initial screen of *Legionella* ssp	[3, 117, 118, 119]
Mallory iron	Hemorrhage	Can detected hemo-siderin-laden macro-phages (not specific for diffuse pulmonary hemorrhage)	[3, 120]
Oil red	Lipid	Can detect lipid vacuoles in macro-phages	[3, 121]

Measurements of BAL fluid concentration are, by necessity, simplifications. It is likely then, that the epithelial lining fluid of the lung is heterogeneous with respect to anatomic distribution and is likely divided into separate phases. Attempts to sample "airways" material, noted above, have consistently demonstrated differing composition of the epithelial lining fluid. IgA, lactoferrin, and lysozyme, which are all airways secretions, for example, are higher in bronchial-enriched bronchial fluid than alveolar samples of lavage fluid [44, 46, 59, 122–126]. The supernatant fluids contain a variety of chemical species which also can be assessed by varied methods. Some molecular species are quite stable and can easily be assayed on frozen samples. Others are quite labile and must be assayed immediately either with or without the addition of special preservatives [30]. Depending on the molecular species of interest and the assay to be used, it may be necessary to concentrate the lavage fluid. A number of methods have been used. Pressure dialysis has been widely applied, but can result in losses of material up to 50%, presumably due to sticking to the membrane [127–129]. The technique cannot be used, moreover, for low molecular weight species. Lyophilization is an alternate method, but results in concentration of the salt present in the lavage fluid and of other molecular species [3]. For lipid soluble mediators, lipid extraction has been used followed by air drying and resolubilization. Each method has advantages and disadvantages which must be tailored for a specific application.

The BAL samples the fluid contents of the lower respiratory tract, but results in a dilution of that fluid. Consequently, there are difficulties in expressing the results of measurements made on BAL samples. The simplest technique is to present the results as concentration/ml of recovered BAL fluid [18]. While this does not correct for the potentially variable dilution which may occur, it is simple and easy for various investigators to compare. Albumin is a plasma constituent which diffuses into all body fluids. Many investigators have quantified albumin in BAL fluid in order to "normalize" the results of one BAL to another [44, 46, 51, 59, 125, 130, 131]. The assumption made, of course, is that the lower respiratory tract albumin content in various individuals is constant. This, however, is clearly not the case. Increases in lower respiratory tract albumin occur regularly with disease through two mechanisms. First, increased concentration of albumin can result from increased leakage from the circulation [132, 133]. Second, accumulations of increased amounts of epithelial fluid, i.e., edema, regularly form in disease [133–135]. The recovery of this increased volume of epithelial lining fluid results in increased BAL concentrations. Finally, albumin may be both actively transported and produced within the lung, thus introducing yet other confounding variables [136–139]. Despite these limitations, "normalization" to albumin has proved very useful to a large number of investigators.

In order to have a better handle on the dilution which occurs during BAL, various investigators have attempted to use endogenous markers of dilution. Methylene blue, when added to the saline instillate in a known concentration, has been used as an external marker of BAL fluid dilution. A dilution factor derived from the difference in concentration of methylene blue in the instilled saline from that in the aspirated lavage fluid allows calculation of recovered epithelial lining fluid (ELF) [140].

The usefulness of this method has been questioned because the volume of ELF recovered was felt to be greater than expected, possibly secondary to binding of the dye to pulmonary epithelial cells [42, 141]. As a marker of dilution, urea has proved most useful. Urea is freely diffusible into the lung, and the assumption is made that BAL urea is the same as plasma urea. By measuring the plasma urea simultaneously with the BAL urea, the "dilution factor" by which the BAL urea is reduced can be calculated [141]:

Dilution factor = plasma urea/BAL urea (note the units must be the same)

The same dilution factor can then be applied to any constituent measured in the BAL to estimate concentration in the lung epithelial lining fluid:

$$\text{ELF concentration} = (\text{BAL concentration}) \times \left(\frac{\text{plasma urea}}{\text{BAL urea}} \right)$$

While the urea method provides an estimate of ELF concentrations, it has several limitations. First, urea can diffuse into the BAL during the procedure [42]. The time to 50% equilibration is estimated to be about 12 min, so the procedure must be completed rapidly. If done within 90 s, it is estimated to be within a factor of 2 of the "true" concentration. Clearly, if the method will be used for comparison among individuals, great care must be used to have a standard technique performed in a standard manner.

One method which has been widely applied to suggest local production (or concentration) of a BAL component within the lung is the "ratio of ratios." A protein is measured both in plasma and in BAL and its concentration is compared to albumin both in plasma and in BAL. A ratio of ratios can then be calculated [141]:

Ratio = (prot. in BAL/alb. in BAL)/(prot. in plasma/alb. in plasma).

The assumption is then made that the protein is less likely to diffuse into the BAL than is albumin. A ratio greater than one implies local production (or concentration). This method, unfortunately, is also limited by the ability of the lung to both produce and actively transport albumin [136–139].

A number of complex techniques have also been developed to improve estimation of BAL dilution and plasma transudation. These include the measurement of multiple protein species of varying molecular weight to estimate partition coefficient, and the use of repeated lavage of the same segment to determine sampling efficiency [142].

The standard technique for processing BAL specimens used at the University of Nebraska Medical Center is detailed in Appendix B.

Many centers have found it exceedingly useful to routinely collect and save standard information on all subjects undergoing a BAL. Examples of the BAL data sheets used at the University of Nebraska Medical Center are shown in Fig. 2.

UNMC #: _____

MC #2_____   DATE: ___/___/___   NAME: _____

BAL PROCEDURE —
VOL INFUSED: VOL RETURNED:
    BR   AL   BR   AL
RUL
RML
RLL
LUL
LING
LLL
EXTRA

TOTAL

CELLS x 10^6
BR _____   % VIABILITY _____ %
AL _____
SC COUNT _____

PULMONARY DIFFERENTIAL

          TECH _____   TECH _____

	N	E	L	M	C	S			N	E	L	M	C	S
BRONCH #1	___	___	___	___	___	___		BRONCH #1	___	___	___	___	___	___
ALVEOLAR #2	___	___	___	___	___	___		ALVEOLAR #2	___	___	___	___	___	___

AREA BRONCHED: _____   BR INFUSED: _____   BR INFUSED: _____
                          AL INFUSED: _____   AL INFUSED: _____
CELLS x 10^6
BR _____   VIABILITY _____ %
AL _____
SC COUNT _____

PULMONARY DIFFERENTIAL

          TECH _____   TECH _____

	N	E	L	M	C	S			N	E	L	M	C	S
BRONCH #1	___	___	___	___	___	___		BRONCH #1	___	___	___	___	___	___
ALVEOLAR #2	___	___	___	___	___	___		ALVEOLAR #2	___	___	___	___	___	___

AREA BRONCHED: _____   BR INFUSED: _____   BR INFUSED: _____
                          AL INFUSED: _____   AL INFUSED: _____
CELLS x 10^6
BR _____   VIABILITY _____ %
AL _____
SC COUNT _____

PULMONARY DIFFERENTIAL

          TECH _____   TECH _____

	N	E	L	M	C	S			N	E	L	M	C	S
BRONCH #1	___	___	___	___	___	___		BRONCH #1	___	___	___	___	___	___
ALVEOLAR #2	___	___	___	___	___	___		ALVEOLAR #2	___	___	___	___	___	___

PUL-39 (4/92)

Fig. 2. Routine BAL data sheets in use at the University of Nebraska Medical Center

UNIVERSITY OF NEBRASKA MEDICAL CENTER
UNIVERSITY HOSPITAL & OUTPATIENT SERVICES

Patient Identification (Stamp)

NAME

REG. NO.

BAL SCORE SHEET

LOCATION

MC #: _____   DATE: ___ / ___ / ___

DATE

LOCATION _____

PROCEDURE/STUDY: BMT: SURVEILLANCE: N Y   DATE OF BMT: ___ / ___ / ___
                  LIVER
                  HIV+
                  STUDY: _____
                  OTHER: _____

DX: 1. _____

    2. _____

BRONCHOSCOPIST INITIALS: 1. _____ 2. _____   TECH: _____

PRE-OP MED 1. ATROPINE   ____ . ____ MG/IV   LIDOCAINE HCL:

           2. DEMEROL   ____ . ____ MG/IV   4% _____ CC

           3. VALIUM   ____ . ____ MG/IV   2% _____ CC

           4. _____   ____ . ____ MG/IV   1% _____ CC

SMOKING HISTORY

SMOKING: U — UNKNOWN   Y — SMOKES   Q — QUIT   N — NEVER

PACK/DAY: _____   # OF YEARS: _____   DATE QUIT: ___ / ___ / ___

COUGH: N Y   SPUTUM: N Y

BRONCH SCORE

	RUL	RML	RLL	LUL	LING	LLL
C-3 ERYTHEMA						
C-3 EDEMA						
C-3 MUCUS						
C-3 FRIABILITY						

TOTAL BRONCHITIS SCORE _____

COMMENTS:

SIGNATURE: _____
PUL-27 (Rev. 5/91)

Fig. 2. Routine BAL data sheets in use at the University of Nebraska Medical Center

Applications in Asthma

It is beyond the scope of this manuscript to review all applications of BAL in asthma. BAL has been used in an attempt to characterize the inflammatory cell populations present within the lower respiratory tract of stable allergic asthmatics (Table 2). Increases in all inflammatory cell types have been shown in the BAL fluid from asthmatic subjects (19, 20, 79, 143, 144). However, the most consistent increase recovered in BAL fluid has been in eosinophils and mast cells (23, 143, 146, 149, 152). These lavage findings are nonspecific and are not necessarily "diagnostic" of asthma (20, 23, 28, 31, 79). Studies of various other subtypes of asthma are currently in progress. In addition, acute changes in asthmatic BAL cell populations following allergen challenge have been described [22, 75–78, 143–146]. It has been possible, moreover, to quantify increases in albumin in BAL fluid, suggesting increased leak following challenge, and it has been possible to quantify a number of potential biochemical mediators ([22, 75–78, 145, 147–151], Table 4). Interestingly, there have been correlations observed between hyperresponsiveness and inflammatory cell populations and certain mediators present in the lavage fluid of asthmatics [151, 152]. It seems very likely, therefore, that the ability to sample the lung in asthma will be an important means in contributing to future studies of asthma.

Preparation for Bronchoscopy, Bronchoscopy, and Bronchoalveolar Lavage Procedure

Preparation

1. Determine whether the patient has any known allergy to lidocaine or other topical anesthetics. Confirm that the patient has had no food or liquids for at least 8 h prior to procedure.
    2. Clotting studies are routinely performed prior to the bronchoscopy.

Table 4. Biochemical mediators found in bronchoalveolar lavage fluid of asthmatics

Biochemical mediator	References
Histamine	[22, 76, 149, 150, 151]
Major basic protein	[23]
Prostaglandin D_2	[22, 76, 147]
Thromboxane B_2	[76]
LTB4	[22, 148]
LTC4	[76]
LTD4	[148]
LTE4	[148, 150]
15-HETE (15-hydroxyeicosatetranoeic acid)	[147]

3. Insert intravenous catheter. Connect ECG monitor to patient and observe for tachycardia or other cardiac abnormalities.

4. Finger or ear probe continuous pulse oximetry should be initiated. Record heart rate and initial arterial oxygen saturation of patient. Oxygen via nasal prongs is initiated at 2 liters/min. A greater FiO_2 can be used as needed.

5. Equipment and supplies used in local anesthesia for flexible bronchoscopy:

- Aerosol set-up (Airlife Misty-Neb nebulizer)
- DeVilbiss Model 15 atomizer (hand held)
- Alupent (0.25 ml) or albuterol (0.5 ml)
- Topical lidocaine HCL 4% solution (40 mg/ml)
- Topical lidocaine 2% solution (20 mg/ml)
- Topical lidocaine 1% solution (10 mg/ml)
- Topical cetacaine anesthetic (benzocaine 14%)

6. Patient preparation:

(a) Patient receives a nebulized aerosol with β_2-agonist 20 min prior to bronchoscopy (3 ml of 4% topical lidocaine plus 0.25 ml alupent or 0.50 ml albuterol); anesthetize oropharynx, base of tongue, and upper airway.

(b) Measure amount of lidocaine remaining and record amount given to patient on bronchoscopy worksheet.

(c) Place 20 ml of 4% topical lidocaine solution into DeVilbiss atomizer. Spray into the patient's mouth as the patient slowly inhales and exhales. Initially, spray no more than 10–12 ml of 4% lidocaine from atomizer, then check for patient's gag reflex.

(d) If patient has a very strong gag or cough reflex, a total of more than 15 ml of 4% lidocaine may be needed for local anesthesia (lidocaine in nebulizer and atomizer).

(e) Preoperative vital signs are taken and recorded on bronchoscopy worksheet (temperature, pulse, respirations, blood pressure). Vital signs and oxygen saturation should be obtained every 15 min or more frequently as indicated.

(f) Preoperative intravenous medications administered at this time are recorded.

Bronchoscopy Procedure

1. Dentures or partial plates are removed. A bite-block is put in place and secured with tape. A towel is placed over patient's eyes.

2. Bronchoscope is inserted through bite-block, with mouth and oropharynx examined.

3. Bronchoscope is passed down to area above the vocal cords. Vocal cords are examined; 1–2 ml 2% topical lidocaine is given above vocal cords. Additional 2% lidocaine can be given if cough or gag reflex is still present.

4. Bronchoscope is passed through the cords and trachea is examined. Additional 1–2 ml 1% lidocaine is given below cords for gagging and cough.

5. Bronchoscopic examination is made of the main carina, and then of the right bronchial tree down to subsegmental level. A Bronchitis Index score is called out by bronchoscopist and recorded by technician for right upper lobe, right middle lobe, and right lower lobe (RUL, RML, and RLL) bronchial mucosa.

6. Examination of the left-sided bronchial tree is then done. Again, a Bronchitis Index score is recorded now for left lower lobe (LLL), lingular and left upper lobe (LUL) bronchial mucosa.

Bronchoalveolar Lavage Procedure

1. Three lobes are lavaged for bronchial and alveolar samples. Usually RML and lingula are two of the three lobes lavaged.

2. Three additional bronchial samples are taken from other lobes.

3. Bronchoscope is wedged into subsegmental or segmental bronchus with care not to overwedge tip of scope.

4. Inject 20 ml warmed (37°C) normal saline into bronchoscope with immediate aspiration of fluid into specimen trap (specimen trap, Cheeseborough-Ponds, Greenwhich, CT) by finger occlusion of suction port of bronchoscope. This is the bronchial specimen for that lobe.

5. Excessive suction pressures can cause collapse of airway mucosa distal to suction channel of bronchoscope. This can decrease optimal lavage fluid returns.

6. This bronchial specimen is transferred to a labeled conical specimen container for later processing and storage.

7. A new specimen trap is repositioned in the suction line system.

8. Aliquots of 20 ml normal saline (37°C) are sequentially injected into bronchoscope and aspirated while the bronchoscope is still in wedged position. A total of 80 ml saline is used for each site lavaged (four × 20 ml).

9. The fluid returned from each 20 ml aliquot is collected in the same specimen trap. This represents the alveolar sample for that lavage site.

10. The alveolar sample is transferred to a separate, labeled conical container.

11. The specimen trap is changed in the suction line system.

12. Ten ml 37°C normal saline is instilled into wedged bronchoscope. This is collected into a specimen trap. This sample is used for culture. The specimen container is used for subsequent culture specimens.

13. This process is repeated at a total of three separate lobes within a subsegmental or segmental bronchus. A culture sample (10 ml of saline above) is taken from each site and pooled in original culture specimen trap.

14. Three lobes that have not been previously lavaged are used for separate bronchial lavages. The scope is again wedged into segmental or subsegmental bronchus.

15. A 20 ml aliquot is infused with the aspirate collected in a specimen trap as previously described.

16. Fluid returned from the three sites is pooled in a labeled cone.

17. Bronchial samples from each lobe are all pooled together as Bronchial Specimen or Fluid. Alveolar samples from each lobe are all pooled together separately from bronchial samples as Alveolar Specimen or Fluid.

Appendix B: Bronchoalveolar Lavage Processing Procedure

1. Record patient data and volume returned from bronchoscopy on BAL worksheet on clipboard attached to laminar flow hood.

2. Filter #1 fluid through nylon mesh and pool (bronchial fluid).

3. Filter #2 fluid through nylon mesh and pool (alveolar fluid).

4. Use glass pasteur pipet, pipet a quantitative amount of fluid from fluids #1 and #2 on to the hemocytometer.

5. If BAL fluid hemoglobin is ordered, remove 1 ml of fluid #2 and place in a 1.2 ml vial and send to chemistry

6. Remove 5 ml of fluid #2 and place in 5 ml vial; save for slides and filters. (Besure to label this vial "Slides and Filters.")

7. Place remaining fluid from both samples into 50 ml conicals and put tubes into centrifuge and spin at 5000 rpm for 5 min. (Besure opposite conicals have the same amount of fluids, to maintain balance during spinning cycle.)

8. Do differential cell counts on hemocytometer. Clean fluids from hemocytometer and cover with alcohol.

9. Calculate the amount of fluid needed for making slides and filters by using the following calculation:

A. $\dfrac{\begin{array}{c}(\text{Total \# of cells counted} \div 10)\\ \times (\text{Total volume of fluid} \div 10)\end{array}}{\text{Total \# of cells per million}} = \text{Total \# of cells per million or } 10^6$

B. $\dfrac{(\text{Total volume of fluid} \div 10)}{\text{Total \# of cells in millions}} = \text{ml volume used to make slides}$

Note: For slides never use more than 0.5 ml or less than 0.06 ml; for filters never use more than 1.0 ml or less than 0.12 ml.

10. When samples are done spinning remove supernant from the conicals containing the samples and aliquot out:

Fluid #1: 5 small tubes containing 1 ml; remaining fluid in 50 ml conicals

Fluid #2: 5 small tubes containing 1 ml; 1 orange capped tube containing 5 ml; remaining fluid into 50 ml conicals

11. Take cell pellets from both samples. Resuspend the fluid #1 cells in Hank's balanced salt solution (HBSS). Use the same amount of fluid as the original volume of fluid obtained.

Resuspend the fluid #2 cells with 10 ml HBSS and put a side for further use.

12. Prepare slides and filters for both samples, using the 5 ml of fluid #2 cells and the resuspended fluid #1 cells.

13. Prepare slides and filters according to the following instructions.

14. Pipet a small amount of fluid from fluid #2 cells which have been re-suspended in HBSS and place on hemocytometer for a second cell count; record this number.

15. Pipet a small amount of fluid from fluid #2 cells which have been re-suspended in HBSS on a slide; then pipet a small amount of (20 μl) erythro-sin onto the slide. The cells that are alive will stain green and dead cells will stain red. Count the red and green cells to 100 and record number of live cells present.

16. Place the remaining fluid #2 cells into the centrifuge and spin at 5000 rpm for 5 min.

17. Stain one fluid #1 and one fluid #2 slide in Diff-Quik stains, 1 min per solutions, blue first, orange second, and last purple.

18. When slides are dry count a cell differential and record on work-sheet.

19. If cell differentials have a >15% lymphocyte count, then surface cell marker testing should be done. Take $5–10 \times 10^6$ μl from fluid #2 which is left over and before cell culture procedure put in 1.5 ml tube.

20. If the second cell count for the fluid #2 cells is greater than 6×10^6 and the viability is greater than 70%, culture cells. See separate procedure for culture (Appendix C).

21. Spin down blood and pipet the serum and plasma into separate tubes and place in freezer with other samples.

Preparation of Filter for Cytology

1. Soak SM filter in 95% ethanol and put on top of the filter holder.

2. Add 10 ml normal saline. Do not let this run dry.

3. When 2–3 ml of the saline remains add the cells at a concentration of 200 000/filter.

4. Fix with 10–15 ml of isopropyl alcohol. Do not let this run dry.

5. When the alcohol has almost all run through remove the filter and place in 95% ethanol.

Appendix C: Cell Culturing

The following is all completed using steriley technique in the laminar flow hood.

1. Cells are obtained from BAL processing lab, usually at a concentra-tion of 1 million cells/ml.

Table C1. Cell culture methods

Total number cells	Procedure		Number of culture wells
6×10^6	A, B	24 h	3 each
8×10^6	A, B	4–24 h	2 each
	A, B	24 h	
12×10^6	A, B	4–24 h	3 each
	A, B	24 h	
15×10^6	A, B	4–24 h	3 each
	A, B, C	24 h	
18×10^6	A, B, C	4–24 h	3 each
	A, B, C	24 h	
21×10^6	A, B, C	4–24 h	3 each
	A, B, C, D	24 h	
24×10^6	A, B, C, D	4–24 h	3 each
	A, B, C, D	24 h	

Cells plated in a 6-well culture plate.
Procedure A: cells (100 μl/ml/well).
Procedure B: cells (100 μl/ml/well) + zymosan (5 μl/well).
Procedure C: cells (100 μl/ml/well) + fetal calf serum (FCS) (100 μl/well).
Procedure D: cells (100 μl/ml/well) + zymosan (5 μl/well) + fetal calf serum (FCS) (100 μl/well).

2. Use Table 1 to determine how to culture cells:
3. Steps to use in culturing:

(a) Place 1×10^6 cells/well (in RPMI) to be cultured.
(b) Add 5 μl zymosan/well where needed.
(c) Add 0.1 ml/well FCS where needed.
(d) Make sure total cell suspension covers the entire surface of each well (i.e., swirl plate gently to cover all of surface).
(e) Place in 5% CO_2 incubator, 37 °C.
(f) At 4 h, remove appropriate plates marked 4–24 h; place in hood.
(g) Sterilely, remove about 0.8 ml media, place in centrifuge.
(h) Add about 0.8 ml fresh media to all wells from which 4 h sample is taken. Add zymosan and FCS to appropriate wells, if needed.
(i) Return to incubator till 24 h time period the next day.
(j) Sample from step 7 above spun 5 min at 1000 rpm; media transferred to labeled blue capped tube for freezing in −80 °C.
(k) Label contents and date.

4. Next day (24 h harvest; no need to be sterile):

(a) Remove plates at 24 h time period.
(b) Place media in centrifuge tube, spin 5 min at 1000 rpm.
(c) Alcohol down each well, discard plates.
(d) After centrifuging media, place media in labeled blue capped tube, ready for freezing in −80 °C.
(e) Label contents and date.

References

1. Dunnill MS (1987) Pulmonary pathology, 2nd edn. Churchill Livingstone, Edinburgh
2. Naylor B (1962) The shedding of the mucosa of the bronchial tree in asthma. Thorax 17:69–72
3. Linder J, Rennard SI (1988) Bronchoalveolar lavage. ASCP, Chicago
4. Reynolds HY (1987) Bronchoalveolar lavage. State of the Art. Am Rev Respir Dis 135:250–263
5. Soboyna RE (1984) Quantitative structural alterations in long-standing allergic asthma. Am Rev Respir Dis 130:289–292
6. Jeffery PK, Wardlaw AJ, Nelson FC, Collins JV, Anokay AB (1989) Bronchial biopsies in asthma: an ultrastructural, quantitative study and correlation with hyperreactivity. Am Rev Respir Dis 140:1745–1753
7. Laitinen LA, Heino M, Laitinen A, Kaua T, Hauntela T (1985) Damage of the airway epithelium and bronchial reactivity in patients with asthma. Am Rev Respir Dis 131:599–606
8. Ikeda S, Yanai N, Ishikawa S (1968) Flexible broncofiberscope. Keio J Med 17:1–16
9. Sahn SA, Scoggin C (1976) Fiberoptic bronchoscopy in bronchial asthma. Chest 69:39–42
10. Zavala D (1978) Complications following fiberoptic bronchoscopy. Chest 73:783–785
11. Credle WF, Smiddy JF, Elliott RC (1974) Complications of fiberoptic bronchoscopy. Am Rev Respir Dis 109:67–72
12. Pereira W Jr, Kounat DM, Snider GC (1978) A Prospective cooperative study of complications following flexible fiberoptic bronchoscopy. Chest 73:813–816
13. Zavala DC (1978) Transbronchial biopsy in diffuse lung disease. Chest 73 (5): 727(s)–733(s)
14. Strumpf IJ, Feld MK, Cornelius MJ, Keogh BA, Crystal RG (1981) Safety of fiberoptic bronchoalveolar lavage in evaluation of interstitial lung disease. Chest 80:268–271
15. Rankin JA, Snyder RRT, Schacter EN, Mathay RA (1984) Bronchoalveolar lavage: its safety in subjects with mild asthma. Chest 85:723–728
16. NHLBI Workshop Summaries (1985) Summary and recommendations of a workshop on the investigative use of fiberoptic bronchoscopy and bronchoalveolar lavage in asthmatics. Am Rev Respir Dis 132:180–182.
17. Kirby JG, Hargreave FE, Gleich GJ, O'Byrne PM (1987) Bronchoalveolar cell profiles in asthmatic and nonasthmatic subjects. Am Rev Respir Dis 136: 379–383
18. Effensohn DB, Jankowski MJ, Redondo AA, Duncan PG (1988) Bronchoalveolar lavage in the normal volunteer subject: 2) safety and results of repeated BAL, and use in the assessment of intrasubject variability. Chest 94 (2):281–285
19. Bousquet J, Chaniz P, Yves Lacoste J, Barneau G, Ghavarian R, Enander I, Venge P, Ahlstedt S, Simony-Lafontaine J, Godard P, Michel F-B (1990) Eosinophilic inflammation in asthma. N Engl J Med 323:1033–1039
20. Foresi A, Bortorelli G, Pesci A, Chetta A, Olivieri D (1990) Inflammatory markers in bronchoalveolar lavage and bronchial biopsy in asthma during remission. Chest 98:528–535
21. Paggiaro P, Bacci E, Paoletti P, Bernard P, Dente F, Marchetti G, Talini D, Menconi GF, Giuntini C (1990) Bronchoalveolar lavage and morphology of the airways after cessation of exposure in asthmatic subjects sensitized to toluene diisocyanate. Chest 98:536–542
22. Miadonna A, Tedeschi A, Brasca C, Folco G, Sala A, Murphy RC (1990) Mediator release after endobronchial antigen challenge in patients with respiratory allergy. J Allergy Clin Immunol 85:906–913

23. Wardlaw AJ, Dunnette S, Gleich GJ, Collins JV, Kay AB (1988) Eosinophils and mast cells in bronchoalveolar lavage in subjects with mild asthma (relationship to bronchial hyperreactivity). Am Rev Respir Dis 137:62–69
24. Metzger WJ, Nugent K, Richerson HB, Moseley P, Lakin R, Zavala D, Hunninghake GW (1985) Methods for bronchoalveolar lavage in asthmatic patients following bronchoprovocation and local antigen challenge. Chest 87 (1): 16(s)–19(s)
25. Smiddy JF, Ruth We, Kerby GR, Renz LE, Raucher C (1971) Flexible fiberoptic bronchoscope. Ann Intern Med 75 (6):971–972
26. Kounat DM, Schaaf JT, Rath GS, Snider GL (1974) Bronchoscopy in perspective. Chest 65 (6):606–607
27. Sackner MA (1975) State of the art: bronchofiberscopy. Am Rev Respir Dis 111:62–88
28. Goldstein RA, Rohatgi PK et al. (1990) ATS statement of clinical role of bronchoalveolar lavage in pulmonary disease. Am Rev Respir Dis 142:481–486
29. Fulkerson WJ (1984) Current concepts: fiberoptic bronchoscopy. N Engl J Med 111 (8):511–514
30. Klech H, Pohl W et al. (1989) Technical recommendations and guidelines for bronchoalveolar lavage (BAL): report of the European Society of Pneumology Task Group on BAL. Eur Respir J 2:561–585
31. Klech H, Hutter C (1990) Clinical guidelines and indications for bronchoalveolar lavage (BAL): report of the European Society of Pneumology Task Group on BAL. Eur Respir J 3:937–974
32. Djukanovic R, Wilson JW, Lai CKW, Holgate S, Howarth PH (1991) The safety aspects of fiberoptic bronchoscopy, bronchoalveolar lavage and endobronchial biopsy in asthma. Am Rev Respir Dis 143:772–777
33. Smiddy JF, Ruth WE, Kerby GR (1971) A new technique of bronchial visualization with fiberoptics (abstract). J Kans Med Soc 72:441
34. Hodgkin JE, Rosenow EC III, Stubs SE (1975) Oral introduction of the flexible bronchoscope. Chest 68:88–90
35. Zavala DC, Rhodes ML, Richardson RH, Bedell GN (1974) Fiberoptic and rigid bronchoscopy. The state of the art. Chest 65:605–606
36. Rees PJ, Hay JG, Webb JR (1983) Premedication for fiberoptic bronchoscopy. Thorax 38:624–627
37. Prakash UB, Offort KP, Stubbs SE (1991) Bronchoscopy in North America: the ACCP survey. Chest 100:1668–1675
38. Patterson JR, Blaschke TF, Hunt KK Jr, Meffin PJ (1975) Lidocaine blod concentrations during fiberoptic bronchoscopy. Am Rev Respir Dis 112:53–57
39. Thompson AB, Rennard SI (1988) Assessment of airways inflammation utilizing bronchoalveolar lavage. Clin Chest Med 9 (4):577–590
40. Pingleton SK, Harrison GF, Stechshulte DJ, Wesselius LJ, Kerby GR, Ruth WE (1983) Effect of location pH and temperature of instillate in bronchoalveolar lavage in normal volunteers. Am Rev Respir Dis (1983) 128:1035–1037
41. Burns DM, Shure D, Francoz R, Kalafer M, Harrell J, Witztum K, Maser KM (1983) The physiologic consequences of saline labor lavage in health human adults. Am Rev Respir Dis 127:695–701
42. Marcy TW, Merrill WM, Rankin JA, Reynolds HY (1987) Limitations of using urea to quantify epithelial lining fluid recovered by bronchoalveolar lavage. Am Rev Respir Dis 135:1276–1280
43. Kelly CA, Fenwick JD, Corris PA, Fleetwood A, Hendrick DJ, Walters EH (1988) Fluid dynamics during bronchoalveolar lavage. Am Rev Respir Dis 138: 81–84
44. Reynolds HY, Fulmer JD, Kazmierowsky JA, Roberts WC, Frank MM, Crystal RG (1977) Analysis of cellular and protein content of bronchoalveolar lavage fluid from patients with idiopathic pulmonary fibrosis and chronic hypersensitivity pneumonitis. J Clin Invest 59:165–175

45. Venet A, Clavel F, Israel-Biet D, Rouzioux C, Dennewald G, Stern MV, Vitticoq D, Regnier B, Cayrol E, Chretien J (1985) Lung in acquired immune deficiency syndrome: infectious and immunological status assessed by bronchoalveolar lavage. Bull Eur Physiopathol Respir 21:535–543
46. Reynolds HY, Nesball HH (1974) Analysis of proteins and respiratory cells obtained from human lungs by bronchial lavage. J Lab Clin Med:559–572
47. Merrill W, O'Hearn E, Rankin J, Matthay RA, Reynolds HY (1982) Kinetic analysis of respiratory tract proteins recovered during a sequential lavage protocol. Am Rev Respir Dis 126:617–620
48. Davis GS, Giancola MS, Costanza MC, Low RB (1982) Analysis of sequential bronchoalveolar lavage samples from healthy human volunteers. Am Rev Respir Dis 126:611–616
49. Dohn MN, Baughman RP (1985) Effect of changing instilled volume for bronchoalveolar lavage in patients with interstitial lung disease. Am Rev Respir Dis 132:390–392
50. Finley TN, Swenson EW, Curran WS, Huber GL, Ladman AJ (1967) Bronchoalveolar lavage in normal subjects and patients with obstructive lung disease. Ann Intern Med 66:651–658
51. Low RB, Davis GS, Giancola MS (1978) Biochemical analysis of bronchoalveolar lavage fluids of healthy human volunteer smokers and nonsmokers. Am Rev Respir Dis 118:863–874
52. Ettensohn DB, Jankowski M, Duncan PG, Lalor PA (1988) Bronchoalveolar lavage in the normal volunteer subject. 1.) technical aspects and intersubject variability. Chest 94 (2):275–280
53. Martin TR, Raghu G, Maunder J, Springmeyer SC (1985) The effects of chronic bronchitis and chronic air-flow obstruction on lung cell populations recovered by bronchoalveolar lavage. Am Rev Respir Dis 132:254–260
54. Albertini R, Harrel JH, Moser KM (1974) Hypoxemia during fiberoptic bronchoscopy. Chest 65 (1):117
55. Dubrawsky C, Awe RJ, Jenkins DE (1975) The effect of bronchofiberscopic examination on oxygenation status. Chest 67 (2):137–140
56. Albertini RE, Harrel JH, Moser KM (1975) Management of arterial hypoxemia induced by fiberoptic bronchoscopy. Chest 62 (2):134–136
57. Gurney JW, Harrison WC, Sears K, Robbins RA, Dobry CA, Rennard SI (1987) Bronchoalveolar lavage: radiographic manifestations. Radiology 163:71–74
58. Stover DE, Zaman MB, Hajdu SJ, Langem M, Gold J, Armstrong D (1984) Bronchoalveolar lavage in the diagnosis of diffuse pulmonary infiltrates in the immunosuppressed host. Ann Intern Med 101:1–7
59. Reynolds HY, Chretien J (1984) Respiratory tract fluids: analysis of content and contemporary use in understanding lung disease. DM 30:1–103
60. Crystal RG, Raynolds HY, Kalica AR (1986) Bronchoalveolar lavage. The report of an international conference. Chest 90:122–131
61. Eschenbacher WL, Gravelyn TR (1987) A technique for isolated airway segment lavage. Chest 92:105–109
62. Zehr BB, Casale TB, Wood D, Floerchinger C, Richerson HB, Hunninghake GW (1989) Use of segmental airway lavage to obtain relevant mediators form the lungs of asthmatic and control subjects. Chest 95:1059–1063
63. Kelly CA, Kotre CJ, Ward C, Hendrick DJ, Walters EH (1987) Anatomical distribution of bronchoalveolar lavage fluid as assessed by digital subtraction radiography. Thorax 42:624–628
64. Lam S, LeRiche JC, Kijek K, Phillips D (1985) Effect of bronchial lavage on cellular and protein recovery. Chest 88 (6):856–859
65. Chafouri MA, Rasmussen JK, Sears K et al. (1985) Use of sequential bronchoalveolar lavage to enrich for "bronchial" and "alveolar" material. Clin Res 33:464A

66. Thompson A, Ghafouri M, Stahl M et al. (1986) Assessment of neutrophilic bronchial inflammation by bronchoalveolar lavage in bronchitis. Am Rev Respir Dis 133:A325
67. Thompson AB, Robbins RA, Shoji S et al. (1986) Chronic bronchitis is associated with enrichment of airways epithelial lining fluid with C_3. Chest 89:499(s)
68. Lam S, LeRiche J, Phillips D, Chan-Yeung M (1987) Cellular and protein changes in bronchial lavage fluid after late asthmatic reaction in patients with red cedar asthma. J Allergy Clin Immunol 80:44–50
69. Rennard SI, Ghafouri MA, Thompson AB, Linder J et al. (1990) Fractional processing of sequential bronchoalveolar lavage to separate bronchial alveolar samples. Am Rev Respir Dis 141:208–217
70. Cherwick WS, Barbero GJ (1959) Composition of tracheobronchial secretions in cystic fibrosis of the pancreas and bronchiectasis. Pediatrics 739–745
71. Keimowitz RI (1964) Immunoglobulins in normal human tracheobronchial washings. J Lab Clin Med 63:54–59
72. Falk GA, Okinaka AJ, Siskin GW (1972) Immunoglobulins in the bronchial washings of patients with chronic obstructive pulmonary disease. Am Rev Respir Dis 105:14–21
73. Mandell MA, Dvorak KJ, Worman LW, de Cosse JJ (1976) Immunoglobulin content in bronchial washings of patients with benign and malignant disease. N Engl J Med 295:694–698
74. Wiggens J, Hill SL, Stockly RA (1983) Lung secretion solphase proteins: comparison of sputum with secretions obtained by direct sampling. Thorax 38:102–107
75. Metzger WJ, Moseley P, Nugent K, Richerson HB, Hunninghake GW (1985) Local antigen challenge and bronchoalveolar lavage of allergic asthmatic lungs. Chest 87:155(s)–156(s)
76. Wenzel SE, Westcott JY, Larsen GL (1991) Bronchoalveolar lavage fluid mediator levels five minutes after allergen challenge in atopic subjects with asthma: relationship to the development of late asthmatic response. J Allergy Clin Immunol 87:540–548
77. Fick RB, Metzger WJ, Richerson HB, Zavala DC et al. (1987) Increased bronchovascular permeability after allergen exposure in sensitivie asthmatics. J Appl Physiol 63 (3):1147–1155
78. Beasley R, Roche WR, Roberts JA, Holgate ST (1989) Cellular events in the bronchi in mild asthma after bronchial provocation. Am Rev Respir Dis 139:806–817
79. Rossi GA (1986) Bronchoalveolar lavage in the investigation of disorders of the lower respiratory tract. Eur J Respir Dis 69:293–315
80. Pirozynski M, Silwinski P, Polubiez M, Zielinsk J, Radwan L (1988) Atropine influences bronchoalveolar lavage-induced arterial oxygen desaturation. Eur Respir J 1 [Suppl]:312
81. Schmidt RM, Rosenkranz H (1970) Antimicrobial activity of local anesthetics: lidocaine and procaine. J Infect Dis 121:597–607
82. Wimberly N, Willey S, Sullivan N, Bartlett JG (1979) Antibacterial properties of Lidocaine. Chest 76:37–40
83. Von Essen SG, Robbins RA, Spurzem JR, Thompson AB et al. (1991) Bronchoscopy with bronchoalveolar lavage causes neutrophil recruitment to the lower respiratory tract. Am Rev Respir Dis 144:848–854
84. Kazmierowski JA, Gallin JI, Reynolds HY (1977) Mechanism for the inflammatory response in primate lungs. J Clin Invest 59:273–281
85. Cohen AB, Batra GK (1980) Bronchoscopy and lung lavage induced bilateral pulmonary neutrophil influx and blood leukocytes in dogs and monkeys. Am Rev Respir Dis 122:239–247
86. Saltini C, Hance AJ, Ferrans VJ, Basset F, Bitterman PB, Crystal RG (1984) Accurate quantification of cells recovered by bronchoalveolar lavage. Am Rev

Respir Dis 130:650–658
87. Chamberlain DW, Brande AC, Rebuck AS (1987) A critical evaluation of bronchoalveolar lavage: criteria for identifying unsatisfactory specimens. Acta Cytol 31 (5):599–605
88. Fleury-Feith J, Escudier E, Pocholle MJ, Carre C, Bernaudin JF (1987) The effects of cytocentrifugation on differential cell counts in samples obtained by bronchoalveolar lavage. Acta Cytol 31 (5):606–610
89. Thompson AB, Robbins RA, Ghafouri MA, Linder J, Rennard SI (1989) Bronchoalveolar lavage fluid processing: effect of membrane filtration preparation on neutrophil recovery. Acta Cytol 33 (4):544–549
90. Rankin JA, Naegel GP, Reynolds HY (1986) Use of a central laboratory for analysis of bronchoalveolar lavage fluid. Am Rev Respir Dis 133:186–190
91. Costabel U, Teschler H, Ziesche R, Guzman J et al. (1989) Transport of bronchoalveolar lavage cells in appropriate medium for 24 hours does not affect cell differentials and lymphocyte subsets. Am Rev Respir Dis 139:(A) 472
92. Thorpe JE, Baughman RP, Frame PT, Wesseler TA, Staneck JL (1987) Bronchoalveolar lavage for diagnosing acute bacterial pneumonia. J Infect Dis 155 (5):855–861
93. Guerra LF, Baughman RP (1990) Use of bronchoalveolar lavage to diagnose bacterial pneumonia in mechanically ventilated patients. Crit Care Med 18: 169–173
94. Kahn FW, Jones JM (1987) Diagnosing bacterial respiratory infection by bronchoalveolar lavage. J Infect Dis 155 (5):862–869
95. Chastre J, Fagon J-Y, Solber P et al. (1988) Diagnosis of nosocomial pneumonia in intubated patient undergoing ventilation: comparison of usefulness of bronchoalveolar lavage and the protected specimen brush. Am J Med 85:499–505
96. Meduri GU, Beals D, Majjab G, Buselski V (1991) Protected bronchoalveolar lavage: a new bronchoscopic technique to retrieve uncontaminated lower distal airway secretions. Am Rev Respir Dis 143:855–864
97. Meduri GM, Baselski V (1991) The role of bronchoalveolar lavage in diagnosing nonopportunistic bacterial pneumonia. Chest 100:179–190
98. Chastre J, Fagon JY, Soler P, Domart Y, Pierre J, Dombret MC et al. (1989) Quantification of BAL cells containing intracellular bacteria rapidly identifies ventilated patients with nosocomial pneumonia. Chest 95:190(s)–192(s)
99. Grocott RG (1955) A stain for fungi in tissue sections and smears. Am J Clin Pathol 25:975–979
100. Chalvardijian M, Grave LA (1963) A new procedure for the identification of pneumocystis carinii cysts in tissue sections and smears. Am J Clin Pathol 16: 383–385
101. Mahan CT, Sale HT, George E (1978) Rapid methenamine silver stain for pneumocystis and fungi. Arch Pathol Lab Med 102:351–352
102. De Garcia J, Curull V, Vidal R, Riba A, Orriols R (1988) Diagnostic value of bronchoalveolar lavage in suspected pulmonary tuberculosis. Chest 93:329–332
103. Xavier R, Henn L, Costa R (1990) Bronchoalveolar lavage in pulmonary tuberculosis. Chest 98:97(s)
104. Baughman RP, Dohn MN, Loudon RG, Frame PT (1991) Bronchoscopy with bronchoalveolar lavage in tuberculosis and fungal infections. Chest 99:92–97
105. Peterson EM, Lu R, Floyd C, Nakasone A et al. (1989) Direct identification of *Mycobacterium tuberculosis*, mycobacterium avium, and mycobacterium intracellulare from amplified primary cultures in bactec media using DNA probes. J Clin Microbial 27:1543–1547
106. Kohorst WR, Schonfeld SA, Macklin JE, Witcomb ME (1983) Rapid diagnosis of Legionnaire's disease by bronchoalveolar lavage. Chest 84:186–190
107. Edelstein PH, Meyer RD (1984) Legionnaire's disease: a review. Chest 85: 114–120
108. Pasculle AW, Veto GE, Krystofiak S, McKelvey K, Vrsolovic K (1989) Labora-

tory and clinical evaluation of a commercial DNA probe for the detection of Legionella ssp. J Clin Microbiol 27:2350–2358

109. Brigati DJ, Meyerson D, Leary JJ et al. (1983) Detection of viral genomes in cultured cells and paraffin-embedded tissue sections using biotin-labeled hybridization probes. Virol 126:32–50

110. Myerson D, Hackman RC Meyers JD (1984) Diagnosis of cytomegalovirus pneumonia by in-situ hybridization. J Infect Dis 150:272–277

111. Kahn FW, Jones JM (1986) Bronchoalveolar lavage in the rapid diagnosis of lung disease. Lab Management 24:31–35

112. Paik G (1980) Reagents, stains and miscellaneous test procedures. In: Lennette EH, Balows A, Hausler WJ, Traunt JP (eds) *Manual of Clinical Microbiology*, 3rd Ed. American Society for Microbiology, Washington DC, Chapter 98

113. Brinn NT (1983) Rapid metallic histological staining using the microwave oven. J Microtechnol 6:125–129

114. Stover DE, White DA, Romano PA, Gellene RA (1984) Diagnosis of pulmonary disease in acquired immune deficiency syndrome (AIDS). Role of bronchoscopy and bronchoalveolar lavage. Am Rev Respir Dis 130:659–662

115. Lennette EH, Balows A, Hausler WJ et al. (1980) Manual of clinical microbiology, 3rd edn. American Society for Microbiology, Washington DC, p 1023

116. Richards OW, Miller DK (1941) An efficient method for the identification of tuberculosis bacteria with a simple fluorescence microscope. Am J Clin Pathol Technical [Suppl] 5:1–8

117. Edelstein PH, Beer KB, Sturge JC, Watson AJ, Goldstein LC (1985) Clinical utility of a monoclonal direct fluorescent reagent specific for *Legionella pneumophila:* comparative study with other reagents. J Clin Microbiol 22:419–421

118. Edelstein PH, Edelstein MA (1989) Evaluation of the Meriflour-Legionella immunofluorescent reagent for identifying and detecting 21 Legionella species. J Clin Microbiol 27:2455–2458

119. Dalquen P, Bittel D, Gudat F et al. (1986) Combined immunoreaction and Papanicolaou's stain on cytologic smears. Pathol Res Pract 181:50–54

120. Drew WL, Finley T, Golde D (1977) Diagnostic lavage in occult pulmonary hemorrhage in thrombocytopenic immunocompromised patients. Am Rev Respir Dis 116:215–221

121. Mallory RF (1938) Pathological technique. Saunders, Philadelphia, pp 118–121

122. Warr GA, Martain RR, Sharp PM, Rossen RD (1977) Normal human bronchial immunoglobulin and proteins: effects of cigarette smoking. Am Rev Respir Dis 116:25–30

123. Merrill WW, Goodenberger D, Strober W, Matthay RA, Naegel GP, Reynolds HY (1980) Free secretory component and other proteins in human lung lavage. Am Rev Respir Dis 122:156–161

124. Merrill WW, Naegel GP, Reynolds HY (1980) Reagenic antibody in the lung lining fluid: analysis of normal human bronchoalveolar lavage IgE and comparison to immunoglobulins G and A. J Lab Clin Med 96:494–500

125. Bell DY, Haseman JA, Spock A, McLennan G, Hook GER (1981) Plasma protein of the bronchoalveolar surface of the lungs of smokers and nonsmokers. Am Rev Respir Dis 124:72–79

126. Merrill WW, Naegel GP, Olchowski JJ, Reynolds HY (1985) Immunoglobulin G subclass proteins in serum and lavage fluid of normal subjects: quantitation and comparison with immunoglobulin A and E. Am Rev Respir Dis 131:584–587

127. Olsen GN, Harris JO, Castle JR, Waldman RA, Karmgard HJ (1975) Alpha-1-antitrypsin content in the serum, alveolar macrohages and alveolar lavage fluid of smoking and non-smoking normal subjects. J Clin Invest 55:427–430

128. Villiger B, Brockelmann T, Kelly D, Heymach GJ, McDonald JA (1981) Bronchoalveolar fibronectin in smokers and nonsmokers. Am Rev Respir Dis 124:652–654

129. Lam S, LeRiche JC, Kijek K (1985) Effect of filtration and concentration on the composition of bronchoalveolar lavage fluid. Chest 87:740–742
130. Hook GER, Bell DY, Gilmore LB, Nadeau D, Reasor MJ, Talley FA (1978) Composition of bronchoalveolar lavage effluents from patients with pulmonary alveolar poteinasis. Lab Invest 39:342–356
131. Hunninghake GW, Gadek JE, Kawanani O, Ferrans VJ et al. (1979) Inflammatory and immune processes in the human lung in health and disease: evaluation by bronchoalveolar lavage. Am J Pathol 97:149–206
132. Davis WG, Rennard SI, Bitterman P et al. (1983) Pulmonary oxygen toxicity: early reversible changes in human alveolar structures induced by hyperoxia. N Engl J Med 309:878–883
133. Buchalter S, Rennard SI, Fulmer J et al. (1984) Evidence for alveolar edema and capillary leak in the lower respiratory tract of patients with sarcoidosis and idiopathic pulmonary fibrosis. Am Rev Respir Dis 129 (2):(A)64
134. Rossman MD, McDonald JA, Broekelman T, Dauber JH, Daniele RB (1983) Protein leak in pulmonary sarcoidosis: assessment of bronchoalveolar lavage fluid and plasma albumin and fibronectin. Am Rev Respir Dis 127 (2):90(A)
135. Daniele RP, Elias JA, Epstein PE et al. (1985) Bronchoalveolar lavage: role in the pathogenesis, diagnosis and management of interstitial lung disease. Ann Intern Med 102:93–108
136. Shasby DM, Shasby SS (1985) Active transendothelial transport of albumin: interstitium to lumen. Circ Res 57:903–908
137. Péterson MW, Stone P, Shasby DM (1987) Cationic neutrophil proteins increase transendothelial albumin movement. J Appl Physiol 62:1521–1530
138. Bonomo L, D'Addabbo A (1964) ^{131}I albumin turnover and loss of protein into the sputum of chronic bronchitis. Clin Chim Acta 10:214–222
139. Jacquot J, Dupuit F, Benali R, Spilmont C, Puchele E (1990) Modulation of albumin-like protein and lysozyme production by bovine tracheal gland serous cells: dependence on culture conditions. FEBS Lett 269 (1):65–68
140. Baughman RP, Bosken CH, Loudon RG, Hurtubise P, Wesseler T (1983) Quantitation of bronchoalveolar lavage with Methylene Blue. Am Rev Respir Dis 128:226–270
141. Rennard S, Basset G, Lecossier D, O'Donnell K, Martain P, Crystal RG (1986) Estimations of the absolute volume of epithelial lining fluid recovered by bronchoalveolar lavage using urea as an endogenous marker of dilution. J Appl Physiol 60:532–638
142. Peterson BT, Idell S, McCarthur C, Gray LD, Cohen AB (1990) A modified bronchoalveolar lavage procedure that allows measurement of lung epithelial lining fluid volume. Am Rev Respir Dis 141:314–320
143. DeMonchy JGR, Kauffman HF, Venge P et al. (1985) Bronchoalveolar eosinophils during allergen-induced late asthmatic rections. Am Rev Respir Dis 131:373–376
144. Fabri LM, Baschetto P, Zacca E, Milani G, Piverotto F, Plebani M, Burlina A, Licata B, Mapp CE (1987) Bronchoalveolar neutrophilia during late asthmatic reactions induced by Toluene Diisocyanate. Am Rev Respir Dis 136:36–42
145. Calhoun WJ, Bush RJ et al. (1990) Enhanced reactive oxygen species metabolism of air space cells and airway inflammation follow antigen challenge in human asthma. J Allergy Clin Immunol 86:306–13.
146. Rossi GA, Crimi E, Lauterno S, Gianiorio P, Oddera S et al. (1991) Late-phase asthmatic reaction to inhaled allergen is associated with early recruitment of eosinophils in the airways. Am Rev Respir Dis 144:379–383
147. Murray JJ, Tonnel Ab, Brash AR (1986) Release of prostaglandin D_2 into human airways during acute allergen challenge. N Engl J Med 315:800–804
148. Lam S, Chan H, LeRiche JC, Chan-Yeung M, Salari H (1988) Release of leukotrienes in patients with bronchial asthma. J Allergy Clin Immunol 81:711–717
149. Wenzel SE, Fowler AA, Schwartz LB (1988) Activation of pulmonary mast cells

by bronchoalveolar allergen challenge: in vivo release of histamine and tryptase in atopic subjects with and without asthma. Am Rev Respir Dis 137:1002–1008

150. Chan-Yeung M, Chan H, Tse KS, Salari H, Lam S (1989) Histamine and leukotrienes release in bronchoalveolar fluid during plicatic acid-induced bronchoconstriction. J Allergy Clin Immunol 84:762–768

151. Casale TB, Wood D, Richerson HB, Trapp S, Metzger WJ et al. (1987) Elevated bronchoalveolar fluid histamine levels in allergic asthmatics are associated with methacholine bronchial hyperresponsiveness. J Clin Invest 79:1197–1203

152. Wardlaw AJ, Dunnette S, Gleich GJ, Colli NS et al. (1988) Eosinophils and mast cells in bronchoalveolar lavage in subjects with mild asthma. Relationship to bronchial hyperreactivity. Am Rev Respir Dis 137:62–69

Subject Index